MAN EATING PLANTS

MAN EATING PLANTS

How a Vegan Diet Can Save the World

Jonathan Spitz

6th

Sense

Press

Man Eating Plants: How a Vegan Diet Can Save the World

Published by 6th Sense Press
P.O. Box 1087
Laytonville, CA 95454

plantbased.js@gmail.com

Cover Art "Winter" by Italian Renaissance painter Giuseppe Arcimboldo (1527–1593).
Earth from space photo from NASA. Photoshop by Dave Williamson.
Cover design by Jonathan Spitz.

Library of Congress Control Number: 2022945773

ISBN (paperback): 9781662932885
eISBN: 9781662932892

Dedicated to

… my parents Hillel and Elinor Spitz who
instilled in me a sense of curiosity.

… my life partner Toni Elizabeth Leet who
taught me compassion for all beings.

… the billions of animals who suffer at the
hands of humans.

Acknowledgments

*M*an Eating Plants: How a Vegan Diet Can Save the World is a work of synthesis, that is to say, I myself did not do any of the original research in support of my thesis, but rather, I have drawn together research published by the world's leading experts on subjects as diverse as botany, biology, ecology, archaeology, anthropology, agronomy, nutrition, medicine, geology, geography, history and economics. As the saying goes, I stand on the shoulders of giants. I hope I have not misrepresented their works in the interest of concision.

I would like to give a special thanks to the trailblazing nutritional scientists who, over the past 40 years, have exposed the disease pathologies of an animal-based diet and the health promoting nutrition of a whole-food, plant-based diet. To these nutritionist practitioners I literally owe my life, were it not for their tireless advocacy of a healthy plant-based diet, I probably would not have made it to the ripe old age of 70 (men in my family tend to die young), and this book would never have been written. When the Nutritionist Hall of Fame is opened, these luminaries will be charter members: Dr. Neal Barnard, MD, Dr. T. Colin Campbell, PhD, Dr. Caldwell Esselstyn, MD, Dr. Joel Fuhrman, MD, Dr. Michael Greger, MD, Dr. Michael Klaper, MD, Dr. John McDougall, MD, and Dr. Dean Ornish, MD.

I would also like to give a special thanks to the visionary writer, John Robbins, author of *Diet for a New America* and many other truly enlightening books. It was upon reading *DNA* in 1990 that I made the transition to a plant-based diet. Smartest thing I've ever done.

And finally, I would like to give a personal thanks to my longtime friend, fine artist, and author of *Greekscapes: Journeys With an Artist*, Pamela Jane Rogers, who first encouraged me to get my ideas down on paper and stuck with me over the long years of writing even when the finish line was nowhere in sight. Also, a personal thanks to my brother Jerry who lent his enthusiastic support throughout, to his friend and editor, Cathie O'Connor Schoultz, who helped me smooth out my unwieldy manuscript into a readable book that is accessible to the uninitiated, to my friend Dave Williamson for his masterful Photoshop work on the book cover, and to my Author Manager, Trinity Nirenberg, and all the support staff at Gatekeeper Press for their superb job of formatting my book into a physical reality.

Although writing is by nature a solitary act, a book is always the product of a larger community.

CONTENTS

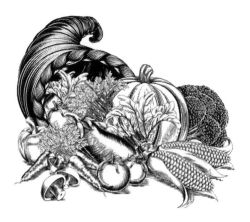

INTRODUCTION

"There is no love sincerer than the love of food."
– George Bernard Shaw, playwright, social critic and inveterate vegetarian (1856 – 1950)

Nothing in life is more intimate than food, not only do we take it into our bodies, it actually becomes our bodies. Considering this unparalleled level of intimacy, it is quite natural for people to develop strong emotional attachments to their food. But the foods we choose to eat have a far greater impact on our lives than simply to salve our emotions. Over the past several decades, nutritional scientists have proven conclusively that plant foods promote health and vitality while animal foods promote chronic disease and morbidity. Also over these decades, ecological scientists have documented the devastating environmental impacts of livestock production to supply our global appetite for meat, dairy and eggs.

As glorified apes, we humans evolved to efficiently process a diet of fibrous fruits, vegetables, tubers, nuts and seeds, not a diet of high saturated fat, high cholesterol, high protein meat, dairy and eggs. With animal foods now a significant part of the diet of billions of people around the world, our naturally herbivorous species has become the world's top carnivorous apex predator species. As a result of this unnatural diet, people living in affluent countries where diets are laden with animal foods suffer from epidemics of chronic degenerative diseases such as atherosclerosis, diabetes and cancers.

Depending on how it is calculated, animal agriculture emits anywhere from 18% to 51% of anthropogenically generated greenhouse gasses. This makes the shift in diet from herbivore to carnivore by the planet's most populous large mammal species the single largest contributor to global warming and runaway climate change. Due to human generated greenhouse gas emissions, the average global surface temperature is expected to rise by 7.2 °F (degrees Fahrenheit) above pre-industrial times by the year 2100. As global temperatures rise, there is an increase in water evaporation from the land and oceans which causes the land to dry out from extended droughts and the atmosphere to contain more water vapor and energy that leads to more frequent and severe storms and floods. Extreme weather conditions are now challenging farmers to produce more food with less fresh water and arable land. Global temperature rise is also causing the polar ice caps and major world glaciers to melt which is leading to sea level rise that is beginning to inundate heavily populated coastal areas. Current climate models project average sea level rise for the contiguous United States to be 7.2 feet (2.2 meters) by 2100 and 13 feet (3.9 meters) by 2150.

Animal foods require many times more natural resources than plant foods to produce nutrients for people. Half the world's habitable land is used for agriculture, but grazing livestock and growing animal feed accounts for 77% of global farmland while producing only 18% of the world's food calories and 37% of total protein. As a result of this enormous ecological footprint, animal agriculture is the primary driver of the sixth great mass species extinction since life began on Earth 3.7 billion years ago. Today, in the early 21st century, 25% of species face extinction and unless urgent action is taken that number will rise to 50% by 2100. This rate of species extinction is up to 10,000 times higher than the natural, historical rate. It is likely that within the next 15 to 40 years, these iconic animal species will become extinct in the wild: chimpanzee, mountain gorilla, orangutan, elephant, rhino, tiger and giant panda, koala and polar bears. As I write, the long term prospect for species diversity on this planet looks bleak.

The modern human diet loaded with animal foods is an aberration from the natural herbivorous diet that our species evolved to thrive on over millions of years foraging in the tropical forests of equatorial Africa. How did this obscure herbivorous species from tropical Africa become the most populous carnivorous apex predator species in the world? How did this change in human diet lead to epidemics of chronic degenerative disease, catastrophic climate change and mass species extinction? How can a change back to our natural herbivorous diet of fruits, vegetables, tubers, nuts and seeds save the world? It is to answer these fundamental questions about the human place on the food chain, that I have written this book.

The story of *Man Eating Plants: How a Vegan Diet Can Save the World,* is told in seven parts:

Part I: Evolution of the Human Diet, reviews groundbreaking research in the late 1990s by a breakaway group of anthropologists led by Dr. Richard Wrangham, who proposed an alternate explanation for human brain development that soundly refuted the generally accepted meat eating hypothesis. Spoiler alert: the evidence they unearthed indicates that humans actually evolved to eat a fibrous whole-food, plant-based diet. Further anthropological evidence indicates that the anatomy and physiology of modern humans is perfectly adapted to thrive on a diet of fibrous plant foods.

Part II: Agriculture & Civilization, traces the natural history of the invention of agriculture and reviews the development of the major civilizations it spawned in both the Old (Africa and Eurasia) and New (the Americas) Worlds. Human population growth propelled by the domestication of staple crops of grains and tubers is what achieved the critical mass of people necessary to build the social institutions and physical infrastructure of civilization.

Part III: The Columbian Exchange, reviews the groundbreaking work of eminent historian, Dr. Alfred Crosby, who changed the study of history forever by showing that human events are shaped more by ecology and biology than by politics. Through meticulous historical research, Dr. Crosby explores how the exchange of germs, plants and animals between the Old and New Worlds that took place after the voyage of Christopher Columbus in 1492, completely reshaped the global distribution of the human population by wiping out millions of indigenous people in the Americas with contagious diseases, while increasing food production and population in Eurasia and Africa with high yield maize (corn), potato and manioc crops originally domesticated in the New World.

Part IV: Rise of the Global Animal Industrial Complex, traces the history of how human exploitation of five animals – sheep, pigs, cattle, chickens and fish – went from small-scale localized operations with limited production and distribution capacity before the 1830s, to a handful of giant, multinational, vertically integrated, agro-corporate behemoths that dominate the entire global food production system today. Before the mid-19th century, most of the calories in the average human diet came from starchy vegetables, whereas now, in the early 21st century, animal foods are central to the diets of billions of people.

Part V: Man Eating Animals: How Animal-based Diets Are Destroying Our Planet, reviews the six most prominent studies and reports published since the turn of the 21st century that have quantified the enormous greenhouse gas emissions and land-use footprint of the global livestock industry. Climate scientists tell us that even if we were to end our reliance on fossil fuels to power our economies, it would not be enough to hold global temperature rise below the 1.5 °C (degrees Celsius) that will threaten the very existence of complex human civilization. Changing the human diet from animal-based to plant-based is the only realistic way to accomplish that.

Part VI: Man Eating Plants: How a Vegan Diet Can Save the World, reviews six groundbreaking studies published since the turn of the 21st century that quantify how human nutritional needs can be met on a plant-based vegan diet using a fraction of the land, water and energy resources it takes to provide an animal-based diet. The only practical way for us to feed our growing population while at the same time mitigate our greenhouse gas emissions and land-use footprint, is to change back to our natural plant-based diet.

Part VII: A Diet for the 21st Century, defines the optimal human diet as prescribed by Dr. Michael Greger MD, one of the world's leading specialists in clinical nutrition. Part VII also includes chapters on how to grow enough food sustainably to feed our growing population a healthy plant-based diet even as arable land and fresh water resources diminish over the coming decades. The book concludes with chapters that offer some practical suggestions on ways to facilitate this back to the future change in the human diet.

That our current animal-based diet and agriculture cause chronic disease and environmental breakdown are no longer matters of serious dispute in the medical and ecological sciences. That adopting a plant-based vegan diet and agriculture would produce a well population and stable ecosystems is also no longer in doubt. The title of this book, *"Man Eating Plants: How a Vegan Diet Can Save the World"* is not hyperbole, the very survival of complex life on Earth literally depends upon the dietary choices we make today.

• • •

The brilliant atomic physicist, Dr. Niels Bohr (1885 – 1962), once wrote, "*Every great and deep difficulty bears in itself its own solution. It forces us to change our thinking in order to find it.*" To paraphrase Dr. Bohr: the great and deep difficulties of chronic degenerative disease, catastrophic climate change and mass species extinction bear in themselves their own solutions. They force us to change our thinking about the human diet in order to find them.

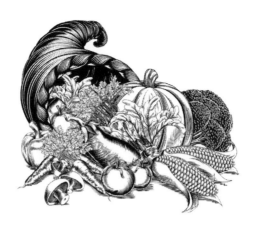

PART I

EVOLUTION OF THE HUMAN DIET

• • •

"We admit that we are like apes, but we seldom realize that we are apes."
– Richard Dawkins, evolutionary biologist (born in 1941)

1
THE FIRST HOMO

(Full disclosure: I am of the genus Homo, so please excuse my occasional use of the pronouns we, our and us.)

Modern humans evolved from a long line of great apes that lived in the tropical forests of equatorial Africa and thrived on a diet of fruits and leaves. Our earliest ancestors, called Australopithecus, diverged from our closest great ape relative, the chimpanzee, around six million years ago and by two million years ago had become widely dispersed throughout eastern and southern Africa. It was during this time interval that Australopithecus evolved an upright posture and bipedalism which made them distinct from all of their knuckle walking great ape relatives (orangutans, gorillas, chimpanzees and bonobos). What adaptive advantage did walking upright give Australopithecus to prompt this major change in posture?

Anthropologists hypothesize that bipedalism was likely an evolutionary adaptation made by this arboreal species to a more terrestrial life. During this geological time period the tropical forests of equatorial Africa were fragmenting and dry open savannas were expanding. Locomotion studies have shown that walking upright is a far more energy efficient mode of transportation on the ground than knuckle walking. Since food on the ground was more widely dispersed than in the forest canopy, expanding their foraging range by more efficient ground locomotion became a significant adaptive advantage for Australopithecus to find food on the open savanna.

Australopithecus had brains slightly larger than modern day chimpanzees and also had very large jaws and molars indicating a diet of tough fibrous plant foods that required a lot of grinding and chewing. By around 1.9 million years ago, the fossil record of Australopithecus disappeared to be replaced by fossils of the first Homo species called Homo erectus (H. erectus). H. erectus had markedly smaller teeth and jaws than Australopithecus with distinctly larger bodies and brains. What could have caused these major anatomical changes that would give rise to this completely new genus called Homo?

2
THE MEAT HYPOTHESIS

The most widely accepted theory among anthropologists for these anatomical changes is called "*The Meat Hypothesis*." One of the leading exponents of *The Meat Hypothesis* is Dr. Katharine Milton, Professor of Physical Anthropology at the University of California, Berkeley. In her paper, "*A hypothesis to explain the role of meat-eating in human evolution,"* published in the journal *Evolutionary Anthropology (1999)*, Dr. Milton explains:

> *"Humans, who are believed to have evolved in a more arid and seasonal environment than did extant apes, illustrate a third dietary strategy in the hominoid line. By routinely including animal protein in their diet, they were able to reap some nutritional advantages enjoyed by carnivores, even though they have features of gut anatomy and digestive kinetics of herbivores. Using meat to supply essential amino acids and many required micronutrients frees space in the gut for plant foods. In addition, because these essential dietary requirements are now being met by other means, evolving humans would have been able [to] select plant foods primarily for energy rather than relying on them for most or all nutritional requirements. This dietary strategy is compatible with hominoid gut anatomy and digestive kinetics and would have permitted ancestral humans to increase their body size without losing mobility, agility, or sociality. This dietary strategy could also have provided the energy required for cerebral expansion."*

There is no anthropologist in the world today who has contributed more to the understanding of the primate diet than Dr. Katherine Milton, and I have nothing but the utmost respect for her as an exceptional scientist. But I must say that her meat eating hypothesis runs completely contrary to the most basic principles of evolutionary biology. In effect, Dr. Milton is saying that humans evolved the gut anatomy of an herbivore while eating the diet of a carnivore. In terms of evolutionary biology, this simply doesn't make sense; in evolution, anatomical body parts become *more* adapted to perform their function, not less.

If meat eating (and we're talking raw meat here) had become a significant source of food energy for early humans, then our teeth would have evolved to become sharper and more serrated like those of carnivorous animals for cutting through tough muscle tissue, not flatter and more rounded like those of herbivores adapted for processing fibrous plant foods. With large amounts of raw meat in the diet, our stomachs would have evolved to have a higher stomach acid like that of carnivores to kill the harmful bacteria in raw putrefying meat, not mildly acidic like that of herbivores to break down plant carbohydrates. And with large quantities of meat in our diet we would have evolved shorter colons like those of carnivores for faster transport of putrefying animal protein, not long colons like those of herbivores for slow passage of hard to break down plant cellulose. If raw meat had become a significant food source for early humans, we would not have evolved the bodies of herbivores; the evolutionary process of natural selection just doesn't work that way.

Dr. Milton's assertion that meat in the early human diet provided *"nutritional advantages"* that *"permitted ancestral humans to increase their body size"* and *"provided the energy required for cerebral expansion"* does not stand up to nutritional scrutiny. Dr. John Speth, Professor of Anthropology at the University of Michigan, is a leading researcher studying the use of food energy resources by modern day hunter-gatherer societies. In his paper, *"Early hominid hunting and scavenging: the role of meat as an energy source"* (*Journal of Human Evolution,* 1989), Dr. Speth notes that the meat of most African ungulates (hoofed animals) is very low in fat and high in protein. Though all great apes including humans typically derive their energy from plant carbohydrates, animal fat can also be used as an alternative energy source, but since wild meat contains so little fat, it is actually a very low source of food energy. And since hunting, eating and digesting meat is a very high energy consuming activity, low-fat meat is actually a net energy loss for modern hunter-gatherers living in arid environments similar to that of early humans. Dr. Speth has found that modern day hunter-gathers in arid environments reduce their use of meat during frequent periods of food scarcity even when meat is readily available, instead relying on plant foods to meet their energy needs.

Dr. Milton's assertion that *"Using meat to supply essential amino acids and many required micronutrients frees space in the gut for plant foods"* also does not stand up to nutritional scrutiny. In the paper, *"Relating Chimpanzee Diets to Potential Australopithecus Diets"* (14th *International Congress of Anthropological and Ethnological Sciences,* 1998), Harvard anthropologists Nancy Lou Conklin-Brittain clearly demonstrated that all great apes including humans have very low requirements for essential amino acids and micronutrients that could easily have been met with the variety of plant foods that were available in the arid environments similar to that of early humans. Rather than *"free space in the gut for plant foods,"* significant meat eating would have taken up space in the gut and reduced the intake of plant foods as is the case in modern day humans on a western meat-based diet. In fact, modern nutritional science has proven conclusively that meat eating confers no nutritional advantages to primates like humans as Dr. Milton herself noted in a study she conducted on the diets of four frugivorous (fruit eating) monkey species on the Barro Colorado Island of Panama. She found that the monkeys' diets of leaves and fruits were *"amazingly rich in nutrients,"* containing the full complement of essential amino acids, a good balance of essential fatty acids, and were high in glucose, calcium, potassium, iron, phosphorus and vitamin C. Dr. Milton was so impressed with the nutritional profile of the monkey's plant-based diet that she remarked:

> *"This information suggests that, for their size, many wild primates routinely ingest greater amounts of many minerals, vitamins, essential fatty acids, dietary fiber and other important dietary constituents than most modern human populations."*

So, if Dr. Milton's hypothesis on the role of meat-eating in human evolution fails to explain what caused the change of the small bodied, small brained, large toothed Australopithecus into the larger bodied, larger brained, smaller toothed H. erectus around 1.9 million years ago, then what does explain it?

3

THE COOKED TUBER HYPOTHESIS

A group of highly distinguished anthropologists including Drs. Ernst Mayr, Richard Wrangham, David Pilbeam and Nancy Conklin-Brittain of Harvard University have explored a new hypothesis that gives a much more plausible explanation for these major anatomical changes from Australopithecus to H. erectus than the meat hypothesis. In his book, *"What evolution Is"* (2002), the legendary evolutionary biologist, Dr. Ernst Mayr, sets the scene:

> *"Human history always seems to have been vitally affected by the environment. Beginning 2.5 mya [million years ago], the climate in tropical Africa began to deteriorate, correlated with the arrival of the ice age in the Northern Hemisphere. As it became more arid, the trees in the tree savanna suffered and gradually more and more of them died and the environment slowly shifted to a bush savanna."*

It was in this increasingly dry and treeless environment that Australopithecus developed its distinct new food niche much different from its forest dwelling past. In the paper, *"The Raw and the Stolen"* (*Current Anthropology*, 1999), anthropologists, Drs. Wrangham, Pilbeam and Conklin-Brittain, et al., describe this food niche:

> *"In line with niche theory and empirical evidence from primates, we propose that these characteristic dental features [large molar surfaces, thick enamel and microwear patterns in Australopithecus] represent adaptation to fallback foods, eaten during periods of food scarcity. Fallback foods are particularly important components of the diet because they represent the kinds of foods to which anatomical and foraging specializations are expected to be adapted (see Boag and Grant 1981, Schoener 1982, Robinson and Wilson 1998). Periods of food shortage would have been frequent (e.g., annual) in all hominid [great ape] habitats, as they are even in rainforests (e.g., Conklin-Brittain, Wrangham and Hunt 1998a, Wrangham, Conklin-Brittain and Hunt 1998). Seasonal shortages mean that preferred foods such as fruits and seeds would not have been consistently available (Peters and O'Brien 1994), and dental and ecological considerations easily rule out the herbaceous leaves and piths that make up the fallback foods of modern African apes such as chimpanzees (Wrangham et al. 1996). In contrast, underground storage organs such as tubers, rhizomes and corms are likely to have been important for australopithecines because of their availability and hominid dental morphology (Hatley and Kappelman 1980), and we propose that they were the major type of fallback food. This hypothesis is supported by ecological, botanical, paleontological and anthropological considerations.*

"*First, underground storage organs occur at higher biomass at drier sites because they store food and/or water during periods of climate stress (Anderson, 1987). In Tanzanian savanna woodland for example, Vincent (1984) found densities of edible tubers averaging 40,000 kg per km2 [kilograms per square kilometer] compared with only 100 kg per km2 found by Hladik and Hladik (1990) in a rainforest of the Central African Republic.*"

So it is easy to imagine that Australopithecus learned how to take advantage of tubers as a new food source on the dry open savanna which enabled them to survive in their changing environment. But as the trees slowly disappeared and the bush savanna took over, Australopithecus must have faced another major problem, as Dr. Mayr describes here in "*What Evolution Is*":

"*[The loss of trees] deprived the australopithecines of their retreat to safety, for in the treeless savanna they were completely defenseless. They were threatened by lions, leopards, hyenas and wild dogs, all of whom could run faster than they. They had no weapons such as horns or powerful canines [teeth], nor the strength to wrestle with any of their potential enemies successfully. Inevitably, most australopithecines perished in the hundreds of thousands of years of this vegetational turnover.*

"*More important for human history, however, is the fact that some australopithecine populations survived by using their wits to invent successful defense mechanisms. What these were we can only speculate about. The survivors could have thrown rocks, or used primitive weapons made from wood and other plant material. They might have used long poles like some chimpanzees from West Africa, swung thorn branches, and perhaps even used noise-making instruments like drums. But surely fire was their best defense, and not being able to sleep in tree nests, they most likely slept at campsites protected by fire.*"

According to Dr. Ralph Rowlett, Professor Emeritus of Anthropology at the University of Missouri, who specializes in lithic (stone) technology and materials analysis, there is ample evidence that by 1.9 million years ago, the larger brained H. erectus had learned how to control the use of fire:

"*Although anthropologists have been reluctant to allow the control of fire by such early humans, a number of sites indicate that H. erectus had the ability to produce and control fire. In addition to the African sites of Chesowanja, Gadeb and Swartkrans, Koobi Fora on Lake Turkana presents extremely good evidence of the use of fire by H. erectus, even in the early phase sometimes called H. ergaster. These ostensible fireplaces have been extensively scrutinized independently by Randy Bellomo and Michael Kean (1991, 1994) and by me working with several different colleagues...*"

It is not at all farfetched to think that by 1.9 million years ago, H. erectus had reached the mental capacity necessary to produce and control fire, after all, by then, stone flaked tool kits had been in use for over 500,000 years (Leakey, M. 1976, Keely and Toth 1981, Toth 1985).

What could have accounted for the increased brain size from Australopithecus to H. erectus? In the research paper, *"Chimpanzee and felid diet composition is influenced by prey brain size"* (*Biology Letters*, 2006), biologists Susanne Shultz and R.I.M Dunbar of the School of Biological Sciences at the University of Liverpool, explain their theory for increasing brain size:

> *"...large-brained prey are likely to be more effective at evading predators because they can effectively alter their behavioral responses to specific predator encounters. Thus, we provide evidence for the hypothesis that brain size evolution is potentially driven by selection for more sophisticated and behaviorally flexible anti-predator strategies."*

Certainly, H. erectus needed to develop very sophisticated anti-predator strategies (what Dr. Mayr referred to as "*defense mechanisms*") to protect themselves and their young from predation on the open savanna and that this put tremendous selective pressure on brain size development. The bigger the brain, the greater the chances of outsmarting their predators and leaving more offspring; what more direct method of natural selection could there be? And with constant exposure to wild fires started by lightning strikes, eventually some H. erectus Einstein reached the cerebral threshold necessary to produce it on demand. This advance in technology must have been a critical juncture in pre-human evolution. Again, Dr. Mayr from "*What Evolution Is*":

> *"Early Homo seems to have relied on fire not only for protection but apparently also for cooking. The reduction in tooth size in Homo has traditionally been ascribed to an increased reliance on meat in their diet. But Wrangham et al. (2001) believe that softening of tough plant material by cooking was a more important cause."*

In "*The Raw and the Stolen*," Dr. Wrangham et al. put forth their hypothesis of how the technology of cooking changed the small brained, small bodied, large toothed Australopithecus into the larger brained, larger bodied and smaller toothed H. erectus:

> *"With the appearance of H. erectus, there are indications that 'early humans were able in some manner to greatly improve their intake and uptake of energy apparently without any decrease in dietary quality' (Milton 1987:106). Particularly strong signals are an increase in body mass (McHenry 1992 1994), reduction in molar size and enamel thickness (Wood 1981, Isaac 1983), and increase in brain volume (Holloway 1979, Milton 1987, Leonard and Robinson 1994, Aiello and Wheeler 1995, Kappelman 1996). Comparative data on primate energetics suggest that total daily energy expenditure rose from australopithecines to H. erectus by a factor of at least 40-45% and probably (assuming a human-style foraging strategy in H. erectus) by 80-85% (Leonard and Robinson 1997).*
>
> *"The dominant hypothesis for the significant dietary change has been an increase in meat intake. We propose that whatever the changes in meat intake, plants would have remained critical, especially during times of resource stress. Among tropical African hunter-gatherers plant items always compose the majority of the diet (Hayden 1981, Hill 1982, Keeley 1988)*

and are vital during periods of food stress (Lee 1968, Silberbauer 1981, Bailey 1991). When plant food is scarce, hunters are probably less willing to risk energy and time in a failed search for meat. In addition, wild meat is a low-fat food which may have low nutritional quality during lean periods (Speth and Spielman 1983, Speth 1989). We therefore suggest that early humans, including H. erectus, continued to rely on plant foods most of the time and especially during the periods of food shortage in which natural selection would have been intense.

"EFFECTS OF COOKING ON PLANT FOOD DIGESTIBILITY

"Cooking makes food more available and digestible by (1) cracking open or otherwise destroying physical barriers such as thick skins or husks, (2) bursting cells, thereby making cell contents more easily available for digestion or absorption, (3) modifying the three-dimensional structure of molecules such as proteins and starches into forms more accessible for digestion by enzymatic degradation, (4) reducing the chemical structure of indigestible molecules into smaller forms that can be fermented more rapidly and completely, and (5) denaturing toxins or digestion-reducing compounds [Stahl 1984]. In its own way each of these mechanisms makes food more available, either rendering it more palatable or increasing its digestibility (defined as the proportion of dry-matter intake not present in the feces).

"The combined importance of these mechanisms can be characterized broadly as enlarging the diet and improving its quality. Both of these benefits are relevant for the use of underground storage organs. First, these organs are often chemically protected, apparently as a result of co-evolution with mammalian herbivores (Lovegrove and Jarvis 1986). In our survey of underground storage organs eaten by African foragers, 21 (43.8%) of the 48 edible species identified required cooking to become palatable. This suggests that cooking can substantially broaden the range of edible species. Furthermore, underground storage organs are frequently considered to be improved by roasting (e.g. Silberbauer 1981). This may be partly a matter of macronutrient availability. For instance, Ayankunbi, Keshinro, and Egele (1991) found that three modes of preparing cooked cassava led to a mean increase in gross energy available of 76.1% over the value of raw cassava (306 kcal/g compared with 174.0 kcal/g). Potato starch, the principle source of digestible energy in potatoes, is highly resistant to digestive amylase (the enzyme primarily responsible for converting complex carbohydrates into usable energy) when raw but rapidly digestible when cooked (Kingman and Englyst 1994). Similarly, the apparent digestibility of soybeans was found to increase linearly with duration of cooking, partly because of the reduction of trypsin-inhibitor activity and the proportion of tannins (Kaankuka, Balogun, and Tegbe 1996). Underground storage organs frequently contain both non-starch polysaccharides and starch, which occurs in a variety of forms, some of them slowly digestible and resistant (Periago, Ros, and Casas 1997). In a comparison of starchy foods, Trout, Behall

and Osilesi (1993) found that the method of preparation was a more important influence on the glycemic index (a measure of the speed of digestion) than the chemical composition of the raw food, although the type of starch and starch granule was also critical. The consistent finding in such studies is that cooking increases digestibility markedly, up to 100% or more.

"In view of its substantial effect on the availability and digestibility of critical food items, we can expect the adoption of cooking to have been rapid. Increased digestibility of ingested food is expected to have left a variety of signals directly or indirectly in the fossil record, including smaller teeth (partly because total chewing time would have been enormously reduced, e.g., from 50% to 10% of the day), by inference smaller guts (since food spends less time in the gut to be digestible), higher body mass in females (e.g., Altmann et al. 1993) and possibly in males, depending on the nature of sexual selection, and an increase in the size of relatively expensive organs (such as brains)."

Where Dr. Milton's "*Meat Hypothesis*" explanation for the anatomical changes between Australopithecus and H. erectus goes against the most basic principles of evolutionary biology, Dr. Wrangham's "*Cooked Tuber Hypothesis*" makes perfect evolutionary sense. By controlling fire H. erectus was not only able to protect itself from predators, but also to make use of an abundant food source on their dry savanna homelands especially as a fallback food during periods of scarcity. And cooked tubers were not only soft and easy to chew resulting in smaller tooth and jaw size, they also provided significantly more carbohydrate energy than raw tubers to power their larger brains. Of course, the reason H. erectus was originally attracted to cooked tubers was not because they understood its nutritional value, the attraction was simply that cooked tubers were easier to chew and tasted better. Natural selection quickly favored those smarter individuals who learned how to cook their tubers.

Dr. Wrangham further points out why it is very doubtful that meat, even more chewable and palatable cooked meat, was a major component of the early H. erectus diet:

"Attributing the signal of increased energy availability for H. erectus to increased meat intake rather than to cooking has several problems. First, because of its low energy value during periods of climatic stress, meat appears unlikely to have been a fallback food (Speth 1989). Its adaptive significance would therefore be as a food type superior to those eaten during periods of food abundance, when selection has reduced effects because populations are less stressed. Second, nonhuman examples do little to support the idea that additional meat in the diet has major effects on energy availability. For example, a highly carnivorous population of chimpanzees [at Gombe] also has the smallest known body weight among chimpanzees (Stanford et al. 1994, Uehara and Nishida 1987), and polar bears, which are much more carnivorous than brown bears, have only 7% more female body mass (which itself may be less than expected simply because of latitudinal differences between the two taxa) and smaller neonates (Oftedal and Gittelman 1989). Third, for ecological reasons human meat intake would presumably have

varied in importance over evolutionary time, just as it does among living populations. For these reasons the fossil signals left by an increase in meat intake are expected to be weaker, less immediate, and more reversible than those left by the adoption of cooking. Fourth, we have tried to compare the amount of energy gained by adding meat to a prehuman plant diet versus maintaining the same plant items in the diet and cooking them. Our (necessarily crude) estimates suggest that cooking raises energy intake substantially more than substituting meat for plant items (tables 1 and 2).

"Accordingly, while we conclude that the signals of increased energy expenditure at the origin of H. erectus were strongly linked to the adoption of cooking, the contribution to energy intake from increased meat intake is less certain. We suggest that the presumed increase in meat consumption in later hominids was a dietary adaptation related to cooking plant material. Specifically, the increased energy availability allowed by cooking plant materials played a permissive role in the intensification of hunting—a high risk, high gain, activity—much the way periods of fruit abundance seem to allow intensification of chimpanzee hunting (Wrangham and Bergmann-Riss 1990, Stanford 1996)."

Besides explaining how cooking tubers reduced the jaw and tooth size of H. erectus and increased energy consumption to grow larger bodies and brains, Dr. Wrangham's "Cooked Tuber Hypothesis" also explains how the H. erectus gut evolved to hold less volume than that of Australopithecus. Breaking down raw plant starch in the intestines is a very time and energy consuming metabolic process which requires slow transit times and large storage capacity in the intestines for adequate time to break down and absorb the nutrients. When starches are cooked, however, heat energy from the fire begins the process of breaking down the starch before the food is ingested. As Anthropology Professor, Dr. Leslie Aiello, of the *Wenner-Gren Foundation for Anthropological Research* notes in *"The Expensive Tissue Hypothesis"* (*Current Anthropology*, 1995), cooking can be thought of as *"a technological way of externalizing part of the digestive process"* that *"not only reduces toxins in food but also increases its digestibility."* Eating partially pre-digested cooked food greatly reduced the amount of time and energy necessary to digest and absorb nutrients from starchy tubers which resulted in the evolution to smaller gut volume and faster transit times. As the gut evolved to be smaller and less energy consuming, this made more energy available to power the evolution of larger brains.

4

THE SHELLFISH HYPOTHESIS

Between 1.9 million years ago and 900,000 years ago, H. erectus made several migrations out of Africa into Eurasia, south Asia and Europe which resulted in genus Homo splitting into many different isolated sub-species. Fossil remains from some of these subspecies have dated migrations back to 1.75 million years ago into southern Eurasia, 1.6 million years ago and again 1 million years ago into south Asia, and 900,000 years ago into western Europe. This period of Homo speciation coincides with the hunter gatherer period of human evolution. But despite the addition of meat to their diet, the size of the brain, jaw and teeth of the H. erectus subspecies in South Africa that would later evolve into modern humans, underwent little change for over 1.7 million years.

Then suddenly, around 200,000 years ago, there began a second period of rapid brain growth and reduction in jaw and tooth size to that of modern humans, and the new subspecies "Homo sapiens" (Latin for "wise man") was born. As with the change in brain, jaw and tooth size that occurred from Australopithecus to H. erectus, the change from H. erectus to H. sapiens was also spurred by a dramatic change in the environment. As of this writing in the early 21st century, the precise time and place of this transition from H. erectus into H. sapiens is not a settled question among anthropologists, but in the paper *"Early human use of marine resources and pigment in South Africa during the Middle Pleistocene" (Science,* 2007), Dr. Curtis Marean, Professor of Anthropology at Arizona State University, appears to be honing in on the answer. In this interview about his findings, Dr. Marean sets the scene:

> *The world was in a glacial stage 125,000 to 195,000 years ago, and much of Africa was dry to mostly desert; in many areas food would have been difficult to acquire. The paleoenvironmental data indicate there are only five or six places in all of Africa where humans could have survived these harsh conditions." (ScienceDaily, 2007).*

Evolution speeds-up when organisms are under conditions of extreme environmental stress. This is because less fit organisms do not survive and subsequent generations are stocked by the more fit survivors. It was the drying out of the African savanna that spurred the evolution of Australopithecus into H. erectus 1.9 million years ago. From his findings, Dr. Marean postulates that the extremely dry and cool climate of the African continent around 200,000 years ago again spurred a similar evolution of H. erectus into H. sapiens. Dr. Marean continues:

> *Generally speaking, coastal areas were of no use to early humans – unless they knew how to use the sea as a food source. For millions of years, our earliest hunter-gatherer relatives only ate terrestrial plants and animals. Shellfish was one of the last additions to the human diet before domesticated plants and animals were introduced. Our findings show that at 164,000 years ago in coastal South Africa humans expanded their diet to include shellfish and other marine resources, perhaps as a response to harsh environmental conditions. This is the earliest dated observation of this behavior." (ScienceDaily, 2007).*

According to Dr. Marean's hypothesis, the introduction of shellfish to the diet was a critical factor in human evolution for several reasons. First, shellfish provided a far more reliable source of food than land animals since they were much easier to catch and they were somewhat higher in fat calories. With a diet of shellfish complimented by tubers which were also plentiful in their dry habitat, food energy was not only abundant, but also required relatively less energy expenditure to acquire. But as Dr. Marean describes, local food abundance had another significant effect:

> *"So, this is an extremely rich marine environment and one of the big impacts that shellfish has on hunter-gatherer economies is that when people began to exploit shellfish they can reduce their mobility so that they become less nomadic. The reason being is that shellfish are easy to capture and they are predictable and abundant. So, people do not have to chase the food so much and one of the things that happen when people reduce their mobility and they have a regular abundant source of food is then the group size can increase and that is often when we see the general culture and particularly symbolic expression in the tree of culture become more complex." (Nature International Weekly Journal of Science, October 2007)*

H. erectus is thought to have lived in small groups of between 30 and 50 individuals as they foraged nomadically on the African savanna. But caught between the desert and the sea on the southern tip of Africa 200,000 years ago, they became more sedentary with an abundant food source. Dr. Marean estimates that a colony of around 1,000 breeding individuals developed. At their archaeological site at Pinnacle Point, South Africa, Dr. Marean's team found evidence of advanced tool making using heat treated stone and also the production of pigments from heated, crushed stone. Dr. Marean postulates that higher population density required H. erectus to begin developing more complex communication skills which enabled them to teach and refine these more advanced technologies:

> *"Finding evidence of the use of pigments like red ochre, in ways that we believe were symbolic, is evidence of cognitive reason. Symbolism is one of the clues that modern language may have been present, and was important to their social relations." (Chrisroper.co.za; 2009)*

The human brain has the same general structure as other mammals, mainly: a brain stem that connects the brain to the central nervous system, a cerebellum that coordinates bodily movement, and a cerebrum that processes thought. Relative to body size, the human brain stem and cerebellum are about the same size as other mammals, but the human cerebrum is over three times as large as that of other mammals of equivalent body size. Dr. Marean makes a plausible argument for a shellfish driven culture in South Africa where the adaptive advantage of cognitive reason is what drove the growth in brain size from H. erectus to H. sapiens.

5
THE SEXUAL SELECTION HYPOTHESIS

On the open savannas of Africa two million years ago, through the evolutionary process of "natural selection," the smaller brained Australopithecus was replaced by the larger brained H. erectus due to the adaptive advantage a larger brain conferred upon H. erectus to develop defensive strategies to protect itself and its young from being killed by predators. But there is another selective process that drives the evolution of species called "sexual selection," first identified by Charles Darwin in his last book published in 1871 titled, *"The Descent of Man and Selection in Relation to Sex."*

Darwin postulated that sexual selection worked in two main ways: either through competition among males for sexual access to females, what he called "combat," or through a choice made by females for attractive male mates, what he called "display." As a classic example of display, Darwin pointed to the flamboyant tail of the peacock. The peacock's tail appears to serve no function in terms of survival, indeed, it may actually be a handicap, as it makes the peacock more visible to predators and less able to flee. Darwin explained this seeming contradiction in terms of sexual selection: the peahens simply found the gaudy tails to be more attractive. Darwin hypothesized that the peahens were attracted to the ornate display as it was a sign of good health and of the peacock's fitness to survive despite its burdensome handicap. Darwin reasoned that in the distant past, when peacocks had ordinary color and length tails, peahens showed a preference to mate with males that had slightly longer and more flamboyant than average tails. Over many generations of this sexual selection, peacocks' developed tails that were longer and brighter. In this way, the ornate tail display bestows such an advantage in mating success that it is selected for despite being a disadvantage in terms of survival. In the final chapter of *"The Descent of Man and Selection in Relation to Sex,"* Darwin discusses sexual selection in humans. To explain why it is the females that display overt signs of attractiveness instead of the males like most other species, Darwin believed that in humans it is the males who sexually select for females, (not likely, as we shall soon see). Darwin's sexual selection hypothesis was not well received in sexually repressed Victorian England, and for many decades after its publication, *"The Decent of Man and Selection in Relation to Sex"* dropped out of favor in the anthropological literature.

This remained the state of debate on sexual selection in human evolution until the book, *"The Mating Mind: How Sexual Choice Shaped the Evolution of Human Nature,"* was published in 2001. Written by evolutionary psychologist and Associate Professor of Psychology at the University of New Mexico, Dr. Geoffrey Miller, the book argues that the spurt in growth of the human cerebrum between 200,000 and 125,000 years ago may have been the result of sexual selection:

"Human language evolved to be much more elaborate than necessary for basic survival functions. From a pragmatic biological view point, art and music seem like pointless wastes of energy. Human morality and humor seem irrelevant to the business of finding food and avoiding predators." (p. 2)

"As we shall see, one of the main reasons why mate choice evolves is [to] help animals choose sexual partners who carry good genes. By comparison, natural selection is a rank amateur. The evolutionary pressures that result from mate choice can therefore be much more consistent, accurate, efficient and creative than natural selection pressures… As a result of these incentives for sexual choice, many animals are sexually discriminating. They accept some suitors and reject others. They apply their faculties of perception, cognition, memory, and judgment to pick

the best sexual partners they can. In particular, they go for any features of potential mates that signal their fitness and fertility." (p. 9)

"Scientists became excited about social competition because they realized that it could have become an endless arms race, requiring ever more sophisticated minds to understand and influence the minds of others. An arms race for social intelligence looks [like] a promising way to explain the human brain's rapid expansion and the human mind's rapid evolution." (p. 12)

If you combine Dr. Marean's shell fish hypothesis of a small colony of 1,000 H. erectus clinging to existence at the southern tip of Africa, with Dr. Miller's sexual selection hypothesis of an endless arms race for social intelligence, then sexual selection by females for males that were more adept at expressing themselves with body painting and expanded vocabulary becomes a plausible explanation for how H. erectus suddenly grew cerebrums to the size of anatomically modern humans starting around 200,000 years ago. Since characteristics of abstract thought are associated with larger cerebrums, it was this sexual selection by females for more clever males that resulted in the rapid evolution to the larger brain and more complex culture of H. sapiens. And as the cerebrum became larger, the mind of H. sapiens became more inventive developing more advanced technologies such as heat treating stone for better tool making. These early H. sapiens became what Dr. Marean called *"masters of fire"* (*ASU Research and Economic Affairs*, 2009). From this earliest evidence of human culture found on the southernmost shores of Africa, Dr. Marean postulated that it may have been this rare and obscure species of ape that eventually came to dominate the globe:

"This evidence shows that Africa, and particularly southern Africa, was precocious in the development of modern human biology and behavior. We believe that on the far southern shore of Africa there was a small population of modern humans who struggled through this glacial period using shellfish and advanced technologies, and symbolism was important to their social relations. It is possible that this population could be the progenitor population for all modern humans." (ScienceDaily, Oct. 2007).

6

FAT HEADS

It was around 200,000 years ago that the human brain started to evolve to its present day average adult size of 1,350 cubic centimeters. The human brain is composed of 60% fat as measured by calories, and there are two types of fat, omega-3 and omega 6 fatty acids, that are essential for brain growth and function. Since fish and shellfish are high in the omega-3 fatty acid "DHA," which is absent from terrestrial plant foods, some anthropologists have hypothesized that it was the introduction of sea animals into the human diet that provided enough of this essential nutrient for the exceptional brain growth of early H.

sapiens. But this hypothesis fails to explain how some modern human populations where sea animals are not part of the diet, are able to supply their large brains with enough DHA for healthy brain growth and function.

The explanation for this seeming contradiction is that plants provide plenty enough omega-3 fats for healthy brain growth and function. The human body has evolved metabolic pathways to synthesize adequate amounts of DHA from the omega-3 fats found in plant foods for healthy brain development even for pregnant and lactating women who have higher requirements, as Dr. John Langdon, Professor and Chair of Biology at the University of Indianapolis explains in his paper, *"Has an aquatic diet been necessary for hominin brain evolution and functional development?"*:

> *"A number of authors have argued that only an aquatic-based diet can provide the necessary quantity of DHA to support the human brain, and that a switch to such a diet early in hominin evolution was critical to human brain evolution. This paper identifies the premises behind this hypothesis and critiques them on the basis of clinical literature. Both tissue levels and certain functions of the developing infant brain are sensitive to extreme variations in the supply of DHA in artificial feeding, and it can be shown that levels in human milk reflect maternal diet. However, both the maternal and infant bodies have mechanisms to store and buffer the supply of DHA, so that functional deficits are generally resolved without compensatory diets. There is no evidence that human diets based on terrestrial food chains with traditional nursing practices fail to provide adequate levels of DHA or other-3 fatty acids. Consequently, the hypothesis that DHA has been a limiting resource in human brain evolution must be considered to be unsupported."* (British Journal of Nutrition, 2006)

No, DHA was not the limiting factor in the development of the larger H. sapiens brain, the limiting factor was energy. Brain cells use twenty times the calories of muscle cells at rest, and though the brain represents only 2% of the body's weight, it uses 25% of the body's total calories at rest. This means that as the brain increased in size relative to the rest of the body, a proportionately larger increase in daily food energy was needed to maintain it. Adding shellfish to the diet solved this energy problem in two ways: first, the fat in shellfish was a consistent secondary source of energy that supplemented the primary energy source that came from plant carbohydrates, and second, since shellfish could not run away like terrestrial animals and did not require digging-up like tubers, they expended significantly less energy to acquire, energy that could then be diverted to brain growth. H. sapiens are subject to the same laws of energy supply and demand as all other animals, and it was shellfish that enabled early H. sapiens to balance that energy equation while growing larger brains.

7

H. SAPIENS

As the cerebrum of H. erectus grew to the size of H. sapiens (anatomically modern humans), the cranium (brain case) became elongated to house the larger brain, causing the palate (roof of the mouth) and mandible (lower jaw bone) to become shorter and the teeth proportionally smaller. This restructuring of the oral cavity caused the tongue to move into the pharynx (back of the mouth). These anatomical changes facilitated the required physiology necessary for speech, a talent shared by none of our great ape relatives.

By around 60,000 years ago modern H. sapiens had fully manifest the four characteristics that in combination are what make us uniquely human: 1) bipedalism, 2) control of fire, 3) complex technologies and 4) symbolic thought and speech. Armed with these extremely powerful tools, this once rare and obscure great ape species was now poised to take on the world. Dr. Marean argues that with cooked shell fish a staple of their diet, traveling the coastlines became H. sapiens primary route out of Africa:

> *"Coastlines generally make great migration routes. Knowing how to exploit the sea for food meant these early humans could now use coastlines as productive home ranges and move long distances.*
>
> *"[Sometime around 50,000 to 60,000 years ago] these modern humans left the warm confines of Africa and penetrated into the colder glacial environment of Europe and Asia, where they encountered Neanderthals.*
>
> *"By 35,000 years ago these Neanderthal populations were mostly extinct, and modern humans dominated the land from Spain to China to Australia.*
>
> *"The command of fire, documented by our study of heat treatment, provides us with a potential explanation for the rapid migration of these Africans across glacial Eurasia - they were masters of fire and heat and stone, a crucial advantage as these tropical people penetrated the cold lands of the Neanderthal." ("Early Modern Humans Use Fire to Engineer Tools", US News & World Report, 2009)*

One hundred thousand years ago, there were four known remaining subspecies in the genus Homo: 1) H. sapiens that lived in Africa and the Middle East, 2) H. neanderthalensis that lived in Europe, 3) H. floresiensis that lived in southern Asia, and 4) H. Denisova that lived in Siberia. As H. sapiens migrated out of Africa around 60,000 years ago, these early modern humans came into contact with these other Homo subspecies and DNA analysis indicates that there was some interbreeding between them, but ultimately, H. sapiens dominated these other archaic Homo subspecies driving them into extinction, and by 28,000 years ago, H. sapiens remained as the only Homo subspecies left on Earth.

By 50,000 years ago H. sapiens had spread across Europe, Asia, Indonesia all the way to Australia. By 13,500 years ago they had migrated into the Americas and by 2000 years ago had colonized most of the Pacific Islands. These dates corresponded closely to the "Quaternary Megafaunal Extinction Event" in which many species of large terrestrial mammals went extinct including woolly mammoths, mastodons, ground sloths, giant beavers and cave bears. The *Quaternary Megafaunal Extinction Event* did not occur all at once or worldwide, but in a continent-by-continent sequence. Australia was the first to be affected losing 88% of its megafaunal species in the period between 50,000 and 32,000 years ago. Next affected was Eurasia where 35% of species went extinct. The Eurasian extinctions occurred in two pulses, the first between approximately 48,000 and 23,000 years ago, and the second between 14,000 and 10,000 years ago. North America saw 73% of its megafauna go extinct between 14,000 and 10,000 years ago, and South America lost 83% of its megafaunal species between 12,000 and 8,000 years ago.

In the study, *"Megafauna biomass tradeoff as a driver of Quaternary and future extinctions"* (PNAS, 2008), Dr. Anthony Barnosky, Professor Emeritus at the Department of Integrative Biology at the University of California, Berkeley, presented *"The Overkill Hypothesis"* to explain this wave of megafaunal extinctions. Dr. Barnosky proposed that H. sapiens killed off the megafauna as they migrated into new territories, over hunting these species to feed their growing populations. The dates and locations of megafaunal extinctions provide support for this hypothesis. In Australia, Eurasia, and North and South America, the megafaunal populations began to decrease and genera-wide extinctions began to occur within a few hundred to a few thousand years after modern humans first arrived into each new territory. Humans first arrived in Australia an estimated 50,000 years ago, which exactly corresponds to the dates of the initial stages of the Australian megafaunal extinction event. The two pulses of the Eurasian extinction events are correlated to, first, the initial wave of humans, and, second, to a dramatic increase in the human population. The megafauna of North and South America were the most vulnerable to the human onslaught, likely due to the advanced stone tools and big-game-hunting methods used by the Clovis hunters, and the megafauna's inexperience with human predators.

The correlating dates and locations of human arrival and megafauna extinctions also explains why Africa and Eurasia experienced fewer megafaunal extinctions than the other continents. As the birthplace of H. sapiens, African megafauna evolved with humans so these large mammals adapted their survival techniques to live successfully alongside humans instead of being completely at their mercy. This is why very few species of African megafauna went extinct during the global Quaternary Megafauna Extinction Event. In Eurasia, subspecies of H. erectus had inhabited the same areas for approximately 1.75 million years, so the Eurasian megafauna had time to adapt to proto-human hunting behaviors and therefore suffered fewer extinctions when modern humans arrived.

The Quaternary Megafaunal Extinction Event was completed shortly after humans had inhabited every continent with the exception of Antarctica. In all, 178 species of megafauna went extinct during the period between 40,000 and 8,000 years ago accounting for two-thirds of all mammalian species. The Quaternary Megafaunal Extinction Event was the first wave of the sixth great mass extinction event that is still underway as a result of the human turn toward carnivory. As we shall see in Part V, *Man Eating Animals: How Animal-based Diets Are Destroying Our Planet*, the second ongoing wave of mass extinctions is a result of the human creation of the global animal industrial complex over just this past century and a half to provide meat, dairy and eggs to billions of people.

Over the relative few thousands of years of the Quaternary Megafaunal Extinction Event, as our early ancestors were gorging themselves on the meat of megafauna, the primate anatomy and physiology we inherited over the prior 85 million years of our evolution to thrive on plant foods, underwent very little evolutionary change. This makes perfect evolutionary sense: humans didn't need to evolve sharp claws and teeth and high stomach acid to hunt, chew and digest meat, since we were able to use stone tools and fire to do the work for us. Over the past 60,000 years of human migration, isolated populations have evolved tremendous variations in skin color, height, build, hair and facial characteristics, but we all still share the same herbivorous primate anatomy and physiology that we inherited from our humble great ape ancestors.

8
Tϸᴇ Inuiᴛ Anᴅ Tϸᴇ Hunᴢᴀ

As anatomically modern humans migrated into new ecosystems that offered food resources distinctly different from their African roots, these new settlers had to modify their diets in order to take advantage of the food resources that were available. Some people who moved into areas with unremittingly harsh climates and limited food resources developed diets as distinctly different from our own modern diets as they are from each other. From the total animal-based diet of the "Inuit" people who live in the frigid Arctic North, to the near vegan plant-based diet of the "Hunza" people who live at an altitude of 8,000 feet (2,438 meters) above sea level in the Himalayan Mountains, their remarkable tales of human survival are a testament to the amazing flexibility of the human digestive system. Let's take a closer look at these extremes of human dietary adaptation.

The Inuit

The Inuit are considered by anthropologists to be a group of culturally similar people who inhabit the Arctic regions of Alaska, Canada and Greenland. They all descended from the Thule whaling culture that developed around 1000 AD in the Bearing Strait region of Alaska and spread eastward across the Arctic. Extremely cold icy weather conditions make it impossible to cultivate plant foods in the Arctic, so the Inuit developed a traditional diet based entirely on hunting and eating animals, mostly whales, walrus, caribou, seal, polar bears, muskoxen and birds.

This diet that contains no carbohydrates would seem to be deficient in vitamin C, an essential nutrient that comes from fruits and vegetables, but the Inuit show no signs of the tissue wasting disease, scurvy, which is caused by vitamin C deficiency. Researchers (Fediuk, 2002) measured the vitamin C content of samples of foods eaten raw by Inuit women living in the Canadian Arctic: caribou liver, seal brain, and whale skin, and they found adequate vitamin C content to meet minimum daily requirements to avoid scurvy. Unlike humans, caribou, seal and whale (and virtually all other mammals) produce their own vitamin C in their livers, and when their flesh is eaten raw, the residual vitamin C in their tissues is absorbed through the human intestinal wall. The meat must be eaten raw, however, because cooking destroys the vitamin C.

Vitamin D that is derived through direct exposure of our skin to sunlight, is essential for development of our bones and for many other metabolic processes. In the winter months of December and January, there is virtually no sunlight to be had in the Arctic, which puts the Inuit at severe risk for Vitamin D deficiency, but they show no signs of the bone deforming childhood disease, rickets, which is caused by vitamin D deficiency. Preformed vitamin D in the flesh of their prey animals provides the Inuit with just enough vitamin D to avoid rickets.

Most of the energy received by humans from their food comes in the form of carbohydrates, but the Inuit who have no carbohydrates in their diet expend enormous amounts of energy to survive their harsh environment, so where does their food energy come from? Unlike the ungulates eaten by early human hunters in Africa, all of the prey animals that evolved to survive in the frigid north have significant fat stores in their bodies to provide energy and insulation to stay warm. As a result, 75% of the calories in the 3,100 calories/day diet of the average Inuit adult come in the form of fat, and 25% comes from protein. Like all modern humans, the Inuit inherited a digestive system that is ideally adapted to processing starchy carbohydrates for food energy, but with no carbohydrates in their diet, nearly all of the energy in the Inuit diet comes from fat through the digestive process of ketosis where the liver turns fat into fatty acids and ketone bodies that substitute for glucose as an energy source. In humans, unlike in true carnivores (cats and dogs), ketosis is ordinarily a secondary source of energy supply only tapped into when the body is starved of carbohydrates, but for the Inuit who eat no carbohydrates, fat is always their primary source of food energy. With fat processed through the liver as their primary source of energy, the Inuit evolved larger livers than all other modern human variants. Generally, when the human body goes into the digestive state of ketosis, it indicates an unhealthy dietary condition (usually starvation), but the Inuit prove that the human body can survive even under very harsh conditions in a sustained state of ketosis.

There is also a metabolic cost to the Inuit's high animal protein diet. The breakdown products of animal proteins that circulate in the blood are acid forming. In order for the blood to accomplish its circulatory functions it must remain Ph neutral, so to neutralize the acid forming animal protein byproducts, our bodies naturally take calcium from our bones. This bone calcium is circulated through the liver and kidneys and excreted in the urine, resulting in a condition of calcium deficit and brittle bones called "osteoporosis." The June 1987 issue of *National Geographic* magazine reported on the medical examination of two Inuit women, one in her 20s and the other in her 40s, who's bodies had been entombed in ice for 500 years; both showed severe signs of osteoporosis.

In late winter when game animals are lean from winter starvation, the percent of fat in the Inuit diet goes down and the percent of protein goes up. If the percent of protein in their diet gets too high, they can go into the digestive state of gluconeogenesis in which protein is then converted directly into glucose by the liver for energy supply. If protein goes above 40% of their diet, a medical condition called "protein poisoning" sets in where feelings of low energy result in symptoms including diarrhea, headache, fatigue and low blood pressure and heart rate. The only cure for protein poisoning is eating more fats and/or carbohydrates.

There is a persistent claim among the medical establishment that due to the high omega 3 fatty acid content of aquatic animal foods, Arctic dwelling people, despite eating enormous quantities of animal fat, were immune from heart disease. This claim has been definitively proven false. The medical examination of the two 500 year old frozen Inuit women in the *National Geographic* article cited above, also showed severe signs of atherosclerosis, as did the medical examination of the 2,000 year old mummified remains of three out of five native Alaskan Aleuts on a similar diet, ("*Atherosclerosis across 4000 years of human history: the Horus study of four ancient populations,*" *Lancet*, 2013).

There are no medical records on the physical health of traditionally-living Inuit populations before contact with Europeans that began around the 1600s. Europeans brought new fatal diseases including tuberculosis, measles, influenza and smallpox that took their toll on the Inuit population. But autopsies of Inuit bodies near Greenland in the early 1900s show that common natural causes of death were pneumonia, kidney disease, trichinosis (from eating raw meat), malnutrition, and degenerative disorders. Studies conducted by anthropologists Knud Rasmussen and Franz Boas in the early 1900s also indicate that death by suicide was a common practice when people were no longer able to fen for themselves. Mortality records kept by a Russian mission in Alaska between the years 1822 and 1836 showed an average age of death (not including infant mortality) of only 43.5 years.

The Inuit have made the most of their seemingly impossible situation and their tale of survival is truly remarkable. But survival as a culture does not necessarily translate into a healthy, long lived population. As much as the Inuit all-animal diet enabled them to survive in their frigid Arctic North habitat, such a diet cannot reasonably be recommended as appropriate for the great majority of people on Earth.

The Hunza

Around 2,000 years ago, 1,000 years before the Thule culture developed in Alaska, a small band of people managed to edge their way over treacherous high passes through the Himalayan Mountains into the Hunza River Valley of Northern Pakistan which sits at over 8,000 feet above sea level. In virtual isolation from the rest of the world over the next two millennia these Hunza people turned what was a steep, barren, rocky, treeless terrain into some of the world's most productive farmland that has sustained a population of around 30,000 people for many centuries.

The Hunza accomplished this food producing miracle by hauling topsoil up from the river thousands of feet below and placing it behind stone retaining walls to form thousands of terraces on the mountainside. These terraces are so well designed and constructed that none of this precious top soil is ever lost to erosion. The terraces are irrigated with mineral water that is diverted from glacial runoff from the Himalayas through over sixty miles of channels and aqueducts.

On these fertile terraces the Hunza grew many varieties of fruits including melons, grapes, mulberries, figs, cherries, pears, peaches, apples, plums and most of all, apricots. They would eat raw fruits picked fresh when in season and sun dry lots of apricots to store and eat during the long frozen winter months. High quality vegetable oil was obtained from the apricot pits and also from ground flax seeds. Nuts which were another good source of fat included walnuts, almonds, pecans and hazelnuts. Grains included wheat, barley, millet, buckwheat and Job's tears which they made into a quick bread called "chapatti." Cultivated vegetables included mustard greens, spinach, lettuce, carrots turnips, potatoes, radishes, squash, lentils and chickpeas eaten raw or very lightly cooked. Dried beans were stored and eaten as sprouts over the winter as a high energy source of fresh greens. There is little fuel for cooking high in the Himalayas, so 80% percent of vegetables and 100% of the fruit in the Hunzan diet was eaten raw. Grass was very limited at that altitude and as a result the Hunza raised very few grazing animals for meat or milk. They also had no fish. In Hunza farming, all residual organic matter, including human manure, was composted and reapplied to the terraces creating a closed loop nutrient cycle.

By the early 1900s, the British had colonized India and Pakistan and had taken military control over the Hunza Valley and soon a persistent rumor that a very long-lived, healthy culture of people were living in the Himalayas started to leak out to the Western world. To find out if the rumor was true, the British army assigned Dr. Robert McCarrison, who was their director of nutritional research in India, to establish a hospital in Hunza where, in the 1910s, he lived among the Hunza for seven years. Dr. McCarrison was amazed by what he found:

> *"My own experience provides an example of a (people) unsurpassed in perfection of physique and in freedom from disease in general...The people of Hunza...are long lived, vigorous in youth and age, capable of great endurance, and enjoy a remarkable freedom from disease in general...Far removed from the refinements of civilization, [they] are of magnificent physique, preserving until late in life the character of their youth; they are unusually fertile and long lived, and endowed with nervous systems of notable stability...Cancer is unknown."*

In 1960 the United States National Geriatric Society sent Dr. Jay Hoffman to conduct a study of the health and longevity of the Hunza. In his subsequent book "*Hunza: Secrets of the World's Healthiest and Oldest Living People*," Dr. Hoffman wrote:

> "*Down through the ages, adventurers and utopia-seeking men have fervently searched the world for the Fountain of Youth but didn't find it. However unbelievable as it may seem, a Fountain of Youth does exist high in the Himalayan Mountains...Here is a land where people do not have common diseases, such as heart ailments, cancer (cancer is unknown), arthritis, high blood pressure, diabetes, tuberculosis, hay fever, asthma, liver trouble, gall bladder trouble, constipation, or many other ailments that plague the rest of the world.*"

Also in 1960, Dr. Allen Banik, an optometrist with a long interest in health, aging and longevity, was sent to investigate the Hunza by the famous TV personality Art Linkletter. In his book "*Hunza Land: The Fabulous Health and Youth Wonderland of the World*," Dr. Banik remarked:

> "*...the Hunzan's eyes were notable. I found them unusually clear; there were few signs of astigmatism. Even the oldest men had excellent far- and near-vision – an indication that their crystalline lenses had retained elasticity.*"

Dr. Banik further noted more generally:

> "*This race, which has survived through centuries, is remarkable for its vigor and vitality... In 2,000 years of almost complete isolation, the Hunzans seemed to have evolved a way of living, eating, thinking and exercising that has substantially lengthened their life span...*
>
> *The Hunzans are a hardy, disease-free people unique in their enjoyment of an unparalleled life span... It amazed me to see the number of older citizens going about their work and showing none of the signs of decrepitude that are so evident in the United States...*"

In 1964, Dr. Paul White, a prominent American cardiologist who had treated President Eisenhower, visited Hunza to check for himself the reputed fitness of the people and he too was amazed by what he found. Dr. White reported in the December 1964 *American Heart Journal* that of 25 Hunza men he studied who were "*on fairly good evidence, between 90 and 110 years old*":

> "*Not one showed a single sign of coronary heart disease, high blood pressure, or high cholesterol levels. They have 20-20 vision and no tooth decay. In a country of 30,000 people, there is no vascular, muscular, organic, respiratory or bone disease.*"

In the early 1970s, *National Geographic* magazine dispatched Dr. Alexander Leaf, who was professor of clinical medicine at Harvard University and Chief of Medical Services at Massachusetts General Hospital, to study the Hunza. In the January 1973 issue of the *National Geographic*, Dr. Leaf extolled on the remarkable health of their elders:

> "*Coming up the hill from our guest house we were overtaken by three elders who walked up the twenty-or-thirty degree incline without pause or difficulty while we stopped every few steps to catch our breath and quiet our pounding hearts... [Another elder] served as our porter,*

shouldering a heavy box of photographic equipment and bounding with it over the forbidding terrain like an agile mountain goat."

Needless to say, the verdict of Western science is in that the rumors were true, the Hunza were an unusually long-lived people who remained vigorous and healthy into their 90s and 100s. So what is it about Hunza life that predisposed these people to such longevity and health? By most accounts, there were three major reasons: 1) they had a very close knit social fabric in which everyone was cared for, 2) in order to survive in their extremely harsh environment they led a physically demanding lifestyle, and 3) due to the constraints of their environment they ate a diet almost exclusively of plant foods. According to Dr. Leaf, who took careful records of the Hunza diet, 99% was of plant origins with only 1% from animals. Nutritionally this diet broke down to 73% carbohydrates (all complex), 17% fat (mostly unsaturated) and 10% protein (mostly plant). Also, most amazingly of all, the Hunza maintained their extremely active lifestyle on only 1,900 calories per day; this compares to today's average sedentary American at just under 2,700 calories per day (***usda**.gov/factbook/chapter2.pdf*). It takes all three of these living conditions working in combination for optimal health; missing any one leads to suboptimal health over time. The Inuit had strong family bonds and a very active lifestyle, yet their diet, though well adapted to their environment, was not conducive to good health into old age.

While the basic Inuit and Hunza diets may both be considered extreme relative to our modern day more omnivorous diets – in terms of optimal human health – the Hunza plant-based diet is anything but extreme, it is actually pretty close to our natural herbivorous diet.

The human digestive tract is perfectly adapted for processing the Hunza plant-based diet high in complex carbohydrates and low in fats and proteins. This diet of mostly raw, fresh, whole, plant foods grown in organically rich soils provides more nutrition per calorie consumed than any other diet in the world and is why the Hunza have so much energy on so few calories.

Earlier in this discussion on the evolution of the human diet, I cited anthropologist, Dr. Richard Wrangham, who argues convincingly that it was the cooking of wild tubers that resulted in human evolution toward smaller teeth, less gut volume and an increase in food energy availability, so how is it that the Hunza diet of mostly raw plant foods produces the optimal food energy equation? The answer is agriculture. First, since agriculture greatly concentrates the food source, it requires much less energy per calorie to acquire food, and second, human selected cultivars of fruits and vegetables contain much higher concentrations of starches, vitamins and minerals and are much easier to chew than the wild tubers eaten by H. erectus and early H. sapiens. Our small teeth and guts are perfectly suited for processing these cultivated raw plants.

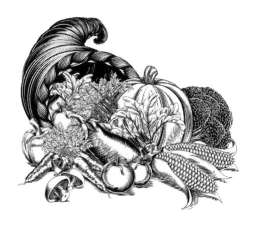

PART II

AGRICULTURE & CIVILIZATION

...

"In this food I see clearly the presence of the entire universe supporting my existence."
– Thich Nhat Hanh, Buddhist monk (1927 – 2022)

9

DⱯMESⱫICAⱫIⱯꝶ ⱯF PLAꝶⱫS

In the 1920s and 1930s, in the early years of the Soviet Union, the prominent Russian agronomist, botanist and geneticist, Nikolai Vavilov, was the director of the *Lenin All-Union Academy of Agricultural Sciences* where he conducted a series of botanical-agronomic expeditions that collected the seeds and specimens of cultivated plants and their wild relatives from many parts of the world, including Iran, Afghanistan, Ethiopia, China, and Central and South America, amassing samples of 250,000 varieties of wild plants including 31,000 wheat specimens. The specimens, which Vavilov collected himself, became the basis of the *Vavilov Institute* gene bank in Leningrad (now Saint Petersburg), which houses the largest collection of genetic resources of cultivated plants in the world. Observations Vavilov made from meticulous study of this vast trove of plants led him to postulate that a region in which the wild relatives of a cultivated plant showed maximum diversity of species represented the cultivated plant's "center of origin." Vavilov noted that the centers of origin of cultivated plants occurred mostly in mountainous regions between the Tropic of Capricorn (23°28′) south of the equator and about 45°N of the equator in the Eurasia and Africa, and between the Tropics of Cancer and Capricorn in the Americas. He also noted that in all cases, agricultural origins and primitive diversity occurred in high and complex mountain regions. As Vavilov obtained new data, he revised his list of centers of origin from 3 in 1924, to 5 in 1926, 6 in 1929, 7 in 1931 and 8 in 1935. In his 1935 paper entitled *The Phytogeographical Basis for Plant Breeding*, Valvilov summarized all the data from the hundreds of cultivated plants from all over the world that he had systematically collected, thusly:

> *"We can now speak with a considerably greater accuracy than dreamed of ten years ago about the eight ancient and basic centers of agriculture in the world, or, more accurately about the eight independent areas where plants were initially taken into cultivation."*

The first plants to be domesticated were grass species – wheat, rice, barley, oats, rye, teff, millet, sorghum, maize (corn), and amaranth – since grass seed is nutrient dense and conveniently broadcast and harvested. Legumes (beans) and tubers (potatoes) were also early domesticated staple crops. Vavilov identified the eight centers of origin as follows:

1) Chinese Center – rice, legumes

2) Indian Subcontinent Center (India, Pakistan) – barley, oats, wheat, legumes

3) Inner Asiatic Center (Tadjikistan, Uzbekistan) – wheats, rye, legumes

4) Asia Minor Center (Georgia, Azerbaijant, Armenia and Turkmenistan) – wheats, rye, oats, legumes

5) African Center (Ethiopian, Sudan and the Sahel) – teff, millet, sorghum

6) Mediterranean Center (Iran, Iraq, Israel, Jordan, Syria, Turkey – emmer wheat, einkorn wheat, hulled barley, legumes, flax

7) Central American Center – maize (corn), quinoa, amaranth, legumes

8) South America Andes Center (Bolivia, Peru, Ecuador) – potatoes, sweet potatoes, manioc, amaranth

As a historical note, Vavilov was a distinguished member of the *Academy of Natural Scientists Leopoldina zu Halle (Saale)*, received the prestigious *Lenin Prize* in 1926 as the highest award of his country, and from 1931 to 1940 was president of the *Geographical Society of the USSR*, but his life came to a tragic end in 1943 at the age of 55 when the brutal anti-science regime of Joseph Stalin sentence him to prison where he died from the extremely harsh conditions. Miraculously, the *Vavilov Institute* gene bank he founded in Leningrad survived the Nazi siege of World War II, and remains as the world's largest seed library of domesticated plants. In 1955, after Stalin's death, the verdict against Vavilov was reversed posthumously and in the 1960s his reputation was officially restored and he was once again revered as a giant of Soviet science.

While Vavilov was basically a geneticist and plant breeder whose primary interest was in improving plant genetics to increase crop yields, he was not particularly concerned with speculating on why the people in those 8 centers of origin made the profound change from nomadic hunter-gathers to sedentary farmers; he left that to others, who have proposed a number of different theories. In my opinion, the "Marginal Zone Theory," proposed by Dr. Lewis Binford, Professor of Archaeology at the University of New Mexico, and Dr. Kent Flannery, Professor of Anthropology at the University of Michigan, best takes into account the relationships between population pressure, change in environment, and human subsistence strategies. At the end of the last Ice Age around 11,700 years ago, hunter-gatherer groups began to inhabit the optimal food resource zones around the globe. Over the 6,000 year period between 10,000 and 4,000 years ago, at varying times human populations began to reached the carrying capacity of the land for hunter-gatherers in these optimal resource zones. This population pressure forced migration into areas of less optimal food resources, or marginal zones, that were located on the hilly grassy flanks of the optimal zones. This move caused a change in foraging strategy that resulted in a shift to grass seed as a new major food source. This foraging strategy led to the seasonal selection of various wild grasses which ultimately led to seed planting and the shift to a new system of village agriculture. Archaeological cites from this period confirm that the earliest villages were located in the marginal zones outside the boundaries of the optimal resource zones.

To grow plants in marginal areas, early agriculturalists had to select seed from wild plants that were naturally well adapted to harsher environments and propagate them. The earliest plants to be propagated in this way – wheat, barley, peas and flax – (known as the "founder crops") were first domesticated in Mesopotamia 10,000 years ago that would later become the basis for systematic agriculture in the Middle East, North Africa, India, Iran and Europe. Agriculture developed independently in other parts of the world at different times. *(Current Anthropology* Volume 52, Supplement 4, October 2011) On the African continent, teff and finger millet were domesticated in the Ethiopian highlands 6,000 years ago and sorghum and pearl millet in the Sahel region 8,000 to 9,000 years ago. Maize (corn) and quinoa were domesticated in Mexico around 7,000 years ago and rice was originally cultivated in China around 5,000 years ago. Amaranth, arrowroot, sweet potato, potato, peanut and manioc were first domesticate in South America.

Besides these "staple" grains, pulses (sometimes called "grain legumes") and tubers that provided the bulk of calories necessary for human populations to expand, many of the vegetables, fruits and nuts we commonly eat around the world today were also first domesticated by ancient agriculturalists. Due to the fact that plants do not preserve well in archaeological deposits there is very limited archaeological evidence as to the precise time and location of the first domestication of specific plant cultivars, but despite this handicap, below is an abbreviated list of some of the most common vegetables, fruits and nuts we know today with their approximate dates and places of origin:

Vegetables

Artichoke – probably first cultivated by the Greeks and Romans who obtained them from North Africa. They have been grown in England for at least 500 years.

Asparagus – originated in Europe predating Ancient Greece.

Beans – wild beans as a basic human dietary staple can be traced back more than 20,000 years in Asia. Ten thousand-year-old lentil remains have been uncovered on the banks of the Euphrates River in what is now Northern Syria. The common bean, lima bean and pinta bean were first cultivated in the very earliest Mexican and Peruvian civilizations more than 5,000 years ago. Chickpeas first appeared around 2,700 years ago in Europe and the Middle East and fava beans were widely cultivated in ancient Greece.

Beet – indigenous to the Mediterranean and the Atlantic seaboard of Europe. Eaten in Roman times at which time it was a long, white root. The swollen red root originated about 500 years ago.

Brassicaceae Family – broccoli, Brussels sprouts, cabbage, cauliflower, kale and kohlrabi all first domesticated in Europe over 2,500 years ago.

Carrot – originated in present day Afghanistan about 5000 years ago. Early varieties had anthocyanin pigments in them giving the carrot a red, purple or black color. A yellow variety without anthocyanin arose 400 years ago and the familiar orange variety 300 years ago.

Celery – indigenous to Europe and Asia. Cultivation was undertaken by the ancient Chinese and Egyptians.

Cucumber – originated in India and was domesticated more than 2,000 years ago.

Eggplant – originated in India and was grown in China as early as 2,000 years ago. Introduced into Spain and northern Africa by Arab traders in the Middle Ages.

Garlic – *Allium sativum*, the domesticated species, is thought to have originated from *Allium longicuspis* which is native to Central Asia. Evidence from Egyptian tombs shows that domestication of garlic goes back to at least 5,200 years ago.

Onion – thought to have been domesticated from one or more species in Central Asia. Onions were being cultivated by the Egyptians by 5,200 years ago but their domestication probably goes back a lot further than that although evidence is lacking because onion remains do not preserve well in archaeological deposits.

Pepper – originated in Central America where most of the main varieties were developed by local Indians. Seeds have been found in archaeological excavations dating back over 7,000 years ago in the Tehuacan Caves at Puebla, Mexico.

Summer squash – native to the Americas. Remains have been found in Central America dating as far back as 9,000 years ago. From its southern origin, squash spread throughout North America. The name squash is apparently derived from the Algonquin "askoot asquash," meaning "eaten green."

Tomato – the 10 or so species of *Lycopersicon* are native to the western coast of South America from Ecuador to Chile, but it appears that domestication took place in Mexico. It is thought that once agricultural fields had become established in Mexico, tomato seeds dispersed by birds were able to become established and it was from these wild tomatoes that Mexicans produced domesticated varieties. It is not known when first domestication took place but it is known to have predated Spanish arrival 500 years ago.

Winter squash – was domesticated in North America from wild *Cucurbita texana*, occurring in the southern North America, and *Cucurbita fraterna*, occurring in northeastern Central America. From archaeological excavations in Mexico, domestication can be dated back to about 10,000 years ago, predating maize.

Fruits and Nuts

Almond – native to the Middle East from the Mediterranean to Pakistan. It was first domesticated around 5,000 years ago and spread along the shores of the Mediterranean into northern Africa and southern Europe.

Apple – originated in the Tien Shan mountains of eastern Kazakstan. Archeological evidence shows that humans have been eating apples for at least 8,500 years, and historical evidence shows domestication by at least 7,000 years ago.

Apricot – originated in the high mountainous region of Hindu Kush – Tien Shan in Central Asia, where the borders of modern day China, Tajikistan, Afghanistan and Pakistan meet. The ancient Tajiks from Sogdain were most likely the ones who first domesticated this fruit at least 4,000 years ago.

Banana – cultivation dates back to 10,000 years ago in Papua New Guinea.

Cashew – native to the American tropics of Brazil, Peru, and Mexico. It is also native to the Islands of the West Indies. In the 1500s the Portuguese found the cashew growing along the coast line and they exported the seed to their colonies in East Africa and India. India is now the dominant producer of cashews in the world.

Fig – remains of figs found in an 11,400 year old house in Gilgal 1, an early Neolithic village in the Jordan Valley, Israel, came from a type of fig tree that could only have survived with the help of human propagation. This places fig domestication before grains.

Grape – it appears that domestication of the grapevine first took place in the region between the Caucasus and Armenia, dating back to at least 5,000 years ago.

Hazelnut – native to an area that stretches from Europe to south west Asia. Pollen studies have shown that the hazel quickly colonized large parts of Europe after the end of the last Ice Age. Modern humans in the temperate zones have had a long and productive association with this highly productive food resource.

Olive – there is clear evidence of domestication of olive trees in the Mediterranean region dating back to 5,500 years ago.

Orange – native to southern Asia, the name "orange" comes from the Sanskrit word naranga, not the color of the fruit. Records of domestication of the orange goes back to about 2,500 years ago. Oranges were cultivated in the Mediterranean by 600 years ago and Europeans spread them around the world 400 years ago.

Pear – archeological evidence shows that pears were eaten from the wild long before they were cultivated. Reliable evidence of pear cultivation first appears in Greek and Roman times.

Pecan – large trees native to Mexico and south central United States. In the south central area, the pecan was a staple of the indigenous people. It is believed that the indigenous tribes planted pecan seeds at their camps as an investment in their future.

Plum – originated in the Caucasus Mountains near the Caspian Sea. Luther Burbank detailed evidence that the prune (dried plum) was a staple food of the Tartars, Mongols, Turks, and Huns, *"who maintained a crude horticulture from a very early period."*

Walnut – native range is from southeast Europe and across to China. The Kashmiri/Northern Pakistan area is a particularly important area of biological diversity for walnuts. The nuts were a premier food for the earliest humans to inhabit these areas. Walnuts were never domesticated, but gathered in season. Even the very recent development of grafting didn't at first result in domestication of the walnut, because walnuts are one of the most difficult trees to graft, and because they were slow to start bearing and are very space demanding trees. Nevertheless, walnuts were spread by humans into Western Europe in prehistoric times and were cultivated in France around 1,600 years ago.

10

DOMESTICATION OF ANIMALS

The first wild animal to be domesticated by humans was the grey wolf possibly as far back as 15,000 years ago, probably not for food though, but for companionship. Humans and wolves share a pack mentality that enables us to socialize well together. The grey wolf was eventually bred by different human cultures into all the modern breeds of dogs that exist today.

In the Near East around 10,000 years ago when human population densities began to increase beyond the forage capacity of the land (estimate by Dr. Paul Martin, Emeritus Professor of Geosciences at the University of Arizona, to be about one person/square mile in high quality foraging grounds), the natural reproductive rates of wild animals could no longer keep pace with human predation. Populations of once abundant prey species began to crash and could no longer be depended upon as a reliable food source. But even as their prey was vanishing, these hunter-gatherers must still have considered these prey animals as a source of highly prized meat as they had done for thousands of years before; so it behooved them to start managing the diminishing herds through a process of selective cull. Over time these managed wild herds were bred for characteristics that made them more attractive for human exploitation. The most common hypothesis states that sheep were the first animal to be domesticated in this way from a wild species called "mouflon" that naturally possessed many characteristics such as lack of aggression, manageable size, early sexual maturity, social nature, and high fecundity (reproductive rate), that made them ideal for domestication. As the practice of domesticating animals spread rapidly to other regions where human population densities were putting pressure on available prey animals, other wild species that had suitable characteristics for domestication soon came under the human hand. All the major domesticated food animals we know today – sheep, goats, pigs, chickens and cattle – were originally domesticated between 11,000 and 8,000 years ago:

Sheep – domesticated between 11,000 to 9,000 years ago, sheep were first herded in a rotation over wild grasslands. Sheep domestication for meat and wool quickly spread to Africa and Europe. Small amounts of sheep milk probably also entered the human diet around this time becoming the first human exposure in all the millions of years of our evolution to the milk of another species.

Goats – wild goats were first domesticated in the Near East over 9,000 years ago for their meat and milk. As browsers of shrubs instead of grazers on grass like sheep, goats did not compete with sheep for the same food.

Pigs – the socially oriented wild boar was also first domesticated around 9,000 years ago into the very friendly and meaty pig in both the Near East and China independently. From the Near East the domesticated pig spread to Europe and eventually the Americas, and from China to Indonesia and eventually to remote Pacific Islands.

Chickens – first domesticated in Southeast Asia about 8,000 years ago by crossbreeding wild birds called red and grey junglefowl (*Gallus gallus and Gallus sonneratii*). Their sociability and prolific egg laying made these birds ideal candidates for domestication. Domesticated chickens then spread to the Near East and Western Europe by about 5,000 years ago, India by about 4,500 years ago, North Africa by 3,400 years ago, the Polynesian islands by 3,300 years ago and Eastern Europe by 3,000 years ago.

Cattle – cattle are also thought to have been first domesticated around 8,000 years ago in the Near East. Due to their ability to interbreed with other closely related species the exact wild ancestor of domesticated cattle has been hard to pin down, but DNA evidence supports the hypothesis that there were multiple domestication events with Near Eastern breeds being introduced into Africa where they were bred with locally domesticated African breeds, and also into Western Europe where they were bred with the wild aurochs. Their mild manner, herd mentality, large size and prodigious milk production made them excellent candidates for domestication. While exploiting other mammals for their milk first started with sheep and goats, archaeological evidence indicates that it wasn't until domestication of the cow that dairy became a significant dietary component. It is thought that the first true dairying culture called the "Linearbandkeramik Culture" (named after its distinct "Linear Pottery") began in the Danube river basin of central Europe around 7,500 years ago and spread into western and northern Europe and eventually to Scandinavia, where they displaced Europe's first early modern human hunter-gatherers known as Cro-Magnons (the Neanderthals were long gone). Genetic evidence suggests that the trait of lactose (milk sugar) tolerance in adults co-evolved with the Linearbandkeramik Culture since raw milk was an essential source of calories for their survival through the long lean winter months when few other food sources were available. The Linearbandkeramik survived by storing loads of hay to feed the cows over the winter and by drinking their fresh raw milk. Before developing this trait of lactose tolerance, humans, like all other mammals, would lose their ability to digest lactose after being weaned from their mothers breast milk. But a genetic mutation occurred that enabled the Linearbandkeramik to continue to produce lactase (the enzyme necessary to digest the lactose in milk) past weaning into adulthood which conferred a survival advantage upon those with the mutated Lactase Persistent (LP) gene. The LP gene spread throughout Europe along with the Linearbandkeramik Culture. (*"The Palaeopopulationgenetics of Humans, Cattle and Dairying in Neolithic Europe"*) The first domesticated cattle were grazed in small herds on local grasslands much the same as sheep, but then about 7,000 years ago a small band of nomadic people far to the north called Kurgans began to herd cattle over the vast grasslands of the Eurasian steppes. Approximately 6,000 years ago the Kurgans domesticated the wild horse for riding as a means to drive their mobile food supply over long distances. Their nomadic culture was organized into a male hierarchy social structure with three distinct classes: a small number of priests at the top, a larger warrior class in the middle, and a mass of commoners at the base. This cultural organization was very different than that of the egalitarian societies to the south where people subsisted in small villages by tilling the soil and shepherding small flocks. The Kurgans ranged in a huge area bounded by the modern-day Ukraine to the west and Mongolia to the east but as climate change pushed them to the edges of this territory they began to range south and invade these small village communities. This invasion came in three successive waves between 6,000 and 2,800 years ago, and by its end, the local grasslands of the original small herding village cultures had been transformed into a new culture dominated by male hierarchies and a warrior class.

As H. sapiens migrated out of Africa 60,000 years ago, they relied exclusively on their nomadic hunter-gatherer way of life for survival as they colonized new habitats. But then around 10,000 years ago starting in Mesopotamia, (the area of the Tigris-Euphrates river systems corresponding to modern-day Iraq, southwestern Iran, southeastern Turkey, and northeastern Syria), a new method of food production appeared in the human repertoire, agriculture, that is: directly raising plants and animals for food instead of merely relying on the natural availability of wild plants and animals. Over the next 6,000 years, agriculture developed independently in such distant places as Asia and the Americas, and by 4,000 years ago, agriculture had become the predominant means of food production for expanding human populations around the world. The great majority of these people subsisted on staple plant crops of grains (grass seeds) and tubers, while nomadic hunter-gatherer societies represented a dwindling fraction of the world's total human population.

11
CIVILIZATION

In the study, *"Global genetic positioning: Evidence for early human population centers in coastal habitats,"* (*Proceedings of the National Academy of Sciences* (**PNAS**) **2005**), researchers William Amos and Andrea Manica of the Department of Zoology, University of Cambridge, UK, traced modern day people back to their roots of origin through the use of genetic regression analysis. They identified 5 main clusters of early human population growth:

Old World (Eastern Hemisphere)

1) **Near East/North Africa** (modern-day Iraq, Turkey, Syria, Lebanon, Jordan, Cyprus, Israel, Palestine and Egypt)

2) **Asian Subcontinent** (modern-day Pakistan, India, Bangladesh, and Sri Lanka)

3) **Far East Asia** (modern-day China, Japan, Korea, Vietnam, Laos, Cambodia, Thailand and Burma)

4) **Eurasia** (Eastern and Western Europe)

New World (Western Hemisphere)

5) **South & Central America** (Peru and Mexico)

Researchers Amos and Manica noted that:

"The placement of many populations near centers of agriculture makes good genetic sense. Our method depends on genetic gradients that take time to establish. Such gradients are expected to be weak when populations are nomadic and relatively insular, but should become much stronger during periods of stasis, when populations remain for long periods in the same place while trade and conflict cause gene flow between neighboring groups. Equally, genetic drift operates slowly and, once formed, gradients are likely to take a long time to degrade, even in the face of modern travel. Thus, genetic gradients are likely to fall behind migration and to reflect the past better than the present. It is, therefore, perhaps not surprising that the inferred locations are consistent with the time when humans first gained the means to form large, stable, long-term communities."

The first major human population centers in the Near East/North Africa, the Asian Subcontinent and Far East Asia all developed in very fertile river basins not far north of the Earth's equator where the climate had remained relatively mild and stable since the end of the last Ice Age around 11,700 years ago. The cultivars listed above (along with many others) were specifically bred to produce large seeds, fruits and tubers that contained much higher yields of starchy carbohydrates and sugars than the wild plant species from which they were bred. As increased starch production fueled human population growth in early civilizations, the natural limits of pastureland to sustain increased meat production meant that meat had to be rationed, and the primary use of domesticated animals shifted to the value they could provide while still alive – milk, eggs, wool, muscle power and manure – and they were only eaten after their productive lives were spent.

As civilizations developed in different parts of the world with different wild plants and animals suitable for domestication and under diverse ecological and climactic conditions, the diets of these various peoples were necessarily very different from one another. In order to examine just what these ancient peoples of the world actually ate and how their diets and agriculture developed, I am now going to trace the development of the most prominent of these civilizations over the course of human history. I apologize in advance to the descendants of the many fascinating and resourceful cultures that I have omitted from this narrative, but the purpose of this exercise is not to be exhaustive, it is to examine the dietary and agricultural practices of people in the world's largest population centers as human beings colonized the Earth. As a further note to readers, for ease of understanding, I have chosen to use the names of places, people and cultures that are in most common usage today though many of these names were not used by the peoples themselves; again my apologies. This historical overview is loaded with specific dates many of which are best estimates. As a matter of convenience, I use the year 2000 AD as my reference year and back date all events from then, for example: 1,500 BC = 3,500 years ago (1,500 BC + 2,000 AD). Please keep in mind as you read, however, that obsessing over particular dates is far less important than following the chronology of events and recognizing the historical trends. So let's take a closer look at the diets and agriculture of Old and New World civilizations.

Old World

Near East/North Africa

Mesopotamia

The geological time period between the end of the last Ice Age around 11,700 years ago to the present day is called the "Holocene Epoch." During this period the general climate trend around the globe was for higher average temperatures and greater precipitation than during the preceding glacial period, although there have also been several multi-century cooling and drying periods over the course of the Holocene. As the continental glaciers retreated northward and upward into higher elevations, groups of human hunter-gathers followed expanding herds of wild grazing animals as they moved into formerly ice-covered areas that had turned into temperate forests and grass savannas. Due to these favorable climactic and material conditions, by around 10,000 years ago in northern Mesopotamia (modern-day Iraq), the population reached a point where the people who lived in drier regions were depleting the prey animals in the geographical area they depended on for food. It was here in the semi-arid mountains of the Near East that humans first began to exploit a series of adjacent but contrasting climatic zones to domesticate wild grasses and wild sheep and goats to create a more stable food supply (*"The Ecology of Early Food Production in Mesopotamia", Science*, March, 1965). These first Neolithic (stone age) farmers were semi-nomadic people who continued to forage for wild species while also occupying areas for months at a time during the spring rainy season to sow and reap their cereal grains of einkorn, emmer (types of wheat) and barley. This pattern fits in with the "Marginal Zone Hypothesis" in which agriculture first developed in marginal food production areas because there would have been no reason for it to develop in places where hunting and gathering still provided an adequate food supply.

This early period of agriculture was interrupted by a major drought period that occurred around 8,200 years ago (6200 BC) in which large villages that had developed in northern and central Mesopotamia became small hamlets as water necessary for agriculture was reduced (Weiss, 1978, Valladas et al., 1996). By 7,500 years ago (5500 BC) with the return of greater precipitation, the people of northern Mesopotamia began to settle down and farm on a permanent basis. In order to farm during the dry season water from the Tigris and Euphrates Rivers was diverted with ditches to flood the rich alluvial (sedimentary) soils of the river valleys marking the beginning of irrigation agriculture. Irrigation allowed the cultivation of flax which is rich in essential dietary fatty acids and is also a valuable source of plant fiber to weave into linen. Over the next two thousand years numerous other plants were domesticated in this region including the date palm, onion, garlic, leek, lettuce, cabbage, carrot, radish, beans, peas, chickpeas and the herbs coriander, fennel, fenugreek, marjoram, mint, mustard, rosemary, rue, saffron, thyme and cumin. Small flocks of adult domesticated sheep were kept for wool and a few cows for plowing. Young sheep and goats and old cows were culled to manage the herds, their meat being dried, smoked, salted or cooked. Surplus milk from the adult herds was made into butter and cheese. Domesticated pigs and wild fish also supplied meat and domesticated ducks and geese supplied eggs and meat to the ancient Mesopotamian diet. ("*Handbook of Life in Ancient Mesopotamia,*" Facts on File:New York NY, 2003)

The first sedentary farmers in northern Mesopotamia were named the "Samarran." The Samarran lived in settlements with populations of several hundred people. The Samarran appear to have developed a highly organized social structure and were the first people to make pottery to store surplus grain which enabled them to greatly enhance their food security and availability. With these more plentiful and consistent food supplies the Samarran population grew and began to spread its influence southward towards the delta wetlands of the Tigris and Euphrates Rivers (in Ancient Greek Mesopotamia means "land between rivers") at the shores of the Persian Gulf.

As irrigation technology spread down river to the mouths of the Tigris and Euphrates Rivers, the Samarran farmers gradually displaced the relatively sparse population of hunter-gatherer-fisher groups who had been foraging in the wetlands there. By 7,300 years ago (5300 BC) these Samarran settlers had developed into a distinctive new culture called the "Ubaid." The Ubaid are considered the first of four succeeding "Sumerian" cultures. The first Ubaid settlements were confined to the shores of the Persian Gulf where they pioneered growing grains in the extreme arid conditions of southern Iraq by making use of the high water table for irrigation. Between 6,800 and 6,500 years ago (4800 BC and 4500 BC) the Ubaid developed extensive irrigation canal networks that radiated from the major settlements. The construction and maintenance of these canals indicates that the Ubaid mobilized, coordinated and fed large labor forces to work on projects that served the collective interests. During this period, Ubaid canal irrigation spread rapidly throughout the wetlands. The period between 6,500 and 6,000 years ago (4500 and 4000 BC) saw an intense urbanization. The Ubaid culture also saw the invention of the potters wheel and the establishment of small craft industries including pottery, weaving, leatherwork, copperwork and masonry as well as trade networks that extended northwest into modern-day Syria and south along the coastline of the Arabian Peninsula as far as modern-day Oman. The Ubaid culture lasted an astonishing 2,500 years from start to finish, until the beginning of the second Sumerian culture called the "Uruk" around 6,000 years ago (4000 BC).

The archaeological transition from the Ubaid to the Uruk is marked by a gradual shift from painted pottery domestically produced on a slow wheel to a great variety of unpainted pottery mass-produced by specialists on fast wheels. By the time of the Uruk the volume of trade goods transported along the canals and rivers of southern Mesopotamia facilitated the rise of many large, stratified, temple-centered cities with populations of over 10,000 people where centralized administrations employed specialized workers. There is little evidence of institutionalized violence or professional soldiers during this period and towns were generally unwalled, though there is clear evidence in Uruk iconography (pictorial representations) that captured slaves from the hill country were used as workers. During this period the city of Uruk became the largest in the world with over 50,000 inhabitants. The decline of the Uruk coincided with another major climate event called the "Piora oscillation" which was a three hundred year drought period between 5,200 and 4,900 years ago (3200 BC and 2900 BC). Archaeological evidence suggests that the social effects of this extended drought period included colony collapse across northern Mesopotamia from the Zagros Mountains in western Iran to Syria where rain fed cereal agriculture became unsustainable (Weiss, 1986, 2003).

The record picks up again around 4,700 years ago (2700 BC) with the "Early Dynastic Period". The epic story of the king Gilgamesh (who lived between 2700 BC and 2600 BC) suggests that this period was associated with increased violence as cities became walled and increased in size and undefended villages disappeared. Semitic speaking nomadic tribes of sheep and cattle herders from the Arabian Peninsula to the south and Jordan and Syria to the west developed a cultural symbiosis with the Sumerians and eventually under the leadership of Sargon the Great, Semites from the city of Akkad in northern Mesopotamia conquered all of Sumer by around 4,350 years ago (2350 BC) and established the fourth cultural period of Sumer. Considered to be the world's first empire, the Empire of Akkad was short lived collapsing around 2150 BC due to yet another extended drought period (Weiss et al., 1993). As the drought wore on nomadic pastoral tribes (sheep, goat and cattle herders) called Gutians from the eastern Zargos Mountains and Amorites from northern Syria drove their herds closer to reliable water sources near the Tigris and Euphrates rivers, bringing them into conflict with the native Akkadian farmers. This was the period when the Akkadians built the monumental fortress like temples called Ziggurats at the centers of their major cities but such costly defensive projects only led to increased political instability. Texts written in Cuneiform (Akkadian wedgeshaped characters impressed on clay tablets) suggest that the Gutians showed little regard for maintaining irrigation canals for agriculture and they let their flocks roam freely in the fields which caused mass starvation among the Akkadians. Another consequence of this severe drought was the salinization of the major agricultural lands of southern Sumer. Due to higher levels of evaporation caused by the drought dissolved salts built up in the intensively irrigated fields, eventually reducing agricultural yields severely. During this period there was a shift from the cultivation of wheat to the more salt-tolerant barley, but this adaptation was insufficient to provide enough food to feed the existing population and during the period from 2100 BC to 1700 BC it is estimated that the population of southern Sumer declined by nearly 60%. (*"Salt and Silt in Ancient Mesopotamian Agriculture, Progressive changes in soil salinity and sedimentation contributed to the breakup of past civilizations." Science,* November 1958). It has also been suggested that the rapid climatic collapse, marking this Akkadian "Dark Age," may have been responsible for the religiously prescribed prohibition against the raising and consumption of pigs that spread through the ancient Middle East since pigs, unlike sheep, goats and cattle, required increasingly scarce wallows to stay cool and hydrated.

The southern part of Mesopotamia appears never to have recovered fully from the disastrous general decline which accompanied the salinization process. While never completely abandoned, cultural and political power passed permanently out of the region with the rise of Babylon to the north under the Amorite King, Hammurabi, around 1700 BC and many of the great Sumerian cities dwindled to villages or were left in ruins. Within two generations of Hammurabi's death the region was again overrun by herding, migrating peoples, this time arriving from the mountainous regions of northern Iran. These invaders included the Kassites and Aryans who were led by a warrior class that was armed with horses and chariots. These tribes spoke Indo-European languages which has led scholars to believe that they originally came from the steppes of Russia and were migrating southward due to climate changes. By 1100 BC the Mesopotamian region had become a political backwater with power and influence having shifted to the Egyptians of the Nile, the Hittites of Anatolia (Turkey), and the Mycenaeans of the Aegean (Greece).

The Levant

The Levant region consists of present day Israel, Jordan, Lebanon, Palestine and Syria on the eastern shores of the Mediterranean Sea located south of Mesopotamia and north of Egypt. The inland Jordan River cuts through the middle of the Levant from its headwaters in the Sea of Galilee flowing south emptying into the Dead Sea. Precipitation amounts and patterns in this predominantly arid to subarid region result from complex interactions between the region's topography and the high and low-pressure systems that come in off the Mediterranean Sea. Climate variability over the millennia played a significant role in the rise and fall of civilizations in the Levant.

The story of the early settlement of the Levant is contained in the "Old Testament" which is the canonical text for both the Jewish and Christian religions. The Old Testament was written and edited by many different people over a two hundred year period between 538 BC and 332 BC. The 39 books of the Old Testament tell the origin story of the Jewish people from the time of creation of the universe to approximately 450 BC.

In book one, "Genesis," god gives to the first humans, Adam and Eve, a plant-based diet:

"Then God said, 'I give you every seed-bearing plant on the face of the whole earth and every tree that has fruit with seed in it. They will be yours for food.'" (Genesis 1:29)

In the Genesis story of Cain and Abel (Adam and Eve's two sons), even as god had given all seed bearing plants to humans for food, he reserved the offering of animals to himself:

"Now Abel kept flocks, and Cain worked the soil. In the course of time Cain brought some of the fruits of the soil as an offering to the LORD. And Abel also brought an offering—fat portions from some of the firstborn of his flock. The LORD looked with favor on Abel and his offering, but on Cain and his offering he did not look with favor." (Genesis 4:2 – 5)

These passages from Genesis suggest the authors believed that in the beginning, plants were for people and meat was for the Lord.

Meat eating was not sanctioned by god in the Old Testament until many generations later when in a fit of rage god destroyed wicked humanity with a great flood, leaving only the good man Noah and his sons to repopulate the Earth:

> *"So God blessed Noah and his sons, and said to them: 'Be fruitful and multiply, and fill the earth. And the fear of you and the dread of you shall be on every beast of the earth, on every bird of the air, on all that move on the earth, and on all the fish of the sea. They are given into your hand. Every moving thing that lives shall be food for you.'"* (Genesis 9:2 – 3)

Written as myths by ancient peoples to establish their tribal identity, these stories of Genesis cannot be taken literally, but they do shed light on the authors' beliefs about human origins. It is interesting to note that even these ancient herding peoples, without benefit of modern evolutionary science, seemed to know instinctively that humans started out as a plant eating species, and that meat eating entered the diet later.

Near the end of Genesis, the Old Testament begins to transition from mythology to the historical era that corresponds to the time period from 2100 BC to 1800 BC when there was a mega-drought in the Middle East and a great famine swept across the land. Even though this period was long after Noah and god's sanctioning of meat eating, the story of Joseph, who led the Israelites from Canaan to Egypt, suggests that livestock were considered distinct from food:

> *"When the money of the people of Egypt and Canaan was gone, all Egypt came to Joseph and said, 'Give us food. Why should we die before your eyes? Our money is all gone.'*
>
> *"'Then bring your livestock,' said Joseph. 'I will sell you food in exchange for your livestock, since your money is gone.' So they brought their livestock to Joseph, and he gave them food in exchange for their horses, their sheep and goats, their cattle and donkeys. And he brought them through that year with food in exchange for all their livestock."* (Genesis 47:15 – 17)

These passages suggest that livestock were primarily used for purposes other than food such as wool, milk, traction (plowing) and transport.

Books two, three, four, five and six of the Old Testament, "Exodus," "Leviticus." "Numbers," "Deuteronomy," and "Joshua," describe the Israelites exodus from slavery in Egypt and their conquest of the Levant region from 1400 BC to 1200 BC. During this time period, the rains had returned to the Levant and its grassy hills and plains once again were prime grazing land for livestock. Though these books were written centuries after the events they describe, and are thus political documents rather than contemporaneous historical accounts, they do appear to have some basis in actual events.

In books two and three, Exodus and Leviticus, while the Israelites were wandering in the Sinai Desert after fleeing Egypt and before invading the Levant, many restrictions were put on the eating of meat: Exodus 29:29-34 restricts the eating of rams (adult male sheep) to priests; Leviticus 11:1-47, prohibits anyone from eating rabbit, pig, all water creatures that do not have fins and scales, all birds of prey, bats, weasel, rat, lizards and snakes; Leviticus 17:1-6 requires that all ox, lamb and goats must be slaughtered by priests in front of the holy tabernacle with transgressors punished by banishment from the tribe; Leviticus 7:19-20 prohibits eating meat that is "ceremonially unclean" or by persons who are "unclean" with transgressors also punished by banishment. These restrictions undoubtedly had a depressing effect on the consumption of meat during the time when the Israelites were living in the desert.

One important function of the Old Testament was to keep an accurate genealogy of the Israelite people. In book four, Numbers, Moses is commanded by the Israelite god to take a census of all the men in the Israelite tribes over the age of twenty who were eligible to serve in the Israelite army (Numbers 26:1-51). Later, after the conquest of the Levant, this census would be used as the basis for dividing up the grazing lands among the Israelite tribes (Joshua 14 – 21). Moses came up with a total of 601,730 men of military age. If older men, woman and children are added to this number, the Israelite population at the time of Moses would have been well over 1.5 million people. Considering that the Israelites were one of the smaller groups in the area, the population of the Levant around 1200 BC was probably upwards of 10 million people.

In book five, Deuteronomy, as the Israelites were preparing to invade the Promised Land (the Levant), Moses in a speech to the assembled Israelites revoked the exclusive franchise of priests to slaughter animals that had been granted in Leviticus:

"When the LORD your God has enlarged your territory as he promised you, and you crave meat and say, 'I would like some meat,' then you may eat as much of it as you want. If the place where the LORD your God chooses to put his Name [the holy tabernacle] is too far away from you, you may slaughter animals from the herds and flocks the LORD has given you, as I have commanded you, and in your own towns you may eat as much of them as you want. (Deuteronomy 12:20 – 21)

Presumably, meat eating was more common among the Israelites after their conquest of the Levant.

In book six, Joshua, the authors make it unequivocally clear that the Israelite conquest of the Levant was for the purpose of controlling grazing rights over the land. Here, Joshua is explicitly commanded by god to kill the current inhabitants and seize their livestock:

"Then the LORD said to Joshua, 'Do not be afraid; do not be discouraged. Take the whole army with you, and go up and attack Ai. For I have delivered into your hands the king of Ai, his people, his city and his land. You shall do to Ai and its king as you did to Jericho and its king, except that you may carry off their plunder and livestock for yourselves.'" (Joshua 8:1 – 2)

Joshua carried out this same command on cities throughout the Levant:

"Joshua took all these royal cities and their kings and put them to the sword. He totally destroyed them, as Moses the servant of the LORD had commanded. Yet Israel did not burn any of the cities built on their mounds—except Hazor, which Joshua burned. The Israelites carried off for

themselves all the plunder and livestock of these cities, but all the people they put to the sword until they completely destroyed them, not sparing anyone that breathed." (Joshua 11:12 – 14)

King Nebuchadnezzar of Babylon conquered the Levant from 605 BC to 562 BC. Near the end of the Old Testament, in the book of "Daniel," Nebuchadnezzar is said to have chosen four Israelites to be trained as his servants. They were to be taught the language and literature of the Babylonians and were assigned a daily amount of food and drink from the king's table to eat. One of the four servants named Daniel protested to the guard appointed to oversee him:

"Please test your servants for ten days: Give us nothing but vegetables to eat and water to drink. Then compare our appearance with that of the young men who eat the royal food, and treat your servants in accordance with what you see." So he agreed to this and tested them for ten days.

"At the end of the ten days they looked healthier and better nourished than any of the young men who ate the royal food." (Daniel 1:12 – 15)

This diet of vegetables and water, known as the "Daniel Diet," indicates that even as early as the 6th century BC the authors of the Old Testament knew that a simple plant-based diet provided superior nutrition to the rich royal diet of meat and wine.

By the 5th century BC, political power in the Mediterranean had shifted to Greece, and by the 1st century AD to Rome. In 70 AD, after the Romans destroyed the Jewish Temple in Jerusalem, the Jewish people dispersed into the diaspora.

Egypt

The Nile River Basin in northeastern Africa is very different than the basins of the Tigris or Euphrates Rivers in Mesopotamia. The Tigris and Euphrates drain a much smaller area than the Nile, and they have dramatic spring flooding events from snow melt in the highlands of Anatolia (Turkey) that carry with them very high loads of silt. The Nile receives all of its water from the tropical highlands of equatorial Africa and has no tributaries for the last 932 miles (1500 km) of its course running through the desolate Sahara Desert to the Mediterranean Sea. The Nile has no sudden rush of floodwaters, but rather steadily rising water that begins in June with snow melt supplemented by summer rains to reach a peak flow in late September and early October, then gradually receding by the end of December. The Nile is known to be one of the most predictable rivers in the world, and its annual flood period averages more than a hundred days. Where the Tigris and Euphrates River basins of southern Mesopotamia are very flat and poorly drained which has caused persistent problems with catastrophic flooding, siltation and soil salinity, the Nile River basin is well drained and has consistent water flows that have prevented excessive siltation and salinization.

The lifeline of the Nile began to sustain modern human nomadic hunter-gatherer groups as far back as 120,000 years ago on their initial route out of Africa. In the early Holocene (11,700 years ago to present) the climate in the Nile River basin was much less arid than it is today and large regions of Egypt were prime savanna hunting grounds traversed by herds of grazing ungulates and vast flocks of waterfowl ("Geology 115" UC Davis). But as the climate of Northern Africa became increasingly drier due to the extreme drought period that occurred 8,200 years ago, the human population of the Nile River basin was forced to congregate closer to the river. By about 7,500 years ago (5500 BC) domesticated strains of Mesopotamian wheat and barley had migrated down to the small tribes living in the Nile valley. In what is called the "Predynastic period" (5500 BC to 3150 BC, before the dynasties of the pharaohs) these early Egyptian farmers developed into a series of cultures demonstrating firm control over irrigation technology and animal domestication. One of the largest of these early cultures in northern Egypt that is now called the "Badari" produced high quality ceramics, stone tools, and copper objects.

Early Egyptian agriculture along the Nile was based on single season winter crops after the annual floods had subsided, but later the development of passive irrigation systems built along the river banks that trapped water during peak flood periods allowed for two to three crops per year. The Nile river valley is very narrow, only 16 miles (25 km) at its widest until it reaches the delta plain below modern-day Cairo, and it is very steep sided. Short irrigation ditches from these elevated reservoirs controlled by simple gates gravity fed water to the crops on the valley floor below. These irrigation schemes were small in scale and highly localized. Sediments that settled in the river basin with each year's floods naturally fertilized the soils. The Egyptians adapted many of the same cultivars developed in Mesopotamia including barley used for making bread and beer, wheat, garlic, onions, lentils, peas, beans, cucumbers, lettuce, and cabbage. Fruits included dates, figs, grapes, plums and pomegranates. Fruits were commonly preserved by drying. The main herbs and spices were salt, cumin, sesame, fennel, dill, and coriander (experience-ancient-egypt. com).

In southern Egypt around 4000 BC a Predynastic culture called the "Naqua" began to expand along the Nile, and over the next 1,000 years they developed from a few small farming communities into a powerful civilization whose leaders were in complete control of the people and resources of the Nile valley. Around 3100 BC to 3000 BC, the Naqada began using written symbols that eventually evolved into the hieroglyphics system of writing used by the ancient Egyptians to record their history.

Around 300 BC an Egyptian priest named Manetho was commissioned by pharaohs during the Ptolemaic dynasty to write a history of Egypt. Manetho's chronology of the 30 dynasties of Egyptian pharaohs dating from 3100 BC to 300 BC is still considered the most authoritative history of ancient Egypt during this period. Like the civilizations of Mesopotamia, Manetho's chronology divides the development of Ancient Egyptian civilization into several distinct phases. There are three highly prosperous periods when Egyptian wealth and power flourished each followed by a period of economic and population stagnation characterized by social, military, and artistic decline. The three periods of prosperity are called the "Old Kingdom" (2686 BC to 2181 BC), the "Middle Kingdom" (2055 BC to 1650 BC), and the "New Kingdom" (1557 BC to 1069 BC) and the three periods of decline are called the "Intermediate Periods".

It was during the first several dynasties of the Old Kingdom that the pharaohs established a well-developed central administration that collected taxes, coordinated irrigation projects, drafted peasants to work on construction projects, and established a justice system to maintain peace and order. As agricultural productivity increased due to major advances in irrigation systems the population of Egypt also increased providing the massive labor force necessary to build some of Ancient Egypt's crowning architectural achievements including the Great Sphinx and Pyramids of Giza. Along with the rising importance of a central administration arose a new class of educated scribes and officials who were granted estates by the pharaoh in payment for their services. On these temple estates the wealthy classes raised domesticated ducks, geese and pigs for meat, but as this was expensive, meat eating was largely the preserve of the wealthy classes. Cattle were kept primarily to provide oxen for plowing fields but were also slaughtered for meat when no longer serviceable. Average Egyptian farmers ate meat only occasionally as part of religious festivals when offerings of sacrificed animals were distributed to the people. It is thought that beef was eaten exclusively by the priests whose job it was to sacrifice the animals (Ancient Egypt online). The administration of the early Egyptian Old Kingdom began to break down around 2200 BC as the great drought that also brought down the Akkadian civilization of Mesopotamia began to reduce agricultural production. Over the next 140 years came a time of great strife and famine known as the First Intermediate period. A civil war ensued for territorial control and political power and by 2055 BC, the Theban forces defeated the Herakleopolitan rulers reuniting Egypt and inaugurating the next period called the Middle Kingdom.

The pharaohs of the Middle Kingdom (2055 BC to 1650 BC) initiated land and irrigation reclamation projects to increase agricultural production which again resulted in population increases. The pharaoh's powerful military reconquered southern territory in resource rich Nubia from where they imported gold, copper, amethyst, carnelian, feldspar, oils, resins, ebony, ivory and exotic wild animals. Due to the Egyptians' highly advanced embalming processes developed during the Middle Kingdom and the natural very dry climate of Egypt, there are many very fine specimens of extremely well preserved flesh from wealthy people who lived at this time. Stephen Macko, professor of environmental science at the University of Virginia, has studied hair samples preserved in these mummified remains and by observing changes in the amounts of carbon, nitrogen and sulfur in the hair, he could determine whether the diet of these high status individuals came from plants or animals and differentiate between terrestrial and marine animals. As Macko notes, *"Unlike bones and flesh which decay and change chemically, hair seems to stay the same. It is a terrific archive of information about the nutrition of ancient peoples."* (ScienceDaily – Oct. 26, 1998) According to Macko's findings wealthy ancient Egyptians ate a fairly restricted diet that was highly concentrated in terrestrial animals.

During the Middle Kingdom the pharaohs organized an enormous labor force to build a line of fortifications called the "Walls-of-the-Ruler" in the north around the eastern delta region of the Nile to defend against foreign attack from the eastern approaches to Egypt. But despite these efforts Semitic herding tribes from the Levant including the Amorites and Israelites (Joseph and the tribes of Israel in the Old Testament) began to migrate into the Nile delta region due the severe ongoing drought of this period. Even during this catastrophic drought the broad flood plain of the Nile delta remained green and suitable to pasture their herds. Archaeological evidence indicates that these migrating Semitic tribes eventually made war on Egypt and subjugated the Egyptian pharaoh to vassal status paying tribute to Semitic rulers. Manethos referred to the Semites as "Hyksos" which translated into English means "rulers of foreign countries". Manethos (as quoted by the 1st century AD Jewish Roman historian Josephus) describes the conquest and occupation of Egypt by the Hyksos:

> *"...during the reign of Tutimaos a blast of God smote us, and unexpectedly from the regions of the East, invaders of obscure race marched in confidence of victory against our land. By main force they easily seized it without striking a blow; and having overpowered the rulers of the land they then burned our cities ruthlessly, razed to the ground the temples of the gods, and treated all the natives with a cruel hostility, massacring some and leading into slavery the wives and children of others... Finally, they appointed as king one of their number whose name was Salitis. He had his seat in Memphis, levying tribute from upper Egypt and always leaving garrisons behind in the most advantageous positions. In the Saite nome he founded a city... and called it Auaris"*

Thus began the Second Intermediate Period around 1650 BC.

Herbert Eustis Winlock was an American Egyptologist who became the Director of the Metropolitan Museum of Art in 1932. During the great era of American museum-sponsored Egyptian excavations between 1912 and 1939 Winlock made major contributions to the study of Egyptology with his extensive excavations at Thebes. In his book *"The Rise and Fall of the Middle Kingdom in Thebes"* (1947) Winlock detailed the new military hardware employed by the Hyksos in their occupation of Egypt including the composite bow, recurve bow, improved arrowheads, various kinds of swords and daggers, a new type of shield, mailed shirts, metal helmets and most importantly the horse-drawn chariot. As horse-drawn chariot technology made its way south from Eurasia during this period it was quickly adopted as a symbol of power by warlords throughout Mesopotamia, the Levant, Egypt, India, China, Mycenaea and Eastern Europe. After many decades of Hyksos rule, the Egyptian pharohs at Thebes rearmed with the latest weaponry finally counterattacked and in a thirty year war drove the Hyksos out of Egypt by 1550 BC destroying their cities of Avaris and Memphis along the way. Thus was the beginning of the New Kingdom.

After expelling the Hykos, the Egyptian pharaohs became emboldened militarily and extended their influence to the largest empire Egypt had ever seen. By 1425 BC the Egyptian New Kingdom stretched from northern Syria to southern Nubia. In the November 18th issue of the *Journal of the American Medical Association* (JAMA) an international team of scientists published the results of their study on the mummified bodies of people who lived in Egypt between the years 1500 BC and 500 AD (from the New Kingdom on). These researchers conducted whole body CT scans on 20 mummies whose tissues were preserved well enough to see the condition of their arteries. All the mummies whose identities could be determined were of high socioeconomic status, generally serving in the court of the pharaoh, or as priests and priestesses. Of the 16 mummies that had identifiable arteries or hearts, 9 had calcified arteries (atherosclerosis) including 7 of the 8 who were older than 45 years old at the time of their death. Dr. Gregory Thomas, associate clinical professor of cardiology at the University of California, Irvine, and co-author of the study, commented in Medical News Today (11/18/2009):

> *Atherosclerosis is widespread among modern-day humans and – despite differences in ancient and modern lifestyles – we found that it was rather common in ancient Egyptians of high socioeconomic status living more than three millennia ago.*

Though it is true that modern lifestyles are certainly different than those of ancient Egyptians, the modern western diet of feasting on animal foods every day is actually not so different than that of the upper classes in ancient Egypt. Another disease that afflicts modern cultures where the general population eats an animal based diet similar to that of the nobles and priests of ancient Egypt is type 2 (adult onset) diabetes. Diabetes is a disease that is difficult to diagnose from bones and mummies, but there is some archaeological and historical evidence that suggest it may have been common among the upper classes in ancient Egypt. Skeletal remains of an adult male Egyptian dating to around 2000 BC from an archaeological site at Dayr al-Barsha display many pathological conditions that, when considered together, likely indicate type 2 diabetes. The same is true of the mummified remains of Queen Hatshepsut, a rare female Pharaoh who reigned around 1500 BC. And around 1550 BC the official physician of the pharaoh, a man named "Hesy-Ra", wrote the "Ebers Papyrus" in which he described a condition now known as "polyuria" or frequent urination, a common symptom of diabetes. This symptom was apparently prevalent enough among high status animal gorging Egyptians to be diagnosable.

Around 1350 BC the stability of the New Kingdom was threatened when a new pharaoh ascended the throne who attempted to institute a monotheist religion to the polytheistic Egyptians causing great disruption in the empire. After his death succeeding pharaohs reestablished polytheism and order in the Egyptian empire. By 1279 BC the Egyptian military was on the march again retaking Canaan, Lebanon, and in the "Battle of Kadesh" in 1274 BC defeating the Hittites in Syria. The Battle of Kadesh is the earliest battle in recorded history for which details of tactics and formations are known and it was probably the largest chariot battle ever fought, involving perhaps 5,000–6,000 chariots. Egypt's expansion and wealth made it a target for invasion, particularly by the Libyans across the desert to the west and the Greeks across the Mediterranean Sea. Egypt eventually lost control of Syria and Palestine and the impact of external threats was exacerbated by internal civil unrest. High priests in Thebes accumulated vast tracts of land and wealth and their concentrated wealth divided the country leading to the Third Intermediate Period.

Between the end of the New Kingdom around 1069 BC and the reestablishment of Egyptian rule with the help of Greek mercenaries in 653 BC, Egypt was conquered and ruled variously by the Libyans Bubastites, the Nubian Kushites and the Assyrian Semites. After evicting the Assyrians in 653 BC the

Egyptians and Greeks established a sea trade alliance with Egyptian grains, flax linens and papyrus paper being exchanged for Grecian silver, timber, olive oil and wine. In the 5th century BC a powerful new Persian culture from modern-day Iran began their conquest of Egypt and at the battle of Pelusium in 525 BC captured the pharaoh thus ending the last native dynasty to rule Egypt. It was not until this "Late Period" of Egyptian history that the camel was domesticated and used as a beast of burden. It was also during this period of Persian rule that the Greek historian Herodotus (484 BC – 425 BC) visited Egypt. Herodotus studied ancient Egyptian texts (that no longer exist) and used them as source materials for his masterwork "*The Histories*" in which he chronicled the ancient traditions, politics, geography, and wars of the various cultures living around the Mediterranean and Western Asia at that time. In *The Histories* Herodotus made special note of Egyptian food customs that seemed peculiar to him. According to Herodotus, Egyptians who raised and ate pigs were shunned and pork was considered "unclean"; priests were not allowed to eat fish and fish was rarely given as an offering to the dead; in certain areas at certain times eating certain kinds of fish was proscribed and apparently at one point the Ethiopian pharaoh of the Kush dynasty (747 BC - 656 BC) refused to dine with the fish-eating noblemen of Lower Egypt because of their diet. Herodotus also noted that quail, ducks, smaller birds and fish were salted and eaten uncooked but that all other kinds of birds and fish, except for those that were sacred, were eaten roasted or boiled. (Ancient Egypt online) These religious and social proscriptions limiting the consumption of certain animals suggest that a system of rationing was necessary to deal with environmental limits on production.

In 332 BC "Alexander the Great" of Macedon, a state in northern ancient Greece, conquered Egypt with little resistance from the Persians and was welcomed by the Egyptians as a deliverer. Alexander's successor Greek administrators, the "Ptolemies", were based on an Egyptian model and established the new capital city of Alexandria on the Mediterranean coast. This city became a seat of learning and culture in the ancient world centered at the famous library of Alexandria. It was during this period that the famed multilingual "Rosetta Stone" was carved which, when rediscovered by a French soldier in 1799, provided the key to the modern-day understanding of Egyptian hieroglyphs. The Greeks did not supplant native Egyptian culture, as the Ptolemies supported time-honored traditions in an effort to secure the loyalty of the Egyptian natives, but despite these efforts the Ptolemies were eventually weakened by internal conflict, family rivalries and external threats from powerful Syrian forces to the north. As the expanding Roman Empire centered in modern-day Italy became more food dependent on imports of grain from Egypt during the 1st century BC, they began to send military legions to stabilize the situation and by 30 BC Egypt was annexed as a province of the Roman Empire. According to the highly regarded Historical Demographer, Dr. T. H. Hollingworth of the University of Glasgow, the human population of Egypt at the time of Alexander the Great reached about 16 million people, fell to about 7 million by around 100 AD only to rebound spectacularly to about 30 million by 600 AD (in Roman times), crashing again spectacularly to about 2 million by 1750 AD not to recover to 30 million again until 1950 AD (modern times). (Historical Demography, Cornell University Press, 1969)

Asian Subcontinent

Around 7,000 years ago another civilization rivaling that of ancient Egypt began to develop independently on the fertile soils of the Indus River Valley in present-day Pakistan. The staple crops of the first settlers were wheat and barley and they also grazed domesticated zebus (a breed of local cattle), water buffalo, sheep and goats on the lush natural grasses. These early settlers built highly sophisticated irrigation systems to capture monsoon rains for use during the long dry season and they developed sophisticated agricultural implements and cropping techniques. By 4,500 years ago (2500 BC) as the human population grew into the millions these initial settlements coalesced into the Harappa civilization which consisted of two major cities that served as capitals for a complex of villages that covered an area twice the size of ancient Egypt. The great cities and towns of the Harappan complex were supported by a highly advanced agricultural system that included a large capacity for surplus grain storage. As amazing as this Harappas civilization was, it literally disappeared from the archaeological record for thousands of years before being rediscovered by British colonizers in the 1850s while building a railway line through the Indus Valley. These ancient ruins indicate a gradual decline in the Harappa civilization over a five hundred year period between 3,500 and 3,000 years ago (1500 BC to 1000 BC) due to an influx of Aryan cattle herders from the Caucuses who were an offshoot from the Kurgan culture. R. A. Guisepi, Dr. of Ancient History and Antiquities at Canterbury University, and a leading scholar on Indus antiquities, interprets the evidence this way:

> "*Between about 1500 and 1000 B.C., as the great cities of the Indus region crumbled into ruins, nomadic Aryan invaders from central Asia moved into the fertile Indus plains and pushed into the Ganges River valleys to the east. It took these unruly, warlike peoples many centuries to build a civilization that rivaled that of the Harappans. The Aryans concentrated on assaulting Harappan settlements and different Aryan tribal groups. As peoples who depended primarily on great herds of cattle to provide their subsistence, they had little use for the great irrigation works and advanced agricultural technology of the Indus valley peoples. Though they conserved some Harappan beliefs and symbols, the Aryan invaders did little to restore or replace the great cities and engineering systems of the peoples they had supplanted*" (The Indus Valley And The Genesis Of South Asian, Civilization, A project by History World International).

By 300 BC, this Aryan culture based on cattle grazing and meat eating had fully established itself in the Indus Valley and the Ganges River basin in present-day Northern India and the human population of the region was approaching 100 million people. Seven hundred years (1000 BC to 300 BC) of intensive cattle grazing to provide meat to this burgeoning population had turned the once fertile soils of these river systems into arid and depleted plains that could no longer provide enough food for everyone. As civil unrest spread against the priestly caste of "Brahmans" who were in charge of cattle slaughter and distribution, the Brahmans realized they couldn't sustain both a cattle culture and a large population at the same time, so they initiated the Hindu religious taboo against eating cattle meat as the solution to this problem.

As land formerly used to graze large herds of cattle was converted to growing wheat, millet, sesame, lentils and peas that could provide food for many more people, the cattle population diminished significantly with the remaining bulls being used as oxen to pull plows and the heifers being used for their milk. Leading theoretical cultural anthropologists, Dr. Marvin Harris, Graduate Research Professor of Anthropology at the University of Florida and former Chair of the General Anthropology Division of the American Anthropological Association, explains this Hindu proscription against cattle meat with his now widely accepted theory of "cultural materialism":

> *"The whole system in larger perspective turns out not to be simply a matter of whim on the part of the theologians who were responsible for elaborating the documents of Hinduism. On the contrary, it turns out that the doctrines of Hinduism reflect the material realities and necessities which the people of the Indian subcontinent face in their struggle to provide sufficient amounts of food for their ever-increasing numbers."* (Marvin Harris Explains The Unexplainable, Interview by Barbara Spronk, Aurora Online, Issue 1987)

From the archaeological record it is clear that the people of the Indus and Ganges civilizations once ate large quantities of beef, but since the Aryans did not mummify their dead as did the Egyptians, there are no well preserved hair or soft tissue samples to analyze to determine their exact diet or prevalence of heart disease.

Far East Asia

A third civilization coalesced around 3,500 years ago (1500 BC) in the Yellow River flood plain of present-day Northern China. A ruling elite established the Shang Dynasty, China's first dynasty that developed towns and cities and engineered sophisticated irrigation systems to grow rice as their staple crop. As the population grew it spread south into the immense Yangtze River system where rice grew well in the marshy wetlands and became widely cultivated. Animal food production and consumption was limited to small amounts of domesticated chickens and pigs that could be fed with kitchen scraps. As for cattle, the bulls were trained as oxen to plow fields and the heifers were impregnated to produce replacement bulls as needed; there was no surplus population of cattle raised for meat or milk, there simply wasn't enough pasture for that.

Rice is different than other grains in that it can be grown in wet environments that are common across Far East Asia. As a result, rice cultivation spread rapidly from China into what are now the modern countries of Vietnam, Laos, Thailand, Cambodia and Burma, as well as the Indonesian archipelago.

By 1 AD the human population of China had reached 60 million people. Over the next two centuries the Buddhist religion in the Mahāyāna tradition began to spread in China which discouraged the killing of sentient beings and encouraged a vegetarian diet. While Buddhism does not place an outright ban on meat eating, a primarily plant-based diet persisted in China well into modern times.

By 1200 AD the population of China had reached 120 million people, but catastrophe lay just ahead. The area around modern-day Mongolia and Manchuria on the Northern perimeter of China was under constant attack from nomadic Mongol tribes who were another herding culture Kurgan off-shoot, and by the early 12th century the Mongolian Chieftain, Genghis Kahn, had united all the loosely organized nomadic tribes of Mongolia, Manchuria, and Siberia into a fighting force of unparalleled mobility and ferocity. Genghis Kahn invaded and overthrown the Chinese dynasty going on an expansionist tear like none seen before or since, culminating in the largest empire in terms of contiguous land area ever established. By the 14th century the Mongol empire stretched from Eastern Europe to the Sea of Japan, from Siberia to Southeast Asia, and from the Indian subcontinent to the Middle East spanning 6,000 miles (9,700 km) and covering an area of 12,741,000 square miles (33,000,000 km²). By comparison, the area of the continental United States is 3,120,000 square miles, less than one fourth the size. The Mongols had developed a nomadic culture based on horseback riding to herd cattle, sheep and goats over vast, sparsely vegetated rangelands, and it was these finely honed skills that enabled them to cover such long distances and wage war so decisively against other preexisting pastoral cultures. The Mongol army could travel without a cumbersome supply train by milking and slaughtering their animals as they went and supplementing their diets with hunted wild animals or looted food from their victims. A dried milk paste was their staple food with strips of dried meat and horse blood drawn from their live horses to round out their diet.

As fearsome as they were, the Mongol fighting force that conquered and ruled over populations numbering in the tens of millions actually numbered only into the tens of thousands of highly mobile warriors. Due in part to the Mongol's tactic of killing all the residents of any city that resisted them, and the Mongol's tactic of destroying irrigation systems to cause mass starvation, the human populations of Iran, Iraq and China underwent significant declines during this period of Mongol occupation. In China, the Mongol conquest disrupted traditional farming and trading practices which caused widespread famine and mass starvation. The population of China is estimated to have fallen by half during this time back to around 60 million people.

But most of the peoples conquered by the Mongols surrendered without a fight and the Mongols strongly supported trade between the far flung cultures of its empire. The Mongols established official relay stations to facilitate movement of goods over the long trade routes from China to Europe and they also developed a pony express mail system to speed communications and enable centralized control over their vast empire.

Though the Mongols practiced a type of religion called "shamanism", a belief that "shamans" are intermediaries between the human world and the spirit world, their military conquests were not religiously motivated and they were completely tolerant of the Buddhist, Christian and Islamic faiths in the lands they conquered. The nomadic herding lifestyle of the Mongols was not adaptable to the densely populated agricultural areas of the lands they conquered and by the end of the 14th century the Mongol minority had either been pushed out of occupied territories by popular revolt or had become assimilated into the cultures of the larger native populations which ultimately marked the end of the Mongol Empire. China was returned to native rule under the Ming Dynasty in 1368 AD.

Crete:

Humans began migrating into Europe from Africa around 50,000 years ago and by 12,000 years ago small widely dispersed groups of migratory hunter-gatherers had occupied most of the continent. Then, between 8,500 and 6,000 years ago (6500 BC and 4000 BC) agriculture spread from the Near East throughout Europe ultimately displacing the hunter-gatherers with agriculturalists who lived in small villages growing grains and herding a few sheep and goats. Unlike the Egyptian, Indian and Chinese civilizations which developed in fertile river basins, the first civilization to develop in Europe began about 4,000 years ago (2000 BC) on the small island of modern-day Crete in the Mediterranean Sea off the coast of modern-day Greece.

The Minoan culture of Crete, like that of the Harappa in the Indus Valley, had literally disappeared from the archaeological record for thousands of years until being rediscovered by British archaeologist, Sir Arthur Evans, at the turn of the 19th century with his excavation of the elaborate palaces of the Minoan city of Knossos. The Minoans developed a highly organized social structure that supported a culture of high art and seafaring trade with no evidence of weapons of war. Minoan agriculture consisted mostly of growing olives which they exported to the mainland. Barley was their staple grain and they also grew figs and grapes. With the rocky terrain of Crete, the Minoans had poor land for grazing domesticated animals so terrestrial meat was not part of their regular diet, though wild caught fish were commonly eaten. Small numbers of goats were kept for their milk to make cheese (drinking milk straight was considered barbaric) and sheep for their wool. The Minoan civilization lasted five hundred years only to be overrun by the warlike, cattle herding, Mycenaeans from mainland Greece. The Mycenaeans brought cattle to Crete and by 1200 BC the Minoan culture collapsed, the population declined substantially and the cities of Crete fell into a state of ruin during the so called "Greek Dark Ages".

Greece

Around 800 BC, a number of city-states began to organize in separated geographical areas on the Grecian peninsula with the largest and most powerful being Athens, Sparta and Thebes. While Greek society was arranged into a male hierarchy class structure of wealthy plebeians, merchants, artisans and slaves, the daily diet even of the rich generally consisted of simple fare. Due to the rocky terrain of Greece, Greek agriculture was very similar to that of the Minoans with wheat and barley the staple grains, and olives the major fruit crop. They also cultivated figs, pomegranates, chestnuts, chick peas, cabbage, onions, lentils, and beans.

Fish, squid, octopus, and shellfish were commonly eaten along the coast and also traded inland. Small herds of goats and sheep were kept for milk to make cheese and wool to weave into fabric. With so little grazing land, very few cattle were kept and meat eating became marginal, restricted to religious sacrifices which took place during civic ceremonies where the meat was distributed among the people. Animal sacrifice was probably a holdover from the meat eating cults of their Mycenaean ancestors.

The Greek religions of Orphicism and Pythagoreanism that stressed a vegetarian diet were established from 600 BC to 500 BC, but most of their adherents came from a relatively small scholarly class. Around 400 BC, at the height of the ancient Greek civilization, Plato, one of the iconic founders of Western philosophy, wrote his master work called "*The Republic*" in which Socrates (Plato's mentor) engages Glaucon (Plato's older brother) in a philosophical debate over the future of their cities. In this debate Socrates argues in favor of a vegetarian diet while Glaucon disdains vegetarianism in favor of meat eating. In this exchange Socrates questions Glaucon:

Socrates: "*And there will be animals of many other kinds, if people eat them?*"

Glaucon: "*Certainly.*"

Socrates; "*And living in this way we shall have much greater need of physicians than before.*"

Glaucon: "*Much greater.*"

Socrates: "*And the country which was enough to support the original inhabitants will be too small now, and not enough?*"

Glaucon: "*Quite true.*"

Socrates: "*Then a slice of our neighbours' land will be wanted by us for pasture and tillage, and they will want a slice of ours, if, like ourselves, they exceed the limit of necessity, and give themselves up to the unlimited accumulation of wealth?*"

Glaucon: "*That, Socrates, will be inevitable.*"

Socrates: "*And so we shall go to war, Glaucon. Shall we not?*"

Glaucon: "*Most certainly.*"

From this dialogue it is evident that even thousands of years ago the ancient Greeks well understood that an animal based diet not only causes disease in humans but that it takes up much more land than does cultivating plants to grow food for people, and that competition for grazing lands was a major cause of war. These were the hard learned lessons from their Mycenaean past history. Interestingly, the warriors of Sparta, the most warlike of the Greek city states, were renowned for their unappetizing animal-based diet of a pig meat stew called "black broth" made from pig meat, salt, vinegar and blood.

With a very long coastline jutting out into the Mediterranean Sea, and a population growing to over 10 million people by 400 BC, the Greeks had turned to seafaring and trade to expand their influence and established hundreds of colonies on many islands of the Aegean Sea and along the Mediterranean coastlines of present-day Turkey, Cyprus, Sicily, Sardinia, Corsica, Italy, France and Spain, as well as the entire coastline of the Black Sea. While the Greek city states of this time developed a highly sophisticated culture making great strides in the fields of literature, government, philosophy and mathematics, they were also almost always at war, either with each other or allied against nearby rival civilizations like the Phoenicians (of present-day Lebanon), the Persians (of present-day Iran) and the Macedonians (of present-day Macedonia). Drained by centuries of war the Greek empire finally fell to the Romans in the Battle of Corinth in 146 BC.

Rome

The Roman civilization first developed into a city-state on the west coast of the Italian peninsula where the Tiber River flows into the Mediterranean Sea around 500 BC. At the peak of its power around 100 AD, Roman legions controlled the entire continent of present-day Western Europe, the Middle East including Egypt as well as the North coast of Africa. The Romans built highly advanced irrigation systems throughout the empire and also spread new plant cultivars to distant territories.

Early on, the class structure of Roman society was similar to that of Greece with a relatively minor disparity in wealth between rich and poor, but as the empire grew and became more prosperous, the exponential increase in material wealth it generated became increasingly concentrated in the hands of a small number of ruling class patricians. A common depiction of the Roman diet is that of a gluttonous feast with course upon course of exotic meat dishes being served, but such extravagant meals were only the province of the very wealthy while the vast majority of Romans relied on a monotonous diet of wheat made into bread or porridge for their sustenance. Grain was so important to the Roman economy that it served as a common measure of value and wages were paid in wheat throughout the Empire. Even the vaunted Roman Legions were largely paid in grain rations. Middle class merchants and artisans could afford to supplement their grain diet with a wide variety of domesticated plants that were being cultivated around the Empire by then such as: fava beans, chick peas, peas, kale, chard, broccoli, asparagus, artichokes, leeks, carrots, turnips, parsnips, beets, green beans, radishes, cauliflower, cabbage, lettuce, onions, cucumbers, melons, apples, pears, cherries, plums, grapes, walnuts, almonds, chestnuts and, most important of all, olives. Meat eating was reserved for religious festivals where domesticated pigs, chickens, ducks and geese were ritually sacrificed as offerings to the gods. Cattle meat was rare since bulls were much more valuable as draft animals for plowing the fields. Unlike the maritime empire of the Greeks which was confined to coastal areas, most of the Roman Empire was inland and fish eating was not common. But like the Greeks, Romans kept flocks of goats to make cheese from their milk. For a period of about two hundred years between 1 AD and 200 AD, an era of relative peace reined over the Empire, the so called "Pax Romana."

The Romans built a remarkable network of roads to unify their Empire and facilitate the movement of goods and troops. The Roman road system spanned more than 250,000 miles (400,000 km), including over 50,000 miles (80,500 km) of paved roads. Historian Henry Moss describes how this road system facilitated a flourishing food economy:

"Along these roads passed an ever-increasing traffic, not only of troops and officials, but of traders, merchandise and even tourists. An interchange of goods between the various provinces rapidly developed, which soon reached a scale unprecedented in previous history and not repeated until a few centuries ago. Metals mined in the uplands of Western Europe, hides, fleeces, and livestock from the pastoral districts of Britain, Spain, and the shores of the Black Sea, wine and oil from Provence and Aquitaine, timber, pitch and wax from South Russia and northern Anatolia, dried fruits from Syria, marble from the Aegean coasts, and – most important of all – grain from the wheat-growing districts of North Africa, Egypt, and the Danube Valley for the needs of the great cities; all these commodities, under the influence of a highly organized system of transport and marketing, moved freely from one corner of the Empire to the other." (Henry Moss, The Birth of the Middle Ages, p. 1.)

Many of the goods being traded in the Roman Empire were luxury items that could only be afforded and consumed by the wealthy few, so the overall volume in these goods was relatively small by today's standards. But the volume of grain traded from Egypt to Europe to feed the masses of people in the burgeoning cities of the Roman Empire was substantial and was by far the single largest commodity in the Roman economy.

Starting with the "Antonine Plague" from 165 AD to 180 AD which caused the death of an estimated five million people, the western part of the Roman Empire began to fall into a steady state of decline. Contemporary descriptions of the disease indicate that it was caused by the small-pox virus which first appeared among Roman soldiers who were at war in what is now modern-day Iraq, but then quickly spread to Europe. As much as one-third of the human population died in some areas and the plague decimated the Roman army. The genes of the small-pox virus suggest that it was once a rodent virus that made its trans-species jump into humans in one of the early agricultural river valleys of China thousands of years ago. Beginning with the Eastern Han Dynasty in 206 BC, China established a sea route from the mouth of the Red River near modern-day Hanoi sailing to Southeast Asia, Sri Lanka and India, and then on to the Persian Gulf and the Red Sea. From ports on the Red Sea goods were transported overland to the Nile and then to Alexandria from where they were shipped to Rome, Constantinople and other Mediterranean sea ports. From the East came silk, satin, hemp, musk, spices, medicines, jewels and porcelain, and in exchange the West sent back saffron, dates, pistachio nuts, frankincense, myrrh and glassware; science, culture and zoological specimens flowed in both directions. Presumably, it was also this trade route that provided the vector for the small-pox virus to spread from China to the Roman Empire. Epidemiologists estimate that the small-pox virus needs a population of around two hundred thousand people living within fourteen days travel of one another in order for the virus to maintain its life cycle. What this means is that the spread of small-pox into human populations was a direct result of the high population densities only made possible through the practice of agriculture. The Antonin Plague was followed by the "Plague of Cyprian" between 251 AD and 266 AD, which was another outbreak of smallpox. According to contemporary sources, approximately 5,000 people a day fell victim in the city of Rome alone and nearly two-thirds of the people died in the city of Alexandria, Egypt.

In 313 AD the Roman Emperor Constantine made Christianity the official religion of the Roman Empire and in 330 AD he moved the capital of the decaying Western Empire from Rome to the thriving ancient Greek city of Byzantium in the eastern part of the empire renaming it Constantinople (what is modern-day Istanbul, Turkey). By 455 AD Germanic tribes from the north called Goths, Vandals and Franks had sacked Rome and destroyed much of the Western Roman Empire and its immense trade network of roads and cities fell into a state of ruin. Due to these multiple calamities it has been estimated that the population of the Roman Empire fell from 65 million to 50 million people between 150 AD and 400 AD, a decline of more than 20%.

While the Western Roman Empire collapsed into anarchy, the Eastern Roman Empire, which was well situated along the overland trade route connecting China and India to the Near East and Europe, continued to prosper. That is, until the "Plague of Justinian" struck in 541 AD with recurring outbreaks through 750 AD. This overland trade route, called the "Silk Road," traversed sparsely populated grasslands through Central Asia that enabled merchants to travel from the shores of the Pacific to Africa and deep into Europe without trespassing on agricultural lands that would provoke local hostility. In addition, the grasslands provided grazing, water, and easy passage for large caravans of domesticated camels, the ideal beast of burden for this arduous journey. Though the volume of trade along the Silk Road was small by today's standards, it represented a significant source of luxury goods for the wealthy classes of all the civilizations involved. But, like the sea route centuries earlier, the Silk Road also provided a vector for a new disease from China, the "bubonic plague," to take root in the Near East and Europe. The bubonic plague is caused by a bacterium called "Yersinia pestis" that circulates between rodents and their parasitic fleas that are native to China. When the rodent host dies the fleas seek other hosts such as humans infecting them with the bacterium. Europe's densely populated cities with no biological immunity or understanding of epidemiology, provided the perfect breeding grounds for this uncontrollable pandemic. It is estimated that the Plague of Justinian ultimately killed up to a 100 million people and reduced the population of Europe by as much as 50 to 60% between 541 AD and 750 AD. As the death toll from the plague weakened its power, Constantinople came increasingly under attack from newly established Islamic Empires emanating from the Middle East, finally falling by the mid 15th century, setting the sun on the Eastern Roman Empire.

Ottoman Empire

While Europe was caught in the throws of the Dark Ages in the 7th century AD, a new religion called Islam was being formed in what is modern-day Saudi Arabia, that, over the course of the next 1,000 years, would develop into the Ottoman Empire that rivaled that of Christian Europe. Through a succession of powerful caliphs (heads of state), by the middle of the 10th century the Ottoman Empire had spread throughout the Arab world and beyond including the entire Middle East, North Africa, Saudi

Peninsula, Afghanistan, Pakistan, India, Malaysia and even to Europe with the Islamic Moors in Spain and Portugal.

Even as the Moors were driven out of Spain and Portugal by Christian armies in the 14th century, the Ottoman Empire was spreading east into the Balkans (modern-day Greece, Macedonia, Bulgaria, Romania, Bosnia, Serbia and Turkey), Hungary, and Central Asia (modern-day Kazakhstan, Kyrgyzstan, Tajikistan, Turkmenistan and Uzbekistan). In 1453 AD the Ottomans captured Constantinople, the last bastion of the Christian Eastern Roman Empire. Centrally located on the Eurasian continent this vast new Ottoman Empire had very long and often contentious borders with its much older, more established neighbors of China and India to the east and Europe to the west. It was during this time period that trade in spice and silk between East Asia and Western Europe was developing into a major source of commerce and all of the goods had to pass through these Ottoman controlled territories.

As the world's new trade center, the Ottoman developed the most advanced forms of business administration, egalitarian economics and natural sciences of its time. The geography of this sprawling empire varied greatly from mountainous to coastal and from river valleys to deserts; climatic conditions ranged from the cold heights of eastern Turkey to the sweltering heat of the Arabian and North African deserts. Rainfall was sparse throughout most of the empire and the grain baskets were in the basins of the Danube, Tigris, Euphrates, and Nile rivers. By developing highly advanced grafting techniques they were able to create many new varieties of fruit trees that were acclimatized to different areas; most notably: orange, lemon, lime, grapefruit, pomegranate, coconut, date cherry, fig, banana, peach, apricot, plum, apple and mulberry. Other plant cultivars common throughout the region included chickpea, asparagus, artichoke, beet, cabbage, leek, cauliflower, carrot and multiple varieties of leafy greens. During periods of adequate rainfall the average person's diet consisted of a much wider variety of fruits, vegetables and grains than in medieval Europe.

According to Dr. Lawrence Conrad, historian of Near Eastern Medicine at the *Wellcome Institute for the History of Medicine*, London, life expectancy in medieval Ottoman society was significantly longer than in the agricultural societies of ancient Rome and medieval Europe which led to a corresponding decrease in birthrates. As with the earlier Middle Eastern civilizations discussed above, raising large numbers of animals for meat was not economically feasible in most of the Ottoman Empire and peasants kept small numbers of goats, sheep and cattle for their milk, wool and motive power so meat was not a significant part of their diet. Pigs were considered unclean animals under Islamic dietary laws and the eating of pork was prohibited. Anthropologist Marvin Harris surmises that the reason for this prohibition was that pigs are not well adapted to living in the desert environment where Islam was founded, so in order to keep wealthy people from using scarce resources to raise pigs as a high status food which would create dissension, they simply banned eating pig meat altogether. Unlike the religious requirements of Jews and various pagan religions of the time, there was no requirement of animal sacrifice in Islam. From the

Christian Crusades in the 11th century to the Mongol invasions of the 13th century, the Ottoman Empire was constantly under attack on both its eastern and western borders.

Medieval Europe

The Goths, Vandals and Franks were cattle herding tribes who had settled in what is modern-day northern Germany. There, they were able to combine cattle and sheep herding with farming barley, wheat, rye, beans and peas to provide enough food for a basic subsistence living, but no surplus to propel population growth so their numbers remained relatively small. As these herding tribes swept through Europe during the five hundred years between 500 AD and 1000 AD, much of the Roman legacy of arts, medicine, government, architecture and science was lost; a period commonly known as the "Dark Ages." During this period the human population of the European continent shrank and became decentralized. Then, starting around 1000 AD, a new system of societal organization began to emerge called "feudalism."

Feudalism revolved around the "manor" which consisted of several thousand acres of land divided into meadow, pasture, forest, and cultivated fields along with a fortified manor house and a few scattered villages of ten to sixty families. A "lord" ruled over the manor by making land grants to "vassals" who were then obligated to protect and defend the lord and the manor. Most of the people on the manor were either "peasants" or "serfs" (peasants had a little more freedom of movement, serfs were attached to the land) who lived in crude huts and tended the fields. By this time in Europe, Christianity had become the dominant religion and the Church which was headquartered in Rome, also owned large tracts of land that were administered locally by Bishops and Abbots. The produce grown in the fields by the peasants and serfs was divided-up with one third going to the lord of the manor, one tenth to the church, and the rest to the farmers. The peasants and serfs relied on barley as their staple grain making a coarse bread and porridge. They also grew and ate most of the vegetable cultivars common in the Roman era although some like cucumbers and lentils were considered suspect. As with all the other hierarchical civilizations discussed above, the poor had limited access to meat. Cattle meat was rarely eaten with bulls being more valuable alive as draft animals to plow the fields and heifers for reproduction and milk production. Goat and sheep meat was also uncommon as these animals were more valuable alive for their milk and wool. Pigs were kept for meat since they could be raised by letting them root in the forest for much of the year where they did not compete for grain fields as did cattle. When it came to the ethics of meat eating, Christianity took a decidedly different turn than either Hinduism or Buddhism where animals became sacred. In the Pagan and Jewish religions that preceded Christianity, animals could only be eaten after they were sacrificed to the gods as spiritual offerings, but in the Christian New Testament Bible story of "Jesus Clears the Temple" (John 2:13 – 22), the sacrifice of Jesus Christ was substituted for the sacrifice of animals as the means for people to have a spiritual communion with God. As Christianity became the dominant religion in Europe the practice of animal sacrifice virtually disappeared and the slaughter and eating of animals became a purely secular affair. However, from their experience during the Dark Ages, the

Christians, as did the Hindus and Buddhists before them, realized that relying on a meat-based diet greatly limited the amount of food they could produced through agriculture which in turn placed severe limits on human population growth. As a way of reducing the amount of meat people ate the Church proclaimed every Wednesday and Friday to be meat-fasting days and they also made meat-fasting a requirement for the 40 days of the holy period known as Lent. This amounted to nearly 40% of the days of the year.

In the 11th through the 13th centuries a vegetarian Christian sect called Catharism flourished in France, Germany, Belgium and Italy. The Cathars refused to eat anything that was the result of "coition" which to their understanding eliminated meat, dairy and eggs. Believing that fish reproduced asexually, they were considered eatable. Due to the Cathars many heretical views to the Catholic Church, the Papacy had them completely exterminated by the end of the 13th century.

While these religious social strategies effectively reduced the amount of meat consumed by the masses, it had little effect on the small percentage of wealthy people at the top of the feudal system who ate a predominantly meat-based diet of both wild and domesticated animals. Fresh vegetables were considered unhealthy by the rich and the only foods they would eat that grew from the ground were garlic, onions, and leeks.

As the grain-based human population again began to increase, growing numbers of itinerant people with nowhere else to go, migrated to new urban centers that were springing up on rivers and crossroads and Europe started to consolidate into nation-states with powerful central monarchies in roughly what are modern-day France, England, Spain, Hungary and Poland. By 1300 AD the population of Europe had reached 70 million people and to feed this large population, forests were cleared and swamps were drained to expand the range of agriculture, while improvements to the plow, the use of draft horses, more advanced crop rotations and cover cropping with nitrogen fixing legumes made agriculture more productive.

In addition, for the three centuries between 1000 AD and 1300 AD, Northern Europe was blessed with an unusually mild climate called the "Medieval Warming Period." In 1965, Professor of Climatology at the University of East Anglia, Norwich, England, and founder of the Climatic Research Unit in the School of Environmental Sciences, Dr. Hubert Lamb, was the first to propose a "Medieval Warming Epoch" in his paper, "*The early medieval warm epoch and its sequel*" (*Palaeogeography. Palaeoclimatology. Palaeoecology, 1965*). Based on historical anecdotes and paleoclimatic data from Western Europe, Dr. Lamb constructed indices of "summer wetness" and "winter severity" and found evidence of warmer, dryer summers and mild winters most pronounced between 1100 AD and 1200 AD. Subsequently, palaeoclimatologists Dr. Raymond Bradley, Distinguished Professor in the Department of Geosciences, University of Massachusetts and Director of the Climate System Research Center, and his colleagues, developed a region-specific climate reconstructions of the Medieval Warming Period from ice cores, tree rings, cave deposits, lake sediments, and documentary records (*"CLIMATE CHANGE: Climate in Medieval Time,"Science*). Their analyses indicated that temperatures from 1000 AD to 1200 AD were almost the same as from 1901 to 1970 and that the last 30 years of the 20th century were on average ~0.35°C warmer than the Medieval

Warming Period. Such favorable climate conditions during the Medieval Warming Period expanded the growing seasons and increased crop yields for medieval farmers.

Also during the Medieval Warming Period the Vikings of Scandinavia (modern day Denmark, Sweden and Norway) developed the "longship" and navigation techniques that enabled them to voyage beyond sight of land into the open sea where massive schools of cod and herring had migrated from the warming southern waters to the cooler waters of the North Sea. Thus started a fishing industry that supplied surplus fish to serve the European demand for fish on Christian days of abstinence from meat (cold blooded fish were not considered meat by the Catholic Church). The fresh water fish of European rivers were being over-fished and the devout Christians provided a ready market for salted cod and herring from the North Sea. It was also during this warming period that the Vikings established colonies on Iceland and Greenland and explored as far west as Newfoundland and North America (Vinland). By the 11th century the warrior cultures of Scandinavia, Hungary and Eastern Europe had been Christianized and formed into powerful state monarchies. With its burgeoning population and large class of armed warriors, Christian Europe felt empowered to try and take back the "Holy Land", the birthplace of Christianity, from its Islamic occupiers. In a series of invasions called the "Crusades" between 1095 and 1291, Christian armies from Europe set out with varying degrees of success to conquer the Holy Land, but in the end they failed to Christianize the Middle East and Islam is still the predominant religion to this day. One unintended consequence of the Crusades was that it exposed many Europeans to new exotic foods and spices from the Middle East which stimulated trade in these products back to Europe.

After finally recovering from the Roman plagues, and after flourishing due to the agricultural abundance of the Medieval Warming Period, the population of Europe had reached its all time high of 70 million people, but this period of prosperity ended abruptly at the end of the 13th century with the beginning of a climate period known as the "Little Ice Age." Based on radiocarbon-dating of 150 samples of dead plant material with roots intact collected from beneath ice caps on Baffin Island and Iceland, Gifford Miller, Professor of Geological Sciences at University of Colorado, and his research team determined that summer cold and ice growth in the North Atlantic began abruptly between 1275 AD and 1300 AD, followed by a substantial intensification from 1430 AD to 1455 AD. Miller dates the beginning of the Little Ice Age to this time. Miller argues that the Little Ice Age, which persisted till around the latter half of the 19th century, coincided with two of the most volcanically active half centuries of the past thousand years which produced abrupt summer cooling that was maintained by sea-ice/ocean feedbacks long after the volcanic aerosols settled from the atmosphere (*"Abrupt onset of the Little Ice Age triggered by volcanism and sustained by sea-ice/ocean feedbacks", Geophysical Research Letters 39, 2012*). The many hardships caused by the Little Ice Age made life a tenuous existence for millions of people around the world.

Periodic crop failures and localized famines have been part of human history for as long as agriculture itself, often causing starvation and localized population decline. But the "Great Famine of 1315 to 1317" was so widespread and long-lasting that its devastating effects on the people of Northern Europe were unprecedented. Starting in the autumn of 1314, unusually heavy rains began in much of Northern Europe that continued without cease until the summer of 1317. By this time, due to widespread crop failures and weakness from malnutrition, millions of people had succumbed to the diseases of pneumonia, bronchitis, tuberculosis and typhoid. Historians debate the death toll but it is estimated that anywhere from 10 to 25% of the population died in many cities and towns. The cause of this unusual weather pattern remains unknown but it is similar to one that occurred after the volcanic eruption of Mount Tambora in April of 1815 that caused the "year without a summer" in Europe.

While Europe was still recovering from the Great Famine, the next purveyor of mass death in the world was fomenting in the embattled regions of central China. At this time China was occupied by Mongol invaders who had destroyed much of the vast irrigation system that the people depended on to grow their crops causing mass starvation and severe malnutrition. In their weakened state, the Chinese people became highly susceptible to contagious diseases, and in the year 1333 AD a second wave of bubonic plague broke-out, the first since the Plague of Justinian 700 years earlier. At this time the Mongols were also in control of the Silk Road, the overland trade route from China to Europe. It is thought that this new wave of plague, called the "Black Death", spread from China to Europe and the Middle East over the Silk Road when in 1346 AD the Mongols besieged a Venetian trading center on the Black Sea and catapulted their own plague infected corpses over the city's walls. Presumably, some of the Venetian traders escaped by sea, carrying the plague with them to Italy, and then, by 1348, on to the Middle East and Europe. By the end of 1350 the Black Death had subsided, but it returned to haunt Europe and the Mediterranean throughout the 14th to 17th centuries. The bubonic plague is estimated to have killed 25 million Chinese and other Asian peoples during the 15 years before it entered Europe, and the Black Death is estimated to have killed half the population of Europe and a third the population of the Middle East in the brief span of 67 years between 1333 and 1400 AD. The world population is estimated to have declined by 100 million people over the 14th Century.

As famine and plague made people feel increasingly insecure, life in Europe took on a tough and violent edge. The effects of this could be seen across all segments of society from an increase in robbery, rape and murder, to popular uprisings against the nobility and the Catholic Church, and to an end to the knightly code of chivalry in warfare in favor of mercenary armies and mass casualties. It is impossible to calculate how many deaths were caused directly by this societal breakdown, but it clearly took place in a social environment where human life had low value and was considered highly expendable. According to contemporary records of the British Royal family, among the well-off in society the average life expectancy in 1276 AD, a few decades before the Great Famine, was 35.28 years, but by 1375, after the Great Famine and recurrent plague epidemics, life expectancy had declined to a mere 17.33 years. What this statistic tells us is that children, the most vulnerable members of society, had an extremely high mortality rate during this period, and that this problem affected all classes of society.

The plunge in human population that occurred during the 14th century had a profound impact on the diet of the peasant classes throughout Europe. Due to a severe shortage of farm labor, many fields that were once farmed for grain production were abandoned to wild grasslands and left to grazing cattle and sheep for meat production. According to French Historian Louis Stouff ("*Meat consumption in 15th century Provence,*" 1969), meat consumption peaked in France and Germany in the 14th and 15th centuries at around 100 kilos (220 lbs)/person/year. But by the time the human population of Europe had finally recovered back to its pre-plague high of 70 million people in the 16th century, meat consumption per person had dropped down to 14 kilos (31 pounds) per year.

As the Little Ice Age progressed and the oceans cooled below 2 °C, the cod and herring fisheries in the North Sea that had been exploited by the Vikings during the Medeival Warm Period (950 AD to 1250 AD) largely moved south to an area off the east coast of modern day England called the "Dogger Bank." While the traditional Viking longboats performed well in the relatively tranquil summer seas of the Medeival Warm Period, the stormier climates of the Little Ice Age (1300 AD to 1850 AD) rendered these vessels outdated and obsolete. Dutch boatbuilders developed a new ship design called a "ketch" that was a short, wide-beamed vessel with a square rigged main sail, a triangular sail attached to a pole (the bowsprit] that extended forward from the prow and a rudder rather than a steering oar. These first ketches were slow but sturdy vessels, capable of plying the rough sea conditions of the Little Ice Age. Even with these more seaworthy vessels, fishing in the frigid stormy waters of the open sea was still a very dangerous occupation and boats were commonly lost at sea, but in an era of very short life expectancies and an imploding medieval population, the risky maritime adventure of cod fishing provided an attractive means of subsistence for many young men. By the late 15th century, English fleets began to sail the western North Atlantic where fish were so plentiful the British port of Bristol became a major city of commerce. English navigation of the western North Atlantic eventually led to the expedition of John Cabot to explore the coast of North America in 1497, just five years after Christopher Columbus had made contact with the New World in the Carribean Islands to the south.

Due to the dry climate and lack of grass for grazing in Andalusia (Southern Spain), the "vaqueros" (the original cowboys), who descended from the herding cultures, drove herds of 1,000 or more cattle over hundreds of miles from the north in the summer south to Andalusia in the winter. It was from these Andalusian vaqueros that the 16th century Spanish explorers Cortés, Coronado, Pizarro, de Soto and **Ponce de León** would later recruit their conquistadors (Spanish for "conquerors") who would make possible their conquest of the New World.

New World

South America

Blood type studies indicate that all modern indigenous people of the Western Hemisphere descended from two migrations of small bands of people from East Asia, the first around 13,500 years ago and the second around 11,500 years ago.

The first migration coincided with the formation of a land bridge from Beringia (the area around the Bering Straight between present day Eastern Siberia and Alaska) to the eastern foothills of the Canadian Rocky Mountains near present day Edmonton, Canada, due to a warming trend and glacial ice melt at the end of the last Ice Age. This land bridge opened up what had been an impenetrable barrier of ice that blocked this migration route during the Ice Age. Over the 1,000 years between 13,500 and 12,500 years ago, the descendants of these migrants moved steadily southward along the eastern foothills of the Rockies down through North America into Central and South America where the earliest human population centers in the Western Hemisphere sprang up several thousands of years later. Some critics of this theory say that it would have been impossible for a primitive Stone Age people to have made this long, arduous, migration in 1,000 years, but Dr. Jared Diamond, Professor of Geography at the University of California, Los Angeles, thinks otherwise:

> *"Could the descendants of the Edmonton pioneers have reached the southern tip of South America in 1,000 years? The overland straight-line distance is slightly less than 8,000 miles, so that they would have had to average 8 miles a year. That's a trivial task: any fit hunter or huntress could have filled the year's quota in a day and not moved for another 364 days. The quarry from which a Clovis tool was made can often be identified by its local type of stone, and we know in that way that individual tools traveled up to 200 miles. Some of the nineteenth-century Zulu migrations in Southern Africa are known to have covered nearly 3,000 miles in a mere 50 years."* ("The Third Chimpanzee" p 340)

The strongest evidence of this early migration route is that modern day indigenous peoples of Central and South America all share the blood Type O which indicates that they all descended from a relatively small group of people (less than 100) who became isolated from their original progenitor population in Asia ("Genes, Peoples, and Languages", North Point Press, 2000).

Dust concentrations, snow accumulation, isotope data from ice cores and fossilized evidence indicate that the Northern Hemisphere underwent a severe cooling trend and rapid return to glacial conditions between approximately 12,800 and 11,500 years ago. This period of geological history called the "Younger Dryas stadial" saw glaciers once again cover much of Alaska and Canada which again created an impenetrable barrier for human migrations from Eastern Siberia to North America. But as warmer weather returned around 11,500 years ago, glacial ice melt reopened the inland corridor which opened up the Americas to a second wave of human migration from East Asia that colonized the North American continent. Differentiating between the first and second wave of migrations is the admixture of blood Type A that is common to the indigenous peoples of North America but completely absent in Central and South America.

Norte Chico

In the mid 1990s, Peruvian anthropologist and archaeologist, Dr. Ruth Shady Solis, principal professor and coordinator of the graduate archaeology program at the National University of San Marcos in Peru, went public with her findings: radiocarbon dating of plant fibers excavated from sites on the north central coast of Peru known as the "Peruvian littoral" (coastal region) indicate that an urban civilization called the "Norte Chico" flourished there by at least 4,090 years ago, concurrent with the Egyptian pyramids. Before Dr. Solis's findings, the earliest civilization known in the Western Hemisphere was the Olmec people on the southern gulf coast of modern-day Mexico at around 3,200 years ago.

Archaeologists have been aware of these ancient sites since at least the 1940s, but it was not until the 1990s that Dr. Shady provided the first extensive documentation of the civilization with her archaeological work at the major urban center of "Caral" located 14 miles (22 km) inland at 1300 feet (400 meters) above sea level. It wasn't until her April, 2001 paper published in the journal *Science* providing a survey of her Caral research that the full archaeological significance of Norte Chico was revealed to the public. Further documentation was published in the December 2004 issue of the journal *Nature* by American archaeologists Jonathan Haas of the Chicago Field Museum and Winifred Creamer of Northern Illinois University with their presentation of radiocarbon dating from 13 additional sites in close proximity to Caral pushing the earliest dates of development back to around 5,200 years ago.

The Peruvian littoral would appear to be an unlikely place for the spontaneous development of a civilization. It is extremely arid being in the cast of two "rain shadows" caused by the Andes Mountains to the east and the Pacific Ocean trade winds to the west. Moisture that sweeps westward across the Amazon rain forest from the Atlantic Ocean falls as snow in the Andes while moisture from the Pacific is swept north by ocean trade winds before it can penetrate inland. This leaves a narrow strip of land along the coast of Peru that gets virtually no rain but is punctuated by numerous short, small rivers that carry Andean snow melt down the western slopes of the Andes to the Pacific Ocean. While these coastal plains receive little to no annual rainfall, the rivers and rich alluvial soils built-up over millennia of siltation have created an ideal situation for the development of irrigation agriculture. The Norte Chico region comprises four such coastal river valleys: the Huaura, Supe, Pativilca, and Fortaleza which share a common coastal plain. While the three principal valleys cover an area only about 26 miles square (42 km square), the Norte Chico civilization consisted of as many as 30 distinct population centers all with monumental architecture and surrounded by irrigation channels.

It was here at Norte Chico in "Early Archaic" times (10,000 to 8,000 years ago) where a band of the original hunter-gatherer Clovis people settled down on the coast by subsisting on the abundant and easily harvested shellfish that lived close to shore and on wild native plants (similar to the first H. sapiens of South Africa some 200,000 years ago). Around 5,100 years ago at a time when the climate turned much drier greatly reducing yields from wild plants these coastal dwelling villagers figured out how to make fishing nets with a species of wild cotton that enabled them to catch the anchovies and sardines that spawn by the billions near shore due to a cold water upwelling called the "Humboldt Current" that flows north-west along the Peruvian coast. This phenomenal technological breakthrough allowed for a greatly expanded food supply resulting in a substantial increase in the human population on the coast. As this fishing technology caught on, the need for net-making material outstripped the available supply of wild cotton and the Norte Chico responded by domesticating the cotton plant and growing it upriver from the ocean on the dry alluvial plains above using simple diversion ditches to irrigate their crops. There are still competing theories much debated among modern-day archaeologists over the exact sequence and relevance of events in this first Western Hemisphere civilization at Norte Chico, but it is clear from the archaeological record that these inland cotton plantations quickly outstripped the coastal villages as the major population centers of the Norte Chico and that most of the people were employed as farmers, weavers and construction workers. Besides cotton, the Norte Chico also domesticated and grew edible plants that facilitated another major increase in food production and human population. Archaeological remains indicate the Norte Chico diet included squash, beans, lucuma, guava, pacay, camote, avocado and achira. Interestingly, maize does not appear to be a significant food source for the Norte Chico making them the rare civilization not based on a staple grain crop. There is also no indication that terrestrial animals provided appreciable subsistence for the Norte Chico.

Dr. Shady estimates the population of the city of Caral at 3,000 people, the population of the Supe valley at around 20,000, and the total population of Norte Chico at possibly 50,000. With a population of this size the Norte Chico people were able to mobilize work forces to build monumental structures including numerous large stepped pyramid mounds – the largest over 500 feet (150 meters) to a side and 60 feet (18 meters) tall – sunken circular amphitheaters and a variety of residential structures. These buildings were constructed out of quarried stone and river cobbles hauled to the sites by workers using bags woven from a reed grass known as "shicra" that was gathered from the highlands above the city. Norte Chico sites are notable for their exceptional urban density and with the possible exception of northern China were likely the densest human populations on Earth at that time. At one Norte Chico site the painted and incised fragment of a gourd bowl dated at 4,250 years old was found featuring a fanged creature with splayed feet whose left arm appears to end in a snake's head and whose right hand holds a staff. This figure appears to be the earliest depiction of the "Staff God" that reappears in various religious guises in Andean cultures over the next three and a half millennia.

Somewhat surprisingly, the very inventive Norte Chico never developed ceramic technology, so unfortunately they left no pottery shards with iconographs (stories in pictures) behind for modern-day archaeologists to divine their history. What the Norte Chico lacked in ceramics though, they made up for in textiles. Cotton fishing nets, clothes, bags, wraps, adornments and "quipu" which were lengths of elaborately knotted and colored string used for keeping records in a still undecipherable language were the most elemental commodities of the Norte Chico civilization. The Norte Chico quipu is also the earliest manifestation of this form of communication that was further developed by numerous Andean cultures over the next 4,500 years culminating 500 years ago with the vast Inca Empire that existed when the Spanish conquistadors arrived. Unfortunately the Spaniards destroyed most of the Andean quipus and few remain today for study by modern archaeologists. That the Norte Chico quipu and staff god were passed on through Andean cultures over great spans of time and distance suggests that the first civilization of Norte Chico had contact and significant influence with people far beyond its own small borders. Indeed, while there are only two confirmed shore sites in the Norte Chico complex (Aspero and Bandurrai), contemporaneous cotton fishing nets and domesticated plants have been found up and down the Peruvian coast. Archaeologist Jonathan Haas surmises that the major inland centers of Norte Chico were at the center of a broad regional trade network centered on these resources. From Dr. Shady's findings at Caral she speculates that the Norte Chico exported their own products to distant communities in exchange for exotic imports like spondylus shells from the coast of Ecuador, rich dyes from the Andean highlands and hallucinogenic snuff from the Amazon.

By around 2,800 years go (1800 BC) extensive irrigation canals were built by other peoples on more fertile plains to the north and south, and Norte Chico became something of a frontier zone between these larger settlements. Eventually warfare broke out and after an astonishing 3,400 year run, Norte Chico was conquered and abandoned. Today Norte Chico is desolate and home to only a few scattered farmers.

Stylized ceramic stew-pots found at the nearby coastal sites of Las Haldas, Caballo Muerto and Ancón, indicate that between 1700 BC and 900 BC – after the demise of Norte Chico – boiling was added as a way to cook food. Las Haldas is located in the Casma Valley which also contains numerous other archaeological sites including Sechin Alto, the largest pre-Columbian (before Columbus) construction in the Western Hemisphere; the Thirteen Towers of Chankillo that mark the 13 lunar months and the winter and summer solstices; and a retaining wall at Cerro Sechin containing nearly 400 granite sculptures depicting a gruesome scene in which a procession of armed men make their way among the mutilated remains of human victims. Considering the shocking nature of these images, it seems likely that some degree of violence and warfare had broken-out among these early coastal peoples. Though little is known about the decline of these cultures, these sites appear to have been abandoned by 800 BC around the same time that the center of Peruvian culture shifted inland to a site called "Chavín de Huántar". Today the Casma Valley supports an agricultural economy that grows a wide variety of produce including avocado, passionfruit, apples, mangoes, pacea, bananas, guayaba, pepino, grapes, maize, cotton, asparagus, chilies and many types of beans.

Chavin

In northern Peru at a site 75 miles (115 kilometers) inland at an elevation over 10,300 feet (3,150 meters) above sea level, where the Mosna and Huanchecsa Rivers merge to carve a high pass through the Andean peaks, an ancient city called "Chavín de Huántar" existed from 850 BC to 200 BC. First excavated in 1919 by archaeologist Dr. Julio Cesar Tello, considered the father of Peruvian archaeology, his findings revealed Chavín de Huántar to be the urban center of a "Chavin" influenced artistic style that became widespread throughout much of Peru at that time. It was during this 650 year period that the cultivation of maize, potatoes and quinoa and the domestication of the llama transformed the economy and social structure of the northern Peruvian highlands from hunter/gatherers to pastoralists and agriculturalists (*"The Importance of Maize in Initial Period and Early Horizon Peru," Academic Press, 2006*) (*"Maize and the Origin of Highland Chavín Civilization: An Isotopic Perspective", American Anthropologist*)(*"Our Father the Cayman, Our Dinner the Llama: Animal Utilization at Chavin de Huantar, Peru", American Antiquity, 1995*).

Through extensive study of bones, hair, pottery, stone sculptures and structural ruins from the archaeological site at Chavín de Huántar and numerous other sites across the Peruvian highlands, archaeologists have managed to piece together the complex living arrangements of these ancient peoples. Maize produces a signature isotope that is very distinct from all the other wild and domesticated plants that were available to the Peruvian highlanders at that time; stable isotope analysis of human bone collagen and hair samples from various archaeological sites scattered around the highlands indicates that maize was a dietary staple only at elevations and ecological zones that were suitable for its cultivation. Most of the land around Chavín de Huántar was too cold and wet to effectively grow maize and stable isotope analysis of bones from the site indicate that maize was not a significant source of food in the Chavin diet. It is likely that cultivars developed from native potato tubers and quinoa grains that thrive in the cold wet weather of Chavín de Huántar were the inhabitants' main source of calories.

Paleontological study of animal bones from in and around Chavín de Huántar indicate the Chavin developed a complex evolving association with llamas over the course of settlement. A preponderance of deer bones dating from the first 350 years (850 BC to 500 BC) of settlement suggests that deer hunting was the primary source of meat for the Chavin with llamas, guanaco, alpacas, and vicuna, guinea pigs, viscachas and small birds of minor dietary importance. In the century between 500 BC and 400 BC there is an almost complete switch-over to llama and alpaca bones suggesting that the depletion of wild deer populations and the domestication of the llama, a practice adapted from herders in the southern highlands where llamas are indigenous, occurred abruptly around this time. By 200 BC, at the end of the Chavin settlement period, the animal bones excavated at Chavín de Huántar are almost exclusively from llamas. The location, type and condition of the bones further indicated that herds of llama were grazed on grasslands at the higher elevations and before winter, when the older underperforming animals were culled from the herd, the llama herders made "ch'arki" (jerky) by "freeze drying" strips of raw llama meat during the frosty nights and sunny days to preserve it for eating throughout the rest of the year. This llama ch'arki was also traded to the valley farmers for potatoes, quinoa, textiles and other goods. Throughout much of the Chavin settlement period llamas were not butchered until after they had productively served their primary function as pack animals and wool bearers, usually between four and seven years of age. But toward the end of the Chavin period, class distinctions developed in living quarters, burial accompaniments and diet with a small upper class consuming the tender meat from young llamas that were sacrificed before achieving their full economic potential; an indication that by the end of the Chavin period the llama had become a status symbol of wealth and power.

Chavín de Huantár is uniquely situated in the Peruvian highlands where there are only two ranges in the Andes instead of three. It is also situated midway between the Amazon jungle and the Pacific coast, on a route accessing the very extensive Marañon River drainage that flows east down to the tropical lowlands and the Santa River drainage that flows west down to the ocean. Via this route it is possible to cross the Andes from jungle to coast by crossing only one high pass over 15,000 feet (4,600 meters) above sea level. With caravans of llamas making it possible to convey heavy loads up and down the steep slopes of the Andes, a trade economy was developed among the many settlements that had sprung-up along this route with Chavín de Huantár at its center. The two primary structures at Chavín de Huantár are the "Old Temple" dating to 850 BC and the "New Temple" dating to 500 BC. These monumental structures were built of white granite and black limestone mined from distant quarries and transported to the site indicating a sizable organized labor force. The temples utilized architectural features adapted from earlier cultures on the north and central coast including sunken circular plazas, U-shaped plazas and what appear to be ceremonial platforms. The temple's design also displays distinct highland innovations including a complex canal system under the temple's foundation to drain high water during the rainy season and avoid flooding. Finely crafted stone artifacts including the Tello Obelisk, tenon heads, Raimondi Stela and the statue of Lanzon are fantastic examples of the Chavin nature-based artistic style depicting exotic jungle animals including caymans (of the alligator family), anaconda snakes, monkeys and jaguars. These mysterious creatures were also expressed in ceramics, metal work and textiles. Many sculptures and carvings show the transformation from a human head to a jaguar head suggesting that the Chavin believed in human transmogrify or "shape shifting". The indigenous psychotropic San Pedro cactus is also frequently depicted in the iconography particularly in the form of the "staff god" who is shown holding the cactus as a staff. It is thought likely that the Chavin religion involved shamans claiming supernatural powers through drug induced hallucinations and shape shifting.

During the formative stage of development at Chavín de Huantár (between 850 BC and 500 BC) the residential area remained relatively small housing only a few hundred inhabitants at most. The site grew appreciably during the subsequent middle and late stages of development reaching around 3,000 people as llama breeding and trade networks expanded, making Chavín de Huantár the largest highland urban center in the Andes at that time. Craft specialization and technological advancements in textiles and metallurgy appear in Chavin households during the final stage of development (400 BC to 200 BC) including the use of dyed llama and alpaca hair in cotton weaves, textile painting, discontinuous warps, warp wrapping, the heddle loom, metal soldering, sweating, welding, silver-gold alloys and three dimensional goldsmithing. These innovations spread widely around Peru through the Chavin trade network and transformed the Andean craft tradition.

During the third century BC, construction at Chavín de Huantár halted and the Chavín trading network began to break down as evidenced by the complete replacement of Chavín style ceramics with local styles by 200 BC. This period of decline is also evidenced by an intensified socioeconomic stratification and the widespread construction of hilltop fortresses in the highlands and coastal valleys. While there is no direct archaeological evidence of conflict, these conditions do suggest that there were hostilities. Today Chavín de Huantár is well off the beaten path and a sorely neglected archaeological site.

Nazca

The Nazca Valley lies on the lowest plateau of the southern coastal plains of Peru which is still over a mile above sea level at 6,500 feet (2,000 meters). On this wide rainless plateau numerous small coastal rivers, the result of summer rains in the highlands, run together to form the Rio Grande de Nazca. Over the course of geological time, the river was blocked on its route to the sea by an upheaval of coastal hills which caused sediments to be deposited on the floor of the Nazca Valley. These rich alluvial soils provided fertile ground for a forest of huarango trees, a specie of mesquite (Prosopis pallida), to grow. It was in this valley that the Chavin influenced Paracas culture developed into the Nazca civilization between 200 AD and 750 AD.

The Nazca civilization produced a distinctive painted multicolored pottery and intricately woven textile patterns but is most renowned for its extraordinary geoglyphs called the "Nazca Lines". The Nazca Lines are large drawings made on the ground by scraping away stones to reveal the lighter soils beneath. The drawings depict various plants and animals as well as geometric shapes, but they are so immense that the images are only discernible from the sky. As with all Andean civilizations, the Nazca created no written language so there are no texts available to explain the Lines. Most archaeologists believe they were drawn as offerings to the gods.

As the Nazca civilization developed they engineered and constructed a remarkable network of underground channels called "puquios" to irrigate their crops on the arid plains of the Nazca Valley. The puquios were dug into the mountainside until they reached an aquifer under the surface. The channels were then lined with river rocks but no mortar so that water could infiltrate into the channels. The water was then transported in these underground channels to above ground canals called "acequias" that irrigated the fields or filled small storage reservoirs called "kochias" for later use. Numerous access holes called "ajos" were placed along the surface of the puquios like modern-day manholes to access the channels for repair and maintenance. (Schreiber and Rojas, 1995) Iconography on ceramics and excavated remains depict a Nazca people with a varied diet consisting of maize, squash, sweet potato, manioc, achira and huarango pods. They also grew several non-food crops such as cotton for textiles, gourds for containers and fishnet floats, as well as coca and San Pedro cactus for hallucinogenic religious purposes. Using stable isotope data from excavated bones in the Nazca region Anthropologists C. M. Kellner and M. J. Schoeninger, of the University of California, San Diego, were able to determine that maize was the staple component of the Nazca diet (*"Wari's imperial influence on local Nasca diet: The stable isotope evidence,"* *Journal of Anthropological Archaeology*, 2008).

The Nazca also raised llamas and stable isotope data from llama bones indicates that their fodder consisted mainly of huarango pods since, unlike the grassy highlands, there was no grassland for grazing in the arid lowlands of the Nazca Valley. Stable isotope data also indicates that over time the llamas' fodder changed from huarango pods to maize. While the Nazca did eat llama meat (Silverman and Proulx, 2002), due to the trophic structure of ecosystems, feeding cultivated grains to large domesticated animals is a very inefficient way to provide food for people when many more people could be fed by eating the grain directly instead of feeding it to the llamas for meat. It was the llamas' utility as a pack animal that made it worth the Nazca's investment of feeding it expensive cultivated grains and, as with the Chavin, meat was a secondary byproduct. The Nazca did domesticate and raise a small native guinea pig for meat, but it does not appear to have been a significant source of calories in the average diet. The southern coast of Peru has no convenient estuaries like Norte Chico for colonization and thus indications are that fish and shellfish were also of little significance in the average diet.

A huge architectural complex called "Cahuachi" covering nearly 400 acres that overlooks the Nazca Lines appears to be the major ceremonial center for the Nazca civilization consisting of over 40 large mounds topped with adobe structures. Limited dwelling quarters suggest there were few full time residents at Cahuachi, but the population of the valley must have been sufficiently large to supply the substantial workforce necessary to build these massive structures and the sophisticated underground irrigation system that served it. Bones found at the Cahuach site indicate that llamas and guinea pigs were used as sacrificial animals. Iconography and human skull collections also indicate that the Nazca ritually practiced "trophy hunting" for human heads. This suggests that there was significant antagonism between the Nazca and neighboring cultures.

The Nazca civilization disappeared around 750 AD. Archaeologists under the direction of Dr. David Beresford-Jones from the University of Cambridge studied ancient pollen samples from the area looking for clues to its downfall (*"Deforestation by the Nazca Civilization of Peru: Environmental Devastation in the Ancient World"*, www.suite101.com). This study revealed a distinct shift in the type of vegetation over time from the natural population of huarango trees to agricultural crops. Dr. Beresford-Jones surmises from this evidence that as the human population increased in conjunction with expanding agriculture, more and more huarango trees were cut down until deforestation was virtually complete throughout the entire valley. With the loss of the huarango, the valley ecosystem lost the tree's leguminous nitrogen fixing quality and over time the soils of the Nazca Valley became nitrogen deficient and unproductive. The huango's canopy and roots that had prevented wind and water erosion were also lost resulting in further soil depletion. Archaeological evidence indicates that as the huarango roots decayed the water table in the valley dropped below the depth of the irrigation canals leading to severe crop failures. Within a few generations massive soil erosion had turned the Nazca Valley into a thirsty desert, and after a 550 year run, the Nazca civilization was gone. Water is still a scarce resource in the Nazca valley to this day.

Moche

As at Norte Chico, for thousands of years, small fisher/forager groups inhabited the deltas of the many small rivers that run off the western slopes of the Andes into the Pacific along the coast of northern Peru. Only fifteen miles (25 km) inland from the Moche River delta the land quickly rises to a coastal plain over a mile and a half above sea level at between 7,900 and 9,200 feet (2,400 and 2,800 meters). Due to double rain shadows, the Moche River Delta is one of the driest places on Earth. Also, like Norte Chico, there is evidence of cotton fishing-net technology being used in these delta regions as far back as 4,000 years ago (2000 BC), but it wasn't until around 100 AD that the fisher/foragers of the Moche River delta established an agriculturally based society on this dry upland plateau transected by the Moche River. Over the next 650 years (until 750 AD), contemporaneously but independently of the Nazca on the south coast, the Moche developed a highly refined and distinctive cultural style that spread to several neighboring river valleys covering a distance of some 250 miles (400 kl) along the Peruvian north coast. (*"Great Journey: The Peopling of Ancient America", London: Thames & Hudson*, 1987)

The Moche built irrigation canals some as long as 60 miles (97 km) extending across these arid coastal plains to make the desert bloom. Their main crops were cotton, gourds, maize, beans, squash, peppers, melons, and peanuts. The Moche also raised llamas on maize (Shimada and Shimada, 1985), but as with the Nazca their primary function was as pack animals with meat a secondary byproduct. Using llama caravans the Moche established an extensive coastal trade network in fish and also nitrogen rich bird guano harvested from island rookeries off the coast to fertilize their fields (*"The Mochica: A Culture of Peru", Praeger Press*, 1972). Wild deer and a domesticated native duck provided some meat, but these resources were very limited and most of the calories in the average Moche diet were derived from domesticated plants and imported fish.

A common artistic style and organizational structure that first appeared in the Moche Valley spread to the other neighboring valleys through conflict and political alliances. Besides its remarkable irrigation systems, this Moche civilization is noted for its elaborate painted ceramics, realistic sculptures, intricate cotton weaves, advanced metallurgy, and monumental constructions of temples and palaces. The adobe pyramid, "Huaca del Sol", on the Moche River was the largest pre-Columbian structure in Peru. Excavated ruins indicate that some large villages were home to 10,000 people surrounded by many smaller outlying farmsteads where the people worked on the canals. The ruling elites lived high atop the pyramids surveying the vast irrigated fields beneath them. Sacrifices to the gods of both nonhuman and human animals are depicted in Moche iconography, and bones of sacrificial offerings have been discovered, but with no written texts, the specific religious context of these sacrifices is unknown. While drinking human blood is also depicted in Moche iconography, depictions of actual cannibalism have not been found. From archaeological remains discovered thus far it appears that human sacrifice did not occur on a mass scale.

Ice cores drilled in 1983 from glaciers in the Peruvian Andes have provided a record of variations in rainfall in northern Peru for the past 1,500 years indicating that between the years 536 AD and 594 AD there was a series of extreme weather events characterized by thirty years of intense rain and flooding followed by thirty years of drought. The year 536 AD was also document in recorded history from the Middle East, Europe and China as being particularly dark, cold and wet suggesting to climate scientists that a worldwide catastrophic event such as a massive volcanic eruption or impact from a giant meteor kicked-up enough dust into the atmosphere to dim the sunlight. Sulfate deposits found in ice cores from glaciers around the world strongly support the volcanic hypothesis; the sulfate spike in 536 AD is even greater than that which caused the "Year Without a Summer" in 1816 after the well documented volcanic eruption of Mount Tambora in Indonesia. Climatologists suspect that this catastrophic event set-off a super "El Niño" (the wet/dry climate cycle on the Pacific coast caused by changes in ocean temperatures) causing the most severe floods and droughts over the past 1,500 years. As the dry river valleys of the Moche civilization became raging torrents, the levees and canals overflowed and collapsed and the arduous labors of generations vanished within a few short years. The floodwaters devastated the valley landscape, burying villages under mud and debris and drowning many of its inhabitants. The floods overwhelmed sanitation systems, polluted springs and streams and stripped thousands of acres of fertile soil. As the waters receded and the rivers went down, typhoid and other epidemics swept through the valleys, wiping out entire communities. With the years of flooding followed by thirty years of drought, crops withered and even more of the already decimated Moche population died of starvation. Remarkably, after more predictable weather returned in 595 AD, the Moche people managed to revive and rebuild their civilization, all be it on a much smaller scale than before. These later settlements were characterized by fortifications and defensive works but, since archaeological evidence of a foreign invasion has yet to be found, many archaeologists suspect internal social unrest, possibly as a result of factional fighting over control of increasingly scarce resources. Around 750 AD, Moche cultural artifacts are suddenly replaced with artifacts from the Huari (a.k.a. Wari) culture from the northern highlands of Peru. It appears that after another severe flood and drought event in the late 7th Century the Moche ruling elite lost their religious authority over the people who welcomed the arrival of the Huari religion and their more advanced irrigation systems, thus ending over 650 years of the Moche civilization (*"Floods, Famines, and Emperors: El Niño and the Fate of Civilizations", New York: Basic Books*, 1999).

Huari – Tiahuanaco

From the remnants of the Chavin Civilization that had flourished centuries earlier (850 BC to 200 BC), a culture called the Huari from the south central highlands of Peru began to expand its influence into the northern highlands around 500 AD. The Huari introduced the concept of the great walled urban center to the Andes, building the city of Huari located 6.8 miles (11 km) north east of the modern-day city of Ayacucho, at an altitude of 9,100 feet (2770 meters) above sea level. This capital city covered 10 square miles (16 square kilometers), and was highly organized into residential, administrative, and religious areas with architecture aligned to conform to the local topography. By conquest the Huari became the first true empire in the Andes establishing architecturally distinctive administrative centers in the central highlands and much of the area that was formerly controlled by the coastal Moche Civilization.

The Huari developed a system of terracing land on slopes at the edges of the valleys that could withstand El Niño floods. They exported this agricultural technique to flood ravaged valley areas while also building irrigation channels that tapped into water from higher-up in the mountains to gravity feed down to their terraced farms. The Huari were also the first in the Andes to develop an extensive road system to facilitate communications and trade in their vertical empire. Roads were constructed to speed the traffic of llama caravans, but were not designed for wheeled vehicles which were never developed in the pre-Columbian Andes. Along with exporting their advanced technologies, the Huari demanded strict adherence to their religious leaders and beliefs. Stable isotope analysis of excavated bones from different regions of the Huari Empire suggest that the Huari did not change the staple crops in areas they conquered which generally meant maize in the lowlands, potatoes and quinoa in the highlands and llamas the essential beast of burden for transporting materials around the far-flung empire.

Also during the post Chavin period between 300 BC and 300 AD, to the south of the Huari, on the border between modern-day Peru and Bolivia near the shores of Lake Titicaca at 12,500 feet (3,800 meters) above sea level, another civilization called the Tiahuanaco (a.k.a. Tiwanaku), was taking root. This area was first inhabited as a small agriculturally based village located between the lake and dry highlands with ready access to wild caught fish and water fowl and herding grounds for llamas. By 400 AD the area around Lake Titicaca is thought to have become a moral and cosmological center to which many people made pilgrimages, and between 600 AD and 800 AD the community grew into the city of Tiahuanaco. The ruins of this ancient city are about 44 miles (72 kilometers) west of modern-day La Paz. The site was first recorded in written history by Spanish conquistador and self-acclaimed "first chronicler of the Indies," Pedro Cieza de Leon, but it has been so pillaged by succeeding Andean cultures and later by Spanish conquistadors that there were few archaeological remains left for modern scholars to examine from excavations made in the late 1970s through the 1990s. The Tiahuanaco are most well known for their precision stone work and the monolithic Gateway of the Sun, which is adorned with the carved central figure of a staff-carrying Doorway God.

In the Lake Titicaca Basin, the Tiahuanaco developed a farming technique using flooded-raised fields called "*suka kollus*" similar to the chinampas of the Aztec on Lake Texcoco. These artificial planting mounds were separated by shallow canals to irrigate crops but also to absorb heat from solar radiation during the day. This heat gradually emitted during the cold nights protected the plants from the frosts that are endemic to such high altitudes. The canals were sophisticated constructions, with a base of cobblestone topped with gravel and impermeable clay, which filtered out salt from the lake's brackish waters and prevented salinization of the topsoil. The canals were also used to raise fish and ducks with the resulting canal sludge being dredged for fertilizer. Though labor-intensive, suka kollus can produce amazing yields. Field trials have shown that while traditional agriculture in the region typically yields 2.4 metric tons of potatoes per hectare, and modern agriculture with artificial fertilizers and pesticides yields about 14.5 metric tons, suka kollu agriculture yields an average of 21 metric tons (*"The Tiwanaku: Portrait of an Andean Civilization"*, *Wiley-Blackwell*, 1993). The Lake Titicaca Basin, unlike the dry desert river basins on the lower western slopes of the Andes, has predictable and abundant rainfall so the Tiahuanaco also grew maize on artificially constructed ponds called "*qochas*" and on irrigated terraced fields.

A precipitous rise in grinding stones and stable isotope analysis of bones indicate that by 400 AD maize production and consumption increased considerably compared to earlier peoples with less consumption of marine and terrestrial animals (Goldstein, 2003; Sandness, 1992). Satellite imaging was used to map the extent of fossilized suka kollus across the three primary valleys of Tiahuanaco, leading to an estimated population carrying capacity of 1.5 million people.

Around 400 AD, Tiahuanaco went from being a locally dominant culture to a predatory state. Archaeologists note the rapid adoption of Tiahuanaco ceramics in the cultures of southern Peru, Bolivia and northern Chile that had all became part of the Tiahuanaco Empire. The Tiahuanaco elites gained their authority by seizing control over maize and coca production from the lower regions of the Empire and by controlling trade between the different cultures within the Empire. Maintaining large herds of llamas was also essential for the Tiahuanaco elites to exercise control as they provided the motive power to transport food, raw materials and finished goods back and forth between the center and the periphery. Key to spreading Tiahuanaco religion from the main site to the satellite centers was the wide distribution of small portable icons made of wood, bone and cloth that held ritual religious meaning.

Despite the fact that the Tiahuanaco and Huari Empires shared a 300 mile (500 kilometer) border between Moquegua and Cuzco, the only evidence found thus far of direct interaction between them is at a unique mesa formation rising 1,968 feet (600 meters) above the valley floor in southern Peru called Cerro Baúl (*"Clash of the Andean Titans: Wari and Tiwanaku at Cerro Baúl,"* *South American Archaeology*, 2003). Around 600 AD the Huari settled the region surrounding Cerro Baúl while the Tiahuanaco settled downstream in the lower reaches of the Moquegua River valley. Later the Huari constructed a city on top of Cerro Baúl complete with their administrative center style of architecture while the Tiahuanaco built an immense temple complex downstream at Omo, the only temple of its kind outside the Tiahuanaco heartland. Interaction was limited at first but over the years there appears to have been some defection of Tiahuanaco settlers over to the Huari religion and economy that weakened the Tiahuanaco hold on the area. But by around 1000 AD, both the Tiahuanaco and Huari had completely abandoned their settlements at Cerro Baúl, and by 1100 AD, both Empires had entirely collapsed. Ice core data from Andean glaciers suggest there was a long drought period between 1000 AD and 1300 AD that coincided with the Medieval Warming Period in Europe causing massive crop failures and population declines of both humans and llamas. As food production diminished the elites lost their source of authority and, as with prior Andean civilizations, broke down into smaller regional kingdoms.

Chimú

The same long drought period that saw the demise of the Huari and Tiahuanaco Empires also saw a new civilization rise from the descendants of the earlier Moche called the Chimú. The Chimú were able to thrive during this long drought due to their location on the north coast of Peru which gave them ready access to one of the most abundant fisheries in the world that was virtually unaffected by the drought. Between 900 AD and 1200 AD, the Chimú built their adobe capital city of Chan Chan on the banks of the Moche River, near its mouth at the Pacific Ocean, rising only 112 feet (34 meters) above sea level. The land outside Chan Chan was farmed on sunken fields called "huachaques" where topsoil was excavated down to the water table to irrigate crops (Moseley and Deeds 1982). Later, in the valleys upriver, the Chimú devised and built even more extensive irrigation systems than their Moche ancestors with large reservoirs to store water and long deep inter-valley networks of canals to irrigate their fields. Their staple crops were maize, beans, sweet potatoes, peppers, papaya and cotton.

As the Chimú dug deep to tap into fresh water to irrigate their crops, they also mined large volumes of clay to build towering 50 to 60 foot (15 to 18 meters) tall adobe walls to surround their triangular city of Chan Chan. The city was composed of ten walled citadels that housed ceremonial rooms, burial chambers, temples, walk-in wells (similar to those of the Nazca) up to 50 feet (15 meters) deep, and residences of the elites. The tallest north facing walls gained the greatest exposure to the sun and served both to block the south-westerly winds off the ocean and to absorb sunlight for heating against the cold frequent fog. The walls themselves were constructed of adobe brick covered with a smooth plaster surface into which intricate designs of realistic and stylized sea animals were carved in relief. Chan Chan was the largest Pre-Columbian city in South America covering an area of approximately 7.7 square miles (20 square kilometers) with a dense 2.3 square mile (6 square kilometer) urban core. It is estimated that at its peak 50,000 people lived in the city. First excavations of Chan Chan began in the mid-1960s attracting the attention of anthropologist, Dr. Michael Moseley, then assistant curator at the Peabody Museum at Harvard, who directed the Chan Chan-Moche Valley Project from 1969 to 1975 to unearth the remains of this vast city and irrigation system.

While farmland was allocated to individual families by local ruling elites, llama herds were managed under centralized control by the elites themselves. Deposits of llama dung indicate that fodder for the llamas came primarily from pods of the algarrobo tree, another specie of mesquite, which was much more common in pre-Columbian times than it is today. Llamas were also fed maize stalks and other plant residues. By examining animal bones found among household effects in Chan Chan and other Chimú villages, it appears to archaeologists that llama meat was a luxury food reserved for the elites except for elite-sponsored religious feasts when it was distributed to the lower classes ("*Between the Kitchen and the Sate: Domestic Parcice and Chimu Expansion in the Jequetepeque Valley, Peru*", Department of Anthropology, University of Pittsburgh, 2009). Animal bones also indicate that small domesticated dogs and guinea pigs were raised at the household level and supplied occasional meat. Fish and other sea animals were a significant component of the Chimú diet, all the more for those who lived closest to the coast.

By 1100 AD the Chimú had consolidated control of the Moche and adjacent river valleys, and then began to expand into a Kingdom that, over the next four centuries, would control a swath of land along the north coast of Peru between the lower slopes of the Andes and the Pacific Ocean 20 to 100 miles (32 to 160 kilometers) wide and 621 miles (1000 kilometers) long. At its height, the Kingdom of Chimor controlled about two-thirds of all agricultural land ever irrigated along the Pacific coast of South America. Archaeologists have noted a large increase in Chimú craft production of metalwork, textiles and ceramics at this time indicating that artisans may have been brought to Chan Chan from other areas as a result of this conquest. The economic and social systems operated through the import of raw materials to Chan Chan where they were processed into prestige goods by artisans. The elite at Chan Chan maintained control of the Kingdom through centralized decision making over organization, food storage, craft production, distribution and consumption. By the thirteenth century more typical weather had returned to the Andes and another powerful culture began its ascension in the southeastern highlands of Peru, the Inca. A war between the Chimú and the Inca resulted in the defeat of the Chimú in 1470 AD and its subjugation into the vast Inca Empire.

Inca

The Inca are by far the most well known pre-Columbian Andean culture in today's popular imagination since it was they who controlled most of the territory at the time of the Spanish conquest in 1532 AD. But as we now know based on archaeological evidence, much of it only uncovered since 1985, the highly advanced and long lived pre-Columbian Andean cultures reviewed above preceded the Inca, and the Inca were relative newcomers in pre-Columbian Andean history. As late as the 12th century AD the Inca people were a pastoral tribe living in the Urbamba River Valley in the highlands of southeastern Peru at an elevation of around 11,200 feet (3,400 meters) above sea level. Then around 1300 AD, they formed the small city-state "Kingdom of Cuzco", but it wasn't until 1438 AD that they began their expansion that would eventually bind most of Peru and Ecuador as well as parts of Columbia, Bolivia, Argentina and Chile into a state comparable to the Roman Empire of ancient Europe.

A team of French, English and American researchers led by Alex Chepstow-Lusty, a paleoecologist from the French Institute for Andean Studies in Lima, Peru, took a core sample from layers of mud on the floor of Lake Marcacocha in the Cuzco region of the Peruvian Andes in the heartland of the Inca people. This record, published in the journal "Climate of the Past" (2009), reveals the climate history of the area for the past 1,200 years dating back to 800 AD. It indicates a period of increased warming from 1100 AD to 1500 AD that coincides with the meteoric rise of the Inca Empire. From pollen, seeds and other environmental indicators in the layers of mud, Dr. Chepstow-Lusty surmises that the increasingly warming climate allowed the Inca to grow maize at higher altitudes by constructing agricultural terraces irrigated by canals with glacial run-off.

Machu Picchu was a royal estate built by Inca rulers outside the capital city of Cuzco in the mid 15th century. The population of Machu Picchu consisted of "yanacona" who were a servant class individually selected by elites and moved about the empire for various services, including permanent residence as retainers at royal estates (Burger et al. (2003) (Villar Cordova 1966). Stable carbon and nitrogen isotope analysis from a large sample of human skeletal remains from these servants at Machu Picchu who came from the far reaches of the Inca Empire would seem to corroborate the importance of maize in the Inca diet. This isotope study indicated that the people's diets varied significantly as children when they lived in different ecozones around the empire, but converged as adults living at Machu Picchu on a maize based diet (*"Variation in Dietary Histories Among the Immigrants of Macchu Picchu: Carbon and Nitrogen Isotope Evidence"* Department of Anthropology, Georgia State University, Atlanta, 2010).

Puruchuco-Huaquerones is one of the largest pre-Columbian cemeteries ever discovered in South America with over 2,200 individuals recovered, most dating from 1476 AD to 1532 AD during the Inca period. Bone, hair, nail, skin and muscle tissues were sampled from 72 partially mummified individuals and analyzed for stable carbon and nitrogen isotopes. Isotope data from all tissues indicated the diet included primarily maize with some lower trophic level animals (e.g., guinea pig, llama) but also included some tubers. Although the site is close to the ocean, isotopic data for most individuals were not consistent with the consumption of marine foods. The isotopic composition of soft tissues demonstrated that tubers were cyclically incorporated into the diet as a wet season crop harvested during the coastal winter. There were dietary differences between males and females; males had greater access to maize, possibly as "chichi" beer, and animal protein relative to females. Isotopic data from all tissues indicated that people buried in rope-encased bundles without weaving tools, assumed to be individuals of high status, consumed a diet rich in marine animals relative to the rest of the population. Comparisons between isotopic data from soft tissues and bone indicate that though the short term diet varied seasonally, isotopically the diet pattern was similar from year to year indicating that the individuals interred at Puruchuco-Huaquerones were native to the coast (*"Investigating Diet and Dietary Change Using Stable Isotopes of Carbon and Nitrogen in Mummified Tissues from Puruchuco-Huaquerones Peru"*, Department of Anthropology, Trent University, Peterborough, ON).

Another record of the ancient Andean subsistence diet comes from the colonial Spanish account of the Jesuit priest Bernabé Cobo who in 1610 AD journeyed through the high valleys of the central Andes, keenly observing the lives of the inhabitants. In his journal first published in 1653, Cobo noted that a handful of goods comprised the bulk of utilized food resources, with broadly distinct but overlapping dietary patterns in the highlands versus the coastal regions. Staple goods included over 20 varieties of maize, 240 varieties of potato, other tubers such as camote (sweet potato), maca, oca, and ulluco and grains such as quinoa (the "mother grain"), kañiwa, and amaranth. Vegetables included squashes, peppers, beans, manioc and peanuts. Maize was eaten fresh (choclo), parched and popped (kollo), made into a hominy (mote), and made into beer (chichi). Coastal populations consumed substantial amounts of crayfish and fresh and dried fish such as sardines and anchovies though there was little evidence to suggest that large pelagic (deep-sea) fish contributed substantially to the diet (Marcus et al. 1999:6568). Sardines and anchovies were also dried and traded for llama ch'arki from the highlands, where they were kept in storehouses (Marcus et al. 1999; Rostworowski 1977). Hunting was strictly regulated by the Inca throughout the empire, while cuy (guinea pig) and llama were consumed primarily in ceremonial or celebratory contexts (Rowe 1946:217); consumption of meat was limited among nonelites in everyday diet. Llama and alpaca were not utilized for their milk, and dairy appeared to have played no part in the diet.

Tamara L. Bray is an archaeology professor at the State University of New York at Binghamton specializing in the study of pre-Columbian societies of the northern Andes and the Inca Empire. In her 2003 review of colonial accounts of Andean diets published by Harvard University online (http://isites.harvard.edu/fs/docs/icb.topic942896.files/Dec%205/Bray.pdf), she notes that the diets of high-status versus low-status groups in the Inca state primarily differed not in their basic components, but in the quantity and quality of resources, the style of preparation and in the variety of accouterments. Thus, the nobility consumed more meat and a greater variety of maize-based dishes, while commoner and servant classes consumed proportionately more tubers and greens.

During the Inca period, the breeding and production of llamas was controlled by state llama herders called "Llama-Michis". Llamas were the property of the government and breeding was closely monitored. The hunting of llamas and alpacas was strictly forbidden. Llama herds were organized into three groups, all of which were tended by peasants. The first group of llamas was given top priority only for use by priests and shrine attendants at religious functions. The second group provided for the royal court and the needs of the government for pack animals. These two groups together were called "capac llama" which means rich herds. The "hucchac llama," which means poorer herds, were of lowest priority and for use by the larger community. Llamas were a source of wealth for the people, but the government would redistribute the poor community's llamas annually based on family size. The Inca maintained a strong commitment to increasing the numbers of llamas and alpacas. Llama-Michis were considered members of nobility and were paid very well to administer the herds. It was against the law to try and cure diseased animals or use them as food, they were to be killed and buried deeply to prevent the spread of disease. Females were not to be killed unless barren and designated for sacrifice. These governmental strategies resulted in a huge increase in numbers of llamas and alpacas during the Inca period. In a study published in the June, 2011 issue of the journal "Antiquity", paleoecologist Dr. Chepstow-Lusty presents findings from a sediment core from Lake Marcacocha in the Cuzco region that show large increases in maize pollens and mites that lived in llama dung both coincident with the Inca period. Dr. Chepstow-Lusty surmises that since maize is a heavy feeder and quickly strips the soil of nutrients that large quantities of llama dung were used as fertilizer and that this nutrient cycle is what made mass scale maize farming possible in the Andean highlands. ("*Did Llama Dung Spur the Rise of Andean Civilization?*" Science**NOW**, 2011)

As food availability increased in the Urbamba River Valley due to the warming climate favorable to agriculture, the human population of the Inca also grew rapidly. While the Inca largely inherited the highly advanced technological achievements of past Andean civilizations including textiles, ceramics, metallurgy and monumental architecture, they scaled them up to new levels of magnitude. The Inca political organization was based upon groupings of ten with records kept on "quipus', an accounting system also inherited from past civilizations using knotted string to keep counts. At the base of the system was the able-bodied tax-paying worker, ten workers had a boss, ten bosses had a foreman, ten foreman had a headman, ten headmen had a district governor, twenty district governors had a provincial governor and four provincial governors answered to the one "Inca" (the term we now use to refer to these pre-Columbian people) who ruled over the entire state. The Inca was also considered god-like in the tradition of the state religion. To maintain control over the expanding Empire, this federal system of government was designed to be top-heavy with management and for every 10,000 people there were 1,331 public officials. With this high level of oversight the Inca were able to direct the labors of their growing population toward the massive construction projects of terracing entire mountainsides with stone retaining walls, digging long irrigation canals to harness glacial runoff, paving hundreds of miles of roads with stairs and provisioned rest stops for faster llama passage, and building monumental stone structures at the capital city of Cuzco, the royal estate at Machu Picchu and many other sites. The Inca also enlisted a large military force through a system of compulsory service called "mita" that required every male to take part in either public works projects or military service. By 1350 AD, through military conquest the Inca had enlarged their territory beyond the immediate area around Cuzco to include all areas close to Lake Titicaca to the south and all the river valleys to the immediate east and north. Around 1350 AD the Inca spanned a deep canyon on the Apurimac River with a bridge 148 feet long (45 meters) using suspension technology unknown in contemporary Europe that opened up access to the western river valleys for conquest. Between 1463 AD and 1525 AD the Inca pushed their conquest into Chile, Bolivia, Argentina, Ecuador and southern Columbia. While the Inca did force mass migrations of conquered peoples to areas where labor was needed for farming, building and mining projects, each geographic area in their long narrow north to south empire was largely self-sufficient in food production and relied on agricultural practices that were adapted to the particular ecological zones. The Inca were also tolerant of local languages and religious customs. Most of the cargo of the llama caravans that connected the periphery of the empire to the capital city at Cuzco consisted of tribute in the form of luxury goods only for use by people at the upper levels of management in the Inca Empire.

Determining the human population of the Andes region controlled by the Inca at the time of the Spanish conquest in 1532 AD has been the subject of great debate among anthropologists. In 1931, American anthropologist Philip Ainsworth Means, after five extended trips to Peru to study the Inca civilization published one of the first books to explain Inca history and culture entitled "*Ancient Civilization of the Andes*" in which he used the Inca decimal-based administrative system as a starting point to surmise that each province in the Inca Empire contained between 200,000 and 400,000 people and with each of the four quarters of the empire containing about 20 provinces he calculated the overall Inca population at between 16 and 32 million people. In 1966, another American anthropologist, Henry F. Dobyns, who had spent eleven years perusing early Spanish mortuary records kept at the Lima cathedral accounting for the deaths of indigenous people by disease epidemics, used a depopulation ratio which he calculated at 25:1 to reach a census figure of 37.5 million people at the time of conquest.

Amazonians

The continental divide of South America, where on one side of the mountain rivers flow east to the Atlantic Ocean and on the other side west to the Pacific, sits atop the ridges of the Andes Mountain Range which runs north to south straddling the west coast of the continent. Due to this topography, rivers that flow west to the Pacific are short in length with relatively low water flows, while rivers that flow east to the Atlantic across the vast expanse of the Amazon River Basin are very long and carry enormous quantities of water.

The Amazon River Basin drains from the highlands of the Andes Mountains in modern-day Bolivia, Columbia, Ecuador and Peru down through the flat plains of Brazil to create the largest river drainage in the world. The shear enormity is staggering: the Amazon basin covers 2,375,000 square miles (6,151,000 sq kilometers) which is four-fifths the size of Australia and three-quarters the size of the continental United States. East to west the river measures approximately 2,240 miles long (3,600 kilometers), second only to the Nile, and the average water flow through the Amazon drainage is 219,000 cubic meters/second which is more than five times greater than the second largest, the Congo River at 41,800 m3/s. The Amazon River drainage accounts for fully 20% of all river flows in the world and at its mouth on the Atlantic coast of Brazil it is 300 miles wide. Most of this vast river network flows across an extremely flat alluvial plain that rises to no more than 328 feet (100 meters) above sea level and is covered with the world's largest tropical rainforest. Throughout most of the basin temperatures range from 60° to 90°F and rainfall averages from 70 to 100 inches per year. There are two basic seasons, "dry" low-water and "wet" high-water when floods inundate low lying areas.

In 1541 AD, not satisfied with the riches from his looting of the Inca Empire, Spanish conquistador Francisco Pizarro sent his half brother Gonzalo on an expedition east into the Amazon jungle in search of the fabled golden city of "El Dorado." Not realizing the scale of his undertaking, Gonzalo's expeditionary force of 243 Spaniards, 4,000 indigenous Andeans and several horses soon met with disaster as they began to run out of provisions and disease killed off 140 of the Spaniards, 3,000 of the Andeans, and they ate the horses. In desperation, Gonzalo sent his second in command, Francisco de Orellana, along with 50 men to continue sailing down river in search of food. While Gonzalo's party ended up returning west back to the Spanish colonies in the Andes. de Orellana's party continued east to complete the first recorded navigation of the Amazon River drainage from the Andes to the Atlantic. A written record of this navigation was made by the party's chaplain, Spanish missionary, Gaspar de Carvajal, in his narratve, "*Relación del nuevo descubrimiento del famoso río Grande que descubrió por muy gran ventura el capitán Francisco de Orellana*" ("Account of the recent discovery of the famous Grand river which was discovered by great good fortune by Captain Francisco de Orellana"). In his account the friar recorded the dates of the expedition and made extensive notes on large populations of indigenous peoples who occupied the banks of the river in major cities and fortified towns with well developed roads and monumental constructions. Carvajal's manuscript remained packed away for over 350 years until finally being published by a Chilean scholar in 1895. But until very recently, Carvajal's stories of ancient civilizations in the Amazon jungle had been largely dismissed as fabrications and propaganda since the natural soils in the Amazon basin are too nutrient depleted to support agriculture which is the pre-requisite for large populations and civilization. Millions of years of rainfall have leached out virtually all the calcium, phosphorus, and potassium from the soil leaving behind a nutrient depleted weathered red clay. The lush Amazon jungle actually subsists on itself by quickly recycling nutrients from decaying leaves and branches. But since the late 1990s, after the careful mapping of extensive deposits of unusually fertile dark soils in the Amazon called "terra preta" (black earth in Portuguese) and "terra mulata" (brown earth), by Southern Illinois University soil geographer William Woods, Carvajal's narrative of a jungle teeming with humans has gained a new credibility. His tales of a lost civilization in the Amazon are now considered the most reliable contemporary chronicle of a pre-Columbian Amazonian civilization that disappeared around 500 years ago with its wooden infra-structure resorbed into the humid jungle.

The peninsula at the confluence of the Rio Negro and Amazon Rivers is one of the Amazon basins most richly biodiverse regions at the heart of the Brazilian rainforest. The first archaeologists to study this area thought the region had been occupied by small bands of hunter-gatherers living in a world of scarcity, but in 2003 archaeologists Eduardo Neves from the University of São Paulo, Brazil and anthropologist Michael Heckenberger from the University of Florida unearthed evidence of a highly sophisticated culture dating back 2,000 years developing into a large urban population that peaked between 1250 AD and 1650 AD. This advanced Amazonian civilization crafted elaborate ceramics, built large mounds and plazas, ringed villages, raised fields, roads and bridges indicating regional trade networks. The researchers also found evidence of extensive anthropogenic (produced by humans) soil modification that transformed the nutrient depleted dirt into "terra preta" and "terra mulata" collectively known as "Amazonian Dark Earths".

Geologist William Denevan from the University of Wisconsin is a prominent researcher of these man made Amazonian Dark Earths. Dr. Denevan observes:

"The black terra preta is associated with long-enduring Indian village sites, and is filled with ceramics, animal and fish bones, and other cultural debris. The brown terra mulata, on the other hand, is much more extensive, generally surrounds the black midden soils, contains few artifacts, and apparently is the result of semi-intensive cultivation over long periods. Both forms are much more fertile than the surrounding highly weathered reddish soil, mostly oxisol, and they have generally sustained this fertility to the present despite the tropical climate and despite frequent or periodic cultivation. This is probably because of high carbon content and an associated high microbial activity which is self perpetuating." (Discovery and Awareness of Anthropogenic Amazonian, Dark Earths (Terra Preta); (2004)

Early Amazonian farmers amended their depleted soils with carbon made from charcoal which was created by slow-burning the woody jungle cover in pits smothered with dirt; every year more carbon would be added by slow-burning brush, weeds and crop wastes. Unlike rotted wood or wood burnt to ash that quickly dissipates its carbon back into the atmosphere, the carbon in charcoal remains locked in the soil for thousands of years. The smaller deposits of terra preta soils Dr. Deneven found near settlements are darker because they contain more organic matter from kitchen scraps and humanure, while the much larger deposits of terra mulata soils found in surrounding agricultural fields are lighter because they were amended only with charcoal and crop residues. These Amazonian Dark Earth deposits are generally from 3 to 6 feet in depth (1 to 2 meters).

Since the early 2000s, modern soil scientists have been studying the soil amending properties of charcoal with astonishing results. Charcoal is a very poros material that substantially improves microbial growth in soil by providing a habitat for bacteria that decompose the biomass in the surface ground cover. As mycellium (fungal roots) grow and spread from the charcoal a process of self-propagation develops fixing additional carbon in the soil as well as increasing retention of nitrogen, calcium, phosphorus, and potassium that then become bioavailable to the roots of nearby plants. University studies cultivating test plots of charcoal amended soils have increased yields of agricultural plants by up to 800%. Because this nutrient cycle is self-perpetuating, Amazonian Dark Earth that was created 2,000 years ago is still fertile today (*"Amazonian Dark Earths: Origin, Properties, Management,"* Department of Crop and Soil Sciences, Cornell University, 2003).

Amazonian Dark Earth is found primarily in the Brazilian rainforest, but it has also been found as far as Ecuador, Peru and French Guyana indicating the technology was widely dispersed. Amazonian Dark Earth deposits generally exist along the main river arteries flowing east through the central basin on the edges of floodplains in plots averaging 49 acres (20 hectares), but some have been found as large as 900 acres (360 ha). Smaller plots averaging around 3.5 acres (1.4 ha) are located on higher ground between the rivers. The Dutch soil scientist, Wim Sombroek, who began his study of these anthropogenic soils back in the 1960s, estimated that they covered at least 0.1% to 0.3% of low forested Amazonia, an area of 2,400 to

7,300 square miles (6,300 to 18,900 sqare kilometers). Soil scientist William Woods, from his studies in the late 1990s, has estimated that they cover at least 10% of Amazonia, an area the size of France.

Early agriculture in the Amazonian basin began with human selection of native fruit and nut trees along pathways through the forest which had the effect of altering the natural floral diversity in their areas of migration. The earliest anthropogenic dark soils began to appear around 450 BC but the area modified by charcoal saw its greatest expansion between 700 AD and 800 AD and suddenly collapse around 1600 AD (*"The timing of Terra Preta formation in the central Amazon: new data from three sites in the central Amazon,"* 2001). With the introduction and spread of Amazonian Dark Earth technology, larger sedentary tribal groups developed. In these settlements the nearby terra preta area was the most fertile soil able to support the cultivation of such exotic crops as maize, squash, beans and gourds as well as sweet manioc tubers. The larger and less fertile fields of terra mulata were devoted to growing more acid tolerant tubers like bitter manioc that were high in starch content and provided the bulk of the calories necessary to grow large human populations. Storing surplus grain in the humid environment of the Amazon rainforest was not possible as in other early civilizations, so tubers were the ideal staple crop for the Amazonians since they could be grown and stored underground throughout the year to the moment of harvest. Tended fruit and nut tree orchards surrounding the periphery of settlements provided a diversity of plant species in the average diet. Fresh water fish and shellfish from the rivers were a significant food source and shell and fish bones provided an important calcium amendment to the terra preta soils. As human populations increased, the population of terrestrial wild prey animals diminished due to over hunting and there is no evidence of animal domestication making it highly unlikely that terrestrial animals provided many calories in the average Amazonian diet (Good 1987). Archaeological sites in Amazonia indicate periodic episodes of abandonment and rehabitation of settlements allowing time for the natural flora and fauna to recover from anthropogenic disturbances (*"The Amazonian Formative: Crop Domestication and Anthropogenic Soils"*, Diversity — Open Access Journal, 2010).

Estimating the human population of Amazonia at the time of European contact in the 1500s is a very problematic exercise due to the extremely limited archaeological and historical record. As more evidence of dark earth is discovered, population estimates based on the carrying capacity of the land have increased. Geographer Dr. William Denevan has proposed a bluff model of human occupation, in which indigenous peoples preferentially settled sandy bluffs alongside rivers and where there were views over wetlands. Dr. Denevan estimates that as many as 10 million people lived in these densely populated riverbank settlements with as few as 400,000 sparsely populating all the rest of Amazonia. Using geophysical techniques of remote sensing that enable archaeologists to look inside sites rather than just excavate them, Anna C. Roosevelt, professor of anthropology at Columbia University, NYC, has documented the existence of a large well developed civilization including monumental earth mound architecture and a rich artistic tradition on the lowland tropical floodplain of Marajo Island at the mouth of the Amazon River from about 400 AD to 1300 AD. Marajo Island is about the size of Switzerland or Belgium. ("*Moundbuilders of the Amazon: Geophysical Archaeology on Marajo Island, Brazil*", 1991)

Central America

Olmec

Six hundred years after the collapse of the first Western Hemisphere civilization in Norte Chico, Peru, South America, a second Western Hemisphere civilization called the Olmec began to develop independently far to the northeast in Central America around 1200 BC. The human population on river drainages on the Gulf Coast of Central Mexico in the modern-day States of Veracruz and Tabasco, reached a critical population density where the hallmarks of civilization including irrigation agriculture, monumental sculpture, urbanism, complex religion, and the beginnings of a written language and a calendar based on astronomical observations began to occur.

The first Olmec artifact was unearthed in 1869 by a farm worker clearing forest land on a hacienda in Veracruz but it wasn't until more extensive excavations in the 1930s and 1940s that a distinctive Olmec civilization was recognized. The Olmec have been called the "mother civilization" of Mesoamerica (a cultural region including central Mexico, Belize, Guatemala, El Salvador, Honduras, Nicaragua and Costa Rica) where large scale maize cultivation provided the basis for a complex state. The two principal Olmec cities of San Lorenzo and La Venta were largely ceremonial centers. Sea level was 13 to 16 feet (4 to 5 meters) lower in 1000 BC than it is today, and there was a coastal plain 7 to 12 miles (12 to 20 kilometers) wide crossed by rivers that developed natural raised levees. Recent research shows that these now-submerged and buried levees along one such river were covered with pre-Olmec and Olmec settlements. The majority of people lived in villages each consisting of several scattered houses. Individual dwellings were comprised of one room, a lean-to and associated storage pits. Herbs, sunflower, avocado and cacao trees were grown in nearby gardens while the river banks were used to plant crops between flooding periods. Fields were located outside the village, and were used for growing maize, beans, squash, manioc, sweet potato and cotton. Sea animals such as fish, turtle, snake, mollusks, crabs and shellfish were also caught and supplemented the average peasant diet. Based on archaeological studies of two villages in the Tuxtlas Mountains, it is known that maize cultivation became increasingly important to the Olmec over time as small prey animals such as peccary, opossum, raccoon, rabbit, and deer became increasingly scarce. Unlike the people of Eurasia with their sheep, goats, cows, camels and elephants, and the people of South America with their llamas, the people of Mesoamerica had no large beast of burden available to them to domesticate for muscle power or meat. Midden surveys in San Lorenzo suggest that a small dog was domesticated for meat production but, as a carnivores, dogs only competed with humans for meat and could have provided little in the way of additional calories or protein for the Olmec population.

Olmec society was organized around a hereditary ruling family who claimed their authority directly from the Olmec gods or supernaturals which provided the legitimacy for their rule. The ruling family along with an elite class of priest and shamans presided over a culture in which complex religious rituals and ceremonies dominated much of public life. While the Olmec culture was the first to develop into a full fledged civilization in Mesoamerica, there were many other distinct cultural groups in the area that were also beginning to develop into city-states at this time. Archaeological evidence suggests that even though Olmec art objects and styles have been found as far as the central highlands of Mexico and over toward the Pacific coast, the Olmec rulers actually exerted no political control over these other territories which operated autonomously under their own ruling families. While prestigious and high-value materials such as greenstone and marine shell had long been traded among the different cultures in the area, the Olmec period saw a significant expansion in interregional trade routes, more variety in material goods exchanged and a greater diversity in the sources from which the base materials were obtained.

The first Olmec center, San Lorenzo, was abandoned around 900 BC at about the same time that La Venta rose to prominence. The reason for this move in cultural center is unknown though the most likely cause is thought to have been a shift in the course of major rivers. Olmec culture continued on at La Venta for another five hundred years until it too was abandoned around 400 BC. It is unknown what caused the eventual disappearance of the Olmec civilization, but the eastern half of the Olmec heartland would not recover until the 19th century. Different reasons proposed by archaeologists for this decline are land subsidence, volcanic eruptions and erosion of the river drainages.

Maya

For the next several centuries after the abandonment of the last Olmec cities, numerous successor cultures continued to inhabit the Mesoamerican region, but none would become as predominant as the Olmec until the emergence of the Maya around 250 AD. Geographically, the Maya civilization developed in an area to the east of where the Olmec had lived in what are the modern-day tropical lowlands of the Yucatan Peninsula and the drier mountainous highlands of Guatemala and Chiapas, Mexico.

Trade between city states was a major feature of the Maya civilization and Maya cities tended to be located in places that controlled trade routes for exotic materials and products. This allowed the elites who controlled trade to increase their wealth and status. Maya cities were designed to mimic the natural landscape, so, on the flat limestone plains of the northern Yucatán they were sprawling metropolises while on the hilly terrain of Usumacinta they were constructed vertically with tall towers and temples. But no matter where they were located, all Maya cities had the same basic layout with large open public plazas and causeways surrounded by massive stone monuments, great stepped pyramids, elaborate government buildings and public ball-courts with careful attention paid to directional orientation of the buildings in accordance with the orbits of heavenly bodies. Classic Maya societies emphasized the centrality of the royal family and these monumental spaces served to embody the aesthetic and moral values of the royal household as a means of defining the wider social realm. Unlike in Olmec cities which were largely ceremonial centers, Maya cities were also population centers and the great public places were surrounded by meandering apartment complexes that were in a continuous state of remodel over the centuries of habitation.

The Maya civilization flourished for over six hundred years between 250 AD and 900 AD, and at its peak supported an estimated population of ten million people (Michael D. Coe, *"The Maya"*). Despite limitations set by the regions poor soils and few natural rivers and lakes the Maya were able to sustain large urban populations by developing a diverse and sophisticated system of food production that was adapted to the different growing conditions of its geography. Though the Maya region is called a rainforest, technically, the area resembles more of a seasonal desert with a thin layer of topsoil and without stable sources of surface water for months at a time. The Maya responded to these fundamental barriers to intensive agriculture by engineering a complex agricultural systems designed to retain water and soils through the use of terraces, dikes, dams, raised fields, ridged fields and canals as well as using swamp muck and human manure to keep the soil fertile. Terraces and dams in hilly areas brought previously unusable lands into cultivation and raised fields in previously swampy areas allowed for year-round cultivation which greatly increased yields. The Maya also practiced a form of slash-and-burn agriculture called "swidden farming." Mayan swidden farming worked by cutting down and burning trees and brush to fertilize the nutrient poor soils of the rainforest and then growing a variety of crops for the next two years until the nutrients were depleted and then letting the land lie fallow for the next eight years (*"Population Crises and Population Cycles,"* 1999). This long fallowing period allowed enough time for the rainforest to recover and the cycle to be repeated sustainably over the long term. Maize, beans and squash (the so called "Three Sisters") were their staple crops but the Maya also cultivated manioc, jícama, sweet potatoes, guavas, and chili peppers. Other fruit tree crops of the Central area were papaya, guavas, avocado, breadnut, Cacao and Zapodilla. They also collect chewing gum from the Chicozapote tree and rubber from the hevea tree, which they used for balls for their ritual Ball Game, and to make water proof clothes and shoes. As with the Olmec, wild prey became scarce and the Maya domesticated a small dog and the turkey for meat production, but overall meat consumption was very limited among the general population. Fish and shellfish were part of the typical diet in the coastal areas of the Northern Yucatan.

The Maya, as did all post-Olmec Mesoamerican cultures, inherited their highly accurate astronomically based calendar from the Olmec, but it appears from the archaeological record that the concept of the "long-count" – that is, counting years from a fixed date in the past – originated with the Maya. The fixed date on which the Maya calendar begins has been calibrated to correspond with the year 3114 BC by our modern calendar. The Maya believed that on this date the universe was created. The Maya also invented a highly advanced writing system that, like the Chinese and Sumerian systems, was a "logographic" system that combined phonetic and semantic elements. Using about 287 symbols they were able to record and transmit complex concepts and ideas. They wrote on stone, murals, and ceramics and in books of folded bark paper and deerskin. Miraculously four of these books somehow survived the ravages of time and their texts have given modern archaeologists a remarkable insight into the complex Maya cosmology that was based on a cult of the dead. Most of the written material recovered from Maya archaeological sites was carved in stone and ceramic on monuments and tombs to immortalize the heroic conquests or eulogize the mortal remains of the ruling families. In Maya society the ruling family along with a small upper class of scribes and priests tended to the religious rituals of the cult and specialized in making the related complex astronomical observations and calculations. Religious rituals involved making offerings to the gods which included acts of blood-letting, self-mutilation, human sacrifice and cannibalism. Subjects for human sacrifice were taken from captives who were enslaved during constant warfare with their neighboring cultures. Serving under the ruling family and their inner circle of religious elite in Maya society were a larger class of artisans such as builders, potters, sculptors, and painters, but the majority of the people were simple peasant farmers whose work in the fields subsidized the elaborate rituals and political lifestyles of the urban elite. With 80% of the Mayan swidden farmer's fields lying fallow at any given time, the Mayan population lived spread out over the land.

Abruptly, in the 8th century AD, Maya rulers stopped erecting large commemorative monuments and buildings and urban populations dwindled. By the 9th century AD, most of the great Maya cities had been completely abandoned and grown over by the rainforest. Evidence of foreign invasion, internal revolt, breakdown of intercity trade and epidemic disease have all been discovered by archaeologists, but none of these causes alone or taken together fully explains the total abandonment of the Maya cities. In their paper, "*Possible role of climate in the collapse of Classic Maya civilization*" (*Nature*, 1995), Dr. David Hodell, Professor of Geologic Sciences, University of Florida, and his colleagues propose the possibility that it was a two hundred year drought that caused the Maya collapse. Dr. Hodell's team used variations in oxygen isotope composition in a sediment core from Lake Chichancanab, Mexico, to reconstruct a continuous record of climate change for the central Yucatan peninsula. Their evidence provides conclusive proof that the interval between 800 AD and 1,000 AD was the driest on record over the past seven thousand years and coincided with the collapse of the Maya civilization. This extreme weather in Mesoamerica also coincides with the extreme weather period in South America that brought down the Tiahuanaco and Huari civilizations and with the Medieval Warming period well documented in Northern Europe suggests there was a worldwide weather event. The drought theory of the Maya collapse provides a comprehensive explanation of the cultural breakdown that took place in Maya society at this time. Since Maya agriculture was totally dependent on stored water, even slight shifts in the distribution of annual rainfall caused severe food shortages and consequent mass starvation. As the food system consistently failed during the drought period, the Maya elite lost their claim of authority from the gods and became vulnerable to external and internal attack while the Maya people became weakened from nutritional deficiencies and subject to disease epidemics. The effects on Maya society were so calamitous that the long-count calendar was discontinued in the 9th Century. As most of the Maya cities fell into ruin, a few Maya cultural centers on the Northern Yucatan survived into the 17th century, presumably due to natural sinkholes in the limestone geology called "*cenotes*" that enabled people to tap into underground water resources to continue irrigating their crops ("*The Great Warming*," 2008).

Aztec

To the west of the Yucatan peninsula in what is modern-day central Mexico lies the Valley of Mexico which rests on the floor of a plateau that is over 7,000 feet (2,200 meters) above sea level and surrounded by a ring of mountains and volcanoes. In pre-Columbian Mesoamerica, this valley contained five lakes with the largest, Lake Texcoco, covering about 580 square miles (1,500 square kilometers) of the valley floor. As the early Olmec and Maya civilizations rose and fell on the Gulf Coast and in the Yucatan, many concurrent independent city-states also rose and fell in the Valley of Mexico including the Teotihuacán from 800 BC to 800 AD, and the Toltec from 1000 AD to 1300 AD. In the year 1428 AD, three of the Valley's independent city-states joined together in what historians call the "Aztec Triple Alliance." The largest city of Tenochtitlan which was built on an island in Lake Texcoco, became the political center of the Aztec Empire which at its peak controlled most of central Mexico from coast to coast with an estimated human population of 25 million. When the Aztec Triple Alliance would conquer other city-states to bring them into the Aztec Empire, they would leave the local rulers in charge demanding only that they pay tribute (luxury items like gold, gemstones or exotic feathers as well as large quantities of food) to the Alliance in return. It was through this system of tribute that the Aztec empire was organized.

The Valley of Mexico is a large closed basin that, before being drained by modern humans, would fill-up with water during the rainy season between May and October becoming one big shallow lake, and then, during the drier winter months as water perked into the ground and evaporated into the air, would separate into individual smaller lakes. Lake Texcoco was the lowest-lying lake and, since there was no way for water to drain outside the valley, all the water in the valley would ultimately drain towards it. To maximize agricultural production from this closed basin water cycle the Aztec developed several sophisticated methods of cultivation. In the hilly areas around the perimeter of the valley they grew crops on terraces during the rainy season. In valley areas a complex system of dams and dikes was used to divert water from natural springs to irrigate fields which allowed for year round cultivation. And in swampy areas along the lakes the Aztec implemented a system called "chinampas" where areas of raised land were created by alternating layers of mud from the bottom of the lake with wild plant matter. These "raised beds" were separated by narrow canals, which allowed farmers to move between them by canoe. The length and complexity of the Aztec canal system far exceeded what the Maya had built centuries earlier. The chinampas were so productive, yielding on average seven crops per year, that they made possible human population densities of up to 580 people per square mile (360 people per square kilometer) which was high even by the standards of ancient Egypt and China. While most of the farming occurred in less dense rural areas, some food was grown within the densely populated cities in small scale garden plots.

As with all Mesoamerican civilizations the Aztec diet centered on maize. Maize was grown across the entire Empire, in the highland terraces, valley farms and also on the chinampas. It was ground into a coarse meal and made into tortillas. Other crops grown by the Aztec were also familiar Mesoamerican cultivars: avocados, beans, squash, sweet potatoes, tomatoes, chia, amaranth and peppers. These crops were also grown everywhere. Crops that were specific to the lowland regions were cotton, fruits, cacao beans and rubber trees. Like the Olmec and Maya before them, the Aztec had no suitable wild animals to domesticate for milk production so there were no dairy products in the Aztec diet. The Aztec did domesticate a small dog and wild turkey but meat production was limited and very little was consumed by most of the Aztec people. From Lake Texcoco the Aztec caught shrimp and harvested an alga that was made into a sort of cake. Insects such as grasshoppers, beetles, ants and larvae were also considered delicacies by the Aztec. Since there were no suitable wild species of mammals to domesticate for draft purposes such as oxen, horses, camels or elephants, it was human muscle power that worked the land and built the cities. In his paper *"Aztec Medicine, Health and Nutrition"* (Rutgers University Press, 1990), anthropologist Bernard Ortiz de Montellano, associate professor of science and technology at Wayne State University, Detroit, Michigan, shows a mean life expectancy of 37 (±3) years for the people of Mesoamerica which compares favorably to contemporary civilizations in Europe, the Middle East and Asia.

While the structure of Aztec society and the design of Aztec cities were similar to that of the Olmec and Maya, due to its much higher population density Aztec society developed into a more rigidly stratified class structure and its architecture was even more monumental in scale than its predecessor civilizations. Another apparent consequence of high population density in the Aztec Empire was a dramatic increase in the practice of human sacrifice and cannibalism. The late Dr. Woodrow Borah, former professor of Latin American history at the University of California, Berkeley, and arguably the world's leading authority on the demography of 15th century Mexico, estimated that the number of people sacrificed in central Mexico at the time of the Spanish conquest in 1519 was around 250,000 per year which was equivalent to 1% of the total population of 25 million. According to Borah, this figure is consistent with the sacrifice of an estimated 1,000 to 3,000 people yearly at the largest temples with lesser numbers sacrificed at the thousands of smaller temples scattered throughout the Aztec Empire. As with the Maya, subjects for human sacrifice were taken from captives who were enslaved during constant warfare with neighboring city-states. While the very thought of human sacrifice and cannibalism is abhorrent to the modern mind, such practices were central to the Aztec culture, and, as with early animal sacrifices in the ancient cultures of the Middle East and Europe, served the essential function of regulating the overall animal population to environmentally sustainable levels. Since the Aztec raised very few animals for food, and their plant-based agriculture was so successful at raising people, virtually all of the large herbivores were humans, so the Aztec had no choice but to use humans instead of domesticated herbivores for sacrifice. Eliminating 1% of the adult population every year would have produced a significant reduction in the demand for food each year and an exponential reduction in demand over the decades. Human sacrifices were justified by the Aztec rulers on religious grounds as ritual offerings to the gods just as nonhuman animal sacrifices were justified as ritual offerings to the gods by the ancient Hebrew and pagan cults of the Middle East and Europe. With no contraceptives available and a fast growing population, human sacrifice was the Mesoamerican solution to population control and living within unyielding trophic limits.

Cannibalism was also part of the Aztec religious ritual of spiritual empowerment just as eating sacrificed nonhuman animals was for the ancient religions of the Middle East and Europe. Ritual cannibalism was also practiced in other ancient cultures around the world where edible terrestrial species had become extinct due to human predation. Such island cultures as the Carib of the Lesser Antilles Islands in the Caribbean Sea, the Fijians of the remote Melanesia Islands of the South Pacific, and the Maori of New Zealand were all practitioners of cannibalism. The Aztec could not eat people living within the Aztec Empire since that would have been socially and politically disruptive, so instead they purposely cultivated nearby "enemy" populations on whom they could prey for captives.

Dr. Michael Harner, former Chair of the Anthropology Department of the New School for Social Research, proposes that the protein derived from eating the sacrificed humans was an important food source for the Aztec and this was their main motivation for cannibalism ("*The Enigma of Aztec Sacrifice,*" *Natural History*, 1977), but this explanation doesn't add up. Eating one person per hundred per year could not have supplied much meat, and besides, human meat was only eaten by a relative few high priests and warriors while most of the population survived almost entirely on plant proteins which produced strong enough bodies for them to build monumental structures and wage war on their enemies.

While anthropologist Dr. Bernard Ortiz de Montellano soundly refutes Dr. Harner's animal-protein theory of cannibalism in his paper, "*Aztec Cannibalism: An Ecological Necessity?*" (*Science*, 1978), his own theory for cannibalism is equally as inadequate. According to Dr. Ortiz de Montellano, "*Sacrificial victims were believed to have become sacred. Eating their flesh was the act of eating the god itself. This communion with superior beings was an important aspect of Aztec religion.*" To say that communion with the gods was the motivation for cannibalism is an inadequate explanation because it begs the question: why did the Aztec religion use the ritual consumption of humans for this purpose while other sacrificial religious cults like early Judaism and paganism used the ritual consumption of nonhuman animals for the same purpose? The answer to this question, according to the "cultural materialism" theory of anthropologist Dr. Marvin Harris, has to be sought in the material conditions of the food production system in Central Mexico compared with the food production systems in other parts of the world. The whole system in larger perspective is not simply a matter of whim on the part of the priests who created the cannibalistic doctrine of the Aztec religion; to the contrary, the doctrine reflected the material conditions in the Valley of Mexico (like on the islands of the Lesser Antilles, Melanesia and New Zealand) where humans were the only large terrestrial herbivore available in sufficient numbers to be used for ritual consumption.

North America

The Clovis People

The earliest ancestors of all modern-day North American indigenous peoples were named the "Clovis" people after their highly distinctive stone tipped weapons that were first found at an archaeological site located near Clovis, New Mexico in 1932. So called "Clovis points" have now been found in south central Canada around modern-day Edmonton, in all 48 of the contiguous United States, Central America, all the way down the Andes mountain range to the southern tip of South America. According to Professor Jared Diamond, Professor of Geography at the University of California, Los Angeles, a small original population of 100 hunter-gatherers could have quickly multiplied into a population large enough to colonize these vast territories:

> *"Populations of modern hunter-gatherers on even their best hunting grounds number only about one per square mile. Hence, once the whole western hemisphere had been settled, its population of hunter-gatherers would have been at most ten million, since the New World's area outside of Canada and other areas covered by glaciers in Clovis times is about ten million square miles. In modern instances when colonists have arrived at an uninhabited land (e.g., when the H.M.S. Bounty mutineers reached Pitcairn Island), their population growth has been as rapid as 3.4 percent per year. That growth rate, which corresponds to each couple's having four surviving children and a mean generation time of twenty years, would multiply 100 hunters into 10 million in only 340 years. Thus, Clovis hunters should easily have been able to multiply to 10 million within a millennium." ("The Third Chimpanzee" pg 344)*

The reason the Clovis people were able to thrive and multiply in the Americas was that they happened upon a landmass that was teeming with unwary, easy-to-hunt megafauna such as mammoths, mastodons, giant ground sloths, horses, camels and buffalo that provided them with an ample, readily available food supply.

Paleontological evidence (animal bones) indicates that by 10,000 years ago all of the easily hunted megafauna of North America had become extinct and a change in animal bones and spear point technology reflects the change over to the hunting of smaller fleet-footed prey species like deer and elk. These early subsistence hunter/gatherers also learned to recognize and eat hundreds of varieties of wild edible native plants that were endemic to the Western Hemisphere. Hunter/gatherer groups subsisted in very low population densities in North America for several thousand years.

Around 9,000 years ago, as descendants of the Clovis began to reach population densities in areas where edible wild plants and small prey could no longer provide for their subsistence, early evidence of plant cultivation by semi-nomadic hunter-gatherers begins to appear in the archaeological record.

Adena and Hopewell

The first evidence of an agricultural based civilization in North America was found in the Ohio River Basin. The Ohio River Basin is formed by the confluence of many rivers flowing off the western slopes of the Appalachian Mountain Range to form the Ohio River which flows into the Mississippi River at modern-day Cairo, Illinois to form the northernmost extension of the "Mississippi Alluvial Plain." Much of the topography of the Basin was sculpted over geological time by several glaciations that left rich soil deposits and a flat to slightly rolling terrain. The northern Mississippi Alluvial Plain is covered with what is generally referred to as "bottomland forest" that is further subdivided into three distinct ecological zones: swamp forest, hardwood bottoms, and ridge bottoms. Due to the ecosystem's central geographical location in the eastern United States, floral species from both the north and south intermix with species common to the central region. The unusually high number of faunal species endemic to this region is a reflection of the ecosystem's diverse geography and unique geological past.

The first of many large earthen mounds discovered in the Ohio River Basin was on the early 19th century estate of Thomas Worthington called "Adena" in Chillicothe, Ohio, thus the name given to this mound building culture. The Adena culture existed from 1000 BC to 1 AD, in a time known as the early Woodland Period. There are around 300 known Adena sites in the central Ohio Valley and another 200 scattered throughout Indiana, Kentucky, West Virginia and Pennsylvania.

As human hunters using spear throwers called "atlatls" gradually increased in the area, they slowly began to reduce the populations of deer, elk and bison, and, since no megafaunal herbivores suitable for domestication were available, the Adena developed a system of burning the forest to create more open meadows for the native wild herbivores to graze. But as the human populations continued to increase, this strategy to produce more food reached its natural limits and the Adena turned to plant domestication as a new strategy to increase food production. The eastern United States is now considered by most ethnobotanists to be one of few regions in the world that was an "independent center of agricultural origin." ("*Initial Formation of an Indigenous Crop Complex in Eastern North America at 3800 B.P.*," *Proceedings of the National Academy of Sciences*, 2009).

The archaeological record suggests that humans were eating seeds from wild varieties of squash, sunflower, pigweed (goosefoot), sumpweed (marshelder), knotweed, maygrass and little barley by 8000 years ago (6000 BC), then gradually modified them by selective collection and cultivation. Archaeologists in the 1970s noticed that seeds found in domestic settings were much larger than in the wild, and these seeds were also easier to extract from the shells or husks; evidence that human cultivators were manipulating the plants to make them more productive and accessible. The Adena never adapted a strain of maize from Central America to the colder North American climate and none of their local seed grains provided the large yields achieved from maize. Today none of the Adena grains are cultivated and most are considered undesirable weeds. Nevertheless, Adena agriculture supplemented their hunting and gathering enough to grow and sustain the population densities necessary to engage in building large earthen mounds.

Adena mounds generally ranged in size from 20 feet (6.1 meters) to 300 feet (91 meters) in diameter and served as ceremonial platforms, burial sites and historical markers. The mounds were built using hundreds of thousands of basketfulls of specially selected and graded earth. Archaeological excavations have shown that the Adena mounds were usually built as part of burial rituals for higher status individuals in which earth was mounded atop a burned mortuary building. New mortuary structures and mounds would be built atop the previous mounds and through many repetitions, a prominent earthwork was raised. The largest of these sites is the Grave Creek Mound in West Virginia. Construction of this mound took place between 250 BC and 150 BC toward the end of the Adena Cultural period. The Cave Creek mound peaks at 69 feet tall and measures 295 feet in diameter. Originally a moat of about 40 feet in width and five feet in depth with one causeway encircled the mound. The building of this mound and moat must have been a massive undertaking requiring the consistent effort of many thousands of laborers to move the over 60,000 tons of earth one basket at a time. The Adena mounds were separated from their domestic living areas. Circular houses from 15 to 45 feet in diameter were built scattered around the mound areas. Wooden posts were joined to form a conical-shaped roof and the roof and walls were covered with bark or mats of woven grasses (*"Mound Builders of Ancient America," New York Graphic Society, 1968)*. The Adena culture is also notable for its pottery, artistic works and extensive trading network which brought them such exotic raw materials as copper from the western Great Lakes, mica from the Carolinas and shells from the Gulf of Mexico.

Around 200 BC a change in the sociopolitical structure of the Adena Culture appears to have occurred marked by the emergence of so called "big-men" who developed influence by creating a network of reciprocal obligations with other important members of the community. Over time the big-men network developed into a more highly organized socially stratified system of "chiefdoms." This higher level of sociopolitical organization began to spread throughout the indigenous populations of the southeastern U.S. and around the Great Lakes region; and along with the chiefdoms came the spread of the Adena Culture. Between 200 BC and 500 AD the mounds built by these widely diverse peoples became larger and more elaborate often built in various geometric shapes. Warren King Moorehead, considered the "Dean of American archaeology" in the late 1890s, explored a group of mounds built during this period in Ross County, Ohio, and named them the "Hopewell Mounds" after the family that owned the earthworks at the time. With the discovery of many other mounds from this time period, this era of cultural expansion in the region became known as the "Hopewell Tradition." Archaeological evidence indicates that there was a significant amount of material exchange between these various regional groups especially along the river and lake waterways that connected them. The Hopewell exchange system was highly advanced with exotic raw material shipped to manufacturing areas and finished goods traded back to far flung localities. Objects from the Hopewell exchange system have been found in burial sites throughout much of the United States and Canada. The plants originally domesticated by the Adena also spread throughout the

Hopewell Tradition in what anthropologist Ralph Linton in the 1940s termed the "Eastern Agricultural Complex".

Around 500 AD the Hopewell exchange system ceased, mound building stopped, and art forms were no longer produced. It was at this time that both North America and Northern Europe experienced the extreme cold weather event of 535–536 that was probably caused by an atmospheric dust veil from a large volcanic eruption in the tropics. As in Northern Europe this most severe and protracted episodes of cooling in the Northern Hemisphere in over 2,000 years caused crop failures and famines throughout the Hopewell Agricultural Complex.

The late Woodland period (500 AD to 1000 AD) was a time of apparent population dispersal although populations do not appear to have declined. Villages dating to this period shifted to larger communities that were fortified with walls and ditches suggesting conflict between neighboring chiefdoms. It was also during this period that the newly introduced bow and arrow technology overtook the use of the spear thrower (atlatl) which had the effect of improved hunting efficiency putting added human stress on populations of small wild animals such as muskrat, raccoon, beaver, duck and turkey. Around 800 AD, likely due to these distinct pressures on food production, a cold weather variety of high yielding maize from Central America was finally bred and introduced into the Eastern Agricultural Complex *("Population nucleation, intensive agriculture, and environmental degradation: The Cahokia example"*, Department of Geography, Southern Illinois University, 2004*)*.

Mississippian Culture

The next great mound building era in the prehistory of indigenous peoples in North America began abruptly around 950 AD in an area of the northern Mississippi River Alluvial plain called the "American Bottom" which consisted of the 10 mile (16 km) wide strip of eastern floodplain found immediately below the confluence of the Illinois, Missouri, and Mississippi Rivers near the modern day city of St. Louis. By this time, according to University of Kansas Geography Professor and leading scholar of Native American prehistory, William Woods:

> *"The effects of many millennia of human occupation of this area had resulted in great landscape change through the extirpation of local animal species; introduction of exotic plants (including domesticates); forest clearance for fuel, construction materials, and agricultural fields with attendant accelerated erosion and downslope deposition; localized enrichment of soils in habitation areas; the maintenance of prairies and removal of forest undergrowth through burning; and, perhaps, managed groves of nut bearing trees on the bluffs and bluff slope environments." ("Population nucleation, intensive agriculture, and environmental degradation: The Cahokia example," Department of Geography, Southern Illinois University, 2004)*

According to Dr. Woods' assessment, this anthropogenically altered riverine landscape:

"...contain[ed] the largest zone in the American Bottom of soils characterized as optimal for prehistoric hoe cultivation (Figure 3)."

Living within this ecosystem the human inhabitants slowly developed a different subsistence pattern than their Hopewell ancestors. Again Dr. Woods:

"For subsistence, faunal recovery indicates extensive use of fish, amphibians, and reptiles, mussels, birds, and mammals, with reliance placed upon small fish, and to a much lesser extent, deer and aquatic birds (e.g., Kelly and Cross, 1984; Kelly, 1997). Floral inventories point to the gathering of a variety of naturally occurring nuts, seeds, fruits, greens, and tubers (e.g., Johannessen, 1984). A number of plants producing masses of small seeds had a long history of regional cultivation and certainly formed a portion of the Mississippian food production system (Lopinot, 1989; Fritz, 2000). Squash and gourds were also present, although not, as widely assumed, domesticated beans. Maize, however, was the predominant produced food and major dietary staple."

It was here on the American Bottom that maize first became a dietary staple in North America. Dr. Woods:

"Here, on the silty alluvial overbank and fan sediments, the large, communally worked, maize outfields would have been located. Additionally, production would have been augmented by multi-crop house gardens within the site itself found on soils highly enriched by the debris from prior habitation activities, as well as from fields situated on vacated ancestral lands further upstream on the Cahokia Creek floodplain."

With the adoption of high yielding maize as their staple crop, a human population explosion occurred in the American Bottom that provided the labor necessary to construct the massive earthen mound city of "Cahokia" and the formation of the "Mississippian Culture".

Although a number of competing settlements containing earthen mounds had been established in the area during the "Emergent Mississippian Period" (800 AD – 1050 AD), by the beginning of the "Mississippian Period" (1050 AD – 1350 AD) Cahokia had become predominant and the other early centers waned through competition or warfare. An overall master plan involving massive labor expenditures was clearly underway at Cahokia by 950 AD and in a relatively short period of time a totally human landscape had been established in the central portion of the site. Over the next three centuries Cahokia grew in size with habitation and ceremonial areas covering at least five square miles (13 square kilometers) including an enormous central plaza and over one hundred and twenty mounds. Dominating the site is Monks Mound, an enormous, multi-terraced platform bigger than the Egyptian pyramids that is the largest prehistoric earthen construction north of Mexico. The community was planned with well defined administrative/ceremonial zones, elite compounds, residential neighborhoods, and even suburbs. Dr. Woods estimates that at its peak the population of Cahokia was around 15,000 individuals, larger than the European city of London at that time.

Symbiotically with Cahokia's rise in food production and population density came a more socially stratified society with institutionalized inequality and the emergence of a more powerful chiefdom where political and religious authority was vested in the hands of one big man. Garbage pits reveal that in elite precincts big fish and choice cuts of venison were commonly fare while Dr. Woods describes the typical Cahokian diet as:

> *"What's for breakfast? Gruel. What's for lunch? Gruel. What's for supper? Gruel and a little fish. You might eat venison sometime in your life." ("The Rise and Fall of the Mound People," Chicago Reader, Arts & Culture, 2000)*

Cold weather varietals of the common bean from Central America were first developed in North America around 1200 AD and with them began the spread of the highly productive agricultural system of the Three Sisters (growing maize, beans and squash together) that had long been practiced in Central America. During the Mississippian Period Three Sisters agriculture spread throughout the entire Mississippi River basin from the Great Lakes to the Gulf of Mexico and from the southeastern Atlantic coast to the edge of the western prairies, but dependence on this agriculture varied considerably by region. In the upper Great Lakes wild rice (*Zizania aquatica*) was a staple food and on the western fringes of the prairies people relied more on hunting the still abundant wild herds of bison. In contrast, residents of the central and southern parts of the cultural area tended to rely heavily upon agriculture. Consequently, human population densities per square mile also varied considerably between these regions being much higher in the central and southern parts where high yielding maize was the staple crop ("Origins of Agriculture," *Encyclopædia Britannica Online, 2012)*. Along with Three Sisters agriculture, the more centralized political power structure of Cahokia spread throughout the Mississippian Culture where large chiefdoms formed into what archaeologists have dubbed the "Southeastern Ceremonial Complex."

Sediment deposits and old-growth tree rings indicate that Cahokia underwent drastic changes starting in the 11th century. The near disappearance of pollen from bottom land trees in sediment cores indicate that as Cahokia's population grew, extensive anthropogenic deforestation took place to clear trees for maize fields and firewood. Sediment cores also indicate that during the 11th century the central United States experience a period of increased rainfall which enabled Cahokia to expand agriculture to nearby upland areas. Old growth tree rings indicate that during the 12th and 13th centuries, a time corresponding to the Medieval Warming Period in Europe, the climate of North America went through decades-long drought periods punctuated by brief periods of heavy rainfall (Larry Benson and colleagues, 2009). By this time anthropogenic deforestation had made Cahokia vulnerable to extensive flooding during these rainy periods. This cycle of flood and drought ate away at Cahokia's maize fields and food base eventually causing the elite class structure to beak down. By 1350 AD Cahokia was completely abandoned. Never again would such a large urban center be constructed in pre-Columbian North America.

The archaeological record over much of the Southeastern Ceremonial Complex during the next 142 years before European contact (1350 AD to 1492 AD), called the "Late Mississippian Period", is characterized by the building of defensive structures at settlement sites to defend winter food stores against raiding parties from neighboring tribes. This warlike behavior suggests these were times of food scarcity due to both climate change and increased human population density. During this period mound building waned and settlements were smaller but maize farming in river valleys continued to provide the staple food in much of the eastern North America. It was also around this time that the people, who had burned undergrowth for centuries to create grassy open meadows to promote deer grazing, began to systematically replant large belts of forestland into orchards of nut trees (hickory, pecan, oak, beechnut, hazelnut, walnut, and chestnut). Within a few centuries humans had transformed the eastern forests from a patchwork of meadows into a mix of farmland and orchards. This change was so sweeping that early European explorers and settlers assumed that these carefully tended orchards were a primeval untouched wilderness.

The Iroquois League, or Haudenosaunee, is believed to have been founded between 1450 AD and 1660 AD, to bring together five distinct nations in the southern Great Lakes area into "The Great League of Peace." The League was governed by a Grand Council, an assembly of fifty chiefs each representing a clan of a nation. Each nation within the League had a distinct language, territory, and function. The Iroquois were constantly engaged in warfare with their neighbors, the Algonquins of the Ottawa River Valley and its tributaries in present day Quebec and Ontario, Canada, and the Huron, also called the Wyandot people, of the north shore of Lake Ontario, Canada. In response to the arrival of the Europeans in the 16th century, the Iroquois Confederacy was formed. At its peak, the Confederacy extended north into present day Canada, and south into the U.S. states of New York, Ohio, Pennsylvania, Kentucky and Virginia, known as the "Six Nations."

Oasisamerica

The desert southwest of modern-day United States and northwest Mexico was the site of another agriculturally driven human population boom to emerge in North America. This area referred to by archeologists as "Oasisamerica" fostered the growth of three major cultures – the Pueblo, the Hohokam, and the Mogollon – surrounded by several other smaller yet distinct cultural groups. *("Archaeology of prehistoric native America: an encyclopedia."* The terrain of this vast region is dominated in the north by the Rocky Mountains of North America and to the south by the Sierra Madre Occidental Mountains of Mesoamerica. To the east and west of these massive mountain ranges stretch the vast arid plains of the Sonora, Chihuahua, and Arizona Deserts. At its height, Oasisamerica cultures settled parts of the modern-day Mexican states of Chihuahua, Sonora and Baja California, as well as the U.S. states of Arizona, Utah, New Mexico, Colorado, Nevada and California. While this land is generally characterized by low annual rainfall, it is also traversed by many small rivers with riparian habitat that was attractive to early human settlers.

Clovis big game hunters passed through this area perhaps as early as 12,000 years ago but the first archaeological evidence of continuous human habitation dates back to about 10,000 years ago near Navajo Mountain, Utah. Archaeological artifacts indicate these people were nomadic hunter/gatherers who traveled in small groups gathering wild plants when in season, and hunting game with stone-tipped spears, atlatls (spear throwers), and darts. By this time the big game mega fauna species hunted by the Clovis had become extinct and prey included smaller animals such as rabbit, deer, antelope and bighorn sheep. For over 6,000 years the population density of the hunter/gatherers in this arid environment remained very low. Then around 1200 BC (3,200 years ago), during a climate interval of above average rainfall, the people began to cultivate gardens of maize and squash using seeds they imported from Central America probably in trade for highly prized turquoise which came from mineral deposits in southern New Mexico and Arizona.

The Pueblo people occupied a geographical area known as the "Four Corners" comprised of southern Utah, northern Arizona, northwest New Mexico, and southern Colorado. Terrain and resources vary widely within this expansive region. The Colorado Plateau has elevations ranging from 4,500 to 8,500 feet (2,600 meters) above sea level with extensive horizontal mesas capped by sedimentary geological layers that supported woodlands of juniper, pinon, and ponderosa pine, each favoring different elevations. Wind and water erosion have sculpted steep-walled canyons with windows and bridges in areas where resistant strata such as sandstone or limestone overlie more easily eroded strata of shale. The southern edge is defined by the Colorado and Little Colorado Rivers in Arizona and the Rio Puerco and Rio Grande in New Mexico. Irregular periods of drought have characterized the region since first human colonization with summer rains undependable and often arriving as violent thunderstorms. While the amount of winter snowfall varies greatly throughout the region, where sandstone overlays shale, snow melt would accumulate to feed seeps and springs that watered lush oases in the desert. The first agriculturalists around 1200 BC were still nomadic part of the year and the women made baskets to collect, transport and store food. They had no pottery.

By 750 AD the Pueblo had constructed deep pit-houses along with some above-ground rooms and had established a sedentary agricultural lifestyle. The bow and arrow replaced the atlatl and spear and painted black-on-white pottery was in use for food storage. The bean was imported from Central America bringing three sisters agriculture to the region. Wild amaranth and pinon pine nuts were also important dietary staples. From 750 AD to 900 AD the Pueblo saw increasing populations, growing village size, social integration, and more complicated and complex agricultural systems.

Core samples from 52 of the oldest sequoia trees in California's western Sierra Nevada Mountains, providing a 3,000-year climate record of the southwestern United States, indicate a period of sustained droughts and frequent fires beginning around 800 AD lasting through 1300 AD (*University of Arizona's Laboratory of Tree-Ring Research*). This time interval corresponds to the Medieval Warm Period in Europe. As water resources became increasingly scarce and irregular the Pueblo began development of a system of reservoirs and canals to maintain their agrarian livelihood. Between 900 AD and 1150 AD as *the droughts wore on, m*ore intensive agriculture was developed utilizing dams, terraces and long irrigation ditches. These irrigation systems were not just built to retain water, but also to retain silt. Intermittent water running down the drainage courses deposited silt accumulating to several feet deep behind the dams which would retain moisture for a considerable period of time. The Pueblo farmers cultivated these moist terraces (*"The Ancient Pueblo (the Anasazi),"* *ICE Case Studies,* American University, The School of International Service, 2003).

During this time the Pueblo also constructed a major regional cultural center called "Chaco Canyon" in New Mexico with an estimated population of 1,500 – 5,000 people. The people quarried sandstone blocks and hauled timber from great distances, assembling 15 major complexes at Chaco Canyon which remained the largest buildings in North America until the 19th century. Chaco Canyon was surrounded by planned towns of "great houses" that were centers of worship built from the wood of more than 200,000 trees. The great houses were immense complexes usually containing more than 200 rooms with some as many as 700. Individual rooms were substantial in size, with higher ceilings than prior ancient Pueblo buildings with great kivas up to 70 feet (21 meters) in diameter. A major road system called the "Chaco Road" that radiated from Chaco Canyon was also constructed at this time. Through satellite images and ground investigations archaeologists have detected at least 8 main roads that together run for more than 180 miles (300 kilometers) and are more than 30 feet (10 meters) wide. These roads were excavated into a smooth leveled surface in the bedrock or created through the removal of vegetation and soil. Large ramps and stairways were cut into the cliff rock to connect the roadways on ridge tops to sites on the valley bottoms. To construct these great houses and roads required a substantial labor force and the agricultural production to feed them.

Tree ring dating indicates that construction of the famous "Cliff Palace" in the southwestern corner of Colorado was continuous from 1190 AD through 1260 AD. The Cliff Palace was constructed in a large crevice on the side of a vertical cliff at the edge of a mesa. Built of sandstone, mortar and wooden beams, it contains 23 kivas and 150 rooms that housed an estimated population of about 100 people. The Pueblo people who built the Cliff Palace and the other cliff dwellings like it in the Mesa Verde area of the Four Corners were apparently driven to these defensible positions due to increasing competition for water and arable land. By the beginning of the 14th century the global cooling period known as the Little Ice Age had succeeded the Medieval Warm Period and brought icy winters and substantially shorter drier growing seasons to the Four Corners region; by 1350 AD the Cliff Palace and Chaco Canyon had been completely abandoned. Archaeologist Steven LeBlanc of the Peabody Museum of Archaeology at Harvard University argues that the Pueblo were forced to give up agriculture in many traditional areas due to extreme cold and drought and migrated to more favorable locations in the better-watered upper Rio Grande River drainage. In some areas archaeological evidence suggests that the Pueblo fought against each other for control over the substantially reduced arable land, water, game and firewood (LeBlanc, 1999; Haas and Creamer, 1997).

The Hohokam and Mogollon cultures each developed over a similar time frame as the Pueblo in different territories of Oasisamerica. The Hohokam culture was centered on the middle Gilla River and lower Salt River drainages in the modern-day Phoenix basin extending north to the Upper Sonoran Desert in Arizona. This area occupied a central position among the many different cultural traditions that developed simultaneously in Oasisamerica. Between the 7th and 14th centuries, the Hohokam built and maintained extensive irrigation networks along the lower Salt and middle Gila rivers that rivaled in complexity those of ancient Egypt and China. Constructed without benefit of advanced engineering technologies, the Hohokam managed to slope irrigation canals with a drop of only a few feet per mile and maintain a delicate balance between erosion and siltation *(Powell 2008, pp. 32, 33)*. Decades of archaeological research have revealed that the Hohokam cultivated varieties of cotton, tobacco, maize, beans and squash, as well as harvested a vast assortment of wild plants. Late in the Hohokam chronological sequence they also used extensive dry-farming systems to grow agave for food and fiber. Hohokam agriculture based on canal irrigation provided for a large population base that built many great houses most prominently "Casa Grande" halfway between modern-day Phoenix and Tucson. The Hohokam, like the Pueblo, finally succumbed to the vagaries of the Little Ice Age weather extremes that destroyed major sections of their delicately balanced irrigation system and by the mid 14th Century the largest settlements had been abandoned leaving only a few small villages concentrated along the Gila River. The O'odham people now living in the area are believed to be the modern descendants of the ancestral Hohokam people.

The Mogollon culture developed to the south of the Pueblo and east of the Hohokum in the high-altitude desert areas of what is modern-day New Mexico, Sonora, Chihuahua and western Texas. With less annual rainfall, Mogollon agriculture was less productive and consequently their population reached less density than their cultural neighbors. By the 14th century the Mogollon had abandoned their major urban centers with some of the people seeking refuge in the Sierra Madre Mountains while others fled to the north where they combined with the ancestral Pueblo. Modern descendants of the ancestral Magollon are believed to be the Hopi and Zuni of the Gila River basin and the Yaquis, Mayos, Opatas and Tarahumara of northeastern Mexico. Much of the original Mogollon territory was later occupied by the nomadic hunter/gatherer Apache who migrated in from the north.

Atlantic and Pacific Coastal Dwellers

(Full disclosure: I live on the Pacific Coast of North America in present day California, so perhaps I have given more attention to these sparsely populated coastal regions than their relative populations deserve. However, in my defense, I will say that these North American coastal dwellers represent an unusual circumstance in human social development whereby they managed to sustain high population densities relative to hunter/gatherer cultures without benefit of agriculture. This makes them particularly interesting ecological case studies.)

The indigenous people of the North Atlantic and the entire Pacific coasts of North America never resorted to agriculture to earn a living; however, due to the exceptional abundance of wild terrestrial and aquatic plants and animals at their disposal, they were able to sustain population densities far in excess of typical hunter/gatherer groups. In 1986 three prominent American anthropology professors, C. Melvin Aikens, Kenneth Ames and David Sanger, published a unique study in which they compared the initial human settlement of the north Atlantic and north Pacific coasts of North America with the Baltic Sea region of northern Europe, and the northeast Pacific region of Japan. *(The University Museum, The University of Tokyo, Bulletin No.27, "PREHISTORIC HUNTER-GATHERERS IN JAPAN—New Research Methods—", Edited by Takeru AKAZAWA and C. Melvin AIKENS, 1986 TOKYO)* While separated geographically by vast distances these areas all share similar ecological characteristics: they are northern temperate lands with much-indented coastlines and backed by wooded hinterlands. This comparison study based on all the relevant archaeological information available at the time found many interesting parallels in how these similar ecological zones were settled by humans, albeit at very different times in human history. Most notably, they all maintained a hunter/gatherer way of life long after the areas around them had adopted agricultural food economies.

According to the authors:

"We suggest that the socioeconomic similarities between the widely separated cultures that are the focus of attention in this paper arise firstly and fundamentally from the need for hunter-gatherers in all of these regions to depend upon storage to some degree. This need is enforced simply by the natural seasonality in biotic productivity that dominates middle and higher latitudes. The natural rhythm requires that at least some resources must be intensively exploited in order to produce stores, and it controls not only the timing of group activity, but also the stability of social aggregations. Groups operating in these regions must be "collectors" sensu Binford (1980). Those discussed here all were characterized-at least in their mature stages-by central residential camps from which specialized task groups exploited particular resources. As Binford points out, this is a subsistence strategy for dealing with resources which are disjunct in space and/or in time. It is therefore a strategy common among hunter-gatherers in middle and northern latitudes. Conceivably, other factors besides global climatic patterns may produce disjunct resource distributions, but it is climate and seasonality-combined with the specific similarities of the regional environments involved-that are basic in the cases to be discussed here.

"The second fundamental factor giving rise to sociocultural similarity between the regions compared is simply that all four of them share highly similar kinds of exploitable resources, which are obtainable in highly similar settings. Those resources include medium-sized to large terrestrial herbivores, marine mammals, resident and anadromous fish, a variety of terrestrial plant foods, and the resources of intertidal zones. As will be shown, the general similarity in

*mode of production shared by the different regions, when combined with specific similarities in
the biotic resource base, determined certain fundamental similarities in the life of all of them."*

So in essence, due to similarities in coastal habitat as well as the seasonal variability of their specific
northern latitudes, coastal dwellers of the north Atlantic and Pacific North America, Baltic Sea region
and North Pacific Japan, though far removed in space and time developed similar food economies that
depended on storing abundant wild resources to feed their dense populations through the lean winter
months. Thus by developing food storage capabilities, these hunter/gatherer populations utilized one of
the main survival strategies that agricultural societies depend on to sustain their high population densities.

North Atlantic Coast of North America

The jagged two thousand mile Atlantic coast of North America from present day Newfoundland
south to Florida is punctuated with hundreds of river estuaries where salt and fresh water meet in so
called "intertidal zones." In these zones that can extend for several miles inland extensive water mixing
and nutrient cycling provides an ideal habitat for the growth of plankton (any drifting plant, animal or
bacterial organism that inhabits water bodies) that forms the base of a highly diverse and productive
marine ecosystem. Such zones generally teem with shellfish as well as anadromous fish like salmon that
migrate from salt to fresh water and catadromous fish like eels that migrate from fresh to salt water to
complete their breeding cycles. From its colder northern-most reaches to its subtropical southern-most
perimeter these coastal aquatic ecosystems provided the first human inhabitants of the east coast with
abundant food resources, but the climate variation from north to south was also a determining factor in
how indigenous people ultimately settled these diverse habitats over time.

By 1000 BC coast dwellers south and west of the Saco River in southern Maine had adopted three
sisters (maize, bean and squash) agriculture that had spread north and east from the inland Mississippian
Cultures as noted earlier. But north of the Saco River along the coastlines of Maine, Nova Scotia and
nearby offshore islands, persistent fog and early frosts made for climate conditions that were unsuitable for
growing these crops and the indigenous people who settled this area never adopted agriculture.

As the glaciers retreated from North America around 12,000 years ago they left behind a landscape
in Maine of rounded gravelly hills, wide, U-shaped valleys, numerous lake bogs, thin soils of clay, silt and
sand, and an abundance of stones and boulders. The first Clovis hunters to enter this area found a boggy
land of sedges and grasses punctuated by scattered stands of birch, willow, alder, and spruce. Recovered
Clovis Points from this time indicate they feasted on the woolly mammoths that grazed on the grassy plains,
mastodons that browsed on the emerging coniferous forests and giant beaver that built dams in the vast
bogs and wetlands. As these mega-fauna were driven to extinction over the next thousand years, recovered
animal bones and smaller stone points indicate that the people turned to following the migrating caribou
herds for subsistence along with hunting other smaller mammals and birds. Starting around 10,000 years
ago, deciduous trees characteristic of a more temperate climate began to fill the landscape increasing the
biodiversity of the Maine forest. By 7,000 years ago, as temperatures continued to warm, oaks had become

the dominant species. The glacier melt also resulted in a sea level rise that stabilized around 5,000 years ago creating new coastal estuaries where marine ecosystems developed increasingly productive biodiversity. Between 4,700 and 3,500 years ago, Maine experienced the effects of another worldwide warming trend that brought butternut and chestnut trees to the interior. These changes are reflected in artifacts found inland like mortars, pestles, and other grinding implements used for processing and preserving seeds, nuts, berries, and roots.

Foraging in this resource dense interior environment, along with the adoption of maize, bean and squash agriculture in southern Maine (south and west of the Saco River) caused the human population to grow quickly which put pressure on terrestrial game populations and gave rise to more intense exploitation of marine and coastal resources. This led to more permanent settlements on the coast, the islands, and along the lower river systems. Shell middens and other preserved organic refuse are evidence of a varied cuisine made up of "... *nuts and berries, waterfowl, deer, moose, bear, beaver, muskrat, porcupine, dog, wolf, fox, otter, marten, fisher, skunk, raccoon, bobcat, alewives, finned fish, shellfish, sturgeon, seal, porpoise, an extinct species of sea mink, and assorted other gleanings from this diverse Maine landscape*" *(Maine Historical Society, 2000)*. By 700 BC these hunter/gatherer coast dwellers were making fired-clay ceramics that replaced wood, bark and woven bowls, a change that meant significant improvements in food cooking and storage capabilities making villages more permanent. Development of the bark canoe extended the hunter's reach into the game-rich upper tributaries and expanded networks of trade and exchange. These coast dwellers also developed new projectile points and cutting, scraping, grinding, and hammering tools of stone and bone adapted for hunting and preparing aquatic prey.

By 1000 AD, the Abanaki (meaning "People of the Dawn") tribe of the Wabanaki Confederation of Maine and the larger Algonquin Confederation stretching from New England to the Great Lakes, populated the tidal basins and the coastal islands of the far northeast coast. Research indicates that the Abanaki had a complex seasonal movement pattern radiating out from year-round village sites near the coast. On the coast, estuaries provided shellfish, waterfowl, lobsters, and weir-trapped fish. This dense array of food resources kept people living near the coast most of the year. But the Maine environment provided no single food resource that could sustain a village coastal or upland through all four seasons, so the Abenaki moved in seasonal rounds seeking subsistence in a constantly changing landscape. The Abenaki summer was a time of maximum mobility, as bands or families dispersed and regrouped for hunting, freshwater and ocean fishing and foraging. During fall women remained in the village smoking lobster for storage and preparing berries by pounding, crushing, boiling, and drying them. In the fall the passenger pigeon and waterfowl migrations filled the larder as well as the harvest of butternuts, chestnuts, and acorns. During late fall men hunted black bear, beaver, deer, moose, and squirrel, and in winter, deer and beaver. In mid-March, anadromous fish were trapped in weirs making their way up river to spawn; in May the people moved to the coast to gather shellfish and catch cod, and in September they withdrew to the "little rivers" where eels spawned. This seasonal rotation varied depending on the availability of resources in each specific area. According to archeologist Stuart Eldridge:

> *"The [Maine] estuarine environment has been construed as an ecotonal patchwork exhibiting high biotic productivities and juxtaposed terrestrial and marine environments, allowing the potential for hunter-gatherers to exercise an option not to move on the landscape as frequently and to have higher population densities. (Abstract, "Archaeology at the Stanley Site, Monhegan Island, Maine: Implications for Modeling Late Archaic Coastal Adaptations" by Stuart Eldridge, THE MAINE ARCHAEOLOGICAL SOCIETY BULLETIN, VOLUME 47 NUMBER 2, FALL 2007.)*

While the Abanaki maintained this semi-sedentary hunter/gatherer subsistence way of life right up to the point of contact by Italian Giovanni Caboto (aka John Cabot), in 1497, agriculture had long before taken hold among the tribes to the south and west of the Saco River. In these agricultural areas the traditional system of defining tribal territories by river drainages had broken down due to demographic pressures and tribes were crossing watersheds as much as traveling up them.

A sediment core drilled into the marsh bed in the lower Hudson Valley near present day New York City in 2005, offered an amazingly detailed history of the northeastern coastal climate going back to 800 AD. Sediment layers from this tidal marsh in the Hudson River Estuary have preserved identifiable pollen and seeds from plants as well as other inorganic materials. These past remnants allowed researchers from Columbia University and NASA to see evidence of a 500 year drought during the Medieval Warm Period from 800 AD to 1300 AD, the cold dry trend of the Little Ice Age from 1550 AD to 1850 AD, and the impacts of European settlers (*"Marshes Tell Story of Medieval Drought, Little Ice Age, and European Settlers near New York City," Goddard Space Flight Center, NASA, 2005*). As the colder temperatures and dry climate of the Little Ice Age began to grip the northeast coast of North America, deciduous nut bearing trees gave way to coniferous forests of spruce and fir along the coastal strip which disadvantaged terrestrial game and reduced the food potential of the terrestrial zone for coast dwellers. The marine ecosystem, however, due to high tidal ranges and increased water column mixing, nutrient recycling, and greater plankton growth reached its maximum potential for productivity resulting in greater human reliance on marine food resources during this period (*The Gulf of Maine.Rockland: Courier of Maine Books,* 1979).

Pacific Coast of North America

The climate, terrain and wild food resources of the Pacific coast of North America are considerably different than those of the Atlantic which resulted in the indigenous peoples of each coast developing their own unique survival strategies. On the Atlantic coast south of Maine, as the population of hunter/gatherers grew beyond the carrying capacity of the coastal environment, all the people eventually adopted agriculture to supplement their diets. But over the entire length of the west coast from Alaska down to southern California into Baja none of the indigenous people ever resorted to agriculture. The question is why?

The Northwest Coast was the most sharply delimited geographical and cultural area of North America covering a long narrow arc of Pacific coast and offshore islands from Yakutat Bay in the northeastern Gulf of Alaska south to Cape Mendocino in modern-day northern California. Its eastern limits were the crest of the Coast Ranges from the north down to Puget Sound, the Cascades south to the Columbia River, and the coastal hills of what is now Oregon and northwestern California. The "Kuroshio", an offshore Pacific Ocean current produces a mild temperature range rarely over 90 degrees Fahrenheit or below freezing. The offshore current also induces precipitous rainfall although it falls unevenly across the region. Annual precipitation averages more than 160 inches (406 centimeters) in many areas and rarely drops below 30 inches (76 centimeters) even in the driest climatic zones. The northern Coast Range averages an elevation of about 3,300 feet (1,000 meters) above sea level, with some peaks and ridges rising to more than 6,600 feet (2,000 meters). In most of the Northwest, the land rises steeply from the sea and is cut by hundreds of narrow channels and fjords. The shores of Puget Sound, southwestern Washington, and the Oregon coast hills are lower and less rugged. The region's temperate rain forests are predominantly dense stands of coniferous tree species including spruce, Douglas fir, hemlock, red and yellow cedar, and, in the south, coast redwood that support a wide variety and great abundance of edible wild flora and fauna.

Most of the northwest coast was deglaciated by 10,000 years ago, and the earliest well-dated coastal human sites are consistently about 10,000 to 9,000 years ago *(Fladmark, 1975, 1982)*. Around 8,000 years ago, the number of dated human sites on the northwest coast increases significantly. Due to glacial ice melt over these millennia, sea level also rose by approximately 200 feet (60 meters) to near its present level which inundated low-lying coastal areas. The people survived through constant mobility exploiting a broad spectrum of different foods from nuts, berries, bulbs, grass seeds and fungi to deer, mollusks, sea mammals, and fish using simple milling stones to process their bounty. Though increasing marginally, human population density remained very low until about 5,000 years ago when large shell midden sites began to appear all along the far northwest coast indicating a sudden intensification of food production and population growth. At this time middens show an intensification of fishing. The hunter/gatherer cultures of the northwest coast reached their peak of social development between 2,500 and 2,000 years ago (500 BC and 1 AD) with village sites consisting of large multifamily plank houses with a highly stratified social structure.

Aquatic food resources were most abundant. Intertidal zones were rich in bivalves, clams, cockles, whelks, barnacles, limpets and sea urchins. Fish species included herring, candlefish (eulachon), smelt, cod, halibut, mollusks, five species of salmon and gray whales. Fisheries were scattered across the region not all equally as easy to exploit. Pink and chum salmon were the most important species for preservation for winter stores as these species had less fat so when smoked and dried would keep for a long period of time. Principal fishing sites in the fall were along rivers and streams in which pink or chum salmon ran to prepare stores for the winter. Sockeye, coho, chinook and king salmon were eaten immediately or dried and kept only for a short period since their high fat content caused the meat to spoil relatively quickly even when dried. In the spring other species of fish became available in tremendous schools: herring came to spawn in coves, candlefish entered certain rivers and farther south smelt spawned on sandy beaches in summer. People also went to sea in longboats carved from single massive logs to hunt marine mammals and to fish for offshore species such as halibut. By the time Europeans arrived in the 18th century the northwest coast was densely populated. Estimating density in terms of persons per square mile has little relevance in a region where long stretches of the coast consisted of uninhabitable cliffs rising from the sea; however, early European explorers noted that many winter villages had hundreds of inhabitants.

On the west coast of modern day California from Cape Mendocino south to San Diego, human settlement of the coast actually occurred much later in the north than in the south. Archaeologists William Hilderbrandt and Valerie Levulett have surveyed the archaeological evidence of many areas of the west coast and they have pinned down the chronology of coastal settlement very convincingly in their paper, "*Late Holocene Emergence of Marine-focused Economies in Northwest California*" (Catalysts to Complexity: Late Holocene Societies of the California Coast, 2002).

On the north coast of California in the King Range area south of present-day Eureka, Hilderbrandt and Levulett discovered sites that chronicle sporadic use of the coast between 500 BC and 500 AD, but it was not until after 1200 AD that intensive shellfish processing took hold on the coast. On the central coast, San Francisco Bay shell midden sites are similarly dated from 600 BC to 1300 AD, whereas large shell midden sites have been reliably dated at 2000 BC on the south coast in the San Diego area. Why such late coastal settlement on the north coast? According to Hilderbrandt and Levulett, the answer may lie in the food resources available in the interior. In the far northwest where deer, elk and other prey abounded in river valleys and forests, shell middens occur no more than half a mile inland. As you travel southward into more arid landscapes, shell middens occur further inland, six miles in Sonoma County, fifteen miles in central California, and as many as twenty miles in the San Diego region. Mollusks assumed ever-greater importance as the hinterland became drier and land mammals became less plentiful. The later move to the coast in the northwest may have resulted from game depletion in the interior ("*Resource Depression and Intensification During the Late Holocene, San Francisco Bay: Evidence from the Emeryville Shellmound Vertebrate Fauna*", Google eBook, 1999), which forced some groups to settle along the shore where access to salmon runs, game and acorns was more limited. Exploiting sea mammals and shellfish, as well as engaging in labor intensive offshore fishing, made sense to people under these material circumstances. In contrast, in southern California, in a far more arid and much less productive inland environment, where salmon runs were fewer the people were forced to consume relatively predictable coastal foods such as shellfish and sea mammals far earlier than their contemporaries to the north.

Sea cores from the San Francisco Bay area and the Santa Barbara channel indicate warmer sea temperatures between 900 BC and 500 AD, cooler sea temperatures between 500 AD and 1500 AD and warmer temperatures to modern times. Warmer sea temperatures cause upwellings that bring plankton close to the surface where massive schools of anchovies feed just offshore. During these periods of abundant anchovy, the indigenous human populations of the San Francisco Bay area and the Santa Barbara channel thrived, but during the cooler period of poor fishing conditions between 500 AD and 1500 AD, the human populations of these areas show signs of stress and violent conflict (*"The Archaeology of War: A North American Perspective," Journal of Archaeological Research, 2002*).

There are fifteen species of oak trees that grew in the coastal mountain ranges from Oregon to southern California and on riverbanks in California's central valley. The oak's ubiquitous seed, the acorn, was utilized by early foraging groups for thousands of years as a fallback food during periods of drought and food scarcity. Acorns are a very labor intensive food requiring gathering, shelling, leaching, milling and storing so they were not a preferred food source during times of abundance and would be passed over until the next food crisis hit. This circumstance underwent dramatic changes between 2500 BC and 1000 BC. As the population gradually increased during this time there were many more groups foraging the landscape and crowding into increasingly more circumscribed territories. As the population density increased to greater than the carrying capacity of the land (1 person/square mile) and easy to forage foods became scarce even in good years due to human over-exploitation, it became contingent upon the people to adopt the labor intensive acorn as a dietary staple year after year. Stone mortar and pestles for processing acorns litter the archaeological landscape of this time and finely woven baskets of grass and reeds were used to wash the acorns in fresh water streams to leach out the harmful tannic acid, and other baskets were woven for dry storage of the processed acorn flour. This move to a more labor intensive food as a staple was similar to the adaptation made by foragers in the Near East who took up the labor intensive task of agriculture around 10,000 years ago. But with acorns so abundant, the west coast foragers of North America didn't need agricultural crops to have plentiful harvests. With their high carbohydrate, protein and fat content acorns are an excellent source of calories and they also store well for long periods without spoiling. Early Californians were not the first people in history to rely on acorns. Foragers in Syria subsisted off acorns 14,000 years ago and Medieval European farmers consumed quantities of acorns as did indigenous people of Midwest North America. As late as the 19th century acorns provided as much as 20% of the calories in some rural areas of Spain and Italy. But acorns were never as important a food source as they were in California, with its highly varied environment and endemic droughts.

As acorns became a dietary staple, the realities of the harvest began to dictate other aspects of group life. Territories shrank as people moved around less and ancestral rights to specific oak groves were what defined a group's boundaries. The land became divided into hundreds of group territories called "tribelets" by Alfred Kroeber of UC Berkeley, one of the first cultural anthropologists to study the indigenous peoples of California. Skeletal remains from this period indicate a larger portion of the population survived to adulthood than before the widespread adoption of the acorn and that the rate of population increase also accelerated after 1500 BC.

Human bones from cemeteries dated 800 AD to 900 AD coinciding with the onset of the Medieval Warm Period indicated people had more pathologies and shorter lives suggesting that by this time the population was so large that the drought ravaged acorn crop was insufficient to provide enough calories and nutrients to avoid widespread famine. *("Bioarchaeological Science: What we have Learned from Human Skeletal Remains,"* Anthropology, San Jose State University, 2009). Human bones from the San Francisco Bay area and the Santa Barbara Channel area dating between 450 AD and 1350 AD also show a marked increase in violent injuries suggesting more aggression between groups likely caused by food scarcity *(Walker and Lambert, 1989).*

UC Berkeley demographic anthropologist Sherburne Cook spent his career studying pre-European populations in California and from his many publications he compiled a map that gives his estimated indigenous population of California by regions in the year 1542 AD. The densest populations were in the acorn rich Central Valley, with much lower densities in the southern deserts and northwest. Cultural anthropologist Alfred Kroeber has estimated population densities at up to 10 people per square mile among tribelets in the Central Valley with territories as small as 50 square miles (picture 500 people living in a square area 7.07 miles to a side). This contrasts sharply with the 6,000 square miles or more required by some desert tribelets in the southeastern California and in the Great Basin (modern-day southeastern Oregon, Nevada and western Utah). Ten people per square mile may seem low by agricultural standards, but it is ten times the carrying capacity for typical hunter-gatherer groups even on good foraging grounds. Sherburne Cook estimated California's total indigenous population in 1542 at 310,000 +- 30,000 people. The acorn harvest around that time has been estimated at about 66,000 tons per year and acorns are thought to have formed as much as half the diet of many groups.

West Indies

At the confluence of the Caribbean Sea and the Western Atlantic Ocean there are three distinct island chains that comprise the West Indies: The Greater Antilles, The Lesser Antilles and The Bahama Archipelago, with a combined land mass of 90,339 square miles (233,976 square kilometers). The entire West Indies spans from Caicos Islands off the coast of Florida in North America, to the island of Trinidad off the north coast of Venezuela in South America.

The West Indies have a tropical maritime climate that is humid year round. Most of the islands experience wet and dry seasons with annual rainfall ranging from 30 to 80 inches (800 to 2,000 millimeters) but reaching more than 200 inches (5,000 millimeters) on the windward sides of the highest peaks. Violent tropical storms called hurricanes (named after the ancient Mayan weather god, Huracan) frequent the area between the months of August and October. Plentiful rainfall, rich soils, a highly variable geography and isolation from humans together made the West Indies island ecosystems exceptionally diverse in plant, fungal, and animal species. The first humans to arrive around 6,000 years ago quickly hunted the largest most vulnerable animals, the giant owl and dwarf ground sloth, into extinction, and later deforestation by the Europeans in the sixteenth and seventeenth centuries to clear land for western style agriculture so altered the natural landscape of the West Indies that today it is impossible to know how many species were destroyed in the onslaught.

The indigenous peoples of the West Indies had no written language so the pre-Columbian period of human colonization has been painstakingly pieced together from carbon dated archaeological remnants discovered on the various islands. The first people to migrate to the West Indies around 6,000 years ago were a group of hunter/gather/fishers called Casmiroids by present day archaeologists and ethnologists who came from the Central American country of Belize on the Yucatán Peninsula. The trade winds and the major ocean currents in the Caribbean generally favor east to west and north to south travel, however there is a phenomenon known as the Cuban countercurrent which is a west to east current south of Cuba, Hispaniola (present day Dominican Republic/Haiti) and Puerto Rico. The Casmiroids took advantage of this current to cross the approximately 125 miles of open water between Yucatán and Cuba known as the Yucatan Passage and later to cross the narrower Windward Passage between Cuba and Hispaniola.

Cuba and Hispaniola are the largest islands in the West Indies and as such had resources that were not available on the smaller islands. On these large islands the Casmiroids were able to survive in small hunter/gather/fishers groups much as their ancestors did on the mainland. The interior of the islands offered hunting and fresh water fishing, the forests and river valleys offered an abundance of wild fruits and vegetables, and sloths, manatees, crocodiles, waterfowl, land crabs and turtles in the mangrove swamps and river estuaries, offered an abundant supply of fish and other sea animals.

Beginning around 4.000 years ago, a second wave of hunter/gatherer/fishers, called the Ortoiroid migrated to the islands of the West Indies. They came from the Orinoco River Delta on the coast of present day Venezuela in South America. Off the coast of Venezuela's neighboring Guyana, the prevailing east to west ocean current is deflected north by the force of the Orinoco River flowing into the sea. The Ortoiroid used this current to travel northward throughout the Lesser Antilles and then followed the easterly trade winds all the way to the Virgin Islands. The Ortoiroid were a coastal people and their settlements were small and widely dispersed and they survived mainly on the resources provided by the sea. These early Ortoiroid settlers became isolated from their mainland roots and over the centuries developed their own distinct culture. By 3,000 years ago (1000 BC) they had reached the island of Puerto Rico where for the first time they encountered another culture, the Casmiroids, on the neighboring island of Hispaniola. The Mona Passage between Puerto Rico and Hispaniola served as a natural barrier separating the Ortoiroid and Casmiroid peoples. The two cultures existed independently until the arrival of a new third wave of immigrants around 2,500 years ago (500 BC).

These new immigrants came from the Arawak tribes of the Orinoco River Basin who were much more technically advanced than their Ortoiroid predecessors having developed terra preta agriculture, more sea worthy canoes and superior weapons. As they made their way north from Trinidad to St. John by around 20 AD, these newcomers easily defeated and replaced the existing population of Ortoiroid whose settlements were sparsely populated and widely dispersed. But when they crossed over the Mona Passage to Hispaniola the preexisting Casmeroid inhabitants possessed better weapons and had a larger population. The Casmeroid were able to defend their culture against the invaders and the two cultures remained in an uneasy stand off on the east coast of Hispaniola for centuries. By around 600 AD the descendants of the Arawak had developed their own distinct culture that was eventually able to expand into Hispaniola and integrate with the Casimiroid culture to create a new mixed culture called the Taino. It was the Taino people of the Greater Antilles who met Columbus upon his arrival in 1492 AD.

Journals kept by the first Europeans to arrive in the West Indies made note of the abundant food available to the Taino. The Taino did not use slash and burn agriculture common to other tropical cultures instead employing a system of mounded soil called *"conuncos."* Conuncos were approximately three feet high and four feet in diameter and laid out in rows to effectively aerate and drain the soil which greatly increased yields. The Taino also practiced crop rotation to keep the soil fertile. Yuca, also known as manioc, cassava or tapioca, and not to be confused with the desert yucca plant, was the staple crop and was so important to the survival of the people that the Taino communities themselves were called *"Yucayeques",* meaning the place where yuca is grown. Yuca is a tuberous root about two inches in diameter and ten inches long with a brown bark-like skin over a white flesh. Yuca produces more calories in the form of complex carbohydrates per unit of land than any other crop in the world. The leaves provide vitamins and some protein. The yuca root can stay in the ground for as long as three years without spoilage providing an easy and reliable means of storage during times of plenty and ready availability during times of need. The most common use of the yuca for the Taino was in the preparation of bread. The roots would be harvested, washed, peeled and grated. The juice would then be squeezed out and stored in a separate container. The remaining pulp was dried and sifted and cooked on an open fire into a cracker-like bread. The juice of the yuca contains many nutrients but is poisonous unless cooked or fermented so the Taino made large pots of boiled yuca juice to which they added seasonal vegetables, meat and fish. This recipe was the origin of the "pepper pot" which is still a traditional food in many parts of the West Indies. Taino farmers also planted sweet potato, beans, peppers, maize, peanuts, squash, pineapple, mamey apple and papaya while gathering wild plants such as palm nuts and guavas and zamia roots from the forests. The high humidity of the tropics made food storage difficult but the Taino constructed storage sheds built so that the interiors were kept in total darkness and packed them full of yuca bread, herbs and dried fish.

Taino villages were usually set up in coastal areas and river valleys where fishermen caught fish with nets, spears, hooks and lines and they also used poisons extracted from plants to stun fish so they could be easily gathered. The Taino hunted sea turtles and manatee and harvested conch, whelk, lobster, and crab. They used underwater pens made of reeds to store live fish and turtles for future consumption. On land, the larger animals had long since been hunted to extinction, but the Taino still hunted hutias (a squirrel like rodent), wild birds and lizards.

The Taíno lived in settlements called "*yucayeques*", which varied in size depending on the location. Those in Puerto Rico and Hispaniola were the largest, and those in the Bahamas were the smallest. Taíno society was divided into two classes: "*naborias*" (commoners) and "*nitaínos*" (nobles). They were governed by chiefs known as "*caciques*" who were male or female and advised by priests/healers known as "*bohiques.*" The commoners lived in large circular buildings that housed 10 to 15 families each constructed with wooden poles, woven straw, and palm leaves and were built around a central plaza. The cacique and his noble family lived in rectangular buildings of similar construction. Taíno home furnishings included cotton hammocks (*hamaca*), sleeping and sitting mats made of palms, wooden chairs with woven seats, platforms, and cradles for children. The Taino fabricated ceramic pottery, made tools and weapons out of shells and stone and carried on extensive trade between the islands and the South American mainland.

Around 1200 AD, nearly three hundred years before Columbus, another tribe of immigrants from the Orinoco River Basin in Venezuela called the Carib began to migrate into the Lesser Antilles. The Carib were skilled boat builders and sailors and archaeological evidence suggests that they displaced the existing Taino population in the Lesser Antilles by warfare, extermination, and assimilation.

Taino agriculture was so productive and sea animals so abundant that by the time of European contact in 1492, the West Indies had become one of the major population centers of the world. In his 1561 multi-volume *History of the Indies,* the Spanish priest, Bartolomé de las Casas, who was living in the Dominican Republic at the time, estimated the pre-Columbian population of the Greater Antilles at over three million people; professor emeritus of history at the University of California at Berkeley, Woodrow Borah, in the most detailed and methodologically sophisticated population estimates ever conducted for the pre-Columbian Western Hemisphere, estimated the population of Hispaniola alone, where Columbus first touched ground, at around eight million people.

Senior Demographer, Carl Haub, of the Population Reference Bureau, a leading demographic research institution, has estimated the total human population of the world 10,000 years ago, right before the beginning of the agricultural revolution, to be about 5 million people, all of whom were hunter/ gatherers. By 500 years ago (1500 AD), as a result of the agricultural revolution, the total human population had swollen to 425 million people, of which less than 2% (6 million) still earned their livings as hunter/ gatherers. As we have seen in the early civilizations examined above, most of the food calories consumed by these burgeoning masses of people came from grains and tubers, while meat, dairy and eggs were relatively minor sources of calories.

Each of these ancient civilizations from around the world developed under very different environmental circumstances, yet they were all bound by the same ecological constraint of having to obtain enough energy from food resources to insure their survival and long term growth. All of these early civilizations went through the same stages of development: first, human hunter/gatherers exceeded the carrying capacity of the land (1 person/square mile in the best hunting grounds) which led to prey animal resources being depleted which led to grain and tuber cultivation which led to massive population increases which led to stratified social structures.

Over the thousands of years that civilizations have come and gone, climate change has played an integral role in their fates. Times of favorable climate produced agricultural abundance which drove population increases, while times of unfavorable climate resulted in crop failures, famines and hostilities which drove population declines. In these modern times of rapid anthropogenic climate change, this is perhaps the most prophetic lesson we can learn from past civilizations.

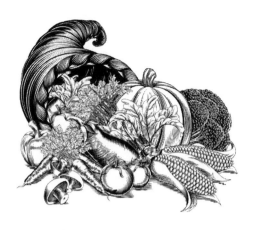

PART III

THE COLUMBIAN EXCHANGE

• • •

"Sharing food with another human being is an intimate act that should not be indulged in lightly."

– M.F.K. Fisher, food writer (1908 – 1992)

12
IMPACTS: OLD WORLD ON NEW WORLD

Anyone who examines human behaviors from an ecological and biological perspective, as I am attempting to do in this book, owes a great debt of gratitude to Professor Emeritus of History, Geography, and American Studies at the University of Texas at Austin, Dr. Alfred W. Crosby Jr., for his groundbreaking book, *"The Columbian Exchange"* first published in 1972. After many years of teaching history strictly in terms of social studies, Dr. Crosby finally came to the realization that human history was shaped more by ecology and biology than politics:

"Sometimes the more obvious a thing is the more difficult it is to see it. I [Dr. Crosby] am 80 years old [born in 1931], and for the first 40 or 50 years of my life, the Columbian Exchange simply didn't figure into history courses even at the finest universities. We were thinking politically and ideologically, but very rarely were historians thinking ecologically, biologically."

("Alfred W. Crosby on the Columbian Exchange: The historian discusses the ecological impact of Columbus' landing in 1492 on both the Old World and the New World"; Interview by Megan Gambino, Smithsonian.com, October 05, 2011)

Using contemporaneous sixteenth century texts written by early European colonists as his main source material and drawing on the early ecological work of the famed American Naturalist, Aldo Leopold (1887 – 1948), Dr. Crosby meticulously pieced together the critical impacts that the exchange of microbes, plants and animals had on both sides of the Atlantic beginning with the first voyage of Columbus in 1492 which united these long separated human and biotic populations. In the preface to the first edition of *The Columbian Exchange*, Dr. Crosby explains his ecological and biological approach to history:

"Nothing can be understood apart from its context, and man is no exception. He is a living entity, dependent on a number of other living entities for food, clothing and often shelter. Many living things are dependent upon him for the same. Man is a biological entity before he is a Roman Catholic or a capitalist or anything else. Moreover, man's history did not start when he first began to keep records, nor is it limited to only the aspects of his existence of interest to the literati. The first step to understanding man is to consider him as a biological entity which has existed on this globe, affecting, and being affected by, his fellow organisms, for many thousands of years.

"Once we have placed man in this proper spatial and temporal context, we can begin to examine single aspects of his history with assurance – or at least the hope – that the results will have a meaningful relationship to that context and will not merely send us off down the weedy little paths that lead from one antiquarian gazebo to another.

"Before the historian can judge wisely the political skills of human groups or the strength of their economies or the meaning of their literatures, he must first know how successful their member human beings were at staying alive and reproducing themselves. He must have some idea of how their efforts in accomplishing these tasks affected their environments. It is to the ecologist and not to the philatelist [stamp collector] that the historians should look for his model of scholarly virtue."

"Tradition has limited historians in their search for the true significance of the renewed contact between the Old and New Worlds. Even the economic historian may occasionally miss what any ecologist or geographer would find glaringly obvious after a cursory reading of the basic original sources of the sixteenth century: the important changes brought on by the Columbian voyages were biological in nature."

When *The Columbian Exchange* was first published in 1972, the magnitude of the devastation wrought by Old World microbes on New World indigenous peoples was little recognized by most traditional historians, and Dr. Crosby's book was generally panned by his peers. Today, after five decades of exhaustive research has revealed irrefutable evidence of mass die-offs of New World peoples, Dr. Crosby's *The Columbian Exchange* has become the standard historical text. Much of the following discussion on this clash of civilizations is based on Dr. Crosby's *The Columbian Exchange*.

The Microbe Exchange

European colonizers brought with them Old World microbes for which New World peoples had no natural immunities causing runaway disease epidemics that decimated indigenous populations everywhere the Europeans set foot:

West Indies

The first consequential European contact with the indigenous peoples of the Western Hemisphere was made by Italian fortune hunter Christopher Columbus in 1492 AD when sailing west for the Spanish crown, he happened upon the island of Hispaniola in the Caribbean Sea. Over the next decade Columbus made three more voyages to the Caribbean to exploit the natural and human resources of the Caribbean Islands for himself and his Spanish sponsor.

At the time Columbus arrived, the indigenous population has been estimated at around eight million people. At ground zero of first contact, of all the peoples of the Western Hemisphere, the "Indians" of the West Indies were the most vulnerable and hardest hit by the European invasion. Warfare, harsh enslavement, resettlement, and separation from families (the "encomienda" system of Spanish rule) all contributed to the dramatic decline of Taino culture only to be finished off by the first recorded smallpox epidemic on Hispaniola in 1518. According to Dr. David Stannard, Professor of American Studies at the University of Hawaii and author of "*American Holocaust*" (Oxford University Press, 1992):

> "*By 1496, we already have noted, the population of Hispaniola had fallen from eight million to between four and five million. By 1508 it was down to less than a hundred thousand. By 1518 it numbered less than twenty thousand. And by 1535, say the leading scholars on this grim topic, 'for all practical purposes, the native population was extinct.'*"

Rape of Taino women was common among the Spanish invaders and as a result, Taino DNA still survives among descendants in the region. The Taino genome project started in 1999 tested mitochondrial DNA of residents throughout the island of Puerto Rico and found that 62% of Puerto Ricans have direct-line maternal Taino ancestry.

The tenacious Carib on a few small islands of the Lesser Antilles managed to maintain autonomy from the Europeans into the 19th century, but eventually they too succumbed to the European invasion.

Mexico

In 1519 the Spanish conquistador, Hernán Cortés, landed on the Gulf Coast of Mexico with steel weapons, fire-arms, horses and approximately 1,000 of Spain's best conquistadors. Cortés quickly allied himself with enemies of the Aztec, the coastal Totonac and the more powerful inland Tlaxcalan, and in 1521 made his assault on the Aztec capitol of Tenochtitlan. By then, a small pox epidemic started on the coast by Cortés' men, had already spread inward and decimated the densely populated Aztec city in 1520, reducing its population by 40% in a single year. A Franciscan monk who accompanied Cortés wrote this gruesome description:

> "*As the Indians did not know the remedy of the disease, they died in heaps, like bedbugs. In many places it happened that everyone in a house died, and as it was impossible to bury the great number of dead, they pulled down the houses over them, so that their homes became their tombs.*"

Over the next 100 years, due to waves of disease epidemics and farmland destruction, the indigenous population of Mesoamerica plummeted. According to leading authority on the demography of ancient Mexico, historian Dr. Woodrow Borah, of the University of California, Berkeley, by 1620 the Aztec population had dwindled to less than one million people, a 95% drop from its peak of 25 million.

Peru

Francisco Pizarro was a Spanish soldier of fortune who had heard of great riches in the New World from tales of earlier explorations by Columbus and Cortés. In 1526, only 34 years after Columbus first landed on the island of Hispaniola in the Caribbean, Pizzaro set sail across the Atlantic to see for himself. After a second trip in 1529, where he encountered the incalculable wealth of the Inca civilization on the

Pacific side of South America, he returned to Spain and convinced the king to finance the conquest of the Inca Empire and to appoint him as viceroy of a new Spanish colony.

When Pizarro returned to conquer Peru in 1532, he found the Inca state in turmoil. A civil war had broken-out between two claimants to the throne, political unrest was festering in the newly conquered territories and perhaps most devastatingly of all, a smallpox epidemic that began to spread from the Columbus expedition of 1498 had moved swiftly through vulnerable native American populations lacking immunity in Panama and Columbia to infect the Andes where it wiped-out as many as half the indigenous population. With just a tiny force of 168 men, 1 cannon and 27 horses, Pizarro used his considerable audacity and cunning to entrap and execute the Inca who had just weeks before defeated his rival in the civil war. This unimaginable turn of events so confused the Inca federalist top down system of governance that it fell into a state of political turmoil and quickly collapsed. Pizarro then adroitly allied himself with the local leaders of the Inca's enemies to establish the new Spanish colony.

The first 40 years of Spanish rule were absolutely catastrophic to the Inca civilization. The Spanish worked them to death in silver mines, destroyed their elaborate irrigation systems causing mass starvation, and started succeeding epidemics of typhus, influenza and a return of smallpox that wiped-out millions more. The Spanish chronicler, Pedro de Cieza de Leon, who traveled Peru extensively during this period, wrote this telling account of a depopulated valley on the coast near present day Lima:

> *"The inhabitants of this valley were so numerous that many Spaniards say that when it was conquered by [Pizarro]... there were ... more than 25,000 men, and I doubt that there are now 5,000, so many have been the inroads and hardships they have suffered."*

Using colonial death records, Dr. Henry Dobyns, University of Arizona anthropologist, ethnohistorian and leading demographer of the Western Hemisphere, has estimated that by 1570 the indigenous population of the Andes region had declined by 93% to around 2.7 million people.

Amazonia

In 1500, only eight years after Columbus's first voyage, Pedro Álvares Cabral, a Portuguese military commander, was commissioned by the King of Portugal to lead an expedition to India following Vasco da Gama's newly opened sea route around Africa. The object of the undertaking was to return with valuable spices and to establish trade relations in India bypassing the monopoly on the spice trade then controlled by Ottoman and Venetian merchants.

Cabral's fleet of 13 ships sailed far into the Western Atlantic Ocean where he made landfall at Porto Seguro in what is now the state of Bahia in present day Brazil. Cabral claimed this new land for the Portuguese Crown. The Portuguese happened to arrive at a time of political turmoil in Amazonia. A mass migration was shifting the population from the south to the coastal regions displacing the residents many of whom moved to the interior. This population shift triggered continuous warfare involving battles that arrayed hundreds and sometimes thousands of warriors in fierce hand-to-hand combat. This struggle over land was politically driven by personal vendettas between tribal Chieftains and the Portuguese adroitly used these vendettas to keep the warring Amazonian tribes from uniting against them and also to obtain slaves.

The Portuguese conquest of Amazonia was not as simple as the toppling of organized empires like the Inca or Aztec, but a drawn out, complicated process that spread over huge distances, many different tribes, and three centuries of time. Also unlike the Spanish whose mission was to spread Christianity among the indigenous population, the Portuguese colony was purely an economic endeavor to obtain natural resources.

After the Spanish Captain, Francisco de Orellana, had accidentally navigated the Amazon River from the Andes end in 1542, the Spanish built numerous missions in the interior of the Amazon basin and over the next two centuries there was competition and conflict between the Portuguese and the Spaniards over control of these territories. Meanwhile, between the enslavement of the indigenous peoples to mine the exotic resources of the tropics, and the exotic European diseases of smallpox, measles, tuberculosis, typhoid, dysentery, and influenza for which the indigenous people had no immunities, the human population of the Amazon plummeted. By the time French geographer, Charles Marie de la Condamine, traveled the Amazon to create the first map of the region based on astronomical observations in 1743, he described a land where isolated bands of people lived as subsistence foragers (Smith 1990). Professor Emeritus of Geography and Environmental Studies at the University of Wisconsin-Madison, Dr. William Deneven, estimates the population collapse in Amazonia at over 90% down to less than one million people (Denevan 1976).

North America

The first European exploration of the North Atlantic coastline of North America was by Italian Giovanni Caboto (John Cabot) who sailed to Newfoundland in 1497, just five years after Christopher Columbus made first European contact in the Caribbean. Cabot was quickly followed by João Vaz Corte-Real in 1500, who first sailed the South Atlantic coastline. A long procession of Spaniards followed with Juan Ponce de León who claimed Florida on the North American continent for the Spanish crown in 1513; Álvarez de Pineda who explored the Gulf Coast to the mouth of the Mississippi River in 1519; Lucas Vázquez de Ayllón who attempted to start a colony on the Atlantic coast of South Carolina in 1526 but was repelled by the indigenous people; Pánfilo de Narváez who attempted to colonize Florida for Spain in 1527 but was also repelled by the natives.

In 1539, Spanish conquistador Hernando de Soto led an expedition through Florida, Georgia, South Carolina, North Carolina, Tennessee, Alabama, Mississippi, Arkansas and Texas to become the first European to explore the interior of the continent and to cross the Mississippi River. By the time of de Soto's exploration nearly fifty years after Columbus's first voyage, Spanish treachery and disease had yet to arrive and one of de Soto's officers noted in his journal:

"The land was very populous and had many large towns and planted fields which reached from one town to the other. It was a charming and fertile land, and grapes along the river on vines climbing up into the trees."

"The next day they went to a palisaded town, and messengers from Mabila came who brought... much chestnut bread, for there are many and good chestnuts in his land." (Translated by James Robertson, Florida State Historical Society – Deland 1933)

Dr. Dobyns estimated the population of Florida at 900,000 people at time of first European contact (*Their Number Become Thinned*, pg 294).

In 1565 Spanish conquistador Pedro Menendez de Aviles, noted for his particularly harsh brand of brutality against the indigenous people, finally succeeded in establishing the first permanent Spanish settlement on the North American continent at what is present day St. Augustine, in northeastern Florida.

Fast in the wake of the Spanish invasion of North America from the south, came the French invasion from the north. In 1524 Italian Giovanni de Verrazano sailing for France explored the north coast of North America from the Hudson River to Nova Scotia, and in 1535 Frenchman Jacques Cartier sailed up the St. Lawrence River as far as present day Quebec and Montreal. Cartier made three voyages down the St. Lawrence River and everywhere he journeyed he found people and villages. At one village he called "Hochelaga" near present day Montreal, he noted that *"...goodly and large fields full of corn such as the country yieldeth"* suggesting that a maize based agriculture supported a large indigenous population. The French, unlike the Spanish, were not in search of gold, but of animal furs, and rather than establish slave colonies to exploit this resource, they developed a trade relationship with the indigenous peoples.

This relatively limited French presence of only a few small outlying trading posts lasted for a little over 70 years until the third voyage of Samuel de Champlain in 1608. Champlain established a small settlement near present day Québec where he managed to forge a political alliance with the Algonquin and Huron tribes and participated with them in raids against their traditional enemy, the Iroquois. Using firearms Champlain succeeded in killing two Iroquois chiefs further ingratiating himself to the Algonquin and Huron even as a small pox epidemic introduced by the French was culling the indigenous population by half. By the 18th century, a weakened Iroquois Federation allied itself with the British in the American Revolution of 1776, and after their defeat, the British ceded Iroquois territory over to the Americans forcing many Iroquois to abandon their lands in the Mohawk Valley and elsewhere and move to the north on lands still retained by the British.

Subsequent French explorers continued pushing farther west down the St. Lawrence River into the Great Lakes region and then south into the Mississippi River Basin. In 1682 René-Robert Cavelier, Sieur de La Salle finally navigated all the way down to the mouth of the Mississippi River claiming its entire length in the name of France. La Salle was the first European since de Soto in 1539 to have traveled this area of the Southeastern United States. Where de Soto found burgeoning populations of settled indigenous peoples, La Salle described a land lightly populated by small tribes of semi-nomadic agriculturalists. In the intervening 143 years between de Soto and La Salle, waves of disease epidemics introduced by the earlier Spanish explorers had decimated most of the indigenous population of the once thriving Mississippian Culture. Dr. Dobyns has estimated the pre-Columbian population of indigenous people in North America from the Great Lakes region south to Tennessee at around four million. Dr. Dobyns further estimated that post-Columbus European introduced disease epidemics ultimately reduced that population by 95% down to around 200,000 (*"Their number become thinned: native American population dynamics in eastern North America", Henry Dobyns, 1983).*

Throughout the 16th century, English, French, Italian, Spanish, and Portuguese mariners were regularly plying the coastline of Newfoundland, Nova Scotia and New England, fishing for cod and occasionally trading with the inhabitants and kidnapping them for slaves. The English fished from small boats close to shore and processed the fish onshore before sailing back to England, while the other Europeans fished and processed aboard their ships at sea not bothering to make landfall. In 1605 Frenchman Samuel de Champlain explored the New England coast making a detailed map of the coastline and describing thriving coastal settlements. But by the time the English Pilgrims landed at Plymouth Rock, Massachusetts in 1620, most of the indigenous people were dead. William Bradford, the first governor of Plymouth Colony wrote, *"died on heapes, as they lay in their houses,"* and the English trader Thomas Morton noted. *"And the bones and skulls upon the severall places of their habitations made such a spectacle."* Archaeologists Arthur Spiess of the Maine Historic Preservation Commission has postulated that an epidemic of viral hepatitis contracted from European traders had wiped out 90% of the indigenous population of coastal New England.

English Captain, John Smith, established the first permanent English colony in North America at Jamestown, Virginia in 1607 with 104 men. Estimates vary of the pre-invasion population of the local Powhatan Indians; one based on Smith's record of about 200 river villages with an estimated forty to fifty per village suggested a population of roughly 8,000 to 10,000 people. A tree ring analysis of 800-year-old bald cypress trees in the area (David Stahle, 1985), indicated that the worst drought in 700 years occurred between 1606 and 1612, so the Powhatan were likely in a weakened state when the English arrived. Less than a century later, epidemics of small pox and measles had devastated the Powhatan. According to sociologist, Dr. Gabrielle Tayac, in her research paper, *"We Have a Story to Tell: Native Peoples of the Chesapeake"* (2006), by 1700 the Powhatan population had decreased by more than 90%:

> *"Although it is difficult to obtain precise population figures, scholars estimate that the Powhatan Chiefdom included about 12,000 people when Jamestown was settled in 1607. Only 1,000 were left by 1700."*

Oasisamerica

The first recorded European contact with the Pueblo of Southwestern North America was by an expeditionary force dispatched by Spanish explorer Francisco Vasquez de Coronado in 1540 during a particularly cold snap of the Little Ice Age. The Spaniards recorded finding four Hopi villages of from 1,500 to 3,000 residents along the Rio Grande River basin whom to this day claim to be direct descendants of the ancestral Pueblo people. At the time of this Spanish intrusion much of the larger Four Corners area had been taken over by the semi-nomadic, hunter/gatherer/gardener, "Hogan" dwelling, Navajo people who had migrated south from the even colder climate of the far north. While the Spaniards made a few attempts to subdue and Christianize the Hopi in the 16th and 17th centuries, ultimately this desert region held little economic promise for the Spanish to expend significant military resources, and the Hopi were able to resist ever succumbing to the Spanish conquest.

Pacific Coast

On the second circumnavigation of the globe in 1579, English explorer, Sir Francis Drake, briefly made landfall on the central California coast, and in 1602 Spanish explorer Sebastián Vizcaíno sailed the California coastline as far north as Monterey Bay, but throughout the 17th and first half of the 18th centuries the English and Spanish were too preoccupied with their colonial aspirations elsewhere to devote resources to the colonization of California. It wasn't until the threat of incursion by Russian fur traders moving down the coast from Alaska in 1765 that Spain began to establish a series of 21 "Missions" along the California coast as far north as the San Francisco Bay.

Run by the Catholic Franciscan Order and protected by Spanish military forces, the Spanish Missions subjugated the indigenous people to Christianity and introduced European livestock, fruits, vegetables, cattle, horses and ranching into the California region. According to Barry Pritzker, author of "*A Native American Encyclopedia: History, Culture, and Peoples*" (*Oxford University Press*, 2000), the Spanish also introduced epidemics of European diseases such as malaria and smallpox that reduced the indigenous human population of California over the next hundred years down to approximately 15,000 people by the end of the 19th Century.

In 1775 the Spanish made a sailing expedition from the west coast of Mexico to the Northwest Coast of North America going ashore and making contact with indigenous people in Northern California, Washington and Alaska. Soon thereafter a smallpox epidemic broke out among the indigenous populations of the Northwest that University of Washington anthropologist, Dr. Robert Boyd, believes was introduced by the Spaniards. Throughout the next century, epidemics of small pox, influenza, measles and tuberculosis would decimate the indigenous population of the Pacific Northwest. In a study of the census data available from that time Dr. Boyd estimated that as a result of these multiple epidemics the indigenous population of the northwest plummeted from a peak of about 180,000 people down to a nadir of 35,000 at the end of the 19th Century. (*The Coming of the Spirit of Pestilence by Robert Boyd, 1999*)

In 1831, English naturalist Charles Darwin set sail on an expedition to map the South American coastline and to carry out chronometer surveys all over the globe. In his chronicle of that journey, *"The Voyage of the Beagle"* (1839), he wrote:

> *"Wherever the European had trod, death seems to pursue the aboriginal. We may look to the wide extent of the Americas, Polynesia, the Cape of Good Hope, and Australia, and we find the same result."*

In his book *"American Holocaust,"* Dr. David Stannard, Professor of American Studies at the University of Hawaii, argues that the European colonization of the Americas after 1492 was the largest genocide in world history. From his methodical research, Dr. Stannard concluded that indigenous peoples of the Americas had undergone the, *"... worst human holocaust the world had ever witnessed, roaring across two continents non-stop for four centuries and consuming the lives of countless tens of millions of people."* Largely due to disease epidemics, Dr. Stannard estimated that almost 100 million people died in the American Holocaust.

The Animal Exchange

Simultaneously with this precipitous decline in the indigenous human population of the Western Hemisphere was a meteoric rise in the population of Old World domesticated animal species introduced to the New World by the European colonists. Dr. Crosby describes this species exchange:

> *"A sensational preview of the impact that Old World livestock would have on the American mainland took place in Espanola and, shortly after, in the other Antilles. One who watched the Caribbean islands from outer space during the years from 1492 to 1550 or so might have surmised that the object of the game going on there was to replace the people with pigs, dogs and cattle. Disease and ruthless exploitation had, for all practical purposes, destroyed the aborigines of Espanola by the 1520s. ...Thus, within a few score years of Columbus's first American landfall, the Antillean aborigines had been almost completely eliminated."*

> *"As the number of humans plummeted, the population of imported domestic animals shot upward. The first contingent of horses, dogs, pigs, cattle, chickens, sheep, and goats arrived with Columbus on the second voyage in 1493. The animals, preyed upon by few or no American predators, troubled by few or no American diseases, and left to feed freely upon the rich grasses and roots and wild fruits, reproduced rapidly. Their numbers burgeoned so rapidly, in fact, that doubtlessly they had much to do with the extinction of certain plants, animals, and even the Indians themselves, whose gardens were encroached upon."* (pg 75)

Dr. Crosby sums up the impacts of larger Old World animals on the dense population centers of the native farming cultures:

> *"By and large, the bigger domesticated animals of the Europeans destroyed rather than enriched the Indians of these areas controlled by the Europeans. The spectacular rise in the population of domesticated animals in these areas was accompanied by an equally spectacular decline in the Indian population; and disease and exploitation do not entirely explain that decline. The Indians were losing out in the biological competition with the newly imported livestock. The people of the high Indian civilization chiefly lived on a vegetable diet, and so anything radically affecting their croplands radically affected them. The Spanish, anxious to establish their pastoral Iberian [Spanish] way of life in their colonies, set aside large sections of land for grazing, a good deal of it land that Indians had formerly cultivate. And the livestock, in this new continent where fences and shepherds were so few, often strayed onto Indian fields, eating the plants and trampling them. As New Spain's first viceroy, Mendoza wrote to his King about the state of affairs around Oaxaca: 'May your Lordship realize that if cattle are allowed, the Indians will be destroyed.' Many Indians went malnourished, weakening their resistance to disease; many fled to the hills and deserts to face hunger in solitude; some simply lay down and died within the sound of the lowing of their rivals. The history of this phenomenon is clear in Mexico, and we have good reason to believe that parallels are to be found elsewhere in the Americas." (The Columbian Exchange, Pg 98-99)*

According to Dr. W.M.S. Russell, founding member of the Department of Sociology at the University of Reading, UK, and a leading researcher on animal agriculture along with his research associate and wife Claire Russell, the decline in the Aztec population of Mexico was not primarily due to epidemic diseases introduced by the Spanish as generally thought, but by the introduction of European domesticated livestock:

> *"... Cortés was himself responsible for the supreme demographic catastrophe, by beginning the import of worse enemies than smallpox – sheep and cattle. Between 1520 and 1620, the Spanish authorities made land grants in Mexico of 44,000 square kilometres for cattle ranches and 31,000 square kilometres for sheep farms, to be stocked at 28 cattle and 257 sheep per square kilometre. The animals roamed freely over native croplands. By 1620, overgrazing had turned large areas to wilderness and caused widespread erosion and valley floods. This drastic decline in land productivity was probably the most important factor of all in the population crash." ("Population Crises and Population Cycles, 9. Central Mexico and the Andes to the Conquests", The Galton Institute, 1997)*

Pigs, sheep, cattle and horses were the primary species the Europeans stocked in the New World. Let's take a closer look at each:

Pigs

During the first two decades of Spanish colonization, the very adaptable pig was the most important food animal imported by the conquistadors. The Spanish pigs were neither like the small peccary native to the Americas, nor the fat slow-footed hog we are familiar with today, but a fast, tough, lean, animal much closer in appearance and personality to a wild boar. The Spanish pigs took up little room aboard ship, survived the long sea passage well, and reproduced prolifically in wet, tropical lowlands and dry mountains alike making them the ideal ambulatory meat supply for the marauding conquistadors. The Spanish bred pigs freely on the islands of the West Indies.

In 1514 Diego Velasquez de Cuellar wrote the King that the pigs he had brought to Cuba had increased to 30,000. Large numbers of pigs also accompanied the conquistadors on their continental exploits. Francisco Pizarro brought pigs to Peru in 1531, and pig meat was the first European meat to be sold in quantity in the Lima meat market. In 1540 Gonzalo Pizarro took more than 2,000 pigs on his expedition in search of the Land of Cinnamon on the east side of the Andes. Hernando de Soto brought 13 pigs with him to Florida in 1539 and using them sparingly for food only in cases of emergency, had 700 only three years later.

Herds of pigs could be found wherever the Spanish settled and the same is true of the Portuguese. The coastal environment of Brazil was not conducive to raising cattle, but the pig thrived on these poor pastures. In the captaincies of Rio de Janeiro and Sao Paulo, pig meat became a major item in the early colonial diet. The Western Hemisphere was so favorable to the Spanish pigs that in many areas they took up an independent existence running wild. By the end of the first decade after the conquest of Mexico, pigs were so plentiful and cheap that stockmen no longer raised them.

Sheep

Sheep were the most common animal herded in Renaissance Spain prized for their wool and meat. The Spanish crown saw in the New World vast sheep grazing potential and Columbus brought the first sheep to the Western Hemisphere on his second voyage in 1493 to start propagation immediately. But unlike pigs, sheep did not do well in the tropical West Indies or in the hot, wet lowlands of Central America and they were much slower to adapt to the New World than pigs. Sheep were not capable of defending themselves against predators requiring the constant watchful eye of shepherds and they could not breed by themselves in the wilderness like pigs which slowed their population growth. A few sheep managed to eke out an existence in the hot Antilles in the early 16th century and as soon as the Aztec resistance was broken in central Mexico in 1521, Hernán Cortés sent back to the Antilles for sheep and other livestock. But it wasn't until 1535 when Antonio de Mendoza, first viceroy of New Spain, imported fine Spanish Merino sheep that their numbers began to increase in central Mexico.

By 1582 it was estimated that 200,000 sheep were grazing on the range just north of San Juan de los Rios in central Mexico which soon gave rise to seasonal migrations where hundreds of thousands of sheep were herded from Queretaro to Lake Chapala and western Michoacan every September, and back again in May, following a sea of grass. Most of the early sheep herding by the Spanish was concentrated in central Mexico with a few ranches as far north as New Mexico in North America. Peru was also a land where sheep could thrive. Sheep were grazed everywhere there was grass, a temperate climate and access to market. Near the end of the 16th century the Spanish Jesuit missionary, Jose de Acosta, wrote of herds in Peru as large as 100,000 sheep. Other areas of South America that favored sheep herding were New Granada in the Andean foothills and highlands and the Portuguese colonies of Rio de Janeiro and Sau Paulo in Brazil. Sheep did exceedingly well in Chile; by1614 the district of Santiago alone contained over 600,000 sheep producing over 200,000 lambs a year. Sheep herding had begun in northern Argentina by 1600 and eventually in Patagonia which later would become one of the chief sheep-herding centers of the Western Hemisphere.

While sheep thrived in the Western Hemisphere in areas where the grass was lush and the climate temperate, they had a decidedly dampening effect on populations of native species as Dr. Crosby explains:

> *"The effect of the sheep and other European livestock on the native herds was not so delightful. The European animals doubtlessly transmitted to the native stock a devastating selection of animal diseases. The llama and alpaca populations diminished as spectacularly as the Indian populations after the conquest; and the reason was largely the same: disease and brutal exploitation."* (*The Columbian Exchange,* Pg. 94)

Cattle

At the time of Columbus's first voyage, Southern Spain was the only part of Western Europe where open range cattle ranching was common. This ranching technique with its dependence on horses, periodic round-ups, branding, and overland drives was perfected by medieval Spanish ranchers. These Spanish *vaqueros* (cowboys) were also experienced in dealing with a frontier threatened by the constant raiding of mounted Moorish enemies; there was no group of Europeans better prepared to deal with the challenges of the New World environment than the vaqueros of southern Spain.

Spanish cattle were carefully bred to be fast, lean and adaptable to varied climates making them fit for long cattle drives that followed the seasonal grasslands and they were armored with long horns for self-defense against predators. The Spanish longhorn was ideally suited for the vast grasslands of the Americas. And for many thousands of years before Columbus, the grasslands of the Americas had grown unchecked by the long extinct herbivorous mammoths, mastodons, sloths, horses and camels. The three greatest of these boundless grasslands in the Western Hemisphere were the prairies of Canada, U.S.A., and Mexico, the llanos of Venezuela and Columbia, and the pampas of Brazil, Argentina and Uruguay.

For the first time in history, by connecting the Old World with the New World, Columbus's voyage of 1492 brought these three critical elements – the horseman, the cattle and the pasture – together, resulting in a biological explosion. The Spaniards went on to embrace the immense grasslands of the Americas, driving their cattle onto them and so multiplying their herds that by the 17th century there were probably more cattle in the New World than any other species of European domesticated animal.

The first cattle in the New World were brought to the Greater Antilles by Columbus in 1493 and by the 1520s Gonzalo Fernández de Oviedo (1478-1557), who wrote the first comprehensive history of Spanish America, (the *Historia general y natural de las Indias*), spoke of herds as large as 8,000. In Spain the biggest herds rarely exceeded 1,000. Cattle hides along with sugar became the chief export of Hispaniola. In the 1560s Hispaniola's income from sugar amounted to about 640,000 pesos annually, and 720,000 pesos from hides.

Cattle were first brought to Mexico for breeding in 1521 and for the first years they lagged behind pigs and sheep in propagation, but after a few decades left them both in the dust. Within a decade there were scores of cattle ranches and by 1568 a traveler recorded over 2,000 were being driven through the town of Vera Cruz every morning. As the European population of Mexico spread north, ranching went along with it. The penetration of Spanish cattle into the rich grass country of northern Mexico in the 16th century set off one of the most biologically extravagant events of all time. In 1579 it was stated that some ranches in the north had 150,000 head of cattle and that 20,000 was considered a small herd. Two ranches on the present day border of Zacatecas and Durango branded 33,000 and 42,000 calves respectively in 1586. According to one witness in 1594 the cattle herds were nearly doubling every fifteen months. At the end of that century Frenchman Samuel de Champlain, on a tour of Mexico for the French king, wrote with awe of the *"great, level plains, stretching endlessly and everywhere covered with an infinite number of cattle."* There were so many cattle that they began to go feral roaming the countryside far beyond the colonists' horizons; their spread north only being checked by the massive herds of buffalo on The Great Plains of North America. When the Spanish began to settle in southern Texas in the early 18th century, they discovered the wild cattle were there before them. These were the Spanish ancestors of the famous Texas longhorns. The English-speaking colonists who moved into Texas in the early 19th century considered these wild cattle as native to the land.

The llanos of Venezuela and Columbia is a great expanse of flat grassland six hundred miles east to west and two hundred miles north to south. The temperature is hotter on average than on the plains of Spain, and the climate is a yearly cycle of drought and flood, but the grass lured the Spaniards anyway. The first Spanish stockmen to pass through the llanos in 1548 were bound for Bogota but it wasn't until the latter half of the century that native resistance had been broken by disease and force of arms that the llanos became open for full exploitation. By 1600, as many as forty-five ranches had been founded on the plains of Venezuela and only half a century later 140,000 head of cattle grazed the llanos. As in Mexico, the cattle tended to move ahead of the stockmen, being quicker to adapt than their owners. Sometimes these "strays" were driven along by slaves imported from Africa who had been brought to Venezuela to replace the dying natives as servants of the Spanish, and who, like the cattle, moved beyond the frontier to escape their captors. The 16th century was a period of bare beginnings, but the time would come two centuries later when cattle on the llanos, domesticated and feral, would number in the millions, and individual ranches would brand ten thousand or more annually. Export of hides to Spain took a prominent place in the economy of colonial Venezuela and from 1620 to 1665 hides accounted for 75% of the total value of exports to Spain.

The pampas of Brazil, Argentina and Uruguay are fertile grassy lowlands with a temperate climate watered by numerous tributaries of the Rio de la Plata River emptying into the South Atlantic at present day Buenos Aires, Argentina. The pampas covers more than 289,577 square miles (750,000 km^2) including the southernmost portion of Brazil, most of Uruguay, and parts of eastern Argentina. Cattle were first brought to the pampas by Spanish conquistadors in 1536 and they multiplied rapidly. By 1619, Governor Gondra of Buenos Aires noted that the number of cattle within the area under his jurisdiction was so great that if 80,000 a year were killed for their hides, natural increase would be sufficient to make up the loss. The herds continued to expand and spread south toward Patagonia. Eyewitness accounts of the cattle herds on the pampas are reminiscent of early accounts of the thunderous herds of wild bison on the North American prairie. Spanish Brigadier General Felix de Azara (1746-1821) explored the region from 1781 to 1801 making extensive field notes of his observations in which he estimated the number of wild cattle in the pampas at an astounding 48 million. Trade in hides, already of some importance by the beginning of the 17th century, accounted for the export of a million hides annually by the end of the 18th century.

There were other areas of South America with grasslands enough to support herds of cattle, though none as spectacularly as the llanos or the pampas. Cattle were brought to Peru by 1539 with herds scattered here and there, wherever the grass was plentiful in the mountains. Cattle spread south from Peru into Chile where they propagated rapidly. In 1614 the residents of Santiago possessed 39,250 head, of which the annual increase was 13,500. Cattle took slowly to the tropical climate of Brazil but by 1590 colonists moving inland from the coastal area of Bahia broke the back of native resistance and soon herds of cattle browsed its grasslands. These back country cattlemen supplied oxen for the sugar plantations that were sprouting laterally along the coast. The oxen supplied the muscle power to haul sugar cane to mills and turn millstones to crush the cane. As the native population declined oxen were also needed to plow the land for food crops. Oxen could pull a plow through thick soil which had always been too heavy for native digging sticks, opening up whole new areas for agriculture that were formerly left fallow. European agricultural use of oxen and plow had a much bigger impact on the natural environment than did the hand tool gardening of native agriculture. As Dr. Crosby notes:

> *"Cultivation of the soil with a plow is much more apt to lead to erosion and destruction of the soil than cultivation with a hoe or digging stick. It is quite likely that soil erosion in the New World accelerated after the arrival of the Europeans. As the number of sedentary Indian*

farmers increased over the centuries in the areas of the high pre-Columbian civilizations, erosion also increased, but not with such rapidity. The Indians did not have the plow, and, more important, their animals were rarely so numerous as to destroy the groundcover." Pg 110

Horses

While horses were never a food animal for the Spaniards, they did play a crucial role in subduing the indigenous peoples of the New World and in the cattle trade that followed. It was the horse that made possible the great cattle industry which, in the final analysis, affected a much larger portion of the New World than did any other European endeavor in that period. A swineherd and even a shepherd could operate effectively on foot, but a *vaquero* (cowboy) needed a horse.

The Spanish conquistadors came from the most equestrian society in Europe. Medieval Spain was the one area of Western Europe where horses were so plentiful and cheap that they were not the exclusive domain of the nobility. Spaniards from all classes were more skilled as riders than any other people along the European Atlantic seaboard. The Spanish horses were the result of crossbreeding between the strong fast horses of Spain and the refined well mannered Arabians brought in by the Moors; the offspring were the finest horses in Europe.

The first horses in the Western Hemisphere since the end of the Paleolithic some 12,000 years ago came with Columbus in 1493. The transatlantic crossing was hard on horses; the sea lane between Spain and the Canary Islands, where most early expeditions stopped on their way to the Americas, was named the *Gulfo de Yeguas*, the Gulf of Mares, and the windless seas of the Atlantic tropics were named the Horse Latitudes because so many horses died and had to be thrown overboard in these areas. But the Spaniards knew the key to their success in conquering the New World was the horse, so stow them they did, and by 1503 Hispaniola had a stock of around seventy horses.

Columbus used the horse to great effect against the Taino as did Cortes against the Aztec and Pizarro against the Inca subduing indigenous populations that outnumbered them by the millions, though in the final analysis it was microbes, cattle and sheep, not horses, that won the day. After the conquest, horses played a major role in keeping the enslaved natives under control.

The horse was slower than the pig to adapt to the tropical climate of the Greater Antilles but their numbers did increase and a few even joined the ranks of feral pigs as free agents. But it was not until the Spanish frontier reached the great grasslands of the New World that the vast herds of horses celebrated in American legend came onto the historical scene. The area first settled and exploited by the Spanish in Central America was the coast and highlands in the general latitude of Mexico City. Large sections of this area offered good grazing for livestock. As of 1531 central Mexico was raising fewer than 200 horses a year but then the Spanish frontier expanded northward to the plains where predators were few and grass plentifull, and by 1550 horses were available for little more than the roping. Within a few years 10,000 were grazing in the pasture lands between Queretaro and San Juan del Rio alone. As the opening of new mines drew the Spaniards further northward, the increase in the number of horses reached the magnitude of a stampede. By the end of the century wild horses beyond counting were running free in Durango. With mounts so plentiful everyone, even the natives were saddling up.

The wild horses continued moving north with only the driest deserts, the snows of Canada, and the eastern woodlands stopping their advance. In 1777 Franciscan friar Fray Morfi wrote that the area between the Rio Grand and the Nueces River in southern Texas was so full of horses *that their trails make the country, utterly uninhabited by people, look as if it were the most populated in the world.* The wild horses never attained such large numbers north of the Nueces in present day United States and Canada, but they ranged widely preceding the westward movement of the English settlers onto the Great Plains providing them and the North American Indians with their mounts.

In South America, the horse was slow to adapt to the hot humid llanos of Venezuela and the tropical climate of Brazil though they did manage to breed enough to supply the vaqueros with mounts to herd their cattle. The horse first arrived in Peru with Pizarro in 1532 and took well to the rich pasture lands around Cuzco and Quito. Within a few years the conquistadors and their mounts moved south into Chile, which by the beginning of the 17th century had become famous for its fine horses. Around this time the first settlers in Paraguay on the east side of the Andes began breeding horses which soon propagated into herds of wild horses. But by far the greatest breeding success story in the Western Hemisphere if not in the entire history of life on Earth was that of the horse in the pampas of Argentina and Uruguay. The first permanent settlers of Buenos Aires at the mouth of the Rio de la Plata arrived in 1580 and found that they had been preceded onto the pampas by enormous herds of wild horses. While it is not known exactly where they came from, it seems most likely that wild horses from Paraguay drifted southward following rivers of grass leading down into the pampas, or that wild horses from Chile found their way through Andean mountain passes. At the beginning of the 17th century the Spanish monk Vazquez de Espinosa wrote of wild horses in the Argentine pampas, *"... in such numbers that they cover the face of the earth and when they cross the road it is necessary for travelers to wait and let them pass, for a whole day or more..."* He wrote in awe of the plains of Buenos Aires being *"covered with escaped mares and horses in such numbers that when they go anywhere they look like woods from a distance."*

These enormous herds of horses, cattle and sheep that the Europeans fostered in the New World did not arise without impacting the environment on a grand scale. Again Dr. Crosby explains:

> *"The European's animals were an even worse threat to the land than the plow, because the plow usually stayed in comparatively level land, where the danger of erosion was not immediate, but horses, cattle, sheep and goats climbed the slopes and destroyed the fragile network of plants and their roots just where the danger of erosion was the greatest. Arroyos and barrancas began to scar the slopes, and trees encroached on the denuded savannas, and the weeds and coarser grasses spread in the steppes. The Europeans and their animals changed the rules of the battle for survival of the fittest.*

"Over a period of generations the civilization of the Americas had accumulated immense treasures of gold and silver, which the conquistadors squandered in a few years. Over the millennia the grasslands of America had been accumulating immense riches in loam, plant and animal life, visible and invisible organisms. The squandering of those riches was already evident in the lifetime of Las Casas [1484 – 1566]. He remarked that there had been a palatable grass, a fine thatch, which he had known as a young man in Española [Hispaniola], but which had disappeared – destroyed, he guessed, by the rapidly increasing livestock herds. In the 1570s López de Velasco remarked that the pastures of that island were diminishing in size as the guava trees encroached along their edges. The disappearance of the Arawak farmers, who had worked constantly to keep the jungle out of their gardens, was probably also a factor in this case. By the 1580s overgrazing in Mexico was becoming apparent, and Father Alonso Ponce saw cattle starving in certain areas. Today the presence of large numbers of palmettos or scrub palms in the regions of Mexico where sheep once grazed in open grasslands is probably due to the fact that the sheep destroyed the other, more palatable plants. Cattle do not crop their grass quite so closely as sheep, but when kept in large herds they have a deleterious effect on the land. The coastal savanna of Sinaloa was giving way to scrub growth within a century of the fall of Tenochitilan.

"The history of this phenomenon is best known in Mexico, but there is sufficient evidence to suggest that a similar sequence of events – expansion of livestock herds and then declines in the size and quality of grasslands – occurred elsewhere, or at least began to occur elsewhere in the Americas in the sixteenth and seventeenth centuries. The accounts of the earliest colonists indicate that the savannas of Central America today are much smaller than they were during Balboa's lifetime [1475 – 1519]. (Here the decline in Indian population was probably more important than the spread of livestock.) No number of animals could bring the forest to the steppes of Rio de la Plata, but in the 1830s Darwin found scores, perhaps hundreds, of square miles in Uruguay impenetrable because they were overgrown with the prickly Old World cardoon (Cynara cardunculus). 'I doubt,' he said, 'whether any case is on record of an invasion on so grand a scale of one plant over the aborigines.' Usually such invasions are so successful only if the original ecology of the area has been shattered – as, for instance, by widespread overgrazing. As for the llanos, no one claims that they are today what they once were, when the seasonal floods were less violent because the ground cover was still thick enough to keep the water from spilling precipitously into the rivers, and the colts could run for hundreds of miles shoulder-deep in the fresh grass at the end of the wet season.

"The awesome initial increase of the herds lasted only a few score years in any given area. There were many factors which slowed the fantastic increase: indiscriminant slaughter of livestock by Spaniards and Indians alike; wild dogs, other predators, insects, and pathogenic

organisms coming in from elsewhere or adapting themselves to European animals as sources of food and hosts. But the most important reason is probably this: when the hoarded riches of the grasslands were gone, the increase of the herds halted or proceeded at a pace now more arithmetic than geometrical. Martin Eriques reported from Mexico in 1574 that the 'Cattle are no longer increasing rapidly; previously, a cow would drop her first calf within two years, for the land was virgin and there were many fertile pastures. Now a cow does not calve before three or four years.'

"This wild oscillation of the balance of nature happens again whenever an area previously isolated is opened to the rest of the world. But possibly, it will never be repeated in as spectacular a fashion as in the Americas in the first post-Columbian century, not unless there is, one day, an exchange of life between planets." (The Columbian Exchange, Pgs 110 – 113)

Other Animals

Though it was Old World pigs, sheep, cattle and horses that played the dominant roles in the colonization of the New World by the Europeans, there were many other imported Old World animals that took root in the Western Hemisphere including dogs, cats, chickens, guinea hens, goats, burrows, donkeys and the honeybee.

In the early 1620s the honeybee, a native of the Mediterranean area and Middle East was first brought to the Americas by English colonists in Virginia and Massachusetts. There are many species of bees that produce honey, but only the honeybee combines high production along with being amenable to human manipulation. Before sugarcane became widely available the main sweetener in the Old World was honey from honeybees. John Josselyn (1638 – 1675) was an English traveler to New England in the 17th century who later wrote books giving some of the earliest and most complete information on New England flora and fauna in colonial times. He noted that in 1663 the European honeybee was thriving *"exceedingly"*. By both human intervention and natural means, honeybees spread west over the Appalachian Mountains to the Mississippi River basin and were sighted in St. Louis, Missouri by 1762. It appears that the honeybee arrived late in Central and South America as there were already honey producing bees in the tropics, but eventually the honeybee was imported from North America and today Argentina is one of the world's top producers of honey, though this is a relatively recent development.

Besides the animals brought intentionally by the colonists, they also brought unintentionally numerous other Old World wild animals that hitched rides across the Atlantic including the "English fly" and the rat. Rat infestations were reported from Port Royal, Nova Scotia down to Buenos Aires, Argentina and everywhere in between. One such graphic report of a rat infestation in 16th century Peru is by Spanish Peruvian chronicler **Garcilaso de la** Vega (1539–1616), *"They bred in infinite numbers, overran the land, and destroyed the crops and standing plants, such as fruit trees, by gnawing the bark from the ground to the shoots."*

The Indians who lived near European settlements, even as their numbers plummeted due to brutal repression and disease epidemics, were quick to adopt the smaller European animals, particularly dogs, cats, pigs and chickens. The Spaniards valued these animals less than the larger herd animals and considered Indian possession of them as no threat. Most indigenous people of the Americas had some experience keeping small animals such as dogs, ducks or pigs, so adopting the Old World breeds of these animals did not require them to drastically alter their way of life. But the larger European herd animals were another story. Examples of Indian sheep, goat and cattle herding in areas under European control are rare. The keeping of such animals called for a radical change in the lives of Indian farmers, and only a few in the Andes highlands and the Southwestern United States ever acquired herds of sheep. Indian herding of cattle was virtually nonexistent.

Prairie Indians

Nomadic Indians who lived on the prairies beyond the boundaries of European settlement were impacted quite differently by the introduction of European livestock than eastern farmers. These Indians received goats, sheep, cattle and horses as valuable new additions to their resources of food, clothing and energy. The animals chiefly involved in this phenomenon were – in ascending order of importance – sheep, cattle, and horses.

Sheep rarely went wild, and with the aforementioned exceptions of the Andes highlands and the Southwestern United States, were only available to nomadic Indians as booty poached in raiding parties.

In the grass country of the North American prairie where vast herds of feral cattle began to replace native bison, the plains Indians became increasingly dependent on cattle for meat and hides. For the most part, these tribes did not become true herdsmen, but obtained their cattle from feral herds.

The story of the horse is similar for all the tribes of the great grasslands, from Alberta Canada down to Patagonia Argentina. Before the arrival of the horse, the grassy steppe lands had few human inhabitants. The tough sod discouraged farming and the plains animals were too fleet of foot to provide a dependable food supply for a large number of pedestrians. Then the horse gave the Indians the speed and stamina needed to take advantage of the immense quantities of food represented by the native buffalo herds of North America and the herds of wild cattle that propagated rapidly in the grasslands of both Americas.

By the middle of the 17th century, the Abipon, Mocovi, Mbaya, and Guaicuru tribes of the South American pampas had acquired large herds of horses and were exploiting the herds of wild cattle. In North America the impact of the horse came later but was similar. By the late 18th century the Great Plains were full of Indians on horseback – the Blackfoot, Arapaho, Cheyenne, Crow, Sioux and Comanche. The horse enabled Indians to kill more animals than they needed for their families, and the surplus hides could be traded for European luxury goods like needles, blankets, firearms and whiskey.

When the only beast of burden was the dog, nomadic Indians could carry few possessions, but the horse enabled them to carry much heavier loads than ever before. The horse also vastly increased the speed with which hunters could move and the area they could hunt increasing their food supply as well as their own populations. Increased wealth and population gave rise to greater social stratification among the nomadic Indians and the egalitarianism of poverty that ruled in the past began to disappear. The number of slaves increased as they could be obtained more easily from neighboring tribes through equestrian warfare. The greatest impact of the horse on the plains Indians was to enhance their ability to resist the advance of Europeans into the interiors of North and South America. Not only did mounted Indians defend themselves more effectively, they were able to raid the herds of the Europeans for food.

The Indian resistance in North America lasted three or four generations, ending finally with the destruction of the bison herds, the catastrophic wars with the United States Army, and the final occupation of the prairies by the Europeans in the last half of the 19th century. The tribes of the pampas also resisted European encroachment through the 18th century. Even as late as 1796 the area around Rio de la Plata that was under European control was no larger than it had been in 1590, but as the Europeans moved into the interior in the 19th century, these mounted tribes were exterminated. As in North America, the horse enriched the tribes of the grasslands and enabled them to resist the advance of the Europeans for a time, only to ultimately succumb to the onslaught.

The Plant Exchange

The Spanish crown realized that the New World would be attractive to Spanish settlers only if familiar European plant foods could be grown there, so on his second voyage in 1493 Columbus was packed off to the West Indies on 17 ships carrying 1,200 men along with seeds and cuttings for the planting of wheat, grape vines and olive trees (the three staple crops of the Spanish diet) as well as cauliflowers, cabbages, chickpeas, onions, radishes, salad greens, melons, stone fruits, oranges, lemons, pomegranates, citrons, figs and sugar cane. Another important plant to arrive in the early years of the conquest was the banana, brought in from the Canary Islands in 1516. Many of these European vegetables and fruit trees grew well in the rich soils and tropical climate of the West Indies, and were later sown wherever there was Spanish settlement and the slightest probability of growing them to maturity. On the other hand, wheat, grapes and olive trees, the holy trinity of Spanish cuisine, fared poorly in the hot, humid lowlands of the Caribbean islands that was so unlike the temperate climate of their native Spain. It wasn't until Cortes and Pizarro brought these Old World crops to the higher altitudes and drier climates of interior Mexico and the Peruvian Andes that they were successfully cultivated in the New World.

Most of the early Spanish farms in the highlands of Mexico raised wheat in accordance with the policy of the viceroys. Farming was not a Castilian strongpoint and the government had to exert constant pressure to assure that Mexico would produce enough wheat to feed itself, but by 1535 Mexico was exporting wheat to the Antilles and Panama and by mid-century wheat bread in Mexico City was as available as it was in Spain. By the last quarter of the century the Atlixco Valley alone was producing 156,200 bushels of wheat per year. In South America, the temperate valleys and highlands near Lima Peru were also producing wheat in quantity by the 1540s and in time Peru became one of the chief sources of wheat exports to Panama. The Spaniards raised wheat every place they settled in the New World where climate permitted; by the late 16th century wheat was being grown in Guatemala, Columbia, Venezuela, Ecuador, Chile and Argentina. A survey taken between 1579 and 1585 of Spanish possessions in the New World commissioned by King Philip II called the *Relaciones Geograficas de las Indias* indicates that by the late 16th century wheat bread was universally available to the Spanish settlers of the New World.

The early records of the Spanish empire are filled with notations of successes and failures in attempts to establish grapevines in the New World. The Mexican highlands, though more temperate than the coastal lowlands, produced little wine because the grapes did not ripen to a high enough sugar content. In the highlands of Peru, however, grapes ripened to perfection and the first Peruvian vintage was bottled in 1551. A hundred years later Peru was producing enough wine to quench not only the local thirst, but enough for export. Grapes also did well in the temperate regions of Chile and Argentina. Records from the diocese of Santiago, Chile, indicate the production of 200,000 jugs of wine in 1614. The size of a "jug" is not clear, but 200,000 of them sounds like a considerable amount.

Few olive trees grew in Mexico, and the total yield of olives and oil there was insignificant in the 16th and 17th centuries. The areas in the New World settled by the Spanish that most closely resembled the dry Mediterranean climate where the olive trees grow best were the coastal valleys of Peru and Chile. The thought that olive trees might prosper there surely occurred to many of the earliest settlers, but it wasn't until 1560 that the first olive trees were planted in Peru. The reason it took longer to establish olives than wheat or grapes undoubtedly stemmed from the fact that the seedlings had to be shipped all the way from Spain because they could not survive in the usual halfway houses of Hispaniola or Panama. Antonio de Rivera, one of the first settlers of Lima, was the first to return from Spain with a number of olive seedlings in 1560, and while only a few survived the journey, it was from these spare beginnings that a flourishing olive oil industry was founded in the dry irrigated valleys of Peru and Chile.

The economic underpinnings of most of the larger European settlements in the New World historically has been the growing of a few large plantation crops for export back to Europe including the Old World endemics of coffee and sugar cane. While neither of these crops are what can be considered the staff of life, sugar cane did provide a tremendous load of calories to a growing European sweet tooth. According to Johns Hopkins University anthropologist Sidney Mintz, by 1650 the English nobility had become "inveterate sugar eaters," by 1800 every English person indulged, and by 1900 sugar supplied nearly one fifth of the calories in the average English diet.

Sugarcane is endemic to tropical South and Southeast Asia. It is theorized that sugarcane was first domesticated as a crop in New Guinea around 6000 BC and was chewed for its sweet juice. The earliest evidence of crystalline sugar production comes from northern India as described in 2,600 year old (600 BC) Sanskrit texts. In the 8th century AD, Arab traders introduced sugar from South Asia to the Arab world as well as Mesopotamia, Egypt, North Africa, Spain and Portugal, and by the 13th century the Spanish and Portuguese were growing it on plantations in the Canary and Madeira island chains off the Atlantic coast of North Africa. These sugar cane plantations that depended on disposable slave labor to function were the prototype for plantations in the New World and also the first example of industrial style mono-crop agriculture.

Columbus's first wife owned a sugar estate on Madeira and he himself had shipped sugar from Madeira back to Genoa, Italy in 1478. Columbus brought sugar cane from the Canary Islands to Hispaniola in 1493 and the cane grew very well in the islands tropical environment. But the sugar industry did not take off in the Greater Antilles until King Charles V intervened, ordering that sugar masters and mill technicians be recruited from the Canary Islands, and loans be made to build sugar mills on Hispaniola. By the late 1530s there were 34 mills on Hispaniola and sugar was second only to cattle hides in the export economy of the island until the latter part of the 16th century when competition from the mainland caused its decline.

During the 16th century the Spanish planted cane wherever the sun was hot and the rainfall sufficient. It became a common crop early after the conquest of Mexico and Peru in the lowlands and deeper valleys of those regions. In the 17th century, from the Gulf of Mexico to the Rio de la Plata sugar was king. Asunción, Paraguay alone boasted 200 sugar mills in the early 17th century. Spanish Jesuit missionary Bernabe Cobo exclaimed, *"there must not be a region in all the universe where so much [sugar] is consumed, and with all this many ships carry it to Spain."* Cobo was mistaken, however, the greatest producer of sugar in the Atlantic world in the 16th and 17th centuries was not the Spanish, but the Portuguese.

Sugar cane from the Portuguese occupied Madeira Islands, which in the 15th century was the largest producer of sugar for the European market, was sent to Brazil soon after first contact. By 1526 duty was being paid on Brazilian sugar at the Lisbon Customs House and by the end of the 16th century Brazil was the largest sugar supplier of the Atlantic world. By one estimate, Brazil had 400 mills producing 57,000 tons of sugar annually by 1610. Later in the 17th century English and French colonies on the Lesser Antilles islands in the Caribbean planted their own cane which in turn caused a decline in Brazil's sugar industry.

From the late 16th century through the early 19th century it was sugar that fueled the "triangle trade" consisting of New World sugar, European manufactured goods and African slaves. Sugar in the form of molasses was shipped from the Caribbean to Europe or New England where it was distilled into rum. The profits from the sale of sugar were used to purchase manufactured goods from Europe which were shipped to West Africa and traded for slaves. The African slaves were then shipped to the Caribbean where they were sold to plantation owners to do the hard labor of growing and milling sugar cane. The slave traders would then use their profits from selling slaves to buy more sugar to haul to Europe or New England thereby completing the triangle. Today sugarcane remains an important part of the economy of Guyana, Belize, Barbados, Haiti, the Dominican Republic, Jamaica, Guadeloupe and other islands.

Other early Old World crops that were of more localized importance were oranges, peaches and rice. In 1829 Charles Darwin found islands near the mouth of the Paraná **River** which runs through Brazil, Paraguay and Argentina thick with orange and peach trees that had sprung up wild from seeds carried downstream from early Spanish settlements. Eighteenth century English settlers of the southeastern section of North America were also met by thickets of peach trees growing wild originally introduced into Florida by the Spaniard in the 16th century. The New World cultivation of rice began in South Carolina in 1696, by English colonist, seaman and planter Thomas Smith (1648–1694) who was the captain of a merchant ship that brought a bag of rice from Madagascar. Smith's experiment growing rice was a success and in three years the people of South Carolina were exporting rice to other colonies where cultivation also began from Georgia to New Jersey. In the 18th century the akee, mango, and breadfruit were imported from Europe to the West Indies.

Many of the Old World plants brought to the New World by the Europeans were what we now think of as weeds. A few species were sown intentionally as forage plants for the European animals to graze on, but most were brought unintentionally mixed in with fodder aboard ship used to feed the animals on their passage across the Atlantic. The story is the same wherever the Europeans touched down in the Western Hemisphere, their animals and all manner of European grasses and weeds quickly became naturalized and invasive. In the West Indies Friar Bartolomé de las Casas wrote of large herds of European animals eating native plants down to the roots in the first half of the 16th century, followed by the spread of Castilian ferns, thistle, plantain, nettles, nightshades and sedge. In Mexico as early as 1555 European clover was so widespread that the Aztecs had a word of their own for it, *Castillan ocoxochitl*, naming it after a low native plant that also prefers shade and moisture. In Peru a European clover they called *"trebol"* took over more of the cool damp country than any other colonizing species, providing good animal forage but smothering Inca crops. Other European weeds in Peru made note of by Spanish nobleman Garcilaso de la Vega and Jesuit Bernabé Cobo, included mustard, mint and chamomile. In the 1780s Spanish military officer, naturalist and engineer, Felix de Azara recorder that in the pampas around Buenos Aires, Argentina, vast numbers of livestock and the practice of burning off the dead grasses annually were eliminating the native tall grasses, and that European exotics were filling in the void. In 1833 Charles Darwin wrote of the wild artichoke (aka, prickly Old World cardoon; *Cynara cardunculus*) being so widespread in Argentina, Chile and Uruguay that *"I doubt whether any case is on record of the invasion on so grand a scale of one plant over the aborigines."* In 1877, Latvian zoologist Carlos Berg published a list of 153 European plants he found in the province of Buenos Aires and in Patagonia, including such familiars as chickweed, clover, curly dock, goosefoot, plantain, red-stemmed filaree, and shepherd's purse. According to field botanists in the 1920s, only one quarter of the plants growing wild on the pampas at that time were natives.

In North America east of the Mississippi the indigenous grasses never had to survive the enormous herds of buffalo that grazed the Great Plains, so they were evolutionarily ill suited for the grazing of European cattle, sheep, and goats and they virtually disappeared from the landscape. The champion pioneers among the European weeds in North America were white clover and Kentucky bluegrass which is in fact native to Eurasia. Spread intentionally by Europeans for forage and by their own aggressive nature, white clover and Kentucky bluegrass soon could be found throughout the thirteen colonies and into Canada along the St. Lawrence. When English settlers crossed the Appalachian Mountains and moved into Kentucky in the last decades of the 18th century, they found white clover and bluegrass there to greet them. In 1832, German-American botanist and mycologist, Lewis D. de Schweinitz, considered by some the "Father of North American Mycology," made a list of 137 Old World weed species in the northern United States including such familiars as chickweed, comfrey, dandelion, dock, henbane, mallow, may weed, mullin, patience, plantain, shepherd's purse, stinging nettle, and wormwood. California, being separated from Europe by a continent and an ocean, and from population centers of the Spanish conquest by inhospitable deserts and unfriendly winds and currents that flow off the California coast, remained one of the most isolated regions of the Americas which served to protect the native flora from the European invasion until the last decades of the 18th century. Starting in 1765 as Spain began to establish Missions on the California coast as far north as the San Francisco Bay, the missionaries intentionally or not introduced black mustard, bromes, chess, common foxtail, curly dock, Italian eyegrass sow thistle, red-stemmed filaree and wild oats that spread along the coastal hills and into the San Joaquin and Sacramento valleys. When American military officer and explorer John Frémont, came down along the American River into the Sacramento Valley in March of 1844, he found red-stemmed filaree, *"just now beginning to bloom, and covering the ground like a sward of grass."* After annexation of California by the United States in the 1848 Treaty of Guadalupe-Hidalgo with Mexico, Anglo-Americans brought European plants with them across the plains from the east. The gold rush of 1849 produced a demand for cattle meat causing severe overgrazing which was followed by extensive floods in 1862 and then an intensive two-year drought. When the rains came again, the introduced Eurasian weeds sprouted first and fastest, and California's grassland flora was transformed into a Eurasian plain. By the 1860s, 91 Eurasian weed species had become naturalized in California. Dr. Crosby remarks on this exchange:

> *"Today an American botanist can easily find whole meadows in which he is hard put to find a single species of plant that grew in America in pre-Columbian times." (The Clumbian Exchange, Pgs 73-74)*

There are numerous accounts by Spanish and English colonists of the Indians not taking the initiative to cultivate Old World crops on their own. In Spanish colonies the Indians were often forced to raise wheat and other European crops, but for their own consumption they preferred to stick with their familiar New World crops. Unlike with the Old World animals, the Indians apparently saw no advantage to adopting Old World crops.

Whereas the indigenous population of the Western Hemisphere plummeted from over 100 million down to around 11.5 million in the first post-Columbian century (McEvedy & Jones, pg 270), and the population of sheep, cattle and horses exploded from zero to countless tens of millions in that first century after European contact, the population of European settlers and African slaves in the New World expanded slowly. Europeans did not flock to the New World and the colonies had to grow from small beginnings.

In the early 1750s, Anglo-American colonial publisher, scientist and statesman, Benjamin Franklin, estimated that there were approximately 1 million Englishmen in North America, most descended from a mere 80,000 who had emigrated from England in the 17th century. Modern-day English demographers Colin McEvedy and Richard Jones in their *Atlas of World Population History* (Harmondsworth: Penguin Books, 1978) estimated that by 1800 North America had a population of fewer than 5 million Europeans plus about 1 million Africans, and South America had less than half a million Europeans. Dr. Crosby's collective name for the Europeans and all the organisms they brought with them is *"portmanteau biota."* He suggests the disparity between the growth of the European populations in North and South America was that in the south *"overweening success of the livestock and forage plants of the portmanteau biota had stymied its human component."* (*Ecological Imperialism The Biological Expansion of Europe, 900 – 1900, pg 297*) In other words, the Spanish livestock and weeds had crowded out the Spaniards themselves.

While the large pre-Columbian Indian populations of the West Indies and Central and South America were sustained on yuca, maize, potatoes and a few other high yielding New World staple crops, the diet of the much smaller Spanish population consisted mostly of Old World imports wheat and meat as Dr. Crosby notes:

> *"By 1600 one of the cheapest foods in the American colonies was meat; the Spanish-American settlers were probably consuming more meat per man than any other large group of non-nomadic people in the world." (The Columbian Exchang,e Pg 108)*

13
IMPACTS: NEW WORLD ON OLD WORLD

Microbes

To this day there is an unresolved controversy over the origins and spread of the venereal disease syphilis. While there are those who argue that the syphilis virus *Treponema pallidum* originated in the New World and spread to the Old World, there is no definitive evidence that proves this. In the first edition of *The Columbian Exchange* in 1972, Dr. Crosby devoted an entire chapter to arguing this point, but in the Forward to the 2003, 30th anniversary edition, he had a change of heart about the significance of syphilis:

> *"We do not know where venereal syphilis started. It could have come from here or there or there or here and there and have leaped in deadlines when mild strains of treponemas met*

and crossed the Atlantic in 1492, or its increased virulence circa 1500 may have had nothing whatsoever to do with Columbus and simply have been a coincidence.

Anyway, I should not have ennobled syphilis with a whole chapter as if it were Montezuma's Revenge. Its Old World debut was spectacular and, like all things venereal, fascinating, but it was not a history maker like the plague in the fourteenth century or smallpox in the sixteenth century. I cast it in a major role because I was uneasy about so many diseases crossing west over the Atlantic and none crossing east. I was like the geographers who believed for generations, before Captain Cook proved otherwise, that there must be a continent, a Terra-Australis, in the far, far south vast enough to balance off all of Eurasia, the bulk of Africa, and North America. Chapter four was my try for a sort of epidemiological symmetry. The aforementioned geographers were wrong and so was I. There was little symmetry in the exchange of diseases between the Old and New Worlds, and there are few factors as influential in the history of the last half millennia as that." (The Columbian Exchange, pg xix)

Animals

As noted earlier, by the time of Columbus in the late 15th century, most of the larger animals of the Western Hemisphere had already been extinct for thousands of years and, with the exception of the llama and alpaca in the Andes, the American Indians had no large domesticatable animals to exploit for food or motive power. Compared to their Old World domesticated pigs, sheep, goats, cattle and horses, the Europeans were unimpressed by the smaller New World animals they found. According to Dr. Crosby:

"The contrast between Old and New World fauna amazed Renaissance Europe... In 1492 [the Indians] had only a few animal servants: the dog, two kinds of South American camel (the llama and alpaca), the guinea pig, and several kinds of fowl (the turkey, the Muscovey duck, and, possibly, a type of chicken). He had no animal that he rode. Most of his meat and leather came from wild game. He had no beast of burden to be compared to the horse, ass, or ox. Except for the minor assistance of the travois-pulling dog, the Indian wanting to move a load moved it himself, no matter how heavy or how far it had to be moved." (The Columbian Exchange, Pg 74)

While the New World held a great diversity of animals that fascinated the European imagination, like monkeys with tails, tiny hummingbirds and giant condors and iguanas, there were no New World animals that could match Old World animals as sources of production, so the Europeans saw no value in taking any New World animals back to the old country for mass propagation.

Plants

According to Nikolai Vavilov, the prominent Russian botanist best known for identifying the centers of origin for cultivated plants and for creating the largest collection of plant seeds in the world at Leningrad (now St. Petersburg, Russia), of the 640 known human cultigens, roughly 500 belonged to the Old World and 100 to the New World. Among the New World cultigens are the familiar maize, bean, peanut, potato, sweet potato, manioc, squash, papaya, guava, avocado, pineapple, tomato, pepper and cacao. After European contact with the New World, all of these crops and more found their way back across the Atlantic to the Old World for cultivation. The first six of these crops were to become staple foods that provided the bulk of calories necessary to sustain population growth over large areas of the Old World. Which New World crops were exploited by Old World cultures depended on the prevailing climate and soil conditions existing on the great land masses of the Old World. Let's now take a post-Columbian agricultural tour of the great land masses of the Old World: Europe, Africa, the Indian subcontinent, the Far East, and Indonesia.

Europe

The impact of maize in Europe was and is restricted almost entirely to the southern half of the continent because it thrives only in areas where there are several months of hot weather. Today maize is a crop of great importance in a band stretching from Portugal through northern Italy, Slovenia, Macedonia, Croatia, Serbia, Montenegro, Bosnia, the Danube Valley, and into the Caucasus. The most valuable characteristic of maize to the European farmer is its high yield per unit of land, on average roughly double that of wheat. Maize also had the benefit of many varieties already developed by the Indians that were adapted to climate extremes so it could be sown in areas too dry for Old World rice and too wet for Old World wheat. But despite these advantages, the Europeans were slow to take up cultivation of maize, possibly because in the 16th and 17th centuries, Europe's population was still recovering from recurrent plagues that had wiped out tens of millions of people since the late Middle Ages and the demand for food could still be met using Old World crops. People then, as now, were reluctant to adopt new foods unless they had to.

By the late 17th century the population of Europe had climbed to 100 million people, well above its former high of 70 million in the early 14th century, and pressure was again mounting on farmers to coax more food from their lands to feed their growing numbers. This population pressure was nowhere more acute than in France. On visiting the south of France in the 1670s, English philosopher and physician John Locke observed *"plots of Maiz in several parts, which the country people call bled d'Espagne, and as they told me, serves the poor people for bread."* Reoccurring disease epidemics throughout Europe during the 17th and early 18th centuries kept a lid on population expansion until a dramatic population increase was experienced between 1750 and 1800 with many countries doubling in size. The reasons for this rapid population growth are many including improved hygiene that reduced the death rate and mechanized farm equipment that increased food production per farmer, but not the least of these reasons was the mass cultivation of high yielding maize.

In the 18th century maize spread widely to become a basic element in the peasant diet of Spain, Portugal, southern France and northern Italy. When the German dramatist, poet and scientist, Johann von Goethe, journeyed to the Po Valley in northern Italy in the 1780s he noted that polenta was the staple of the peasant's diet there. By the mid 18th century in some areas of Spain, northern Italy and France the people had become so dependent on maize that they developed vitamin B3 (niacin) deficiencies causing outbreaks of the vitamin deficiency disease called "pellagra" (literally – sour skin). The main symptoms of pellagra – diarrhea, skin lesions, dementia and death – spring up in extremely poor areas where niacin deficient maize is the only source of sustenance. It wouldn't be until 1937, after severe outbreaks of pellagra in the southeastern United States, that American biochemist Conrad Elvehjem identified niacin deficiency as the cause. There are still pellagra outbreaks today in poverty stricken regions around the world.

The importance of maize in Hungary and the Balkans area of southeastern Europe seem to date to around the beginning of the 18th century. Between 1541 and 1699 the Islamic Ottoman Turks had defeated and dispersed an estimated 3 million Christian Hungarians from their homeland and used the depopulated region to graze and herd cattle to southern Germany and northern Italy. In some years this cattle trade reached as many as 500,000 animals. But by the end of the 17th century the Christian Habsburg dynasties of Europe had driven out the sparsely populated Ottoman pastoralists and thousands of peasant farmers streamed back onto the Hungarian plains repopulating Hungary. By the end of the 18th century the chief product of eastern Hungary was maize. In the 19th century the population of other Balkan states grew so rapidly – both cause and effect of the cultivation of maize – that the Serbs, Macedonians and Rumanians eventually followed the Hungarians in changing from pastoralists to agriculturalists bringing an end to pastoralism in southeastern Europe. In Rumania where maize pairs well with wheat in crop rotations, the Rumanians ate the maize and exported the surplus wheat to become one of Europe's major breadbaskets. In his book, "*A Serbian Village*," Joel Halpern, notes that the poorer peasants of Orasac, Serbia still raise maize rather than wheat on their small plots of land due to maize's superior yield.

Like New World maize, the New World potato was not readily adopted by the Europeans in the first 100 years after its initial introduction in the 16th century. As late as the 18th century avant-garde French philosopher and social critic Denis Diderot wrote in his monumental work, *Encyclopedia*, that no matter how the potato is prepared, "*… this root is insipid and mealy. It cannot be classed among the agreeable food stuffs, but it furnishes abundant and rather wholesome nutrition to men who are content to be nourished. The potato is justly regarded as flatulent, but what are winds to the vigorous organs of peasants and laborers?*" Diderot's critique of the potato notwithstanding, the advantages of the potato as a food crop could not be concealed from the farmers of northern Europe forever. It was the Irish who first wholeheartedly adopted the potato in the last years of the 16th century, recognizing the fact that potatoes could produce more nutrients per unit of land than any other crop. Within a century the Irish were known as "*mighty lovers of potatoes.*" In 1724 Irish satirist Jonathan Swift, described his countrymen as "*living in filth and nastiness upon buttermilk and potatoes.*" The moist, cool climate and deep friable soils of Ireland are perfect for the potato, and the Irish, forced into poverty and hunger under English rule, could have asked for no better gift from the New World than the potato. As the crop spread throughout Ireland, the population grew, which lead to more potato cultivation. No other plant could feed so many people on such small plots of land: a family could survive for a year on one-and-a-half acres planted in potatoes. It was not unusual for an Irishman to consume ten pounds of potatoes a day and nothing else. On this diet the Irish, without benefit of improved hygiene, industrialization, or a benevolent government, increased from 3.2 million people in 1754 to nearly 8.2 million in 1845, not counting the 1.75 million who emigrated to other lands before 1846. Then came the potato blight of 1845 through 1852, the failure of the Irish potato crop and one of the worst famines in modern history. During the Irish Potato Famine approximately 1 million people died and a million more emigrated from Ireland causing the island's population to shrink by nearly 25%.

As the population of England grew and industrialization drew more and more people to the cities, the potato assumed greater importance in the diet of the 18th and 19th century English peasant and laborer. The number of articles in English journals on potato cultivation and potatoes recipes increased noticeably like this one from *The Annual Register* of 1803 entitled, *"Observations on the Means of Enabling a Cottager to Keep a Cow by the Produce of a Small Portion of Arable Land"*, calling for the planting of three-and-one-quarter acres of land in potatoes, turnips, a grain crop, and clover in rotation. The *"potatoes shall go for the maintenance of the cottager and his family'* and the rest for the cow and to sell for cash income."

Peasants on the continent of northern Europe adopted the potato a generation or two after the English as a result of conscious government policies to feed their growing populations. The potato was served at the royal table in France and Marie Antoinette even wore its flower as a corsage to promote its acceptance. A famine and epidemic in 1765 persuaded Catherine the Great of Russia of the importance of the potato and her government launched a campaign to encourage its cultivation. The potato did not become a staple crop in central Russia, however, until many decades later after the famines of 1838 and 1839. By 1900 the Russian potato harvest had increased by 400% and the Russian population by 70%. Today Russia is the world's leading producer of potatoes by a wide margin.

Fredrick the Great of Prussia urged the cultivation of the potato in his country, and in Hungary after the famine of 1772 the government ordered that potatoes be grown. Typically potato production spurted upward throughout Eastern Europe after famines. In the first years of the 19th century Prussian geographer, naturalist and explorer, Alexander von Humboldt (1769 – 1859), referred to the potato as a *"beneficent plant"* that was indispensable for most people living in the colder climates of northern Europe.

The bean family contains over 1,000 species, some of New and some of Old World origins, and since most writers, historians and statisticians have been negligent to differentiate between the two, it is difficult to determine the importance of New World beans in the Old World. The single most important bean in the Eastern Hemisphere is the Old World soybean, but the lima, butter, haricot, pole, kidney, navy, snap, string, common, and many other beans now raised in the Old World originated in the Western Hemisphere. Beans are not only an excellent source of nutrients, they are also important nitrogen fixing plants that are essential for nitrogen fixing in organic farming.

When the Europeans arrived in the Western Hemisphere, varieties of New World beans already existed suitable to almost every climate, and the New World beans were so clearly superior to most Old World pulses that they quickly spread to almost all latitudes of Europe. Because they have often been a private garden crop rather than a field crop, beans escaped the official government censuses and their importance defies statistical description. It is assumed that New World beans were first cultivated in Europe in the 16th century and spread rapidly to become an important part of the diet by the 18th century, but information on where and when the bean became important and just how important it became is scant. The haricot bean was in Europe at least by 1542 when the German botanists Tragus and Leonard Fuchs described and sketched it. It was probably grown in appreciable quantities in France by the end of the century as English poet Barnaby Googe, referred to it as the *"French bean"* in 1572. String beans and lima beans were among the chief products of Spain in the 17th century. While traveling on the continent in 1678, Englishman John Locke advised: *"Take the leaves of kidney beans... and put them under your pillow or some convenient place about your bed. They will draw all the puneses [bedbugs] and keep you from being bit."* A Gallic botanist summed up the bean's significance in a book published in 1701 describing the common bean *(Phaseolus vulgaris)* as *"cultivated almost everywhere because of the use that is made of its fruits in the cuisine."*

Africa

Except for the Americas themselves, nowhere is so great a proportion of the population dependent on New World plants than the people of the African continent. According to the Russian botanist Vavilov, only 50 out of the 640 human cultigens originated in Africa, and they were not of the high yielding species; so the Africans had to import their chief food plants from Asia and the Americas. This was especially true in the rain forest regions where practically none of the jungle food crops are native to Africa. From Nigeria east to the center of the continent, maize, manioc, peanuts, squash, and sweet potatoes have all become primary crops and nearly everywhere else in Africa they are cultivated as secondary crops. Of these crops, maize and manioc are the two that have become dietary staples over large areas of Africa.

Maize was first cultivated in West Africa at least as early as the second half of the 16th century. The chief grains of Africa before the 16th century were millet and sorghum which yielded considerably less than maize in the wet tropics and so maize spread rapidly in the rain forest areas. In the 17th century, Dutch physician and writer, Olfert Dapper, wrote that there was an abundance of maize on the Gold Coast of modern-day Ghana where *"it grows profusely. They bake it, with or without mixing it with millet."* Maize was also recorded to the south on the Congo and Angola coasts. Oral tradition indicates that maize came to the interior Bushongo people of the south-central Congo River basin in the 17th century. By 1900 maize could be found almost everywhere in Africa, exceeding in production all other grains but rice in the jungles, the savanna regions, and along the rivers; and successfully competing with millet and sorghum in many of the drier areas. The Boers, as they colonized South Africa in the early 19th century, found the

Bantu planting and harvesting maize. Today maize is the staple of the Bantu diet. South Africa is one of the world's top producers of maize accounting for about 70% of its total crop. In the 20th century cultivation of maize continued to spread and maize has become a mainstay of the diet for most of eastern and central tropical Africa. Maize reached Egypt early in the 16th century but did not become a staple crop until the 18th. Its cultivation continued to rise in the 19th and 20th centuries along with a steady rise in the Egyptian population. In 1882 Egypt had 6.7 million people, in 1907 11.2 million, in 1935 16 million, and in 1964 28.9 million. There has been some territorial expansion of Egypt in this time and some improvements in health care, but most of this population rise has come from natural increase stemming from the expansion of maize production, without which the present population of Egypt could not exist. The rich soil, plentiful water from the Nile, and hot sun make maize the perfect crop for Egypt. No other grain crop produces such yields in this environment, and the labor costs of cultivating maize in Egypt are lower than those of any other grain. Today a greater area is devoted to maize in Egypt than to any other food crop.

Since Columbus first saw manioc upon his arrival in the West Indies, this productive root has spread around the globe in a band 30 degrees north to 30 degrees south of the equator becoming a staple crop in parts of Africa and Indonesia. Native to Brazil, the yuca plant, now more commonly called manioc, is as important a contribution to the food supply of tropical areas as maize or potatoes are to temperate zones. The manioc plant is a large shrub which is harvested anywhere from 5 to 12 feet tall. Its young shoots and leaves are edible but it is grown primarily for its roots, which, at harvest, are usually 1 to 2 feet in length, 2 to 6 inches in diameter and generally weigh from 2.32 to 11 pounds (1 to 5 kilograms) or more. Manioc grows well from sea level to seven thousand feet in soils too poor to support almost any other important crop, it is drought tolerant, resistant to insect pests, and although it is composed chiefly of starch with little protein or fat, contains significant amounts of calories, vitamins and other nutrients. All manioc requires is a frost-free climate, soil that is neither saline nor swampy, and from 20 to 200 inches of rain a year. Under these conditions manioc produces more food by weight per unit of land than any other tropical plant.

Drought is common in the grasslands that compose most of sub-Saharan Africa and manioc has become a staple or supplemental crop in every area of Africa from south of Ethiopia to north of the Zambezi River. Manioc was probably first brought to the west coast of Congo and Angola by the Portuguese in the 16th century and around the Cape of Good Hope to Madagascar and Mozambique in the 18th century. Manioc was much slower to spread than maize, possibly due to ignorance of how to leech out its poison before eating. Manioc did become established on the west coast of Congo before 1850, and Dr. Crosby hypothesizes a connection to the ensuing African slave trade:

> *"As for the influence of these crops [maize, manioc and others] before 1850, we might hypothesize that the increased food production enabled the slave trade to go on as long as it did without pumping the black well of Africa dry. The Atlantic slave traders drew many, perhaps*

most, of their cargoes from the rain forest areas, precisely those areas where American crops enabled heavier settlement than ever before." (The Columbian Exchange, pg 188)

It wasn't until the last half of the 19th century that manioc spread into the interior and was grown throughout most of its present range by 1900. In the 20th century African production of manioc shot upward, with Nigeria, Africa's most populous country, producing more manioc than any other food.

The population of Africa has risen from 90 million in 1800 to 95 million in 1850, to 120 million in 1900, to 198 million in 1950, to over 1 billion in 2010 (United Nations census). This rapid rise in African population following 1850 coincides directly with the spread of maize, manioc and other New World crops.

Asian Subcontinent

In 1600, the population of the Asian subcontinent (what is now India and Pakistan) was around 100 million people. Over the next 200 years the population grew slowly to approximately 120 million. Then in the 19th century the population began to rise dramatically: 130 million by 1845; 175 million by 1855; 194 million by 1867; 255 million by 1871; over 500 million by 1964; to over 1.21 billion by 2010. This population expansion coincides with the widespread adoption of New World crops in South Asia. New World fruits such as pineapple and guava reached India and were cultivated in significant quantities as long ago as the 16th century, but they probably had little effect on population growth. These foods have never been staples for any large number of people. Maize, manioc, sweet potatoes, white potatoes, peanuts, peppers, lima beans and squash are all now grown on the Asian subcontinent in such quantity as to provide a significant food source for the Indian people. As in Europe and Africa, these New World crops were first cultivated in quantity in the 18th century but did not become major elements in the Indian diet until the 19th and 20th centuries.

There is little evidence of widespread maize cultivation in India at the beginning of the 18th century, but after 1800 it spread rapidly, largely displacing millet as it did during the same time period in Europe and Africa. By the last decades of the 19th century maize was being grown in some quantity throughout the Indian subcontinent. In terms of range and depth the greatest compilation of commercial plants in India ever written is the ten volumes of the *Dictionary of the Commercial Products of India* (1889–90), compiled by British botanist George Watt. In it Watt noted, *"So completely has India now appropriated the Makkal [maize] that few of the village fathers would be found willing to admit that it had not always been with them as it is now, a staple article of diet. They may even cite its supposed ancient names and quote wise sayings regarding it, oblivious all the while that a very few years ago these were universally accepted as denoting an altogether different plant."* In the 20th century India became one of the top maize producers in the world.

Manioc did not arrive in India until about 1850. It soon became a staple in the northeastern state of Assam, where in the 19th century a British military officer, Major Jenkins, wrote of it, *"There is no barren waste or hill land about us in which this plant [manioc] does not thrive.*" Manioc has attained its greatest importance in southern India in the states of Travancore and Cochin, where it has become a principle staple. The reason for its wholesale adoption by the Indians in these areas of dense population is that manioc yields 11.6 million calories per hectare (2.471 acres), as compared with 5.5 million for rice and 5 million for maize.

As the Indians found that sweet potatoes would grow in soil too poor for other crops, its cultivation spread through the hot lowlands and it became a familiar item in the diets of Indians of all classes in the 19th century. The white potato has also been raised in mountain areas or as a winter crop in all suitable areas of India. Sweet and white potatoes never attained the status of staple crops in India but they do provide a significant source of calories and nutrition in specific areas.

India has also become the world's leading producer of peanuts, growing almost 5.3 million metric tons in 1963, and peanuts have become common in the Indian diet, especially in southern India. The chile pepper has become an indispensable ingredient in the most Indian of dishes: chutneys and curries. George Watt noted at the end of the 19th century that the chile pepper, *"ground into a paste, between two stones, with a little mustard oil, ginger and salt…, form the only seasoning which the millions of poor can obtain to eat with their rice."* The lima bean, pumpkin and squash are also grown ubiquitously throughout much of India.

Far East Asia

At the time of European contact at the end of the 15th century, the Far East, including China, Japan, Korea, Vietnam, Laos, Cambodia, Thailand and Burma, was already the most heavily populated area on Earth. By 1650 the Far East with an estimated 327 million people accounted for 60% of all the people on Earth. While Old World wheat and millet were important dry land crops in the Far East, this massive population was largely sustained by the mastery of growing the ancient Asian staple crop of rice. But around the middle of the 19th century the farmers' ability to grow more rice on the available land to feed ever more mouths reached the point of diminishing returns where increased labor no longer produced increased yields. According to Dr. Crosby this food crisis in the Far East was different than in other areas of the Old World:

> *"An examination of the role of crops raised for human consumption in the Far East is more worthwhile than for any other area because the pressure of population on the food supply has been so great for so long that east Asians probably depend less on animals as a source of nourishment than any other large group of people in the world. They cannot afford the extravagant practice of grazing cattle on arable land then eating the cattle. They know that it is much more efficient, in terms of filling human stomachs, to raise food crops on the land, and let the livestock scavenge for that nourishment. For example, about 98 percent of the caloric content of the Chinese diet is of vegetable origin. In the phrase of [French geographer] Pierre Gourou, the Orient has a 'vegetable civilization'."*

Sweet potatoes from South America actually arrived in Far East Asia and Polynesia before the Columbian Exchange. Archaeologists have radiocarbon dated prehistoric remnants of sweet potato found in Polynesia back to between 1000 AD and 1100 AD. How the sweet potato crossed the Pacific remains a mystery, but speculation has it that skilled Polynesian sailors actually made landfall on the South American continent nearly 500 years before Columbus and returned with sweet potatoes. Or it could have floated over on a log. The sweet potato was adopted rapidly because it did not compete with rice and other traditional crops, but thrived in previously unutilized soils, such as the rocky Shantung coast, the rice-deficient southeast provinces and the drought-ridden highlands. By the 18th century the cultivation of the sweet potato had become government agricultural policy and it spread into nearly every climatically hospitable corner of China. After rice and wheat, the sweet potato is now China's most important crop. It is the traditional food of the poorest classes; to be called a sweet potato eater was an insult in pre-communist China. By the 20th century, China had become by far and away the world's largest producer of sweet potatoes, averaging at least 18.5 million metric tons a year from 1931 to 1937.

Peanuts were being grown near Shanghai, in Fukien province of southeast China, by the mid 16th century. Peanuts have taken on an important role in the Chinese diet and agriculture. The plant enabled Chinese peasants to make greater use of the sandy coastal soils than was possible before the New World crop was introduced in the 16th century, and the peanut, as a nitrogen fixing legume, plays an important role in crop rotations with rice in some areas. By the mid 20th century China was harvesting 2.4 million metric tons of peanuts making it second only to India in peanut production. Today peanuts are grown throughout China and are especially common in the north.

It wasn't until the late 18th and early 19th century that maize became a primary food crop in large parts of the uplands of southwestern China. As the valleys of the Yangtze River and its tributaries overflowed with people in the 18th century, the excess population was forced up into the hills and mountains where they found that maize was the key to extracting food from the previously barren highlands. The northern Chinese farmer was slower to take up maize, not cultivating it in quantity until the 19th century, but by the mid 20th century around one-seventh of all the food energy in northern China was being provided by maize. China, which harvested 16,849 million metric tons of maize in 1952-1953, stood second only to the United States in its production at that time. And, as in most countries other than the United States, nearly all of China's maize went to feeding people, not livestock.

China's agricultural production is so great that it ranks high as a producer of crops which are of secondary importance to the Chinese people. In the years 1948 through 1952 China produced over 12 million tons of potatoes annually, about as much as the United States at that time. The potato was grown in Fukien before 1800, but has since become an important food source in the high mountain areas where it is a staple on the high plains of Kansu, Inner Mongolia and Manchuria.

More is known of the impact of New World foods on the population of China than in any other country in the Far East due to Chinese-American historian Ping-ti Ho's monumental book, *"Studies on*

Population of China, 1368-1953" (1959). For as far back as census figures go, China's population has been huge, but by 1900 it had reached an estimated 400 million people; by 1953 there were 580 million Chinese and, according to the United Nations census, 1.3 billion in 2010. This phenomenal growth pattern would not have been possible without the addition of New World crops to the Old World standbys of rice, wheat and millet.

Japan

The islands of Japan lie too far north to grow manioc and its people have never developed a taste for maize, but New World sweet and white potatoes have been an important food crop there for many generations. The sweet potato spread to Japan from China, via the Ryuku Islands, in the last part of the 17th century. In the famine years of 1832, 1844, 1872, and 1896 the sweet potato provided unfailing famine insurance for large numbers of the Japanese people who found themselves depending on sweet potatoes for survival. Japan is now the world's second largest producer of sweet potatoes, which are the staff of life on Okinawa. The white potato arrived no later than 1615 when an agent of the English East India Company visiting Japan wrote, *"I tooke a garden this day, and planted it with pottatos."* Like in most Old World cultures, the Japanese did not take to the potato at first, but during floods and famines in the 1680s they discovered that potatoes could grow in colder climates and higher altitudes than the sweet potato. The Russians introduced the potato into Hokkaido in the latter part of the 17th century and when Japan opened its doors to the rest of the world in the mid 19th century, potatoes were found to be a common food, especially in the north. In the mid 20th century Japan raised far more rice than any other crop – over 8.5 million metric tons – but at over 4.6 million metric tons of sweet potatoes and over 2.2 million metric tons of white potatoes, New World crops contributed significantly to the islands food stuffs, food that could not otherwise have been grown. In the 170 years between 1700 and 1870 the population of Japan rose by only 4 million people from 29 million to 33 million, but by 1900, only 30 years later, the population had risen by 17 million to a total of 50 million, 83 million by 1950 (even after the devastation of World War II), and to 128 million by 2010.

Indonesia

Indonesia is the largest nation of Southeast Asia in terms of population and land area. New World beans first arrived in Indonesia as early as the 17th century and, according to English explorer William Dampier, by 1699 maize was a staple for the people on the coastal plains of Timor. In 1789 as English Navy Captain William Bligh (1754 – 1817) set ashore on Timor after the mutiny of his crew on the H.M.S. Bounty, he was met by obliging Timorese who *"brought us a few pieces of dried turtle and some ears of Indian corn [maize]."* Some time around 1800 the Dutch introduced the white potato into the mountains of Java. But New World crops were not grown extensively in Indonesia until the 19th century when, as in the Far East, most of the land suitable for growing rice, and most of the ways to increase its yield per hectare, had been utilized generations before. In the 19th century New World maize, manioc, sweet potatoes, peanuts, and chile peppers have all increased in importance relative to rice in Indonesia. This is particularly true in the uplands where rice doesn't grow but where population growth has equaled that of the rice growing regions of the coastal lowlands. Of these New World crops, the most important have been maize, manioc and sweet potatoes.

According to Scottish physician John Crawford in his book, *History of the Indian Archipelago* published in 1820, maize may well have become the most important secondary crop on Java by 1800. Maize cultivation pushed by population increase spread rapidly through the islands and by the mid 20th century maize ranked second in importance only to rice among cereal crops in Indonesia as a whole, and is now the staple food in parts of the Celebes, Timor, Lombok, East Java, and Madura.

Manioc made its first appearance in Indonesia as early as the 17th century but, as elsewhere in the world, was adopted slowly by local farmers. Eventually, however, population pressures along with manioc's incredible productivity combined to make its appeal irresistible. One advantage of manioc over rice is that manioc grows back each year from the inedible stalks, so no part of the plant must be saved for planting the next year. Taking into account that a portion of the rice crop must be preserved for the next year's seed, manioc yields nearly twice as many food calories per unit of land in Java as rice. Manioc also grows in areas where rice and maize languish such as on the dry limestone plateau of the Gunung Sewu of Java, where it is the chief crop. United Nations statistics place Indonesia second only to Brazil, its homeland, as a producer of manioc.

There are few parts of the world where the sweet potato is the primary crop, but its high yield – three to four times that of rice – and its resistance to drought and tolerance of poor soils make it a vitally important secondary crop throughout a wide band of land around the Earth's equator. The Indonesian island archipelago, which straddles the equator between the Indian and Pacific Oceans, produced 13.4 million metric tons of rice in 1962-1963 and over 3 million metric tons of sweet potatoes. The sweet potato is especially important as an "in-between" crop in Indonesia, providing nourishment in-between rice harvests.

The population of Indonesia grew rapidly over the 19th and 20th centuries, especially on the larger islands of Java and Madura. In 1815 the population of Java and Madura was around 4.6 million, in 1890 it was almost 24 million, in 1960 approximately 62.5 million, and in 2010 140 million. The total population of Indonesia in 2010 was estimated at 237 million people. Rice production was not able to keep pace with this population expansion, especially in the 20th century and this widening gap was largely filled by cultivation of New World crops in rotation with rice. In 1900 the people of Java had available to them, per capita, per year, 110 kilograms (kg.) of rice, 30 kg. of tubers and three kg. of pulses. By 1940 the proportions had changed: 85 kg. of rice, 40 kg. of maize, 180 kg. of tubers and about 10 kg. of pulses. The difference between the two diets consists almost exclusively of increased quantities of New World plants. As Dr. Crosby notes:

"A connection between the two phenomenon [New World crops and population increases] is as certain here [in Indonesia] as anywhere in the world."(The Columbian Exchange, Pg 194)

Effects of Columbian Exchange on World Population

Before the European conquest of the New World began in 1492, there were approximately 100 million people living in the Americas and another 325 million in the Old World for a total world population of 425 million (*Atlas of World Population History*, Colin McEvedy and Richard Jones, 1978). Two hundred years later by 1700 AD, the world population had grown by an additional 185 million people to a total of 610 million, but the distribution between the Old and New Worlds was quite different than it was in 1500. While the large indigenous population of the Americas was decimated by disease and war and the European colonizers were slow to repopulate the New World, the population centers of the Old World were expanding rapidly due to the introduction of high yielding New World crops. In 1500 the New World represented nearly 25% of the world's total human population, but by 1700 that number had plunged to less than 3%.

As I have already noted in *The Columbian Exchange* discussion above, the populations of both the New and Old Worlds did not truly begin to take-off until the late 18th and through the 19th centuries, adding another 290 million people by the end of the 18th century, and another 725 million people in the 19th century for a total of 1.625 billion by 1900. That is more than a doubling of the Earth's human population in 200 years, and in absolute terms an additional 1 billion mouths to feed. The increased food production made possible worldwide by the widespread adoption of higher yielding New World crops was key to this post Columbian population explosion.

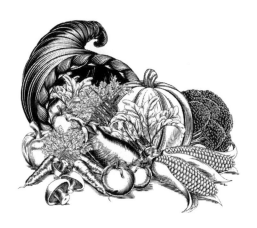

PART IV

RISE OF THE GLOBAL ANIMAL

INDUSTRIAL COMPLEX

• • •

"Now and then a visitor wept, to be sure; but this slaughtering machine ran on, visitors or no visitors. It was like some horrible crime committed in a dungeon, all unseen and unheeded, buried out of sight and of memory."

– Upton Sinclair, writer, muckraker, political activist (1878 – 1968)

Between the mid 19th and early 21st centuries, the production of meat, dairy and eggs transformed from small scale localized operations with a limited production capacity, to a handful of giant multinational corporations that dominate the entire global food production system. As the human population quadrupled over the course of the 20th century, feeding these additional billions of people an increasingly animal food based diet has wreaked havoc on the Earth's natural ecosystems. The history of the rise of the global animal industrial complex is complex, so to make heads or tails of it, I have decided to break down this historical review into separate discussions of the five major food animals – sheep, pigs, cattle, chickens and fish.

14

SHEEP

S heep were first domesticated around 10,000 years ago (8000 BC) in ancient Mesopotamia from a subspecies of wild sheep called *mouflon* (*Ovis orientalis*). Today, ten millennium later, humans have bred sheep into hundreds of meat and wool bearing breeds that are adapted to different climate zones on every continent around the world except Antarctica. While in the early 21st century, sheep meat commands only 6.4% of the world's meat market, in some geographical areas that are dominated by sparsely vegetated range lands, sheep meat is the largest source of meat.

Early Domestication

A study published in the October, 2015, edition of the journal *Molecular Biology and Evolution,* rewrote the genetic history of sheep. The product of an unprecedented collaboration involving scientists in China, Iran, Pakistan, Indonesia, Nepal, Finland, and the United Kingdom analyzed the complete mitochondrial DNA of 42 domesticated native sheep breeds from Azerbaijan, Moldova, Serbia, Ukraine, Russia, Kazakhstan, Poland, Finland, China, and the UK, along with two wild sheep species from Kazakhstan. This data was compared to DNA sequences of 150 breeds from several other countries to complete the most exhaustive maternal genetic analysis of sheep ever undertaken. The DNA of contemporary sheep can now be read like a historical record, allowing researchers to look back 10,000 years to the time when humans first started herding sheep in Mesopotamia.

Jian-Lin Han, a senior scientist working on the project from the Chinese Academy of Agricultural Sciences noted, *"What we found is that sheep in Asia are far more genetically diverse than sheep now common in Europe..."* The study found that the rich genetic heritage of Asian sheep is a product of two distinct migratory waves of domesticated animals, not one as previously thought. The DNA analysis confirmed previous findings that domesticated sheep first emerged in Mesopotamia around 10,000 years ago and then made their way east to what is now China and Mongolia, but the researchers discovered a second migration with evidence that herders in what are now northern China and Mongolia developed their own unique breeds around 5,000 years ago. These animals were later sent back west along the Silk Road, where frequent trading of ewes (breeding females) allowed them to be mixed in with the progeny of their ancestors to produce yet more distinct breeds. The Mongol hordes of Genghis Khan often rode west with live sheep strapped to their horses. Olivier Hanotte, a livestock geneticist and study collaborator from the University of Nottingham in the UK, noted:

> *"What this study shows is that the genetic lineages of modern sheep were shaped by thousands of years of trading and breeding moving first west to east and then back, east to west, which created a unique collection of beneficial traits." ("New study rewrites genetic history of sheep", September 1, 2015 © Phys.org, <u>Science X network</u>)*

First Breeds

Between 3000 BC and 1 AD, sheep and wool spread to Persia (modern day Iran), Greece and Rome where herders contributed to improving breeds for wool and meat. The Romans were responsible for the spread of sheep to North Africa and Northern Europe. The famous Merino wool breed resulted from a crossing of the Tarentine sheep of Rome with the Laodician sheep of Asia Minor by breeders in the provinces of Terraconenis in Spain. After the fall of Rome, the Merino breed deteriorated, but it was later revived by the Muslims when they conquered Spain early in the 8th century. Under the Muslims, a wool export trade was established with North Africa, Greece, Egypt, Byzantium and Constantinople. When the Muslims were expelled from Spain by the Christians in the 14th century, the Merino sheep remained to become a rich source of income for the Spanish Crown. Income from the wool trade helped finance the voyages of Columbus and the Conquistadors. To carefully guard it's source of wealth, Spain refused to export a single Merino ewe under penalty of death until the year 1786 when Louis XVI of France imported 386 Merino ewes from Spain and cross bred them with sheep on his estate at Rambouillet, thereby creating the Rambouillet breed which is now considered one of the most desirable wool and meat breeds in the world.

English Empire

Legend has it that sheep were first brought to the English Isles by the Phoenician sailors from the Middle East sometime between 800 BC and 500 BC, and it was from these sheep that the heavily muscled English meat-breeds descended. The Romans later brought wool breeds to the Isles and established a woolen manufactury in Winchester, England in 50 AD. In 1337 AD, King Edward III of England, decided to make England self-sufficient in wool, so he decreed the importation of woven goods and the wearing of garments made of foreign wool illegal. At the same time, he invited skilled Flemish weavers to settle in England which invigorated the English wool industry by opening new markets at home and abroad, and encouraging English weavers to improve the quality of their products.

During this period, kings and nobles placed bounties on the killing of wolves to protect their herds of sheep, and by the reign of Henry VII (1457 – 1509), wolves had been extirpated from England.

England's woolen empire reached its zenith during the reigns of Henry VIII and Elizabeth I in the 16th century. In the process of Henry VIII's split from the Catholic Church over the issue of divorce, he seized the sheep herds from the monasteries and redistributed them among his court favorites and supporters. The new owners promptly fenced in the sheep which led to mass unemployment of shepherds who had previously tended the herds in open pastures. Unable to pay their debts, many shepherds were imprisoned and it was the political discontent stirred by the injustice of these debtors prisons (among other factors) that created a surge of migrants from England to the new American colonies.

In 18th century England, each region had its own improved meat breeds of sheep that were bred for the specific conditions of that area, but there were no "pedigree" breeds with carefully kept records of their breeding history. In 1780, sheep farmer John Ellman realized the sheep from the "South Downs" district of Sussex had breeding potential and he set out to standardize the breed. Ellman's new Southdown breed was small, polled (hornless), thick in the shoulder, full breasted, round and straight through the abdomen, wide in the loins and hips with fore and hind legs that stood wide, and fast maturing. The soils in the south of England known as the "downs", are chalky and not naturally fertile, but with the introduction of new forage crops that could thrive on alkaline soils such as field turnips, swedes and kohl rabi, the downs became prime sheep pasture and the flocks multiplied. While the Southdown was the first pedigree meat breed, Ellmen was instrumental in disseminating the breed over the entire downs and soon Southdowns were being used as breeding stock for several other well known pedigree meat breeds such as the Suffolk, Shropshire, Hampshire, and Oxford. By 1803, the Southdown had been introduced to Ireland and Scotland and later Ellman's son (also John) sold them to Australia, Portugal, America and the West Indies. In 1822, Jonas Webb, who farmed sheep in the downs near Cambridge, used Ellman stock to develop a larger Southdown type and he achieved nearly as much fame as Ellman himself. When Webb retired in 1861, 1,000 people attended his stock sale and his Southdowns were sold to sheep farmers in nearly every country in Europe, North and South America, as well as Australia and New Zealand.

The United Kingdom's (Great Britain and Northern Ireland) sheep population peaked at the end of World War I (1918), after which cheaper imports from Australia and New Zealand lead to a steady decline. According to Philip Walling, well known sheep farmer, barrister, and author of *"Counting Sheep: a Celebration of the Pastoral Heritage of Britain"*:

"In 1992, there were 44.5 million sheep in the United Kingdom — roughly the same as the number of adult humans. Now [2014] the sheep population has almost halved, to 23 million, and sheep farmers are becoming a rare breed." Walling expounded, "First, the national flock has never recovered from the foot and mouth slaughter of 2001, which reduced it by 5.5 per cent. Also, farmers and shepherds are growing old and retiring with no young people to take

their place." ("*Britain's sheep are vanishing . . . and part of our history is disappearing with them,*" Daily Mail, 1 May 2014)

European Union

According to Eurostat (the statistical office of the European Union), in 2013 there were 87.1 million sheep in the 28 EU countries, with 72% concentrated in five Member States: the UK (which was still a member of the EU at this time) had the largest national flock by far at 23.82 million sheep, followed by Spain – 15.96 million, Greece – 8.74 million, Italy – 7.28 million, and France – 7.16 million. The remaining 24.14 million were divided among the 23 other EU countries.

Northern EU countries had no or limited dairy production whereas dairy ewe sheep farming was significant in the southern EU countries. The farming systems for ovines in the southern countries was similar to that of bovines with both dairy and meat flocks co-existing. Dairy animals in the south were more profitable than meat animals and therefore more likely to be supported by technology, (i.e. advanced breeding, nutritional supplementation, farm equipment, etc.). Meat was produced, either from young animals in the dairy herd (lambs) or from meat herd animals fed on grassland or feedstuffs. Sheep farming is possible in areas with limited agronomic potential (rough grazing), but only at low levels of profitability per animal. The trend is either one of increasing herd size or of turning to dairy production. The EU's 2010 Farm Structure Survey indicated that 7.7% of farms in the EU had sheep and nearly half of the sheep belonged to flocks of over 500 animals. Though there were no EU subsidies designed to support sheep farming, EU Member States Greece, Spain, Italy, the Netherlands, Poland and Portugal have specific national support measures for sheep and goats.

Eurostat statistics on EU meat production in 2014 indicated that sheep and goats together accounted for 0.8 million tons or around 2% of all meat. Sheep and goat meat represented 1.4% of total EU agricultural output. Most of the animals were processed in official EU sanctioned slaughterhouses though a significant number were butchered in so-called "*other slaughtering*" facilities, primarily ritual slaughter at home. Eighty-one percent of ritual slaughter occurred in Member States that joined the EU in 2004 or later. Ritual slaughter accounted for 11.3% of total slaughtering in the 13 newest EU Member States and only 0.4% in the original 15 Member States. Ritual slaughter fell by 44% in the EU-28 between 2009 and 2014, but remained common in Bulgaria and Romania.

Of the 28 EU Member States in 2013, only Greece was among the top ten countries worldwide in per capita sheep meat consumption, ranking seventh at 28.25 pounds (12.8 kilograms) per person per year. The UK was a distant second at 10.38 pounds (4.7 kilograms) followed by France, Romania and Spain. (**Helgi Analytics,** Jaselská 18, Prague 6, 160 00, Czech Republic, Copyright © 2018 Helgi Library) The EU was a net importer of sheep meat at around 212, 000 tons in 2014, mainly from New Zealand and Australia accounting for 23% of total consumption.

North America

The first sheep in the Western Hemisphere arrived in Cuba and Santo Domingo with Columbus on his second voyage in 1493. These sheep were large, coarse-wooled, Spanish "Churros", bred for meat, and were brought for food, not wool. In 1519, Cortez took with him the offspring of Columbus' sheep as a mobile food supply in his conquest of Mexico. It was descendants of these Churros that were later adopted by the Navajo Indians of the North American Southwest.

During the colonial period of North America, England tried to discourage the wool industry in the colonies, but the colonists managed to smuggle in some sheep from England and in 1635 the Pilgrims of Plymouth Rock were able to purchase 40 sheep from the Dutch on Manhattan Island. By1643 the flock had grown to 1,000 and by 1664, the sheep population in Massachusetts had grown to 100,000. By the early 1700s, northern colonists had established an export trade shipping wool to other counties in return for manufactured goods. This contraband wool trade further heightened tensions with England leading up to the American Revolution. During the period following the revolution, the first leaders of the new country, acutely aware of the lack of good wool sheep breeds and fine quality wool, began importing Spanish Merino sheep in the early 1800s. By 1811, about 29,000 Merinos had been imported firmly establishing the breed in the U.S.

As American settlers moved west over the 1800s, they took with them flocks of sheep that were mostly of English meat breeds as a mobile food source. Inventory data on sheep kept by the U.S. government began in 1867, when 45 million animals were counted. During the late 1800s sheep ranching expanded into the plains states of the American west and the national flock size peaked in 1884 at 51 million, then dipped to 38 million by 1921, and then peaked again in 1942 at 56 million. During these years between the end of the Civil War and the beginning of World war II, at the behest of western sheep ranchers, the U.S. government established a predator control program that led to the extermination of the gray wolf from the continental U.S. Most sheep ranching was to produce wool and, while sheep meat has been popular among certain ethnic communities in the U.S., it never gained the market share of cattle, pig or chicken meat among the U.S. population.

From the early 1940s forward, sheep numbers in the U.S. plummeted as competition from Australia and New Zealand drove many sheep farmers out of business. Annual per capita consumption of sheep meat declined from nearly 5 pounds in the 1960s to under 1 pound in the 1990s. In that time U.S. sheep operations declined from around 105,000 to around 80,000 due to shrinking revenues and low rates of return. By the early 2000s, sheep numbers were down to around 6 million and according to the Economic Research Service of the USDA, the sheep industry accounts for less than 1% of U.S. livestock industry receipts *("Sheep, Lamb & Mutton: Background", United States Department of Agriculture, Economic Research Service (last updated May 26, 2012).*

In the U.S., commercial sheep production consists of two main types of operations: 1) range sheep of relatively large flock sizes that graze on native or unimproved pasture, mostly located in the western states, and 2) farm flocks, characterized by smaller numbers (often less than 50 animals) and raised on small improved pastures or in feedlots, mostly located in the Midwestern and eastern states. Sheep production from these operations provide specialty wool and pelts for textiles and milk for specialty cheeses and yogurts, but it is meat from young lambs that sustains the U.S. sheep industry. Lamb meat is primarily marketed through traditional channels, in which lambs move from pastures to higher-nutrient feeding systems where they grow to finish weight and then on to a commercial slaughterhouse.

New Zealand

The modern day country of New Zealand consists of two large islands and a number of smaller outlying islands located in the South Pacific Ocean about 1,250 miles (2,012 kilometers) southeast of the continent of Australia. In total area, the country is slightly smaller than the country of Japan. It's two main islands, North Island and South Island, are separated by a strait that is 14 miles wide (22 kilometers) at its narrowest point. The islands of New Zealand formed at the juncture of tectonic plates and their varied topography from sharp mountain peaks to broad grassy plains is largely due to tectonic uplift and volcanic eruptions.

The South Island's terrain and climate make it particularly adaptable to sheep farming. English explorer, Captain James Cook, realized this potential on his first voyage to New Zealand in 1769 and on his second voyage in 1773 he brought sheep stock with him, but they did not survive their new habitat. Anglican missionary, Samuel Marsden, had more success when he brought sheep from New South Wales, Australia, in 1814 to feed the whalers and sealers who were hunting there, but his flock remained small and did not spread beyond the mission stations.

The real foundations of sheep ranching in New Zealand were laid in 1843 and 1844 when several English settlers shipped 1,600 Merino sheep from Australia where they had already become established. These were the sheep that would stock New Zealand's most suitable ruminant habitat including the Canterbury Plains, now famous for its fine Merino wool. The drier eastern region of the South Island was more attractive to sheep farmers once the shrubs and tall tussock grass had been burned off and sown with herbs, grasses, and clovers ideal for grazing sheep. In 1847, 3,000 sheep were transferred to a huge block of grazing land on the northeast coast of the South Island. After this, running wool sheep on large tracts of land expanded rapidly through the South Island, stimulated by the demand for fine wool from the textile mills of England, Europe and the U.S.

In the second half of the 19th century, large scale pastoralism would dominate the sheep industry on the South Island. By about 1866, sheep farmers had taken up all the suitable land for grazing sheep. While shepherds raised Merinos for their fine wool, the breed was not a good meat producer or well adapted to the heavy soils of small farms, so small farmers began to import British meat breeds such as the Leicester, Lincoln, Romney and Southdown to better provide for domestic meat consumption. In the late 1870s, the population of New Zealand was a little over half a million people, compared with a population of 15 million sheep. Wool was the only product from sheep that could be exported as meat could not survive long sea voyages to England without spoiling. The invention of refrigerated shipping in the late 19th century opened up the export market for New Zealand's surplus sheep meat to the 35.6 million inhabitants of England in 1880. The first shipment of frozen meat from New Zealand to England in 1882 carried more than 4,000 adult and 600 lamb carcasses. By 1900, New Zealand was exporting more than 3 million sheep carcasses annually, mainly to England.

As meat exports increased over the first decades of the 20th century, land was farmed more intensively. Large areas were planted in turnips that were used as winter feed and wetlands were drained, cultivated, and sown in pasture. The total area of occupied land was nearly 45 million acres, on which 5 million acres supported up to 8 sheep per acre per year, and 9 million acres supported from 1/2 to 2 sheep per acre per year. Nearly half of the occupied land was in holdings of over 5,000 acres, with 90 holdings of over 50,000 acres and 18,694 holdings from 50 to 200 acres. By 1896 the national flock size had reached about 19 million sheep with an average individual flock size of 1,081. Grass was the primary crop. Blood-and-bone, a by-product of the meat industry, and superphosphate were more widely used to fertilize pastures.

New Zealand sheep farmers began cross-breeding Merinos with English meat breeds to develop new breeds that were particularly well suited to the different micro-climates and soil conditions of the islands. In 1868, a sheep farmer named James Little, who managed Corriedale Station, began trying to establish a "fixed inbred halfbred" that would be both a good wool and meat producer. At the time, there was much debate about whether an inbred halfbred sheep could be bred, but by the 1890s the dual purpose inbred halfbred known as the Corriedale had become well established. The Corriedale's wool is long and medium-to-fine and the breed is more fecund than the Merino, it is fast maturing and produces a heavily-muscled carcass. The Corriedale was bred for the plains and gentle hills of the drier eastern districts of both the North and South islands.

Soon after the frozen meat trade began, the Merinos became marginalized to the semi-arid and mountainous regions of the South Island. The Corriedale has since spread around the world and in the early 21st century vies with the Merino as the world's most popular sheep breed. There are about 2.8 million Corriedales in New Zealand, and 100 million worldwide. Another crossbred that was well established by the early 1900s was the New Zealand Romney which was a dual purpose breed distinctly different from the English Romney meat breed from which it was bred. The New Zealand Romney is suited to high rainfall and heavy soils, and has the highest resistance to footrot of any breed in New Zealand. It grows a heavy fleece used in carpets, furnishings and knitting yarns. The New Zealand Romney was the single most popular breed in New Zealand through the 20th century making up about 68% of the national flock in the early 2000s with over 25 million sheep. By 1912, 93% of the national flock was defined in government statistics as "crossbreds". This basic system set up in the early 20th century was still in practice into the early 21st century.

By the mid 1950s, wool accounted for 35% of New Zealand's export revenue and red meat (including sheep and cattle meat) accounted for 30%, together representing nearly two thirds of New Zealand's export revenues, with England dominating the export market. Then in 1973, nearly tariff-free access to England for New Zealand sheep meat was severely curtailed by England's entry into the European Economic Community (EEC) sending shock waves through the New Zealand sheep industry. This turn of events forced New Zealand sheep farmers to find and develop new markets, and they began to market their product to countries around the world. In 1971, 87% of New Zealand lamb exports went to England, but by 2009 that number was down to 22% with the rest divided between over 100 countries including China, Germany, France, U.S., Saudi Arabia, Canada, Belgium and Mexico.

Also in 1973, in response to the first major world oil shock induced by the Organization of Petroleum Exporting Countries (OPEC), the government of New Zealand, to encourage the country's two main exports to pay for imported oil, provided incentives to increase sheep numbers including land development subsidies and price supports that farmers would receive for their meat and wool. These government agricultural policies led to significant growth in sheep numbers reaching an all-time high of 70 million in the early 1980s. In 1984, the newly elected Labour Government began deregulation of the economy, including a rapid phase-out of all agricultural support measures. As a result, sheep meat prices collapsed and farmers scaled back production; by 1987, the sheep population was down to 39 million, and by 2014, 29.8 million, still nearly 7 sheep for every human in the country.

With this decline in sheep numbers also came a consolidation in the New Zealand sheep industry. The number of commercial sheep farms declined by nearly 40% after 1984, but the average farm carried 27% more sheep. The average number of sheep per farm by 2007 was 4,250, and most farms were still owned and operated by farming families. New Zealand sheep farmers also began producing more and heavier finishing animals. On-farm productivity gains were largely due to enhanced breeding mixes and improved lambing percentages.

Historically, a large proportion of the meat processing industry was controlled by English interests, which exported most meat as carcasses to butchers in the UK, where it was then turned into retail cuts. However, in the 1970s, new veterinary and hygiene requirements in the U.S. and Europe meant that significant investment would be required in many plants in order for them to continue exporting to these markets. The UK companies, unwilling to make the investment, began to depart the sector, and the influence of New Zealand-owned companies began to grow. The decline in the number of retail butchers and the growing dominance of supermarkets and retail chains, meant New Zealand had to provide pre-packaged, retail-ready products. By the early 2000s, meat processing companies in New Zealand ranged in size from small, single plant operations, to some of New Zealand's largest companies. The four largest meat processing companies in 2007 were ranked in the 40 largest companies in New Zealand (by revenue). With New Zealand's investment in meat processing, productivity in processing plants increased dramatically. A typical sheep processing chain in the 1980s employed more than 50 people and processed 3,000 sheep per day. Newer plants typically employed 30 people and process 4,000 sheep a day. This calculates out to an increase in productivity on sheep chains from 55 sheep per person per day in the 1980s, to nearly 130 per person per day in the early 2000s. Technologies such as yield grading systems, and automated and robotic meat cutting systems have been introduced. Advances in packaging, handling and distribution have seen exports progress from frozen whole carcasses, to further processing into pre-packed frozen and chilled cuts and boneless products. Industry marketing campaigns have positioned lamb as a premium meat at the higher-priced end of the market. New Zealand's lamb exports have moved from primarily frozen carcasses in the early 1970s, to now nearly 95% being further processed, value-added product. By 2007, New Zealand had become the largest sheep meat exporter by volume in the world accounting for 40% of global exports.

Australia

The first sheep to arrive in Australia came with the English First fleet in 1788, but they all died or were slaughtered for food and did not proliferate. More sheep arrived in 1793, but they were used exclusively to feed the penal colonies that the English were establishing in Australia and they too did not proliferate.

The sheep that would become the backbone of the Australian livestock industry did not arrive until 1797 when Captain John Macarthur imported 16 Spanish Merinos from South Africa to his 100 acre farm near the present day city of Sydney on the southeast coast of New South Wales. By 1801, Macarthur had 1,000 head of sheep, and in 1803 he exported 245 pounds (111 kilograms) of wool to England. With wool reaching record prices in Europe, especially during the Napoleonic Wars from 1803 to 1815, there was a large influx of Merinos into Australia.

In 1813, after a period of drought, three settlers – Gregory Blaxland, William Lawson and William Wentworth – went west with an Aboriginal guide and three convicts in search of grasslands for sheep pasture. They surveyed a route inland over the Blue Mountains in the Great Dividing Range where they found a vast expanse of bush and grasslands. Soon after, a team of convicts was set to building a road and settlers began to populate the area, bringing their sheep (and cattle) to graze on the open plains.

In 1824, the Australian Agricultural Company was established through an Act of the English Parliament, with the right to select 1,000,000 acres (404,686 hectares) on the East coast north of Sydney for agricultural development. Cheap labor was sourced through convicts, aboriginals and indentured laborers on seven-year contracts to bring this land into sheep production.

In the late 1820s the English Governor of Australia, Major-General Lachlan Macquarie, had the vast tablelands south of Sydney in New South Wales and Victoria surveyed where they found rich soil and open plains that started a stampede of settlers eager to graze sheep there. These extensive grasslands and open woodlands were largely the result of "fire-stick farming" which had been practiced by the aboriginal people of Australia for centuries before they were displaced by the English settlers and their grazing animals. Huge areas of forest and scrub were cleared for pasture and crop farming along Australia's coast and inland setting-off explosive growth in Australia's sheep industry. In 1820, the continent held 100,000 sheep, a decade later it had one million and by 1840, New South Wales alone grazed 4 million sheep. By the end of the 1850s, sheep numbers across Australia had reached 16 million, or around 39 sheep per person.

Between 1850 and 1880, early Australian pioneer breeders, like Thomas Shaw and George Peppin used Merinos and other breeds from Europe, North America and New Zealand, to re-create the famous short-stapled Spanish fine-wool sheep into completely new domestic sheep strains that were larger bodied and with longer wool. As a result, the present day Australian Merino is not a single homogeneous breed, but rather a number of strains which are uniquely Australian. Most of the Australian sheep flock was (and still is in the early 2000s) either pure or part Merino and the most notable feature of the Australian sheep flock is that it was bred primarily for wool production. With the expansion of sheep and wool industries, sheep meat was still cheap and abundant. In 1903, it was estimated that the average Australian ate 90 pounds (41 kilograms) of sheep meat per year mostly culled from the adult flock, though lamb meat was favored in sparsely populated rural areas.

About two-thirds of Australia's vast land mass is given over to farm production, and about 90% of that farm land is used for grazing sheep and cattle on native pastures, mostly in the arid and semi-arid zones commonly known as the "outback". The development of Australian agriculture relied upon overcoming the long distances that separated farms from their major urban markets. In the 1830s, droving herds of sheep and cattle from distant stations along Traveling Stock Routes was how livestock reached the cities. The exploits of "drovers" and "overlanders" remain vivid in Australian folklore.

The first paddle steamer arrived in Australia in 1831, and paddle-steamers plied the Murray and Darling Rivers with agribusiness supplies and returned cargoes of wool for the next 70 years. The building of railways from the 1850s onward began to connect the more remote farmers with quicker and easier transport of their products to the cities and ports.

The development of steam clipper ships in the 1850s significantly cut the time it took to complete the voyage from Australia to England, taking only 90 days instead of 140. Wool and leather hides were the main cargo of these ships since meat spoiled on the long sea voyage. While sheep meat was an Australian favorite, with so many sheep and so few people, there was a large surplus of sheep meat with no accessible market. This problem was remedied when, in 1881 the steam clipper Dunedin, owned by the New Zealand and Australian Land Company, was refitted with a compression refrigeration machine and successfully delivered a cargo of frozen meats to the UK. Soon thereafter, an extensive frozen meat trade from Australia to the UK developed. Over 16 different "reefer" ships were built or refitted by 1900 and between 1901 and 1906, exports of frozen sheep meat rose by 50%. By 1910 UK refrigerated meat imports had risen to 760,000 tons carcass weight per year.

In the 1850s the Australian government erected a centralized slaughterhouse on Glebe Island out in the Sydney harbor to remove animal slaughter from the center of the city. In 1882 the Royal Commission found that 524,415 sheep, 69,991 cattle, 31,269 pigs and 8,348 calves were slaughtered there. By the 1890s, the Glebe Island slaughterhouse had become a public nuisance, the subject of constant complaints about the smells as well as the pollution of the surrounding harbor and it was finally shut down in 1915, its works transferred to a new government slaughterhouse at Homebush to the west of Sydney. By 1923 the Homebush slaughterhouse was the biggest of its kind in the entire British Commonwealth employing up to 1,600 men with a killing capacity of 20,000 sheep, 1,500 cattle, 2,000 pigs and 1,300 calves per day. The inspiration for the Homebush slaughterhouse was the Chicago meat packing plants in the U.S., with a disassembly line subdividing each task down to very simple operations. Homebush was different than U.S. meat packing plants in one respect: as a government operated facility, it did not trade in meat, and was solely dependent on service fees to maintain the operation.

Though a few other municipal slaughterhouses had been built in other cities, the Homebush plant near Sydney operated as the major centralized slaughtering facility in Australia up into the 1950s when rapid population growth began to strain the meat distribution system. In the 1950s the New South Wales government initiated the building of several decentralized slaughterhouses in major regional centers to reduce the load on Homebush. These were medium-sized, multi-species facilities operated by either municipal authorities or county councils. At that time, the only single species slaughterhouses in Australia were in Queensland to service the meat export trade, but the increasing specialization in the meat industry led to an increasing move toward single species facilities for sheep and cattle. All new slaughter capacity built since the 1990s has been for single species operations. Single species slaughterhouses required a larger stock catchment areas to operate at full capacity so they were conveniently located adjacent to feedlots to keep them fully supplied.

By the late 1800s, much of Australia's native pasture had become overrun with European annual grasses, clovers, and other invasive plants like the deliberately introduced prickly pear which was to eventually occupy 60 million acres. Australian pastures were further depleted by overstocking and overgrazing with introduced European sheep and cattle. In 1859, the European wild rabbit which was brought for the purpose of hunting, also contributed to overgrazing. Wild rabbits multiplied by the millions throughout Australia and their ravenous appetites caused the extinction of many native plant species leading to soil erosion, nutrient loss, siltation of waterways, destruction of aquatic ecosystems and the demise of many native marsupial species such as the bilby and the bandicoot who lost their food supply.

As a result of all these destructive influences, the livestock carrying capacity of the Australian pasture began a precipitous decline; in the major sheep producing regions of western New South Wales, sheep numbers fell from 13.6 million in 1891 to 5.4 million in 1900. The use of fertilizers on pasture had its beginnings in the early 1900s with emphasis on increasing fodder production both by grasses and legumes, but despite higher fodder yields, accelerated soil exploitation saw a further decline in Australia's soil fertility over the first three decades of the 20th century. From the 1930s forward, as

Australian farmers realized that it was the extreme poverty of their soils that was causing the decline in agricultural production, the government launched an ambitious campaign to raise soil fertility over vast areas of poor soils by introducing a new cropping technique called "ley farming" in which large quantities of fertilizers and legume seeds were applied to pasture lands by aircraft. The introduction of phosphorous, sulfur, potassium and trace element fertilizers plus the fixation of nitrogen and carbon with leguminous plants resulted in large and sustained yield increases in Australia's pasturelands over the next several decades. One study documenting the increase in sheep numbers in each of Australia's states in the period between 1947 and 1963 found that each additional improved acre led to an increase of 1.6 sheep and of that increase, 48% was associated with pasture improvement, while 52% was due to all other factors combined including rabbit control, disease control, fodder conservation, fencing, irrigation, improved transportation *("The Progress of Australian Agriculture and the Role of Pastures in Environmental Change," The Australian Journal of Science, January 1965)*. One outcome of ley farming was better nutrition for pregnant ewes and an increase in their lambing rate by as much as 20% over sheep grazed on unimproved pasture. With this increase in lambing rate, lambs became more numerous, and milder tasting lamb meat soon overtook adult sheep meat as the preferred consumer option.

England joined the European Economic Community (EEC) in 1973 and promptly ended their most favored nations trade agreements with British Commonwealth countries including Australia. Australian sheep farmers responded to this economic setback by aggressively marketing Australian lamb in the Middle East, North Africa, Europe, the U.S. and Asia. As market demand grew, the Australian national flock also continued to grow through the 1970s and 1980s, peaking at 172 million animals in the late 1980s. Since 1990, due to difficult economic conditions and severe prolonged drought, the Australian sheep population steadily declined to 98 million in 2004 and to 72.6 million in 2014. In 2014-2015, Australia produced 506,605 tons (carcass weight) of lamb and 214,446 tons (carcass weight) of adult sheep meat.

In 2014-15, Australia exported 56% of their total lamb meat production and 95% of total sheep meat produced. The Middle East was the largest export market for Australian lamb accounting for 28.7% of total Australian lamb exports (by value) in 2014-15, followed by the U.S., China and the EU. In 2014-15 Australia was second only to New Zealand in world lamb meat exports and was the largest exporter of adult sheep meat. Australia was also the world's largest live sheep exporter, exporting 3.1 million live sheep in 2014-15 to major markets in the Middle East including Kuwait, Bahrain, the United Arab Emirates, Qatar and Jordan where they are ritually slaughtered.

Around 81.4% of Australian households purchased lamb in 2014-15 and Australians ate around 21 pounds (9.4kg) of lamb meat and 1 pound (0.5kg) of adult sheep meat per person in 2014-15, placing Australians among the highest sheep meat consumers in the world.

China

As discussed above, sheep breeds in modern China descended from breeds first bred in China around 5,000 years ago from the original domesticated sheep that came from Mesopotamia. Over the next five millennia, Chinese breeders developed hundreds of breeds unique to China. Since there are no recorded historical accounts of this breeding process as in the West, modern genetic studies have been relied upon to untangle the complex web of interbreeding of China's sheep population. One such study, *"… revealed three major clusters in Chinese indigenous sheep (Mongolian sheep, Kazakh sheep and Tibetan sheep), except Zhaotong and Guide Black Fur sheep. They were probably caused by different breeding history, geography isolation and different levels of inbreeding"* ("Genetic diversity of Chinese indigenous sheep breeds inferred from microsatellite markers," *Small Ruminant Research,* May 2010). Another genetic study found that:

> "With the establishment of modern sheep production systems in China, various forms of hybridization with Western breeds and between native breeds have been utilized for genetic improvement. At the same time, the progressive destruction or deterioration of sheep habitat has accompanied urbanization in China. Together these factors have accelerated the loss of genetic diversity, or even resulted in the extinction of some indigenous breeds." ("Phylogeography and Origin of Sheep Breeds in Northern China," *Conservation Genetics,* February 2006)

FAOStat data indicate that in 2014 China was by far the leading sheep raising country in the world with approximately 202 million animals. Most of these sheep grazed on the vast grasslands along China's northern border with Mongolia, Russia and Kazakhstan, in the Province of Gansu and the autonomous regions of Xinjiang and Inner Mongolia.

China's grasslands are diverse environments that are exploited to graze sheep, goats, cattle and yaks, ranging from the high-altitude seasonally frozen plains of the Qinghai-Tibetan plateau to the low-altitude steppes of Inner Mongolia. They cover roughly the same area as Australia's grasslands, about 1,544,400 square miles (400 million hectares), but with far greater temperature variations. Across much of these plateaus temperatures range from -40° F (-40° C) in winter to summer highs of 104° F (40° C). Forage plants grow for only three months out of the year and at higher altitudes upper soil layers remain frozen for much of each year.

The long narrow Province of Gansu that runs southeast to northwest has served for centuries as a vital strategic corridor linking the center of China with the vast territory in the far Northwest. Northern Gansu is squeezed between the autonomous regions of Xinjiang to the west and Inner Mongolia to the east. Plateaus dominate the landscape of northwest Gansu at an average elevation of about 3,000 feet (900 meters) above sea level; in northeast Gansu, hilly terrain gives way to the Gobi Desert. Rainfall is meager with long cold winters and short summers. Traditional Han Chinese constitute the largest ethnic group, but several other minority ethnic groups also live there including the Hui, Mongol, Turk, Uyghur, and Tibetan. Gansu is the poorest province in China with subsistence farming and grazing animals the primary agricultural activity. Sheep constitute approximately half of all animals grazed. In 2010 the human population of Gansu Province stood at 25.6 million people.

To the west of Gansu lies the autonomous region of Xinjiang which has a varied topography including lakes and oases fed by glacial runoff, desert plains, mountain peaks over 16,000 feet (4,877 meters), valleys below sea level, and extensive grassland plateaus. Xinjiang prospered for many centuries as an important region along the Silk Road overland western trade route with Persia (modern day Iran) and Rome, but once shipping became a more reliable form of transportation after the 16th century, the area returned to a more frontier economy. This long history of foreign trade brought many ethnic Muslims to the region such as the Uyghur, Hui, Kazakh, and Kyrgyz. These Muslim cultures have long pastoral traditions of sheep herding. A "fat tailed" sheep variety is raised mainly for meat, but also for milk to make cheese and yogurt. Other varieties are raised primarily for wool which varies in texture and is most suitable for weaving carpets. In 2010 the human population of Xinjiang stood at 21.8 million people.

The autonomous region of Inner Mongolia lies to the east of Gansu and is largely an inland plateau at an elevation of about 3,300 feet (1,000 meters) above sea level, fringed by mountains and valleys. To the northwest the land falls away toward the forbidding Gobi Desert. The Yellow River makes a great loop through south-central Inner Mongolia delineating and providing irrigation water for the arid Ordos Plateau. Rich grasslands are concentrated in this central part of the region. Sheep and goats in roughly equal numbers are by far the most numerous animals grazed on these grasslands. Han Chinese constitute the bulk of the population with Mongols being the largest minority. In 2010 most of Inner Mongolia's 24.7 million people lived in the agricultural belt south of the Mongolian Plateau near the Yellow River and on the eastern slopes of the Da Hinggan Mountain Range.

Trade in grazing animals has a long history in China as age old trade routes connected the grasslands to the northern cities near the herding regions. Well into the 20th century, annual sheep drives were how pastoralists would transport their livestock to the nearby cities. This pastoral economy began to change in the 1950s when projects associated with Communist China's first Five Year Plan from 1953 to 1958 aimed at expanding and developing animal industries across the northern provinces. In a forced settlement of pastoral people into herding communes (*muqu gongshe*), sheep and cattle raising were brought under state control. Through the 1950s, command purchasing by the state encouraged communes to abandon cows in favor of sheep, which breed more quickly, increasing the sheep population commensurately (*"Big Meat: The rise and impact of mega-farming in China's beef, sheep and dairy industries,"* Asia-Pacific Journal: Japan Focus, September, 2017).

China's largest slaughterhouse in Hailar was completed in 1956 which greatly expanded industrial processing capacity. While most of the meat from this plant was sold to foreign markets, local consumption of sheep meat in herding regions remained high, even through the period of severe privation during the Great Leap Forward from 1958 to 1962. But despite this national emphasis on meat production, per capita meat consumption remained very low throughout most of China through the 1950s, 60s and 70s.

Before the 1980s, herds of sheep and cattle were driven by nine-man teams into Hailar from as far away as 92 miles (150km), a process that was arduous and costly because the animals lost significant weight along the way. Reforms in the 1980s built regional slaughterhouses in other cities and shifted the task of transportation to professional middlemen, who purchased and delivered the animals by truck. In an attempt to relieve grazing pressure on grasslands which by then had been severely overgrazed, while also steadily increasing meat production, China began a deliberate policy called the "1985 Chinese Rangeland Law" to establish large-scale, intensive farms and to import animal feed mostly from the U.S. and Brazil. Also to relieve grazing pressure on grasslands, the Ministry of Agriculture in 1988 began to shift cattle and sheep production to agricultural provinces like Henan and Shandong to the south. Despite, or as a result of these policies, China's sheep and cattle populations sustained phenomenal growth rates throughout the 1990s and 2000s and China emerged as the world's leading sheep producing country.

At the invitation of the Chinese Government in 2001, Professor David Kemp, one of the world's foremost scientific experts on temperate grasslands and chair of farming systems at Charles Sturt University in western New South Wales, Australia, traveled through China's northwest to study the deteriorating grasslands. Professor Kemp noted:

> *"'Our estimate is that there would be three to four times the number of animals in China as there would be in Australia on similar grassland types,' Professor Kemp says, explaining that there is consensus that China's grasslands are being considerably overgrazed.*
>
> *It is a phenomenon that began to appear during the past few decades, as stock numbers on the grasslands have more than doubled in response to human population growth and government policies and programs. The problem has been exacerbated by the conversion of some grasslands into croplands.*
>
> *Traditional herd-management practices, largely born of social and community behaviours, can be counter-productive. For example, although the grasslands are green for only three months a year and covered with frost and dead plant remnants for the rest of the time, herdsmen typically graze their animals every day, no matter how inhospitable the weather or sparse the feed supply.*
>
> *'The energy costs that animals expend just walking around are often greater than any nutrition they ever get out of the pastures, and they typically lose 25 to 30% of their bodyweight through autumn, winter and spring before regaining it over summer,' Professor Kemp says.*
>
> *As a result it takes cattle, for example, four to five years to reach the size of 18-month-old animals in Australia." ("Restoring China's grasslands," ustralian Centre for International Agricultural Research, 2008)*

The trend in China's sheep production in the 2010s has been towards factory farming. The most notable example of a factory sheep farm is *Green Grassland*. Founded in 2014, *Green Grassland* had 100,000 sheep at its main facility in Wuyuan, and smaller numbers at production sites in Henan and

Xinjiang. It is also vertically integrated with its own facilities for feed production, slaughtering, processing and distribution.

In 2015, two meat trade associations – the *International Meat Secretariat* and the United Kingdom's *Agriculture and Horticulture Development Board* – issued a joint industry report entitled, *World Sheep Meat Market to 2025, which* analyzed current international sheep market trends and made future forecasts through the year 2025. The report starts out with this declaration, *"The emergence of China is changing the dynamics of the global sheep meat market. China is now the largest producer, consumer and importer of sheep meat."* Overall, the report predicts that despite certain environmental constraints, domestic production will likely continue to increase marginally due to farmers reacting to high market prices relative to cattle and pig meat.

Current per capita annual consumption of sheep meat amounted to only about 3.5 pounds (1.5kg), but the report concludes that an increase in demand from more affluent urban consumers will continue to outstrip domestic supply which will create an expanding market for imports. While the current market for "premium" quality sheep meat was very small, the report saw great potential for growth through market penetration by major U.S. and European multinational supermarket, restaurant and hotel chains:

- Supermarkets – Wal-Mart (more than 380 stores), Carrefour, Auchan, Metro and Tesco
- Restaurants – Pizza Hut and Little Sheep (both owned by Yum! Brands Inc), KFC and McDonalds
- Hotels – International Hotel Group (Intercontinental, Crown Plaza, Holiday Inn), Accor Hotels and Resorts (Sofitel, Pullman), Cendant (Howard Johnson, Wyndham), Starwood Hotels and Resorts Worldwide (Sheraton), Marriott Hotel Group (Renaissance, Marriott), Shangri-la Hotel and Kempinski Hoteliers

This overall bullish report on sheep meat production and consumption in China by the *International Meat Secretariat* and the *Agriculture and Horticulture Development Board* of the UK, makes scant reference to the environmental impacts sheep and cattle grazing on such a large scale has had on China's fragile grassland ecosystems, but on the ground, the situation is dire. An article published by *The Conversation US* in 2016, (a self styled *"independent source of news and views from the academic and research community"*), entitled *"China's desertification is causing trouble across Asia"*, lays out the problem:

> *"Creeping desertification in China is swallowing thousands of square kilometres of productive soil every year. It's a challenge of gigantic and unprecedented proportions.*
>
> *"The rate of desertification increased throughout the second half of last century and, although this trend has since stabilised, the situation remains very serious.*
>
> *"More than a quarter of the entire country is now degraded or turning to desert, thanks to 'overgrazing by livestock, over cultivation, excessive water use, or changes in climate'. The Gobi desert alone gobbles up 3,600km^2 of grassland each year. China's own State Forestry*

Administration has identified land desertification as the country's most important ecological problem, and climate change will only make things worse.

"Ecological disasters have social effects. Desertification threatens the subsistence of about a third of China's population, especially those in the country's west and north, and could pose serious challenges to political and economic stability. It costs China roughly RMB 45 billion (US$6.9 billion) per year.

"Research shows that 'for seriously desertified regions, the loss amounts to as much as 23.16% of … annual GDP'. The fact that one third of the country's land area is eroded has led some 400m people to struggle to cope with a lack of productive soil, destabilised climatological conditions and severe water shortages. Droughts damage "about 160,000 square kilometres of cropland each year, double the area damaged in the 1950s".

"Blaming the desertification on overgrazing and bad cultivation, the state has since 2005 started to reallocate millions of people from dry and barren territories under its controversial and hotly-contested 'ecological migration' programme.

"Despite extraordinary efforts by the government to reduce the rate of erosion, culminating in the largest reforestation project ever undertaken, the government itself conceded in 2011 that the 'desertification trend has not fundamentally reversed'."

This rapid desertification of China's grasslands has greatly exacerbated massive dust storms that emanate from the Gobi Desert. A New York Times article on May 17, 2017, headlined, *"Dust Storms Blanket Beijing and Northern China,"* describes the scene:

"Dust storms enveloped parts of northern China for a second day on Friday, reducing visibility in cities like Beijing and threatening the health of millions of people.

Such storms have become an increasingly common phenomenon for the region, as China's deserts expand by gobbling up roughly 1,300 square miles a year. A half-century ago, such storms happened every seven or eight years; now they are an annual occurrence."

A study published by the *Australian Centre for International Agricultural Research (ACIAR)* in 2008, entitled "Restoring China's grasslands", explains the dust storm phenomenon:

"Dust storms have long been a part of life in Beijing. China's capital can be blanketed during the northern spring by layers of dirt and grit up to two centimetres thick, as winds dump hundreds of thousands of tonnes of eroded soil across the city.

This airborne pollution is carried from the extensive native grasslands that stretch for some 3,000 kilometres across the nation, from the west to the north-east. As these ecosystems have become increasingly degraded, China's infamous dust problem has worsened, drawing complaints from as far away as Japan and Korea.

Dust storms are a consequence of increasing human and livestock populations on China's grasslands, large expanses of which are now characterised by low-income households and deteriorating ecosystems. '*Studying dust problems independently of the way livestock are managed will not bring sustainable solutions,' explains Professor Nan Zhibiao, dean of the College of Pastoral Science, Lanzhou University."*

China's dust storms have major impacts on human health as noted in the 2016, *The Conversation US*, report referenced above:

"Inhaling this dust has devastating effects on the health of animals and humans alike. Asian dust has in the past decade been linked to both cardiovascular and respiratory diseases while more recent research discovered 'a statistically significant association between Asian dust storms and daily mortality'.

Dust storms also transport toxic pollutants, bacteria, viruses, pollen and fungi. Microbiologists looked at a dust storm in South Korea and found big increases in aerial bacteria." (*"China's desertification is causing trouble across Asia", The Conversation,* May 16, 2016.)

China's move towards imported animal feed and factory farms in the sheep industry has its own set of environmental impacts. Local environmental impacts of factory farms include the contamination of land, air and water from the mountains of manure and rivers of urine they generate. And buying feed grown on land reclaimed from the Brazilian rainforest simply transfers the ecological destruction to another part of the world.

Asian Subcontinent

Though the rankings vary from year to year due to changing climatic and economic conditions, FAOStat data from 2014 listed India as the third largest sheep farming country in the world with 63 million animals. India's sheep are direct descendants of the first domesticated sheep from Mesopotamia. Domesticated sheep were already present in the Harappa and Mohanjo-daro civilizations (2500 BC) in the Indus Valley of modern day Pakistan. In 2014, Pakistan was the world's eleventh largest sheep farming country with 29.1 million animals).

While sheep farming is spread across the subcontinent, in India it is most concentrated in the northwestern states of Rajasthan, Gujarat and Uttar Pradesh, and the southern states of Andhra Pradesh, Tamil Nadu and Karnataka, where arid and semi-arid regions are marginal for intensive agriculture. Sheep farming in India is primarily left to landless or land poor people who graze their small flocks on common grazing lands, wastelands, fallow lands, stubble of cultivated crops and tree loppings; rarely are they fed on grain or cultivated fodder.

Indian sheep farmers employ two basic types of shepherding systems: 1) Nomadic flocks with no fixed home location that follow seasonal migratory routes to grazing areas. This system is highly dependent on the availability of natural forage and drinking water resources. In Rajasthan, where flocks are in permanent migration, shepherds relieve one another and return home in rotations. 2) Seasonally migrated flocks are grazed on fallow lands during monsoon and on stubble after the Kharif crops are harvested from September through October; they spend the rest of the year on uncultivated lands where they are non-migratory. In both types of flock management, top feeding by lopping tree branches and shaking of pods is common. In the extreme heat of the summer months, flocks are grazed in the cooler evening hours of the day. They are brought to watering holes around midday and rested during the heat of the day between 12:00 noon and 5 pm.

Most of the breeds of sheep in India evolved naturally (with limited human selection) through adaptation to the agro-ecological conditions of India's arid and semi-arid regions. These breeds have generally been named after their place of origin or on the basis of prominent characteristics. While there has been some cross-breeding with exotic dual purpose breeds, (e.g. Hissardale, Kashmir Merino and Nilgiri), most sheep in India are of nondescript or mixed breeds. Most Indian sheep are well adapted to the harsh climate, long migrations, and lack of vegetation and drinking water of their grazing lands. Among Indian sheep breeds, the most important in number and distribution are the Marwari and Deccani. The Marwari covers the greater part of the arid northwestern region, in both Rajasthan and Gujarat. It is highly migratory, following a nomadic system of management, and has made the greatest impact on other breeds, especially those with very coarse and hairy fleeces such as the Malpura and Sonadi. The Sonadi covers most of the central part of the southern Indian peninsula in the states of Maharashtra, Andhra Pradesh and Karnataka. Current breeding policy for improving wool production and quality and increasing meat production is to cross the better carpet-wool breeds and extremely coarse and hairy breeds with exotic fine-wool and dual purpose breeds. Quality and yields of Indian sheep meat and wool is relatively low compared to more advanced countries largely due to inadequate grazing land, lack of veterinary resources, and limited effort to improve genetics.

While sheep meat is a staple in the diet of India's poor sheep farmers, for the large majority Hindu population of India, sheep meat is not a significant part of their diet. In the far northern States of Jammu and Kashmir, which have been disputed territories between India and neighboring Pakistan since both countries gained independence from the British Empire in 1947, sheep farming and meat eating are long standing cultural traditions.

Middle East

The Middle East, where sheep were first domesticated, is still one of the world's major sheep producing regions. FAOStat data from 2014 ranked Iran as the #4 sheep farming country in the world with over 50 million animals. Other Middle Eastern countries among the top 20 are #8 Turkey with over 31.1 million animals, and #17 Syria with 17.8 million. (An ongoing civil war in Syria starting in 2011 severely downsized Syria's flock size.) Overall, FAOStat 2014 listed 14 Middle Eastern sheep farming countries, including war torn Iraq and Afghanistan which also lost flock size, and not including Egypt which is included with the African continent (see below). Taken together, the Middle East with a combined flock size of over 204 million animals, is roughly the same size as China's.

With the exception of the Jewish State of Israel (which farms the least number of sheep in the Middle East at 574,000), all of the other Middle Eastern countries are predominantly Muslim with long traditions of raising sheep for local meat and milk consumption and for wool to make carpets for export markets. While people living in Middle Eastern countries eat less meat overall (including cattle, pig and chicken) than people in the European Union and Western Hemisphere, most Middle Easterners eat more sheep meat than the 3.75 pounds/person/year (1.7 kilograms/person/year) worldwide average in 2014, with Saudi Arabia at 12.3 pounds/person/year (5.6 kilograms), Turkey at 8.4 pounds (3.8 kilograms) and Pakistan at 7.3 pounds (3.3 kilograms) all well above the world average (OECD-FAO Agricultural Outlook 2015-©, 2012 – 2014 average consumption). Despite being a major producer of sheep meat, the Middle East was also the world's largest importer of live sheep from Australia and New Zealand to satisfy local demand.

While there is considerable climate variation over the Middle Eastern land mass, including a few areas of high rainfall in Turkey, Afghanistan and Pakistan, most of the region is characterized by arid and semi-arid climactic conditions, marginal vegetation, and low meat, milk and wool yields per animal relative to countries with denser forage.

Enumerable local sheep breeds have been naturally adapted in the Middle East over thousands of years that are well equipped to survive in the many varied habitats comprising the region. Similar to India, there are three main types of sheep management systems employed in the Middle East: 1) nomadic, 2) semi-intensive and 3) intensive. Traditional nomadic sheep herding is typical to the dry plateaus and desert areas. As the human population of the Middle East increases, rangeland conversion of these areas to irrigated cropland has reduced the land available for traditional nomadic sheep herding. With less grazing land available to support increasing numbers of sheep, nomadic rangelands have become severely degraded and the animals sickly and undernourished. In semi-intensive systems, sheep flocks are rotated around fallow agricultural fields and then herded to a home base during off seasons where they are fed on fodder. Intensive systems where the animals live their entire lives in confinement are a small but growing segment of the sheep meat and milk market as demand for these products continues to grow along with the human population.

Africa

With 49 countries raising well over 300 million sheep according to FAOStat 2014, Africa is by far the largest sheep farming continent in the world. From Nigeria at #5 in the world with over 40 million animals, to the tiny island nation of Mauritius at #145 in the world with 6,500 animals, African sheep herders raise sheep in all types of climactic and topographic conditions from the vast arid zones of the Sahara Desert covering all of northern Africa, to the moist tropical equatorial zones of sub-Saharan central Africa, to the more temperate zones of southern Africa.

Saharan Africa

The Sahara is the largest hot desert in the world (only the cold deserts of the Antarctic and Arctic are larger) encompassing an area of 3,600,000 square miles (9,200,000 square kilometers), comprising about a third of the African continent or roughly the size of China or the United States. The dust dry Sahara desert is bounded on three sides by water, to the north by the Mediterranean Sea, to the west by the Atlantic Ocean and to the east by the Red Sea. Ten Saharan countries are listed raising sheep in 2014 (FAOStat 2014): Algeria, Chad, Egypt, Libya, Mali, Mauritania, Morocco, Niger, Sudan and Tunisia, with a combined total of over 174.7 million animals. Most of the populations of Morocco, Algeria, Tunisia, Libya, Mauritania, northern Mali, northern Niger and a small part of western Egypt are ethnic Berbers. Their ancestors who were subsistence farmers and herders first arrived in North Africa around 10,000 years ago. The majority of Berbers are Sunni Muslim with long traditions of sheep herding that go back to ancient times when domesticated sheep were first brought to north Africa by the Romans. Berber shepherds bred their sheep to survive the harsh climate of the Saharan landscape.

Across north Africa from west to east the Saharan countries of Morocco, Algeria, Tunisia, Libya and Egypt, where over 66.4 million sheep were raised in 2014, all have lengthy coastlines along the Mediterranean Sea extending from the Strait of Gibraltar in the west to the Red Sea in the east. In parts of Morocco and northern Algeria two ranges of the Atlas Mountains run parallel to the Mediterranean coast. The Tell Atlas and the Sahara Atlas ranges form two natural barriers, the first against the sea to the north and the second against the desert to the south. The northern slopes of the Sahara Atlas receive more rainfall than the high plateaus that lay between the two ranges, watering grasses where sheep are grazed. Sheep are also grazed in the northeast corner of Algeria and across the border into western and central Tunisia where seasonal rains in the eastern Tell Atlas range produce salt marshes that offer seasonal grazing for semi-nomadic sheep herders. To the east of Tunisia, lies the flat desert plains of Libya where only 2% of the land receives enough rainfall to be cultivated. But in the 1950s, while drilling for oil, a massive fresh water aquifer underneath much of Libya was discovered. The water in this aquifer pre-dates the last ice age and the Sahara Desert itself, and is not replenished by rains in the current age. The largest sheep flocks in Libya are grazed in the southeastern district of Kufra, where in the early 1970s, the Libyan government launched an ambitious irrigation project using water from the aquifer to make the desert bloom. As of December 2011, this exploitation of the aquifer has resulted in the complete drying up of the oasis that had been the water source of the Kufra residents since ancient times.

In the northeast corner of Africa lies the storied land of Egypt, where the eternal Nile, the world's longest river, flows north to its final destination at the Mediterranean Sea. Over most of its course cutting through Sudan and Egypt, the Nile is flanked on either side by bone dry desert, but in it's lower reaches as it nears the sea, the Nile fans out into one of the world's largest river deltas rich in fertile alluvial soils from eons of sediment deposits. To the west of the Nile Delta, Egypt's Mediterranean coastline has a hot desert climate, but winds blowing in from the sea moderate the temperatures, making summers tolerably hot and humid while winters are mildly wet. Sheep are grazed on grasses during the wet months and herded eastward to the Nile Delta to graze on agricultural stubble and supplemental feed in the dry summer months. By 1987, overstocking had degraded the grasslands and Egyptian shepherds became increasingly dependent on nutritional supplementation to manage their herds. Sea level rise due to global climate change is also an existential threat to the Nile Delta and the Egyptian Mediterranean Coast.

The five Saharan countries of Mauritania, Mali, Niger, Chad and Sudan form a continuous belt across the widest part of north Africa from the Atlantic Ocean in the west through the heart of the Sahara Desert to the Red Sea in the East. Between them, they raised over 108.3 million sheep in 2014 (FAOStat 2014). Most of the land base of these countries is uninhabitable sand and rock desert, but on their southern borders the Sahara begins a transition from dry desert to the more tropical influences of equatorial Africa. This ecological zone across this southern swathe of north Africa is called the "Sahel". The Sahel is an ecoregion characterized by semi-arid grasslands, savannas, steppes, and thorn shrublands where sheep, goats, cattle and camels have been traditionally grazed. Annual rainfall varies from around 4 to 8 inches (100 to 200 mm) in the north to around 24 inches (600 mm) in the south. During the long dry season, many trees lose their leaves and the predominantly annual grasses die. The Sahel was formerly home to large populations of wild herbivores and carnivores such as the scimitar-horned oryx, dama, Dorcas and red-fronted gazelles, the giant prehistoric buffalo *(Pelorovis)*, the Bubal hartebeest, the African wild dog, the West and East African cheetahs, and the West and East African lions, but these large mammals have all been greatly reduced in number or pushed to extinction by over-hunting and competition with domesticated animals. The Dorcas and red-fronted gazelles, cheetah, lion and African wild dog are all on the brink of extinction, the Scimitar-horned oryx is extinct in the wild, and both the giant buffalo and the Bubal hartebeest are now extinct. Rains in much of the Sahel have been marked by annual variability throughout the 20th century, with the most severe drought on record beginning in the late 1960s and lasting, with one break, well into the 1980s. In the 21st century, drought cycles have become shorter and more frequent with droughts in 2005–2006 and again in 2010.

The World Resources Institute in partnership with Landesa (Rural Development Institute) produced a series of Briefs entitled **"***Focus on Land in Africa***" (2011)."** Brief number three, **"***Mali, Lesson 3, Farmer Herder Conflicts,***"** focused on the agricultural and social effects of these droughts in Mali:

> *"The Malian government has recognized these variations as symptoms of climate change. In 2007, the Ministry of Equipment and Transport published their national strategy for adapting to climate change. Their strategy ranged from equipping boreholes or wells with solar or wind energy-fueled pumps, to developing crops that can be used as animal fodder and the promotion of livestock feed banks. The report mentions that continued degradation of water resources (including sedimentation, pollution, and waste) has led to "significant change in [agricultural] production systems" which in turn has led to land disputes between farmers and herders.*

"In response to these changing conditions, many Malian agriculturalists are resorting to urban migration in hopes of securing wage labor or other sources of income. Some pastoralists take up farming, remain for longer periods of time in fertile zones near water, or become completely sedentary. Farmers have begun raising livestock or increased the size of their herds. These livelihood changes combined with population growth and declining herder mobility have contributed to the increased area of land under cultivation, as well as the increased concentration of human and animals on arable land, and contributed to competition over arable land. Available arable land has become scarce and the arable land that is available is less productive because average fallow periods in recent years have decreased from 10-15 years to 1-2 years, preventing the soil from fully recovering from intense cultivation."

"To the extent that climatic variation leads to increasing frequency and longer periods of drought, Mali and its neighboring countries in the Sahel are likely to witness more extensive and intense conflicts over land, water and food resources." (*"Mali, Lesson 3, Farmer Herder Conflicts", Focus on Land in Africa, Brief, World Resources Institute in partnership with Landesa (Rural Development Institute,* February 2011).

Another area deeply affected by the Sahel droughts is Lake Chad, a critical water source for 30 million people in Chad, Niger, Nigeria and Cameroon. The Lake Chad Basin is the largest closed drainage basin in the world covering over 1.5 million square miles (2.5 million square kilometers), or about 8% of the African continent. The prolonged Sahel drought from the late 1960s to the early 1980s reduced water flow into the lake. The drought combined with population growth pushed people in the drainage basin to expand irrigation, and beginning in 1983 the amount of water used for irrigation began to increase dramatically which further undercut the flow of water into the lake. Ultimately, between 1983 and 1994, the amount of water diverted for purposes of irrigation quadrupled from the amount used in the previous 25 years. Once one of Africa's largest bodies of fresh water, Lake Chad has dramatically decreased in size. According to a 2011 study by University of Wisconsin-Madison researchers working with NASA's Earth Observing System program, the lake is 1/20th the size it was in 1976.

Similar farmer herder conflicts as in Mali have broken out in Chad, Niger and northern Nigeria. The Chad Basin is where the notorious Islamic fundamentalist terrorist organization, Boko Haram, has killed thousands of people in what the corporate media has attributed to long standing and deep seated ethnic conflicts. While the conflict does break along ethnic lines, the actual antagonism is between traditional Muslim herders and modern Christian farmers over the rapidly diminishing water resources in the region. There has been ethnic tension in the Chad Basin for generations, but it had not erupted into open warfare until 2002, when the violent terrorist group Boko Haram was formed in northern Nigeria. In the local Hausa language the name Boko Haram translates to *"Western education is sin,"* and these traditional Muslim herders are in open rebellion against the modern administrative state that has taken over the resolution of herder/farmer conflicts that had traditionally been under control of powerful

Muslim Clerics. In January, 2015, Boko Haram carried out its deadliest attack to date, killing up to 2,000 people in one day. According to the International Organization for Migration, more than 1 million people are thought to have been displaced by Boko Haram violence, moving to refugee camps in neighboring Cameroon, Chad and Niger where they barely survive in desperate poverty.

The UN Environment Program (UNEP) and the Lake Chad Basin Commission, which was established by the leaders of Chad, Nigeria, Cameroon and Niger in 1964 to save the lake and mitigate the impacts of its shrinkage on people's lives, have developed plans to replenish the lake with water by building a dam and 60 miles of canals to pump water uphill from the Congo River to the Chari River that flows into Lake Chad. This ecologically ruinous project to reconfigure the natural plumbing of the Lake Chad Basin that received support from the international World Bank in 2014, is more an indication of just how desperate these people are, than it is a serious proposal to deal with the compounding problems of climate change, recurring drought, and human and domesticated animal overpopulation that plagues the Sahel region.

A third hot spot in the Sahel devastated by drought is the Darfur region of western Sudan. This passage from the April, 2007, *Atlantic* magazine tells the story:

"To truly understand the crisis in Darfur—and it has been profoundly misunderstood—you need to look back to the mid-1980s, before the violence between African and Arab began to simmer. Alex de Waal, now a program director at the Social Science Research Council, was there at that time, as a doctoral candidate doing anthropological fieldwork. Earlier this year, he told me a story that, he says, keeps coming back to him.

"De Waal was traveling through the dry scrub of Darfur, studying indigenous reactions to the drought that gripped the region. In a herders' camp near the desert's border, he met with a bedridden and nearly blind Arab sheikh named Hilal Abdalla, who said he was noticing things he had never seen before: Sand blew into fertile land, and the rare rain washed away alluvial soil. Farmers who had once hosted his tribe and his camels were now blocking their migration; the land could no longer support both herder and farmer. Many tribesmen had lost their stock and scratched at millet farming on marginal plots.

"The God-given order was broken, the sheikh said, and he feared the future. 'The way the world was set up since time immemorial was being disturbed,' recalled de Waal. 'And it was bewildering, depressing. And the consequences were terrible.'

"In 2003, another scourge, now infamous, swept across Darfur. Janjaweed [Arabic for 'a devil on a horse.'] fighters in military uniforms, mounted on camels and horses, laid waste to the region. In a campaign of ethnic cleansing targeting Darfur's blacks, the armed militiamen raped women, burned houses, and tortured and killed men of fighting age. Through whole swaths of the region, they left only smoke curling into the sky.

"At their head was a 6-foot-4 Arab with an athletic build and a commanding presence. In a conflict the United States would later call genocide, he topped the State Department's list of suspected war criminals. De Waal recognized him: His name was Musa Hilal, and he was the sheikh's son.

"The fighting in Darfur is usually described as racially motivated, pitting mounted Arabs against black rebels and civilians. But the fault lines have their origins in another distinction, between settled farmers and nomadic herders fighting over failing lands. The aggression of the warlord Musa Hilal can be traced to the fears of his father, and to how climate change shattered a way of life." ("The Real Roots of Darfur, The violence in Darfur is usually attributed to ethnic hatred. But global warming may be primarily to blame." By Stephen Faris, The Atlantic, April 2007 Issue)

The 2005 and 2010 droughts in the Sahel resulted in widespread famine. This 2010 editorial in *The Guardian* newspaper titled *"Food crisis in the Sahel: unlearned lessons"*, describes the dire situation and the world's response to it:

"Millions in the eastern Sahel are facing famine, just as they did in 2005 – yet the response from some major aid donors has been no swifter than it was then

"A catastrophe is about to unfold for millions of the world's poorest people. It happened five years ago, and this time the international aid agencies were in place when the early warning lights started flashing. But it is nonetheless happening all over again. More than 10 million people in the eastern Sahel, in some of the world's poorest nations such as Niger, Chad and Mali, have exhausted their food supply and all their assets two or three months before the next harvest. Thousands of animals have died, forcing pastoralists to leave their villages. In large parts of Niger and Chad, people are eating wild berries and leaves, while fields of stunted millet stand in the baking heat.

"The World Food Programme (WFP), which had planned to provide for 2.3 million people in Niger alone between March and October, has had to dramatically revise that figure to 7.9 million. It takes between two and three months for food procured internationally to arrive, but with the rainy season under way in a vast landlocked country like Niger, it may well take longer."

Sub Saharan Africa

In the 29 sub-Saharan African countries that straddle the Earth's equator, the arid winds blowing from the Sahara desert to the north give way to the humid tropical weather patterns swirling around the equator that moderate temperature extremes and grow a dense cover of vegetative biomass. Of the 144.3 million sheep raised in these equatorial countries (FAOStat 2014), 116.3 million (81%) are raised in the

5 countries of Nigeria (40.1 million), Ethiopia (29.3 million), Kenya (17.4 million), South Sudan (16.8 million) and Somalia (12.3 million).

With over 40 million sheep, the west African country of Nigeria has the largest national flock on the African continent and the 5th largest in the world. Nigeria is also home to the largest human population on the African continent with over 181.2 million people in 2015 and growing at a steady rate over 2.6% per year. Nigeria's population is diverse with hundreds of languages spoken including Yoruba, Igbo, Fula, Hausa, Edo, Ibidio, Tiv and English. Nigeria is divided roughly equally between Islam and Christianity. The majority of Nigerian Muslims are Sunni and are concentrated in the northern region of the country where sheep herding predominates. From its southern coastline on the Atlantic Ocean, Nigeria's land mass extends north well inland to the Sahel region and Lake Chad basin, which, as discussed above, is where most of the country's sheep are raised and where the terrorist organization Boko Haram operates. There are four main breeds of sheep in Nigeria: Balami, Uda, Yankasa and west African Dwarf sheep. Balami is most predominant in the north east, is fast growing and drought tolerant; Uda are raised throughout the Sahelo-sudan vegetation zone, thriving in a hot, dry environment, it is well adapted to extensive trekking for forage; the Yankasa breed is widely distributed in the north and is intermediate in size between Uda and the west African Dwarf sheep; the west African dwarf sheep is widely distributed in the south, is a small, compact, hardy breed considered tolerant to trypanosomiasis, a parasitic disease carried by the African tsetse fly.

While Ethiopia is at approximately the same latitude as Nigeria, the country lies far to the east on the Horn of Africa close to the Red Sea, Gulf of Aden and the Indian Ocean. Ethiopia is dominated by a vast highland complex of mountains, plateaus and lakes that forms the largest continuous area of its elevation on the African continent, with little of its surface falling below 4,900 feet (1,500 meters). This highland complex of mountains is divided diagonally by the Great Rift Valley that is surrounded by lowlands and steppes. Ethiopia stretches over three different tropical climate zones divided by elevation: 1) Tropical zone (Kolla) – under 6,000 feet (1,830 meters) above sea level, 2) Subtropical zone (Woina dega) – includes the highlands areas of 6,000 – 8,000 feet (1,830 – 2,440 meters) above sea level, and 3) Cool zone (Dega) – over 8,000 feet (2,440 meters) above sea level. The human population of Ethiopia was 98.8 million people in 2015 and the sheep population 29.3 million in 2014. While there are more than 80 different ethnic groups within Ethiopia, nearly 2/3 of the population is Christian (Ethiopian Orthodoxy, Pentay, Catholic), 1/3 is Muslim and there is a small remnant population of Jews said to be direct descendants of King David. There are several varieties of landrace sheep (locally adapted, traditional, domesticated varieties) in Ethiopia. One creative observer classified Ethiopian sheep by tail shape and wool type into 14 distinct varieties, but in 2002, further genetic analysis revealed that there are actually only four distinct varieties: short-fat-tailed, long-fat-tailed, fat-rumped, and thin-tailed. Sheep production is a major component of the livestock sector in Ethiopia. At the smallholder level, sheep serve diverse functions such as food, wool, cash income, savings, fertilizer and cultural identity. Most sheep of Ethiopia's sheep are grazed by pastoralist/agropastoralist in the subalpine highlands where crop production is unreliable. Sheep are also a foreign currency earner for Ethiopia accounting for 34% of live animal exports in 2011.

Just south of Ethiopia bisected by the Earth's Equator lies the east African country of Kenya. From its coastline on the Indian Ocean, Kenya's flat land rises westward into the central highlands to the country's highest point: Mount Kenya, at 17,057 feet (5,199 meters) above sea level. The Kenyan highlands are bisected by the Great Rift Valley that divides Kenya down the length of the entire country. The Great Rift Valley contains a great diversity of landscapes including uninhabitable desert, flat arid plains, fertile farmlands, steep cliffs and slopes, active and semi-active volcanoes, numerous hot springs and a string of alkaline lakes including Lake Turkana, the world's largest permanent desert lake and the world's largest alkaline lake. Located in the far north of Kenya, Lake Turkana is surrounded by volcanoes and ancient lava flows and borders the Chalbi Desert which is the hottest and most arid region of the country. The human population of Kenya in 2015 stood at 47.2 million people the sheep population 17.4 million in 2014. Bantu and Nilotic peoples together constitute around 97% of the nation's inhabitants, while Cushitic peoples form a small minority. The Cushites, who originally came from Ethiopia and Somalia in northeastern Africa, are mostly Muslim herdsmen concentrated in the North Eastern Province bordering on Somalia. The North Eastern Province has a semi-arid and hot desert climate with rainfall usually only around April or October that is sporadic from year to year. Sheep in Kenya are divided into two breeds: "hair", and "wool and dual purpose". The major hair breeds include: Dorper; Nyanza Fat-tail; Persian Black Head; Red Masai and crosses of these four with local stock. The hair sheep are mainly reared in the arid and semi arid areas. Sheep and goats are preferred animals in arid zones where droughts are frequent since they are small and fecund, and flocks can be cut down during drought periods and quickly re-stocked afterwards, which reduces stock losses due to starvation. The major wool and dual purpose breeds include traditional imported breeds such as Merino; Corriedale; Hampshire Down; Romney Marsh and crosses of these breeds with local stock. Wool sheep are primarily raised in higher rainfall areas.

South Sudan is a relatively new country having gained its independence from the Republic of Sudan in 2011 after two civil wars. South Sudan is a landlocked country in east central Africa with many neighbors, bordering on the Republic of Sudan to the north, Ethiopia to the east, Kenya to the southeast, Uganda to the south, the Democratic Republic of Congo to the southwest and the Central African Republic to the west. It includes the vast swamp region known as the Sudd, formed by the White Nile, a main tributary of the Nile River which passes through the country. The Sudd swampland is considered to be one of the world's largest wetlands, and within the Nile basin is the largest freshwater wetland. During the wet season, the Sudd extends some 50,193 square miles (130,000 square kilometers). Situated near the Equator, much of the South Sudanese landscape consists of tropical rainforest, grasslands and protected national parks that are home to a profusion of migrating wildlife. Located in the southeast, and extending into Uganda, the Imatong Mountains contain South Sudan's highest point: Mount Kinyeti at 10,456 feet (3,187 meters). Though most people of South Sudan are of Nilotic origins, much of the political tensions between Sudan and South Sudan were religiously based between predominantly Muslim Sudan and predominantly Christian South Sudan. In September 2017, the United Nations Special Representative for Children and Armed Conflict said that half of South Sudan's inhabitants were under 18 years of age. South Sudan has suffered chronic ethnic violence since 2013. According to statistics from the South Sudan Ministry of Agriculture, Forestry, Tourism, Animal Resources and Fisheries, South Sudan was the world's leading nation in terms of domestic animal wealth per capita, with an estimated 12.4 million goats, 12.1 million sheep and 11.7 million cattle in a country of around 12 million people. Despite this more than 3:1 ratio of domestic animals to people, in 2014 South Sudan imported most of the meat consumed by its people from neighboring countries. The reason for this is that in South Sudan, domesticated animals are raised not for food, but for prestige. Herders are respected in their communities relative to the number of animals they own, so slaughtering them actually diminishes their wealth and prestige. Animals are mostly used to pay dowries or as compensation in cases of murder or adultery. (Ninety-eight percent of the South Sudan economy is based on oil revenues.) This national obsession with hording domestic animals has resulted in a severe animal overpopulation and its resultant negative environmental impacts. In excerpts below gleaned from a May, 2014, article headlined, **"*South Sudan, Where Livestock Outnumbers People and the Environment Suffers*"** published by the *Inter Press Service News Agency,* describes the damage:

> *"While South Sudan's livestock population is estimated to have an asset value of 2.2 billion dollars — the highest per capita holding in Africa — Isaac Woja, a natural resources management consultant, tells IPS that these livestock are not being managed sustainably and are causing both water scarcity and environmental degradation."*
>
> *"According to the African Development Bank, 80 percent of the people here live in rural areas and rely on agriculture, forestry and fisheries for their livelihoods."*
>
> *"'People come to water bodies to water their animals and cause damage to the river beds. The animals and the pastoralists also defecate in the water, which in a way pollutes the water,' adds Miteng."*
>
> *"Woja adds that overgrazing and the resultant soil erosion is also an issue."*

Extending out to the tip of the Horn of Africa, Somalia is the easternmost country on the African continent. Apart from a mountainous coastal zone in the north and several pronounced river valleys, most of the country is extremely flat, with few natural barriers to restrict the mobility of nomadic herders. The landscape consists mostly of thornbush savanna and semidesert. While Somalia has long coastlines on the Gulf of Aden and the Indian Ocean and its southern border dips just below the Equator, its climate is mainly hot and dry. The Somali people are clan-based Muslims, and according to the Central Bank of Somalia, in 2015 about 80% of its 13.9 million inhabitants were nomadic or semi-nomadic pastoralists who raised sheep, goats camels and cattle. Agriculture is Somalia's most important economic sector with animal agriculture contributing about 40% to Gross Domestic Product (GDP) and accounting for more than 50% of export earnings. Most of the 12.3 million sheep in Somalia descended from the Blackhead

Persian which was bred in South Africa between the late 19th century and early 20th century and has been extensively crossbred in many tropical areas. Somali sheep are a fat-tail type with a black head and white body and both genders are polled. The breed is mainly raised for meat and is a major export of the Somali economy, particularly to the Arabian peninsula. With the advantage of being located near the Arabian peninsula, Somali traders have increasingly begun to challenge Australia's long standing dominance over the live animal and meat markets in the Gulf region, offering lower prices. Saudi Arabia and the United Arab Emirates have made strategic investments in Somalia, building animal export infrastructure and purchasing large tracks of farmland. In June 2014, the European Union (EU) and African Union InterAfrican Bureau for Animal Resources (AU-IBAR) launched the joint project "*Reinforcing Animal Health Services in Somalia* (RAHS)" at a cost of $5.4 million dollars (4 million Euros) to promote domesticated animal production for over 250,000 Somali pastoralists. Also in 2014, the Somali government in conjunction with the FAO, made greater investment in animal agriculture infrastructure, vaccination and veterinary services, fodder production and modern slaughterhouse facilities. According to the FAO (2014), Somalia exported a record 5 million animals to markets in the Gulf region including 4.6 million sheep and goats.

Southern Africa

While there are 13 countries in southern Africa where sheep are raised – Angola, Botswana, Comoros, Lesotho, Madagascar, Malawi, Mauritius, Mozambique, Namibia, South Africa, Swaziland, Zambia, Zimbabwe – sheep herding is much less practiced in temperate southern Africa than in humid equatorial or arid northern Africa. Of the 33.1 million sheep raised in southern Africa in 2014, the country of South Africa at # 13 in the world with 25.5 million animals, accounts for 77% of the total.

South Africa lies at the southern tip of Africa, its coastline stretching more than 1,770 miles (2,850 kilometres) from its western border with Namibia on the Atlantic Ocean southward down around the Cape of Good Hope and then northeastward up to the eastern border with Mozambique on the Indian Ocean. South Africa is divided into three major geographic regions, 1) the narrow low-lying coastal plains cut by numerous short rivers and fertile valleys, 2) the Great Escarpment where the elevation and terrain varies with its highest point in the Drakensberg Mountains along the border with Lesotho, and 3) the African Plateau in the country's interior that forms a portion of the Kalahari Basin that is semi-arid and sparsely populated. The African Plateau slopes gently in the north and west but rises to 6,500 feet (2,000 meters) in the east. Two major rivers cross the African Plateau: the Limpopo (a stretch of which is shared with Zimbabwe) and the Orange (with its tributary, the Vaal) which runs with variable flow across the central plain from east to west, emptying into the Atlantic Ocean at the Namibian border. Sheep were first introduced to South Africa around 2,000 years ago by the Khoikhoi people (formerly called Hottentots as a racial slur), a pastoral culture that originated in the northern part of modern Botswana. The Afrikaner breeds of sheep such as the Damara, Black-headed Persian, Pedi and Zulu herded by the Khoikhoi originally came from the Middle East. In South Africa the Khoikhoi took up grazing their sheep in the fertile coastal valleys coexisting with the San people who were the indigenous hunter-gatherers in the region. In the 3rd century AD, Bantu farmers encroached on the Khoikhoi territory and pushed them inland into more arid areas. The Khoikhoi first encountered European settlers around the 16th century who exposed them to smallpox epidemics that decimated their population. The Khoikhoi waged gorilla warfare against the European incursions, but as the Dutch East India Company enclosed traditional grazing land for farms over the following century, the Khoikhoi were steadily driven from their land, effectively ending their pastoral way of life. Harsh laws were implemented in the 19th century to force the remaining Khoikhoi to work as laborers on white farms. This system of black servitude was institutionalized from 1948 to 1991 when the all-white National Party held power in South Africa, strictly enforcing policies of racial segregation under a system of discrimination called "apartheid." Under apartheid, nonwhite South Africans (over 90% of the population) were forced to live in separate areas from whites, use separate public facilities, and have limited contact with whites. Merinos imported from Spain first arrived in South Africa in 1789, and over a century and a half later in 1932, Mutton Merino were imported from Germany that were cross bred with Merinos to create the Dohne Merino and cross bred with Dorsets to create the Dormer. By the early 21st century these breeds along with the Dorper (a cross breed between a Dorset and a Black-headed Persian) had become the major sheep breeds in South Africa. While subsistence sheep herding still existed into the 21st century, the great majority of South Africa's 25.5 million sheep (2014) were being raised by commercial sheep farmers on large scale operations to produce meat, wool and hides mostly for domestic consumption by South Africa's 55.3 million people (2015). Commercial sheep farmers distribute their products to domestic markets through large scale slaughterhouses and wholesalers.

Central and South America

The first Spanish and Portuguese colonists introduced sheep to the Western Hemisphere in the early 16th century, and by the end of the century, hundreds of thousands of sheep grazed the grasslands of Central and South America. Sheep were grazed on the range just north of San Juan de los Rios in central Mexico, the Andes Mountains of Peru, the Andean foothills of New Granada, the highlands of Rio de Janeiro and Sau Paulo Brazil, the Santiago district of Chile, and the Patagonian Pampas of Argentina.

While millions of sheep are still grazed on the grasslands of Central and South America, of the approximately 1.1 billion sheep globally in 2014, only 80 million (7.2%) were produced in Latin America. Of that 80 million, an estimated 71 million were raised in six countries of Brazil (17.6 million), Argentina (14.7 million), Peru (12.4 million), Bolivia (9.5 million), Mexico (8.6 million) and Uruguay (8.2 million). While each of these countries has its own unique history of sheep farming, the means and methods are similar to those already discussed in other parts of the world, so I will spare you the details; besides, I'm getting tired of counting sheep.

The reason sheep are so ubiquitous the world over is that as a small, docile, fast breeding herd animal that can survive on marginal range lands and be exploited for both food and fiber, they are the ideal animal for hundreds of millions of poor and landless people around the world to accumulate some material wealth in their otherwise impoverished environments. Since sheep were first domesticated in Mesopotamia some 10,000 years ago, the timeless rhythm of nomadic herding peoples has been woven into the social fabric of all pastoral cultures thereafter.

Largely due to its status as a cultural rite, sheep herding is generally thought of as at worst, an activity that is benign to the natural environment, and at best, an improvement on nature. These beliefs are plausible only if viewed through the lens of anthropocentrism. When viewed through the lens of ecology, the human herding of domesticated sheep on marginal rangelands can only be seen as highly disruptive to native habitat. Wherever sheep are grazed, they compete with native wild herbivores for forage which reduces habitat available to native species. Also, as native herbivores are replaced by sheep, native predators such as wolves, coyotes, jackals, dingos, lions, tigers, pumas, leopards, lynx and bobcats are left with only sheep to prey upon, thus becoming targets themselves of human predation. By extirpating native predators, herders completely disrupt the finely tuned trophic structure of the natural food chain which profoundly degrades the entire ecosystem. As human and sheep populations grow, rangelands become overgrazed which leads to accelerated erosion and desertification. And as we have seen time and again throughout history, pastoralists and agriculturalists covet the same increasingly scarce land and water resources leading inexorably to armed conflicts.

In the former British colonies of North America, New Zealand and Australia, European diseases such as measles, smallpox and tuberculosis swept the land of indigenous native peoples only to replace them with massive numbers of the non-native exotic species: sheep and cattle. After the first human inhabitants of North America and Oceana hunted the native mega-fauna to extinction, and before the arrival of the first Europeans, for thousands of years low population densities of aboriginal peoples hunted wild native herbivores in relative equilibrium. In the few centuries since Europeans introduced domesticated grazing animals, the finely tuned trophic structure of these complex rangeland ecosystems endowed by evolution with a wide diversity of native species has been lost forever.

15

PIGS

The modern day mammal we call the "pig" (probably from Old English *picg*), was originally domesticate from different subspecies of wild boar native to much of Eurasia with the taxonomical classification *Sus scrofa*. Wild boars were the first animals to be domesticated for food by nomadic people over 15,000 years ago, even before the earliest civilizations. Pigs were a good fit for nomadic peoples because they could forage for themselves in the woodlands that covered much of Eurasia at that time by eating acorns, nuts, seeds, berries, flowers, fungi, roots and grubs, and they didn't need large expanses of open pasture like ruminant cattle and sheep. Pigs could also eat the scraps and feces left over from human food consumption making efficient use of human waste products. One school of evolutionary thought is that pigs actually domesticated themselves by learning to scavenge waste products from roving bands of humans thereby acclimated themselves to the human presence. Another value pigs offered early humans was they reproduce very quickly: a cow gestates for nine months and usually just one calf is born that takes a year or two to grow big enough to slaughter for meat, whereas a pig gestates in just four months and has 6 to 12 piglets each of which grows to slaughter weight in about half the time it takes a cow. From these humble beginnings 15,000 years ago, the pig has become the third most populous large mammal on Earth after humans and cattle, and a major source of food for billions of people around the world.

Early Domestication

Archaeological evidence suggests that wild boar were first being managed in the wild around 15,000 years ago in the Tigris and Euphrates River Basin of the Near East. Remains of domesticated pigs dating back to 13,400 years ago have been found on the Mediterranean island of Cyprus suggesting a second independent European domestication, and bones dating back to 8,000 years ago indicate a third independent domestication event took place in China. DNA evidence from the teeth and jawbones of Neolithic pigs indicate that the first domesticated pigs in Europe were imported from the Near East which stimulated the Europeans to domesticate their own local subspecies of wild boar. In a study of all the genetic evidence of pig domestication published in the April 2010 Proceedings of the U.S. National Academy of Sciences, researchers found a difference between patterns of early domestication and movement of pigs in the Near East, Europe and China. The researchers looked at the DNA sequences of more than 1,500 modern and 18 ancient pigs. Lead author of the study and professor of Archaeology at Durham University, UK, Dr. Greger Larson, noted:

> *"Previous studies of European domestic pigs demonstrated that the first pigs in Europe were imported from the Near East. Those first populations were then completely replaced by pigs descended from European wild boar.*
>
> *"However, despite the occurrence of genetically distinct populations of wild boar throughout modern China, these populations have not been incorporated into domestic stocks.*
>
> *"The earliest known Chinese domestic pigs have a direct connection with modern Chinese breeds, suggesting a long, unbroken history of pigs and people in this part of East Asia."*

Sam White, assistant professor of history at Oberlin College, further noted in his 2011 article *"from globalized PIG BREEDS TO CAPITALIST PIGS: A STUDY IN ANIMAL CULTURES AND EVOLUTIONARY HISTORY"*:

> *"Recent archaeological evidence suggests the first service that pigs provided humans was probably not food conversion but simply food storage. As depositories for surplus calories, pigs provided a unique method of preserving, sharing, and exchanging wealth; their keeping*

*became a marker of status, as found in Neolithic burial excavations in both southern China
and the Near East, where they were separately domesticated.*

*"It would appear, however, that as agriculture developed and as larger human settlements put
increasing pressure on land and resources, pigs were forced to evolve into new roles. In China,
this adaptation took the form of eating human scraps and refuse, first as foragers and later
as true farm animals — a transition they achieved around eight thousand years ago. In this
role, they were separated from their traditional habitats and feeding habits. Raised in sties
and fed at troughs, they were spared the usual evolutionary pressures that had governed the
shape of their wild progenitors and were left instead to the priorities of human breeding. Across
East Asia round, pale, short-legged, and pot-bellied varieties long predominated, with many
traditional regional breeds persisting to the present day." ("from globalized PIG BREEDS TO
CAPITALIST PIGS: A STUDY IN ANIMAL CULTURES AND EVOLUTIONARY HISTORY"
by SAM WHITE, Downloaded from ENVIRONMENTAL HISTORY 16, JANUARY 2011)*

Let's take a closer look at the domestication of pigs throughout history:

China

China's higher population density relative to Europe in ancient times, and China's more intensive
agriculture began to put greater pressure on woodland resources, particularly once the population began
to shift to rice-growing regions of central and southern China in the first millennium AD. This shift to
more intensive agriculture also created more opportunities to raise pigs in stys (small outdoor enclosures)
on kitchen and farm scraps. When pigs were domesticated in various parts of China, each place had its
own locally adapted breed, and most households raised at least one or two pigs each year. Pigs were more
valuable alive than dead, acting as efficient converters of organic matter that was inedible to humans into
nutrient-rich fertilizer, before being butchered for meat that could be given as a wedding gift, used to curry
social or political favor, or eaten at a New Year celebration. For the vast majority of people, pig meat was
a rare treat and the smallholder model of raising pigs defines much of China's 8,000 years of agricultural
history *("The decline of household pig farming in rural Southwest China: Socioeconomic obstacles and policy
implications," Culture & Agriculture, 2010).* After sty raised pigs were bred in China, they migrated with
humans into South East Asia, then to the islands of the Pacific.

Near East

In the Near East, domesticated pigs came to quite a different fate than pigs in China. As human
population density increased in the early settlements of Mesopotamia, farmers cut down oak woodlands
to make way for olive groves and drained marshes to plant crops. The land gradually deteriorated from
forestland to cropland to pastureland to desert, with each successive stage providing less habitat for pigs.

By 1200 BC (3,200 years ago) religious elites in the Near East had begun to shun pigs as filthy animals due to the habits of urbanized pigs that survived by eating human garbage and excrement. By 1000 BC archaeological evidence indicates that the keeping and eating of pigs had sharply declined even among poor people in the Near East. The shunning of pig meat as unclean was later adopted by the Hebrews around 800 BC and again among Muslims with the founding of Islam around 700 AD. As Muslims now predominate in the Near East, pig meat is still shunned there even to this day.

Greece

While pigs became scarce in the semi-arid Near East, they became an iconic animal of the early civilizations on the wetter continent of Europe. Susan Cole, associate professor and chair in the Department of Classics in the University at Buffalo's College of Arts and Sciences, has thoroughly researched the role of pigs in ancient Greek social and religious life. She notes:

"Meat production was always a tricky business in the eastern Mediterranean. In the context of early cities, swine were economical to raise, easy to sell, hard to store and good to eat, and for that reason they were certainly the stars of family dinners and temple feasts. The Greeks didn't waste many resources, however, and upon close inspection, we find that even animals raised for food had other important emblematic and ritual cultural uses."

In ancient Greece, the pig served as a sacrificial animal, an offering to the gods, especially to those gods who preferred pig over chicken or cattle. Demeter, the Greek goddess of abundance who was worshiped by women, was closely linked to the sacrifice of piglets. At "Thesmophoria", the most widespread festival in ancient Greece, priestesses would cast piglets into a pit and later retrieved their rotting carcasses and place them on the altar of Demeter; the rotted carcass would then be scattered in the fields to ensure a good harvest. Demeter symbolized the cycle of life and death, winter followed by the rebirth of spring. Such ritual sacrifices were one function of the religious cults that were ubiquitous in ancient Greek culture. The cults were relatively small circles of individuals united by a particular religious devotion or practice that met to offer sacrifices on behalf of their patron deities. Nearly all Greeks belonged to several cults. Cult members ritually made animal sacrifices in the temples to honor and recognize the principles and powers represented by each god. When a cult presented an animal for sacrifice, only part of the animal was consumed by fire – that part was for the gods – the rest was shared by the sanctuary attendants and members of the cult. This was how meat was distributed in ancient Greece. When a large animal like a sow or a boar was sacrificed, a fairly large dinner party was held for members of the cult that had purchased the animal used in the sacrifice. Dinner menus from sanctuaries and cults indicate that pigs were a commonly sacrificed animal (*"Hog Wild in Athens B.C.E.! Role of Pigs in Social and Religious Life Provides Insights into Ancient Greece: How much can just one trait tell us about a culture? Ask the ancient Greek pig,"* 2000).

Rome

Pigs were important animals to the ancient Romans as well. Romans ate cattle, sheep, goat and chicken, but they preferred pig. There were more Latin words for pig meat than for any other animal, and the trade became highly specialized. In the article entitled *"High on the Hog: Linking Zooarchaeological, Literary, and Artistic Data for Pig Breeds in Roman Italy"* (*American Journal of Archaeology,* October, 2001), University of Alberta archaeologist, Michael MacKinnon PhD, reviewed zooarchaeological, literary, and artistic data from ancient Rome to determine how pigs were used in Roman times. These records show the presence of at least two distinct breeds – a large, fat, short-legged variety and a small, bristled, long-legged variety. Zooarchaeological data indicated that the smaller breed figured more prominently as a source of meat in the Roman diet. Roman texts by Columella, Cato, Pliny the Elder and others suggest that this breed was kept in herds and "pannaged" (the practice of releasing domestic pigs into the forest) to feed on "mast" (the fruit of forest trees like acorns and nuts). The larger breed seems to have been raised in a different manner, being stall fed, and in far lesser numbers than its smaller relative. Because of its large size and the message of social and economic prosperity with which stall feeding was associated, this larger breed predominates among artistic depictions of pigs in the feasts of wealthy Romans. In the most detailed contemporary recipe book on Roman cuisine known as *De re coquinaria,* (or *On Cooking*), pig meat dishes far outnumber those made with other meats: the section called "Quadrupeds" contains four recipes for cattle, eleven for sheep, and seventeen for pig. Roman texts name several regions as key centers of pig production including areas of Gaul (France), Spain and the northern fringes of the Roman Empire (*"High on the Hog: Linking Zooarchaeological, Literary, and Artistic Data for Pig Breeds in Roman Italy," American Journal of Archaeology, October, 2001*) (*"Lesser Beasts: A snout-to-Tail Histoty of the Humble Pig,"* Basic Books, May, 2015).

Middle Ages Europe

After the fall of the Western Roman Empire, pigs remained an important animal to the Celts and other pagan cultures that inhabited Northern Europe in the Early Middle Ages (the 5th to the 10th century AD). Pigs had symbolic meaning in pagan cults: sows (female pigs) were often a symbol of fertility. In Celtic mythology the sow-goddess, Henwen, was the animal form of the goddess of imagination. Boars (male pigs) were considered fierce opponents who fought to the death and were often used as a heraldic device. The coat of arms of King Richard III, whose nickname was "The Hog", featured a boar in recognition of the king's prowess as a soldier. In Ireland, boars were used as war symbols representing their clever, indomitable, and ferocious behaviors. "Swineherds" were important people in these pagan cultures. The swineherds' job was to guard the herds of pigs when they were sent to mast feed on the autumn acorn and nut drop in the forest to fatten up before slaughter. For the swineherd to survive out in the forest alone for months at a time required a vast knowledge of the natural world, and for that wisdom, swineherds were considered holders of visionary and magical powers. For Early Middle Age pagan cults, swineherds represented a supernatural conduit between humankind and the natural world. As Christianity spread across Europe over the course of the Early Middle Ages, magical swineherds played an important role in transitioning pagan culture over to Christianity through borrowed religious symbols and rituals. Saint Patrick of Ireland was originally a swineherd (*"Swineherds: The magical swineherds of Irish Mythology," The Atlantic Religion, June, 2015*) (*"A Short History of English Agriculture," Clarendon Press, 1909*).

In Europe, unlike in China, mast feeding remained the primary means of raising pigs for slaughter well into the Middle Ages. This agricultural practice of "pannage" kept European swineherds from breeding pigs into fully domesticated farm animals as had the Chinese since mast-fed pigs still had to range deep into the woods and fend off predators and competing boars. As long as they ranged freely in the woods, controlled breeding remained difficult if not impossible; in fact, mast-fed pigs often mated with wild boars and European pigs remained fierce agile creatures with long lean legs, ridges of bristles, and residual tusks. Swineherds were not ignorant of ways to select more meat efficient types, but as long as they wished to take advantage of mast feeding, these breeding imperatives competed with evolutionary pressures selecting for more effective ranging and scavenging in the woods. Through the 11th century and beyond pigs remained so closely associated with mast feeding that forests were measured by the number of pigs they could feed.

By the 13th century in England and in the low-lying delta regions of the Rhine, Meuse, Scheldt and Ems rivers of coastal northwestern Europe, deforestation had reached a point where traditional pannage became difficult if not impossible, forcing many land owners to abandon raising pigs altogether, and where pannage was still possible, mast feeding was restricted by range and season. Studies of animal remains from this period indicate that pig meat was increasingly restricted to elite households in the growing urban markets of the High Middle Ages. While subsistence farmers still kept a few pigs as garbage disposals, pig meat consumption plummeted among rural populations.

With the great famines and plagues of the 14th century, however, the tremendous reduction of human and livestock populations took the economic pressure off the remaining forests of Europe and this reprieve on forests resources enabled the practice of pannage to continue in Europe well into the 17th century. Consequently, European pig breeds remained forest scavengers and there was little incentive to breed farm raised meat animals. As the human population finally recovered to pre-plague levels in the 16th century, deforestation again reduced the forest available for mast feeding which again resulted in a major decline in pig meat production. As the price of pig meat rose due to scarcity, pigs were giving way to cattle as the ascendant animal in the agricultural revolution that overtook Europe in the late 17th and early 18th centuries. Without new breeds, pig meat seemed destined to become a minor player in the diet of average Europeans much like goat and rabbit.

But then in the early 18th century, a number of agricultural and economic pressures came to bear in Europe to turn pig farming into a profitable enterprise. New crop rotations, especially pulses to fix nitrogen and restore the soil, provided an ideal fodder to raise pigs. Increased amounts of brewery and dairy waste provided another sources of concentrated pig fodder, and potatoes introduced from South America also became a good source of pig fodder even before most Europeans decided the tuber was fit for human consumption. The ongoing "enclosure" movement eliminated some of the last remaining common pastures and woodlands for pannage and discouraged the promiscuous intermingling of livestock that had undermined previous efforts at breeding. The shift from subsistence farming to commercial "husbandry" created a year-round demand that traditional seasonal mast feeding failed to meet. Once farmers had to think in terms of constant feed conversion rather than periodic mast, they had a strong incentive to develop new breeds of pigs that more efficiently reached slaughter weight at an ever younger age. At the turn of the 18th century, English agricultural manuals suggest that farmers around Leicestershire had managed to produce the first improved breed in Europe which started a trend of raising pigs on peas and beans, supplemented by brewery and dairy waste, especially around cities and in the region of Leicestershire and Northamptonshire. The new breed, while not comparable to a modern hog, was still distinctly rounder and grew more quickly than the medieval scavenger variety. As the English pig changed its shape, it also changed its role in English culture. As the lean, dark, fearsome scavenger of the Middle Ages gave way to a rounder gentler farm animal over the 16th and 17th centuries, by the early 18th century the pig had lost its symbolic and religious associations and year-round breeding and marketing had put an end to the centuries-old seasonal rituals of pannage, slaughter, smoking, and salting.

It was in this context that Chinese sty raised pigs were first introduced to Europe in the early 18th century and crossbred with European pig stocks. This combination would prove decisive in changing the pig into the modern hog we know today. By the end of the 18th century crossbreeds that combined the larger framed European pigs with the rounder body and faster weight gain Asian pigs had revolutionized pig farming in Europe. These improved crossbreeds produced a proliferation of pig varieties in the early 19th century and over the next fifty years the number of local and regional crosses exploded as farmers experimented with the new genetic potential offered by Asian mixes. By the mid 1800s, a few prize breeds had emerged including the modern Yorkshire, Berkshire, Hampshire, and Suffolk hogs, all of which depended on crossing Chinese with improved English varieties. While pure English breeds took well over a year to grow to slaughter weight, the new crossbreeds could be brought to slaughter in as little as nine months. This assured the crossbreeds preeminence in the rapidly expanding pig meat markets. In the 1800s breeders developed exceedingly large and fat varieties, some scarcely capable of walking. This trend led to the development of lard hogs for the specific purpose of producing industrial quantities of oil and grease, before they were replaced by petroleum products at the end of the century.

United States

While the initial steps toward turning the pig into a major world food commodity took place in 18th and 19th century England, the final industrialization of the pig occurred principally in the United States. The first pigs to reach the Western Hemisphere were brought to the Caribbean by Christopher Columbus on his second voyage to the New World in 1493, followed soon thereafter to South America by Francisco Pizarro and southeastern North America by Hernando de Soto. Rapidly expanding pig populations were an essential food source for the early Spanish Conquistadors. Sir Walter Raleigh brought the first English pigs to Jamestown, Virginia in 1607. All of these pigs were of the traditional European type (before Chinese crossbreeds) and ideally suited to scavenge in the vast woodlands of North America and they bred prolifically. Escaped pigs soon turned feral (an animal living in the wild but descended from domesticated stock) destroying the crops of settlers and Indians alike. On Manhattan Island, a long solid wall to exclude rampaging pigs was constructed on the northern edge of the colony; an area now known as Wall Street. With the westward expansion of the frontier over the 18th and 19th centuries, settlers continued to let pigs range free in the woods in expectation of hunting them later, in effect seeding the land with meat. In most cases, however, labor was scarce and land cheap, making the breeding, and management of pigs uneconomical. Left to natural selection, the American pig became notoriously wild in demeanor, fierce, lean, and long-legged. By all appearances, it was one of the world's least likely candidates for modern industrialized pig meat production.

Nevertheless, as in early 18th century England, economic and agricultural forces came to bear in the U.S. in the late 1700s that would reshape the American pig. Greater population density on the East Coast created new economic pressures for agricultural and livestock improvement which resulted in the importation of Chinese breeding stock to Eastern Pennsylvania, probably via Europe. And by the early 1800s the fertile farmlands of the Ohio River Valley began to turn their excess maize production into pig feed to supply the pig meat markets in the Eastern cities. While most farmers just rounded up the regional feral "razorbacks" and fattened them on maize for a few weeks, others began to breed more systematically to meet the growing scale of production. In 1816, the Ohio Valley Shaker Society developed a crossbreed called "Poland China" that was the first major improved breed in America, and the one that would later come to dominate the U.S. pig market in the late 1800s. Getting pigs to market in the 1850s was an arduous task. Drovers with the aid of drivers who handled up to 100 pigs each would drive the pigs along designated trails; a herd could travel 5 to 8 miles a day over a total distances of up to 700 miles. It has been estimated that annually between 40,000 and 70,000 pigs were driven from Ohio to eastern markets. Pig drives were also common from the western Appalachian states to the Southeastern States to feed African American slaves on the tobacco plantations. As pig herds in the Midwest increased, processing and packing facilities began to spring up in major Midwestern cities. Pigs were first commercially slaughtered in Cincinnati, which became known as "Porkopolis" and by the mid 1800s Cincinnati led the nation in pig processing. After the Civil War, the advancing railroads took over livestock transportation and in the late 1800s Chicago, the nation's rail hub, became the center of industrialized meat packing and refrigerated shipping, Chicago became known as the "hog butcher for the world." By the early 1900s, America considered itself a nation of cattle meat eaters, but in fact pigs were the main source of meat among the people. Pig was the meat of poor rural dwellers because unlike cattle meat, when heavily salted and cured, it could be stored in barrels for months at room temperature without spoiling. As working incomes rose among the growing urban population after World War II, more people could afford the higher class cattle meat and home refrigeration to keep it from spoiling. In 1953, for the first time in U.S. history, per capita consumption of cattle meat overtook pig meat at 77.6 pounds per year to 63.5 pounds per year, and pig meat would never regain the top market share of meat consumption.

As the hog butchering and processing industry grew larger and more mechanized in the early 1900s, through a series of buyouts and takeovers the industry consolidated into a few large corporations that came to dominate the market. The Smithfield Packing Company started in 1936 by Joseph Luter, Sr. and his son, Joseph, Jr., in Smithfield Virginia, would, by the end of the 20th century, become the largest hog butcher in the world. But even as the hog processing industry was consolidating well into the mid-1900s, hog farming remained in the hands of many small farmers each producing just a relative few hogs. Concentrated Animal Feeding Operations (CAFOs) came to the pig farming industry much later than to the cattle and chicken industries. Hog CAFOs can be traced back to Wendell Murphy who was a North Carolina state senator in the 1980s. Prior to becoming a state senator, Murphy was a pig farmer and he decided to apply the same principles of industrialized animal husbandry used in the chicken meat industry to raising hogs. In 1960 Murphy went into the hog raising business buying feeder pigs, raising them on dirt lots on his farm, and feeding them maize from his feed grain mill. This venture proved very profitable, but after a cholera outbreak in 1969 shut down Murphy's farm, he contracted with his tobacco-farming neighbors to raise hogs instead. Murphy supplied the pigs, feed, and fences; the neighbors supplied the land and labor. Murphy's horizontal integration of the hog farming business pioneered the modern day factory hog farm. By the 1980s, the most advanced pig farming operations practiced so called "life-cycle housing" in which the pigs lived their entire lives crowded inside large shed like buildings under temperature and light controlled conditions. By the 1990s, hog confinement buildings had become standardized metal structures 300 feet long by 60 feet wide on top of a concrete foundation. During his time in the North Carolina legislature, Murphy helped write state laws that were very friendly to CAFOs helping to propel North Carolina to the #2 hog producing state in the U.S. In 2007, the five largest states for factory-farmed hogs – Iowa, North Carolina, Minnesota, Illinois and Indiana – accounted for about two-thirds of all factory-farmed hogs in the U.S.

Given the pig's natural capacity for rapid weight gain and prolific breeding enhanced by millennia of domestication, they have proven to be remarkably adaptable to industrialized CAFO livestock production. Modern breeding has led to the almost universal adoption of Yorkshire (or "large white"), Duroc, and Hampshire breeds, all of which sprang from Chinese stock. These large bodied, short legged breeds would never be able to pannage for mast in the woods or be herded hundreds of miles to market, but they are specifically bred to live under conditions of extreme confinement where they waste no energy moving around, thereby most efficiently turning feed grain into pig meat. From birth to death "breeder sows" live in wire crates where they barely have enough room to lie down. When sows are old enough to give birth, they are artificially inseminated and over the entire length of their four month pregnancies they lay in "gestation crates", that are cages 2 feet wide and too small for them to turn around or lay down comfortably. Feed and water is constantly made available through mechanized feeding systems. After giving birth, mother pigs are moved to "farrowing crates," that are cages similar to gestation crates except that they have a small concrete pad on which the piglets can nurse. The piglets are weaned from their mothers when they are less than a month old and the mothers are impregnated again in a continuous cycle that keeps them living under conditions of extreme confinement their entire lives. After three or four years, breeder pigs' bodies give out and they are shipped off to slaughter. (Gestation and farrowing crates are considered so barbaric that they have been banned in several U.S. states as well as in the U.K. and Sweden.) After weaning the piglets are moved to a "nursery" where they are kept until they reach from 30-80 pounds. Male piglets have their testicles cut off and both males and females have their tails docked, their teeth clipped in half (to prevent tail biting), and their ears notched for identification, all without any anesthetics. After 8-12 weeks in the nursery the hogs are moved to the "finishing" farm where they are housed in large indoor temperature and light controlled sheds that are divided into smaller "batch pens." There are so many hogs crowded into each batch pen that there is virtually no room for the hogs to move and there is no straw bedding for them to nest in which is their natural instinct. Mechanized feeding and watering systems deliver a steady flow of maize and soy meal supplemented with vitamins and minerals and water at all times. Impeccably clean by nature, hogs on these "growout farms" live on slatted floors where their manure and urine falls through the floor and is flushed away with fresh water into giant open air pits euphemistically called "lagoons." A typical 10,000 pig factory farm produces 130,000 pounds of excrement per day, as much as a town of 40,000 people, but with none of the attendant public health and hygiene regulations. In 1995, the 60 million pigs in the U.S. produced almost as much sewerage as the country's 266 million people. As we shall see, these pig manure pits cause major public health problems and severe environmental impacts.

Extreme overcrowding, poor ventilation, and being forced to live over toxic septic pits all cause rampant disease; by the time the hogs are sent to slaughter many suffer from Porcine Reproductive and Respiratory Syndrome (PRRS) and one-third to half of hog farms have some level of salmonellosis. Up to 70% of U.S. hogs show evidence of infection with bratislava (a type of Leptospirosis bacteria) and 80% to 85% of sows have been exposed to parvovirus. An epidemic of Porcine Epidemic Diarrhoea virus (PEDv) wiped out more than 10% of the U.S. hog population in the first year after it appeared on U.S. hog farms in May 2013, when it also appeared in Canada, Mexico and Japan. Transmission of PEDv is fecal – oral and it is most serious in neonatal piglets where mortality can reach 80% to 100%. The virus was first recognized in the UK in 1971 and had spread throughout much of Europe and Asia by 2013. Hogs are fed sub-therapeutic doses of antibiotics as a growth promoter, but still many die from these infections. Because of illness, lack of room to exercise, and genetic manipulation that causes them to grow too large too quickly, hogs often develop arthritis and other joint problems. As hogs are intelligent, sensitive and social creatures by nature, many literally go insane under these conditions of extreme duress which is manifested in neurotic behaviors such as chewing on their cage bars or obsessively pressing on their water bottles. In the 1930s pigs gained 1 pound of weight for every 4 pounds of food they consumed, in the 1980s that ratio was down to 3.5:1 and by 2000 was below 3:1 – second only to that of meat chickens. The efficiency of turning feed to meat at the modern factory hog farm has resulted in a major shift in the U.S. hog farming industry in the early 21st century. In 1992, less than a third of hogs were raised on factory farms with more than 2,000 animals; by 2004, 80% of hogs were raised on these giant operations and by 2007, 95% of hogs were raised in operations with more than 2,000 hogs. The number of hogs on factory farms grew from 46.1 million in 1997 to 63.2 million in 2012, the equivalent of adding 3,100 hogs to factory farms every day for 15 years. The average size of a hog factory farm in that time increased from 3,600 to nearly 6,100 hogs. In less than two decades the number of hog farms had declined by over 76%, from more than 240,000 in 1992 to fewer than 56,000 in 2012. Despite this collapse in the number of farms, the number of hogs remained fairly constant as the scale of the remaining operations exploded. One hundred million hogs a year are raised in the U.S. for food, nearly all on factory farms.

After six months on the factory farm, workers load the hogs onto 18-wheeler trucks bound for the slaughterhouse by beating them on their noses and backs or sticking electric prods into their rectums to force them to move. The hogs are packed so tightly in the trucks that they cannot move and on the trip to the slaughterhouse they often are subjected to hot and cold temperature extremes and forced to breath ammonia fumes and diesel exhaust. According to a 2006 industry report, more than 1 million hogs die each year in the U.S. from transport alone. Another industry report notes that, in some transport loads, as many as 10% of hogs are "downers," animals who are so ill or injured that they are unable to stand and walk on their own. At the slaughterhouse, these sick and injured pigs are kicked, stuck with electric prods, and finally dragged off the trucks at the slaughterhouse. A typical modern slaughterhouse in the U.S. kills around 1,100 pigs every hour, and most slaughter over one million hogs a year. The slaughter operation is designed to process hogs as efficiently and quickly as possible. The hogs are first rendered unconscious by stunning with electrical current applied with electrodes or with a captive bolt pistol shot to the forehead. They are then hoisted on a rail by one leg and their throats are cut to bleed them out. After bleeding out the carcass is dragged through a "scalding tank" to remove the hair, which is subsequently completed by using scissor-like devices and then if necessary with a torch. The U.S. Department of Agriculture, the government agency responsible for inspecting slaughterhouses, has documented numerous incidents of improper stunning, and bleeding out sending many hogs to the scalding tanks still alive. According to one slaughterhouse worker, *"There's no way these animals can bleed out in the few minutes it takes to get up the ramp. By the time they hit the scalding tank, they're still fully conscious and squealing. Happens all the time."* After scalding, the carcass is scraped and washed, de-gutted, de-larded, decapitated, split in half and finally, chilled in cold storage. From start to finish the whole operation takes about 15 minutes per pig. After cooling down, the carcass is processed further into edible products: the buttocks are cut into hams, the ribcage into bacon and the bulk of the meat is ground into sausages. The remaining fat is made into lard through a heating process.

In 1990, Smithfield Foods, embarked on a business strategy of vertical integration in the hog industry and began buying up hog farming operations. This vertically integrated organizational structure allowed Smithfield to control every stage of the hog production process, from conception and birth to slaughter, processing and packing. As part of this business strategy Smithfield acquired Murphy Family Farms in 2000 to become the largest hog producer in the world. Since the early 1990s, all of the major pig meat producing countries in the world have adopted CAFO technologies as the most efficient business model for large scale meat production, and as hog operations have grown larger and larger, the pig meat industry has simultaneously undergone a consolidation into fewer and fewer vertically integrated hog processing corporations that are increasingly international in scope. Since the 1990s, a wave of mergers has significantly increased consolidation in the pig meat processing industry. In 1995, the top four pig meat packers slaughtered under half of all hogs in the U.S. (46%), but by 2012 the top four firms slaughtered nearly two thirds (66%). These vertically integrated corporations pressed farmers to enter into contracts to raise hogs owned by the processors or to commit to selling to a specific processor. In 1993, 87% of hogs in the U.S. were sold at auction by independent growers to processors, by 2013, 93% were controlled well before slaughter by the processors, either by the processor owning the hogs or by contract to buy the hogs. The use of these contractual arrangements depressed the price of hogs to the actual farmers. In an ironic twist, in 2013, as part of this industry wide consolidation, Smithfield was bought by the Chinese corporation, Shuanghui Group (since renamed WH Group Limited), presently the world's largest hog producer and processor. It was ancient Chinese pig breeds that first inspired the modern Western hog industry, and it has now come to pass that a Chinese company owns the largest hog processing corporation in the West; the international pig has come full circle.

Modern Pig Industry in China

For thousands of years the vast majority of Chinese people lived in rural areas and worked as subsistence farmers. These small farmers who raised fewer than five pigs per year along with crops on about a half acre of land, produced around 95% of China's pig meat. As the availability of pig meat was limited by these small scale production methods, eating pig meat was reserved for special occasions. Before the Communist Chinese Revolution in 1949, the vast majority of the Chinese population received only 1% of their food energy from animal products, while grains made up the bulk of their diets. (*"Food in Chinese culture: Anthropological and historical perspectives," Yale University Press, 1977*). After the communists overthrew the dynastic system of rule in China, agriculture was collectivized under central state control, but raising pigs remained small scale much as it had always been in the past. This ancient regime began to change in 1978 when Premier Deng Xiaoping initiated his "Reform and Opening" program which loosened central control over agricultural production and distribution, increased state purchase prices for grain, and re-introduced selling of surplus pig meat through private markets. The Chinese government also began to subsidize and invest heavily in chemical fertilizers, pesticides, irrigation and high-yielding seed varieties (China's Green Revolution). At the same time, rapid industrialization and urbanization in China created large markets for pig meat among working class people in the growing cities (much like what happened in 18th century Europe and 19th century U.S.), turning pig meat into a commodity that demanded large scale production methods.

Pig meat is now at the center of China's livestock sector, but due to the sheer number of farmers in China, the transition from small backyard farms to mega-industrial farms was slow in the 1980s and 1990s. Then, in the mid-1990s, the Chinese government negotiated China's entry into the World Trade Organization (WTO). To meet WTO protocols for entry, China cut tariffs on soybean imports for use in livestock feed which effectively bypassed the country's natural limitations on pig meat production. This move was crucial to the emergence of industrial livestock production in China. In the 1990s soy imports quickly overtook domestic production, and by 2010, China was the world's leading soybean importer. In 2010, more than 50 million metric tons of soybeans came into China, mostly from the U.S. and Brazil. These imported beans accounted for 73% of soy consumption in China, and were used exclusively in the production of soybean meal for livestock feed and soy oil for cooking (meal and oil are coproducts in the soy crushing process). Unlike China's pig meat production industry which is dominated by a handful of domestic corporations, the soybean crushing industry is dominated by transnational agribusiness corporations including Archer Daniels Midland, Bunge, Cargill, Louis Dreyfus and Wilmar. Soy is particularly important in commercial pig feed mixes, but for smallholders and specialized household farmers in China, maize is the most used feedstuff. Maize is protected as a "strategic crop for food security" in China, as this Western Hemisphere import has become a staple food for human consumption. Increasingly, however, maize is being used in the manufacture of industrial products including commercial livestock feed. In 2010, China became a net maize importer for the first time since 1995 (*"Feeding China's Pigs/Implications for the Environment, China's Smallholder Farmers and Food Security", Institute for Agriculture and Trade Policy,* May 2011).

The most intensified and recent phase of industrialized pig meat production in China began in 2006 after an outbreak of the porcine reproductive and respiratory syndrome (PRRS) virus swept through the country's pig herds. The government responded with measures to increase state support for large-scale, industrialized, and standardized pig meat production in a misguided attempt to address the country's food bio-safety concerns. Throughout the reform era, the number of backyard farmers and their share of production declined as state policies and investments supported industrialized operations; in 2008 alone, the number of rural households that raised pigs dropped by 50%, and in some poor regions only about 35% of households still engaged in the practice of raising pigs. Government policies in 2006 to encourage scaled-up production were so successful that by 2009 farms raising more than 50 pigs a year accounted for almost 60% of total slaughter, up from less than 50% in 2007. The range of annual pig production on Chinese farms varies tremendously from fewer than 10 to as many as 100,000. Between these extremes are so-called "specialized household farms" where pig raising is a professional endeavor based on production for sale instead of self-consumption. These operations are operated by individual families, small-scale companies, or several backyard farmers who come together to focus on pig raising exclusively. Some specialized household farmers sell piglets and meat pigs to local dealers who then sell pigs to processing and retailing operations, but increasingly these specialized household farms are working under contract with large commercial farms in a vertically integrated system modeled after the U.S. hog farming industry. Large scale commercial farms typically range from 500 to 50,000 pigs, but this segment of the industry is growing rapidly in size and capacity; increasingly, single farm capacity is in the hundreds of thousands of hogs per year, either through contracts or in a single production facility. Among China's largest producers, the Wens corporation produces 7 million pigs per year and the CP Group, Zhengbang Technology Co, Chuying Agro-Pastoral Group and Munyuan Foodstuff Co. Ltd all have farms with more than 500,000 pigs. Most commercial operations in China are domestic agribusiness corporations, but transnational corporations play an important role in Chins's pig farming sector, ironically by supplying pig genetics from Western breeds that are specifically bred for factory farming. Transnational agribusiness corporations also supply China with imported feed from the U.S. and Brazil, and advanced factory farm technologies. With the Shuanghui Group's purchase of Smithfield, Chinese corporations are themselves becoming international in scope. Both commercial mega-farms and specialized household farms in China use CAFOs that were pioneered in the U.S. They buy their equipment from international dealers like "Big Dutchman," or from Chinese copycat companies like "Big Herdsman." The Chinese government strongly supports CAFOs seeing them as the solution to China's food safety problems by using standardized methods of feeding, vaccinating and rearing. Of course, actual experience on factory farms shows that just the opposite is true: as more and more animals are confined into cramped filthy spaces, the risk of disease increases.

A consolidation of China's slaughter and meat processing industry has also taken place since 2006 as the government closed down many medium and small pig meat processors and slaughterhouses. The total number of "designated" slaughterhouses decreased from 30,000 in 2006 to 10,000 in 2012. The top meat processors continue to plan for increased capacity, such as Yurun's announced plans to increase slaughter capacity to 70 million pigs by 2015 and Shuanghui's expects to reach a slaughter capacity of 55 million.

Pigs even more than chickens are the most distinctively Chinese food animal. The ancient household practice of raising pigs is even reflected in the Chinese Mandarin language; the word for meat (rou) refers to pig meat, and the written character for home and family, 家 (jia), added a roof over the pig character, literally putting a roof over a pig's head. This cultural and historical significance is key to understanding why the Chinese government chose to promote pig farming as the centerpiece of its agricultural reform program. After the food rationing that occurred during the Cultural Revolution between 1966 and 1976, supplying the population with the food that most symbolized wealth and prosperity in Chinese culture was the government's way of gaining back legitimacy and trust with the people. This government agricultural policy proved to be phenomenally successful at achieving these goals. By 2014, more than half of all the pigs on Earth were raised and eaten in China and Chinese farmers produced 55,620,000 metric tons of pig meat from a domestic herd of 660 million pigs. This was nearly 2.5 times more pig meat than was produced in all 27 EU countries combined (22,390,000 MT), and more than 5 times the U.S. production (10,530,000 MT). On a per capita basis, the average Chinese citizen went from consuming pig meat just a few times a year before 1976, to consuming 73 pounds (33.3 kg) per year in 2012; that compares to 66 pounds (30.3 kg) per year in the U.S. *(FAOSTAT)*.

Modern Pig Industry in Europe

On a per capita basis, the Chinese and Americans are actually far down on the list of pig meat consuming peoples, with the top ten nationalities all coming from European countries *(www.economist. com, Apr. 30, 2012 (courtesy UNFAO)*:

Country	pounds/person/year	kilograms/person/year
Austria	146	66.0
Serbia	143	64.8
Spain	134	60.9
Germany	123	55.6
Denmark	109	49.5
Hungary	104	47.2
Czech Republic	103	46.6
Luxembourg	100	45.5
Portugal	99	45.1
Italy	99	44.7

This large demand for pig meat in the EU (as in the U.S. and China) has led to a changeover from small farmers to large CAFO mega-farms in the late 20th and early 21st centuries. By 2010, 75% of pigs in the EU were raised by just 1.5% of the largest farms. The remaining small producers were mostly found in the 13 member states that joined the EU after 2004. The major production region in the EU extends from Nordhein-Westfalen and Niedersachen in Germany to Vlaams Gewest in Belgium which accounted for 30% of EU sows. Other important production regions include Spain (mainly in Cataluña and Murcia), Italy (mainly in Lombardia), France (mainly in Bretagne) and some areas of central Poland and Northern Croatia. According to the Eurostat 2010 Farm Structure Survey, the distribution of the pig population by size of herd shows that 1.7% of pig farms had at least 400 pigs. In twelve member states – Belgium, Czech Republic, Denmark, Estonia, Ireland, Spain, France, Italy, Cyprus, the Netherlands, Sweden and the UK – the herd size of 400 pigs accounted for more than 90% of all pigs produced, while in Poland and Romania this category represented approximately 33%. Farmers that raised less than 10 pigs were important in Romania (62.8%), Croatia (45.3%), Slovenia (31.4%), Lithuania (28.8%) and Bulgaria (25.8%). In the EU overall, small producers accounted for 73.3% of all the pig farms, yet they raised only 3.8% of the EU's pigs. (*"Pig farming in the European Union: considerable variations from one Member State to another," Pig farming sector - statistical portrait,* 2014). In 2014, the world's 5th and 9th largest vertically integrated pig meat processing corporations – Vion Food Group of the Netherlands which processed 320,000 pigs per week, and Danish Crown AmbA of Denmark, the world's leading pig meat exporter – were based in Europe *(Meat Atlas, Der Fleischatlas report,* 2014).

After recovering from the devastation of World War II, the largest agricultural economies in Western Europe came together in 1962 to establish a strongly interventionist agricultural policy called the Common Agricultural Policy (CAP). The result of the CAP's market interventions was to produce a highly volatile livestock feed market in Western Europe over the second half of the 20th century. The CAP first intervened to support feed grain production by maintaining high domestic prices for unlimited quantities of feed grains produced and by imposing import tariffs that eliminated competition from cheaper imports from abroad. These policies worked, from a net importer in the 1970s, Western Europe emerged as a major net exporter of wheat and other feed grains by the 1980s. But there were unanticipated consequences of these CAP price supports: skyrocketing agricultural budgets for Western European governments and chronic surpluses of feed grains. Western Europe's livestock producers were also saddled with high feed grain prices and European meat consumers with higher meat prices. While tariffs were high on imported feed grains, they were low on so called "Non-Grain Feed Ingredients" (NGFIs) and in the 1980s European livestock farmers began importing large amounts of these alternative feeds as cheap substitutes for expensive European domestically grown grains. These NGFIs included linseed meal, cottonseed meal, and peanut meal from various origins, sunflower seed meal from Argentina, Eastern Europe, and the former Soviet Union, rapeseed meal from Eastern Europe and Australia, copra and palm kernel meal from Indonesia, Malaysia, and the Philippines, distillers' dried grains from the U.S., peas and beans from Canada and Australia, maize germ cake from South America, cassava from Thailand, Indonesia and China, molasses from Pakistan, India, Egypt and the U.S., citrus pulp and other fruit and vegetable wastes from Brazil and the U.S., and sugarbeet pulp from the U.S. From 1984 to 1992, grain feed use in Western Europe declined by 11% while, due to imports of NGFIs, total feed use increased by 9%. CAP policymakers saw this substitution of imported NGFIs for European grains as a serious policy-induced problem that effectively increased Western Europe's grain surpluses and the associated costs of export subsidies to dispose of those surpluses. In 1994, the agricultural trade rules of the World Trade Organization (WTO) established limitations on the quantity of subsidized exports and on the total value of export subsidies. In preparation for the implementation of these new WTO rules, in 1993 the newly created European Union (EU) began to reduce grain prices by 30% over the next 3 years. The EU also raised the quality standards required for wheat to qualify for price support, leaving feed quality wheat without any subsidy. In 2000, further reforms provided another reduction in grain prices of 15% and reduced compensatory payments for oilseeds, field peas and beans. In addition to these reductions, a 30% decline in the value of the euro from 1994 to 2000 led to significant reductions in the gap between EU grain prices and those on world markets. The hoped for result of these grain price reductions was to reduce European imports of NGFIs and to stimulate the domestic market for EU produced feed grains. While the new agricultural policies did result in reduced imports of NGFIs, they did not increase EU production of feed grains, but instead, lower WTO tariffs on imports stimulated EU livestock producers to buy cheaper "feed concentrates" on world markets. Feed concentrates include grains, oilseed and other protein meals, field peas and beans, dehydrated fodders, cassava, skimmed-milk powder (SMP), corn gluten feed (CGF), bran, corn germ meal, citrus pulp, sugarbeet pulp, brewer's and distiller's residues, fruit and vegetable wastes, molasses, animal and vegetable fats, fish meal, and meat and bone meal (MBM). EU pig meat production is largely dependent on these imported feed concentrates.

Pig meat accounted for roughly half of EU meat consumption in 2014. In recent decades, pig and chicken meat consumption grew faster than total meat consumption, in part due to the outbreak of Bovine Spongioform Encephalapathy (BSE), or "mad cow" disease in 1986 which scared people away from eating cattle meat. Pig meat consumption dipped in 1997 when the Netherlands was afflicted with its worst ever epidemic of "swine fever" which spread to several other countries. More than 10 million pigs, including half the Dutch herd, were destroyed and pig meat production was reduced by the epidemic just as demand was rising due to mad cow concerns. With pig meat production down, many consumers switched to chicken in 1997, but pig meat production and consumption fully rebounded over the following two years. The overall shift in EU meat consumption from cattle and sheep towards pig and chicken effectively shifted meat production in the EU from animals that primarily grazed on grass to animals that are fed on feed concentrates. Pigs require more than twice as much feed concentrate per pound of meat than chickens making pig feed by far the largest contributor to the EU's demand for imported feed concentrates.

Worldwide Production and Consumption of Pig Meat

Brazil's agricultural revolution in the 1990s and 2000s saw an explosion in the production of livestock feed as well as cattle, chicken and pig meat, both for domestic consumption and for export. By 2012, Brazil was the world's fourth largest pig meat producer at 3,240,000 metric tons (less than 6% of China's production), and three of the top ten vertically integrated pig meat processing corporations in the world were based in Brazil including the number one processor, JBS SA (also the world's largest cattle processor). Pigs are raised and eaten in many countries around the world; rounding out the top ten producers after China, the EU, the U.S. and Brazil are:

Country	Metric Tons
5. Russia	2,400,000
6. Vietnam	2,220,000
7. Canada	1,820,000
8. Philippines	1,350,000
9. Japan	1,309,000
10. Mexico	1,281,000

*USDA FAS 2013

All of these countries use CAFO technologies to some degree. While most pig meat is consumed in the country of origin, there is a world market for imports and exports that reached 7 million Metric Tons in 2013. Listed below are the world's top five importing and exporting countries in 2013:

Pig Meat Imports:

Rank	Country	Metric Tons
1.	Japan	1,223,000
2.	Russia	868,000
3.	Mexico	783,000
4.	China	770,000
5.	Hong Kong	399,000

Pig Meat Exports:

Rank	Country	Metric Tons
1.	United States	2,264,000
2.	European Union	2,232,000
3.	Canada	1,246,000
4.	Brazil	585,000
5.	China	244,000

*USDA - FAS 2014

Environmental Impacts of Pig Meat Production

In 2011, there were approximately 968.16 million pigs worldwide according to the independent statistical service Statista, and in 2014, total world pig meat production reached over 110 million metric tons according to the USDA – FAS. This massive scale of pig meat production has had far ranging environmental impacts.

In the 20th century, pigs have become a major vector for the spread of the zoonotic (a disease that can be passed from animals to humans) influenza virus. The first appearance of "swine influenza" (commonly known as swine flu) was during the worldwide human influenza pandemic of 1918, when pigs became ill at the same time as humans. Swine flu is now common throughout pig populations worldwide. Its symptoms include: fever, lethargy, sneezing, coughing, difficult breathing and decreased appetite. Though swine flu is not usually fatal in pigs, there is a 1% to 4% mortality rate and the virus also induces weight loss which is a significant economic loss to pig farmers. A study conducted in 2008, published in the journal *Nature*, traced the evolutionary origin of the swine flu virus to before 1918 when the ancestral influenza virus that was of avian origin (bird flu), crossed species boundaries and infected humans as the human H1N1 virus. The human virus later infected pigs leading to the emergence of the H1N1 swine strain. Pigs have acted as an incubator for the influenza virus ever since, and since the 1970s there have been numerous instances of the swine flu epidemics in pig and human populations. In 1998, swine flu was found in pigs in four U.S. states and within a year it had spread through herds across the U.S. Scientists found this virus had originated in pigs as a recombinant form of flu strains from birds and humans. This outbreak confirmed that pigs serve as an incubator where novel influenza viruses emerge as a result of the reassortment of genes from different strains. Pigs have been termed the "mixing vessel" of flu because they can be infected by both avian flu viruses, which rarely infect humans, and by human viruses. When pigs become simultaneously infected with more than one virus, the viruses can swap genes, producing novel variants which can pass to and spread among humans. Genetic components of this 1998 triple-hybrid stain would later cause the flu pandemic of 2009. On June 11, 2009, the World Health Organization raised the worldwide pandemic alert level to Phase 6 for swine flu, which is their highest alert level. This alert level means that the swine flu had spread worldwide and there were cases of people with the virus in most countries. Swine flu spread rapidly worldwide due to its high human-to-human transmission rate and to the frequency of modern air travel. While this new variant was no more lethal than typical flu viruses, unlike most flu epidemics, younger people under 50 were at much higher risk of infection. By mid November 2009, the swine flu virus had infected one in six Americans with 200,000 hospitalizations and 10,000 deaths mostly of people with already compromised immune systems. The potential certainly exists inside the guts of a pig for a much more lethal strain of flu to develop like the one that caused the pandemic of 1918 which killed up to 100 million people.

According to a 2010 report entitled "*Factory Farm Nation: How America Turned Its Livestock Farms into Factories*" by the NGO, *Food & Water Watch*, there were 17 U.S. counties that held more than half a million hogs on factory farms. These counties effectively generated the same amount of untreated manure as the volume of sewage that enters the wastewater treatment plants of some of America's largest cities. The nearly 2.3 million hogs in Duplin County, North Carolina, generated twice as much waste as the entire New York City metropolitan area; Sampson County, North Carolina, generated six times as much waste as greater Philadelphia, Pennsylvania; Sioux County, Iowa produced as much hog manure as the sewage from Los Angeles and Atlanta combined. Before CAFOs took over the pig industry, pigs were raised in stys with a place for the animals to defecate and bedding to absorb urine; this mixture was then composted and used as fertilizer. With the intensive confinement in CAFOs, there is no bedding or place to defecate, all the excrement drops through slats in the floor and is flushed into giant open air pits 30 feet deep and acres wide typically containing 500,000 gallons of "Liquid Manure." The 2010 *Food & Water Watch* report cited above notes that the environmental hazards of hog CAFOs are exemplified by the state of North Carolina, where factory hog farming has been most thoroughly studied:

> *"North Carolina, where intense hog production increased significantly during the 1980s, embodies the risks created by the rapid rise of big pork packing companies and factory farms. In the 1990s, lenient environmental regulations and local zoning exemptions attracted corporations like Smithfield and Premium Standard Farms that transformed the state into a pork powerhouse. After Smithfield and Premium Standard merged in 2007, Smithfield controlled an estimated 90 percent of the hog market in the state... The hog population in North Carolina nearly quadrupled from 2.5 million hogs in 1988 to more than 10 million by 2010... The state's 10 million hogs produce 14.6 billion gallons of manure every year. The burden of these facilities is concentrated in some of North Carolina's most impoverished areas. Nearly two-thirds (61 percent) of North Carolina's factory-farmed hogs are located in five counties in the eastern part of the state. One study found that North Carolina industrial hog operations are disproportionately located in communities of color and communities with higher rates of poverty. North Carolina's waters have been polluted repeatedly by waste from hog factory farms. The public first became aware of problems with the lagoon and sprayfield system when in 1995, a lagoon burst and released 25 million gallons of manure into eastern North Carolina's New River. Hog lagoon spills were responsible for sending one million gallons of waste into the Cape Fear River and its tributaries in the summer of 1995, one million gallons into a tributary of the Trent River in 1996, and 1.9 million gallons into the Persimmon Branch in 1999. Hog waste was also the likely culprit for massive fish kills in the Neuse River in 2003; at least 3 million fish died within a two-month span. Perhaps the most infamous example of the danger hog factories pose to the environment occurred in 1999 when Hurricane Floyd hit North Carolina. The storm flooded fifty lagoons and caused three of them to burst, which led to the release of millions of gallons of manure and the drowning of approximately 30,500 hogs, 2.1 million chickens and 737,000 turkeys."*

Liquid manure from fecal ponds is sprayed onto adjacent fields as fertilizer. While it is a significant cost savings for pig CAFOs to distribute liquid manure locally through piping systems rather than regionally by truck, the tremendous volumes of manure concentrated in local soils is causing a problem called "manure overload." When the application exceeds the ability of fields to absorb the nutrients, the residual nutrients from manure – mostly nitrogen and phosphorus – and bacteria leach off fields and into groundwater and rivers. The long list of contaminants making their way from manure into drinking water includes heavy metals, antibiotics and pathogenic bacteria. Six of the 150 pathogens found in animal manure are responsible for 90% of human food- and water-borne diseases: Campylobacter, Salmonella, Listeria, E. coli 0157:H7, Cryptosporidium and Giardia. Freezing temperatures in the U.S. upper Midwest exacerbates the problem of manure overload as explained in the *Food & Water Watch* report:

> *"Much of U.S. hog production is concentrated in the grain- and soybean-producing Midwest. The tremendous amount of manure produced on hog factory farms is stored in lagoons and applied — often over-applied — to cropland. In the upper Midwest, where farmland freezes solid during the winter, manure applied to frozen fields cannot be absorbed, so it runs off into local waters.*

These open sewers are directly exposed to the air and are a major cause of localized air pollution. Chemicals added to the manure ponds to "reduce odor," change the 'organic' chemistry of the manure and upon entering the air cause acid rain which is a leading tree killer. Dried particles and mist from sprayed fertilizer also enter the air leading to high rates of respiratory diseases such as asthma in populations living near hog manure ponds. An article in June 2013 journal *Environmental Health Perspectives* describes the plight of poor people who live near hog CAFOs in North Carolina:

> *"On the coastal plain of eastern North Carolina, families in certain rural communities daily must deal with the piercing, acrid odor of hog manure—reminiscent of rotten eggs and ammonia—wafting from nearby industrial hog farms. On bad days, the odor invades homes, and people are often forced to cover their mouths and noses when stepping outside. Sometimes, residents say, a fine mist of manure sprinkles nearby homes, cars, and even laundry left on the line to dry.*[1]
>
> *Today's industrial-scale farms—called concentrated animal feeding operations (CAFOs)— house thousands of animals whose waste is periodically applied to "spray fields" of Bermuda grass or feed crops.*[2,3] *The waste can contain pathogens, heavy metals, and antibiotic-resistant bacteria,*[4,5] *and the spray can reach nearby homes and drinking water sources. The odor plume, which often pervades nearby communities, contains respiratory and eye irritants including hydrogen sulfide and ammonia.*[6,7,8] *A growing body of research suggests these emissions may contribute not only to mucosal irritation*[9] *and respiratory ailments*[10] *in nearby residents but also decreased quality of life,*[11] *mental stress,*[12,13] *and elevated blood pressure.*[14]

Although the Midwest is the traditional home for hogs, with Iowa still the top-producing state, North Carolina went from fifteenth to second in hog production between the mid-1980s and mid-1990s.[15] This explosive growth resulted in thousands of CAFOs located in the eastern half of the state—squarely in the so-called Black Belt, a crescent-shaped band throughout the South where slaves worked on plantations.[16,17] After emancipation many freed slaves continued to work as sharecroppers and tenant farmers. A century later, black residents of this region still experience high rates of poverty, poor health care, low educational attainment, unemployment, and substandard housing.[18,19]

The clustering of North Carolina's hog CAFOs in low-income, minority communities—and the health impacts that accompany them—has raised concerns of environmental injustice and environmental racism.[20] As one pair of investigators explained, "[P]eople of color and the poor living in rural communities lacking the political capacity to resist are said to shoulder the adverse socio-economic, environmental, or health related effects of swine waste externalities without sharing in the economic benefits brought by industrialized pork production."[21] Although North Carolina is not the only area with environmental justice concerns vis-à-vis CAFOs, it has become one of the best studied." ("CAFOs and Environmental Justice: The Case of North Carolina", Environ Health Perspect 121:A182-A189 (2013). http://dx.doi. org/10.1289/ehp.121-a182 [online 01 June 2013])

Starting in about 2009, a gray, bubbly substance the consistency of beaten egg whites began appearing at the surface of the fecal soup under hog CAFO hog barns. The foam grows to a thickness of up to four feet and seeps through the slats on the floor of hog barns that are designed to let the manure and urine drop through the floor to be flushed away. As the manure breaks down, it emits toxic gases like hydrogen sulfide and highly flammable methane, that get trapped under this thick layer of foam; sudden releases have resulted in a number of explosions in the U.S. Midwest. A 2012 report from the University of Minnesota noted that by the Fall of 2011, the foam had led to about a half-dozen such explosions, one that destroyed a barn on a farm in northern Iowa, killing 1,500 pigs and severely burning a worker. According to Dr. Larry Jacobson, professor of Agricultural Engineering at the University of Minnesota who has been working on this issue, surveys indicate that around 25% of operations in the hog-intensive regions of Minnesota, Illinois, and Iowa are experiencing foam. The cause of the foam is not fully understood but Dr. Jacobson suspects the practice of feeding hogs distillers grains, the mush leftover from the maize ethanol process, might be one of the triggers. Distillers grains entered hog rations in a major way around the same time that the foam started emerging, and manure from hogs fed distillers grains contains heightened levels of undigested fiber and volatile fatty acids both of which are emerging as preconditions for foam formation. Dr. Jacobson has found that the only thing that works consistently to break up the foam is dumping pounds of the antibiotic, minensin, on the foam which likely works by altering the mix of microbes present. Yet another misuse of antibiotics in factory farming.

The environmental impacts of industrialized hog production are not confined to the U.S. As the factory farming of pigs has proliferated in 21st century China, so have the environmental impacts associated with this industry. In 2011, the *Institute for Agriculture and Trade Policy* issued a report entitled *"Feeding China's Pigs/Implications for the Environment, China's Smallholder Farmers and Food Security"* which examined the environmental and social impacts of large scale pig farming in China. Here are some of the notable findings gleaned from the Executive Summary of that report:

> *"Starting in 1979, pork became the most produced and consumed meat in the world. The reason for its ascent to the top of the global meat heap is simple: China. In 2010 alone, farmers and companies in China produced more than 50 million metric tons of pork, virtually all of which was sold and consumed domestically. This Chinese pork boom, which today accounts for half of all the pork in the world, is the result of a set of policies and trade agreements that liberalized and industrialized Chinese agriculture and enabled enormous production increases... The consequences of these changes in pig production and pig feeding have wide-ranging impacts. In terms of environmental degradation, agriculture in general—and livestock farming in particular—are the most important sources of pollution in China. Livestock farms produce more than 4 billion tons of manure annually, much of which contributes to nutrient overload in waterways and subsequent eutrophication and dead zones. Globally, as more and more land is converted to intensive monocrop production of soybeans and corn (and others in a narrow range of industrial feed crops), pesticide and fertilizers pollute waterways, biodiversity declines, natural carbon sinks are destroyed, and greenhouse gases are emitted in all stages of intensive feed production and transport. Industrial pig feeding also carries a range public health concerns. China is becoming increasingly infamous as a site of food safety scandals, most of which stem from feed additives such as hormones and growth regulators ending up in meat and livestock products. On top of this, the prophylactic administration of antibiotics in confined animal feeding operations (CAFOs) has resulted in antibiotic-resistant and disease-causing organisms emerging in China, just as in the United States and Europe."*

Pig CAFOs are having major environmental impacts in EU countries as well, as this 2016 report from the Organisation for Economic Co-operation and Development (OECD) makes clear:

> *"It is difficult to quantify the specific contribution of pig production to water pollution but an indirect measure — the OECD's soil nitrogen balance indicator — can reveal the potential risks... Countries can be grouped into four distinct groups according to the level of risk as measured by the overall nitrogen balance and the importance of pig manure as a source of nitrogen. The risk is highest in certain regions of Belgium, the Czech Republic, Denmark, France, Germany, Japan, Korea, the Netherlands, Norway and Switzerland. In Australia, Italy, Mexico, Poland, Sweden and the United States the risk of nitrogen pollution from pig production is low at the national level, although studies indicate that the risk at the regional*

level, particularly in the United States, can be just as large as in the high-risk countries... In some countries, the emission of ammonia from livestock housing facilities and from badly managed storage and spreading of manure are also of serious local concern. Livestock accounts for around 80% of total ammonia emissions in the OECD, with the importance of pigs as a source of emissions following a similar pattern to its contribution to livestock nitrogen manure production i.e. the issue is particularly serious in regions of high pig concentration in parts of northern Europe and Asia.

Pig CAFOs account for a significant amount of greenhouse gas (GHG) emissions worldwide. Pig meat production results in the emission of GHGs primarily in the form of methane and nitrous oxide, which are generated by the biological activity that breaks down manure in treatment or storage. Methane (CH_4) has approximately 20 times the greenhouse gas potential of an equivalent quantity of carbon dioxide (CO_2), and nitrous oxide (N_2O) has about 300 times the greenhouse gas potential of CO_2. GHG emissions in the U.S. from pig farming have been well quantified in this 2006 report by eXtension.org, a research service of U.S. land-grant universities:

"The EPA estimated that manure management was responsible for 56 MMT of CO2 Eq in 2006. Methane emissions were 41 MMT [metric megatons] of CO2 Eq, ... Of the 41 MMT of CO2 Eq in the form of methane, swine production was considered responsible for 18 MMT. Methane production occurs when manure is handled under anaerobic conditions such as in liquids and slurries. When manure is handled as a solid, little or no methane is produced. The amount of methane produced is affected by diet, temperature, moisture, manure composition, storage system, and time in storage. Higher energy feed generally have a greater potential for manure methane emissions. However higher energy feeds can be more digestible than lower quality feeds leading to less overall manure produced by the animal. Intensive livestock production, as occurs in the U.S. swine industry, produces less GHG per unit of meat produced than do less intensive production systems. Of the 14 MMT of CO2 Eq in the form of nitrous oxide, swine production was responsible for 1.5 MMT. Nitrous oxide is produced from organic nitrogen in both manure and urine. Solid manure management systems produce nitrous oxide because they have both aerobic and anaerobic decomposition that nitrifies and then denitrifies the nitrogen in the manure and urine.

Manure management from swine production emitted a total of 19 MMT of CO2 Eq in 2006. This equals about 34% of all GHG emissions due to manure management ... in the U.S."
("Pork Production and Greenhouse Gas Emissions" Author: Ray Massey and Ann Ulmer, University of Missouri, eXtension.org)

While pigs are far more efficient at converting feed grains into meat than are cattle, it is simply not possible to produce pig meat as a staple food for billions of people worldwide without causing severe environmental impacts on both a local and global scale. Over most of the 15,000 year relationship between pigs and humans, pigs were raised either by herding them in forests to forage for their natural diet, or by feeding them human agricultural waste products. Herding pigs in the forest has not been sustainable anywhere in the world for well over a century, and there are not enough agricultural waste products in the world to produce the quantities of pig meat necessary to satisfy world market demand. These natural constraints on pig feed have been overcome only by growing vast amounts of maize and soybeans for livestock feed and through an international market in livestock feed that is a major threat to regional biodiversity and ecological integrity.

As we have seen, pig meat has been part of the human diet in many cultures throughout history, but it wasn't until the 18th century that industrialized agriculture began to turn the pig into a food commodity to feed a rapidly growing and urbanizing population. Not only did the number of humans explode over the 19th and 20th centuries (from 1 billion in 1804 to 7 billion in 2011), pig meat consumption per person also climbed dramatically over these two centuries. To satisfy this unprecedented world demand for pig meat, pig meat production had to increase well beyond the capacity of traditional farming practices. Factory farming was the agricultural sector's response to this consumer demand: by using cheap energy in the form of petroleum and cheap fertilizer in the form of synthetic nitrogen to produce vast quantities of feed, and by using extreme animal confinement to maximize the feed to meat conversion ratio – factory farms produce the most meat at the least cost. It is important to note, however, that in this business calculation, the environmental cost imposed on society by factory hog farms is not factored into the cost of production. Economists refer to these industrial costs of production that are borne by the general public as "externalized costs." If these externalized costs were included as a cost of production, the true costs of factory farmed pig meat would make it unaffordable for the great majority of people.

16

CATTLE

Cattle are raised to provide both meat, milk and hides. Though cattle meat and milk are food products derived from the same animal, the meat and milk industries that exist today developed as interconnected, yet separate, highly specialized enterprises. First let's examine the cattle meat industry.

Meat Cattle

All modern day cattle breeds are descended from the "Aurochs" which became extinct in the 17th century. The Aurochs that originally ranged from Europe, North Africa to much of Asia, were first domesticate around 8,000 years ago by nomadic meat eating cultures that herded domesticated cattle over the vast grasslands of Eurasia. As the human populations of agriculturally based early civilizations grew, cattle were primarily used to pull plows and produce milk, only to provide meat and hides when no longer otherwise productive. There were, however, several notable exceptions to this rule.

Around 1500 BC, Aryan cattle herders from present day Iran began to drive their cattle herds across the Hindu Kush Mountains to graze in the verdant Indus Valley of present day Pakistan where the Harappa civilization had flourished for centuries. By 300 BC, this Aryan cattle based culture had fully established itself in the Indus Valley and the Ganges River basin in present-day Northern India. As the human population of this region approached 100 million, intensive cattle grazing to provide meat to this burgeoning population had turned the once fertile soils of these river systems into arid and depleted plains that could no longer produce enough food to feed the people. It was this existential crisis that motivated the Hindu religion to ban the consumption of cattle meat and turn to a sustainable plant-based diet.

Over the course of the 14th century, due to the "Little Ice Age," the "Great Famine of 1315 to 1317," and the "Back Death" bubonic plague epidemics of 1333 and 1346, the human population of Europe plummeted by half. During this time there was a severe shortage of farm labor and many fields that were once farmed for grain production were abandoned to wild grasslands and left to graze cattle and sheep for meat production. Also in the 14th century, vaqueros on the grassy plains of Southern Spain and Ottoman Turks on the grassy plains of Hungary were driving herds of thousands of cattle to markets in cities. As a result of these circumstances, per capita meat consumption in Europe peaked in the 14th and 15th centuries. In France and Germany people were eating around 220 pounds/person/year (100 kilos). By the time the population of Europe had recovered to its previous high of 70 million people in the 16th century, meat consumption per person had dropped to 31 pounds per year (14 kilos).

In the 15th and 16th centuries, the Spanish and Portuguese colonists of Central and South America introduced cattle to the vast grasslands of the New World producing herds the size of which the world had never seen before. At this time in history, meat would spoil on the long sea passage back to the Old World, so it was only the Spanish and Portuguese colonists themselves to eat unlimited amounts of cattle meat. While the Spanish and Portuguese colonists gorged on enormous quantities of meat, the total European population of the New World remained very small throughout this period, so most of the meat went to rot.

United States

The cattle industry we know today which provides meat for hundreds of millions of people, is based on growing crops specifically to feed to cattle. The system of using feed crops instead of forage to raise cattle got its start in the 1830s in the Ohio Valley in the U.S. With its rich soil and favorable climate the Ohio Valley was a premier maize growing region. At the same time Northern Indiana, which was maize poor, had land suitable for pasturing small herds of cattle. Entrepreneurial farmers from these neighboring regions came to realize that fattening cattle on surplus maize before they were shipped to Cincinnati for slaughter was to both of their advantages and the first grain-fed cattle complex was born in America.

The meat from cattle finished on maize has fat marbling throughout the muscle making it distinctive from cattle finished on grass. As the U.S. population grew in the years before the Civil War (1861-1865) this maize fed cattle system moved west into Illinois and Iowa and on the eve of the Civil War cattle were regularly being shipped from the prairies of Iowa to be fattened-up on Illinois maize before being shipped to Chicago or St. Louis for slaughter. During the Civil War these cattle stocks became depleted and to satisfy demand for beef in the Northeast after the war, entrepreneurial northern livestock dealers looked southward to Texas where as many as five million longhorn cattle, descendants of old Spanish stock (see "Columbian Exchange"), roamed wild. Up until then, wild Texas longhorns with horn spans of up to eight feet had only been hunted for their hides since there was no way to transport their meat to eastern markets. But with the building of the first transcontinental railroad commencing in 1863, it became possible to move these cattle by rail to the eastern markets where most of the people lived. As the railroad passed through Abilene, Kansas in 1867, an Illinois livestock dealer named Joseph McCoy (the Real McCoy), saw the potential for making tiny Abilene into a booming cattle town so he bought 250 acres near the railroad and built a stockyard, outbuildings, a hotel, and a bank. He also contracted with cowboys (mostly war veterans, freed slaves and Indians) to drive the Texas longhorns from central Texas to Abilene, a distance of 500 miles, where they were loaded onto railroad cars and shipped live to eastbound destinations. Other cow towns sprang up at Caldwell, Ellsworth, Wichita, and Dodge City. Herds of 1,000 to 10,000 animals were driven over these open ranges; altogether four million longhorn cattle were herded north between 1866 and 1888.

For countless millennia before the 1870s, great herds of American bison had thundered across the western plains from Montana and North Dakota south to New Mexico and Texas. These large bovines that were up to 11.5 feet long and weighed as much as 2,000 pounds grazed on the indigenous prairie grasses that were resilient to drought which provided them with a nourishing source of forage year-round. Humans only began to inhabit the plains around 13,000 years ago, but it wasn't until after the arrival of the horse with the Spanish conquistadors just over 500 years ago that the plains Indians were able to efficiently exploit the bison as a resource for wealth accumulation (see "The Columbian Exchange"). Still, as with all hunter-gatherer societies, the Indian population density on the vast North American plains remained very low. In the 19th century, as the settlers in the eastern States dispossessed the Indian plague survivors of their lands, many were forced to move to the western plains. Eastern settlers had always thought of the western plains as a wild and desolate place, but after the Civil War the US government made westward expansion a national priority, and the bison and the Indians stood in the way. In the 1870s, to clear the plains of these impediments to what the settlers considered to be their "manifest destiny," the US Army teamed up with eastern bankers and the railroads in a systematic campaign to exterminate the bison and thereby deprive the Indians of their sustaining resource. Perhaps it was former Union Civil War General and latter commander of the Armies of the West, Philip Sheridan, who said it most bluntly:

> *"These men [the bison hunters] have done... more to settle the vexed Indian question than the entire regular army has done in the last thirty years. They are destroying the Indian's*

commissary; and it is a well known fact that an army losing its base of supplies is placed at a
great disadvantage. Send them powder and lead if you will; but for the sake of lasting peace
let them kill, skin, and sell until the buffalo [bison] is exterminated. Then your prairies can
be covered with speckled cattle and the festive cowboy who follows the hunter as a second
forerunner of an advanced civilization." ("Beyond Beef", Jeremy Rifkin, pg 78, Dutton, 1992)

US Army Colonel Richard Dodge estimated that in the brief span of four years (from 1871 to 1874)
four million bison were killed. The dead bison were simply left on the ground to rot, and though a brisk
hide tanning business developed over the few years of the slaughter, millions of pounds of bison bones
littered the plains for the next decade. Harvesting these bones became a booming industry throughout the
1870s; commercial scavengers would take their "white harvest" to the nearest railhead where speculators
would buy them and load them onto trains headed back east to manufacturers where they were made
into bone char used in sugar refining, ground into phosphorus fertilizers, or fashioned into bone china;
the horns and hooves were used to make buttons, combs, knife handles and glue. By the end of the 1870s
the bison were gone, bones and all, the Indian resistance had been broken, and the Great Plains had been
made safe for cattle ranchers and homesteaders.

Conditions on cattle trains transporting Texas longhorns back east were brutal, with many of the
animals dyeing along the way and the remainder losing marketable weight. Transporting live animals
also required the costly expense of transporting the 60% of the animal that was inedible over long
distances. In 1869 a Detroit meat-packer (a meat packer handles the slaughtering, processing, packaging,
and distribution of meat animals) named George Hammond began shipping "dressed" (slaughtered
and gutted) carcasses to Boston in refrigerated rail cars using ice from the Great Lakes. This innovation
eliminated the need to ship live animals which greatly improved Hammond's return on investment. In
the early 1870s Hammond moved to northwest Indiana where he built a meat-packing plant along the
tracks of the Michigan Central Railroad and by 1873 the George H. Hammond Co. was selling $1 million
worth of meat a year; by 1875 sales were nearly $2 million with markets extending across the Atlantic. At
that time American consumers came to prefer lean cattle meat from Texas longhorns and the maize fed
"fatted" cattle meat was primarily sold to European markets. American refrigerated fatty cattle meat was a
big hit particularly in England where marbled meat was highly prized by the English gentry and military.
In 1876 U.S. Commissioner of Agriculture, Fredrick Watts, formalized this new relationship between the
plains and the grains:

"Let the vast areas of pasture in the border states and territories be employed with breeding
and feeding the cattle until they are two years old, and then let them be sent forward to the
older sections to be fed a year on corn and rounded up to the proportions of foreign demand."
("*Cow Country*", Edward Dale, University of Oklahoma Press, 1942.)

By the middle of the 1880s, Hammond had built a new plant in Omaha, Nebraska, that was
slaughtering over 100,000 cattle a year, and he owned a fleet of 800 refrigerated rail cars. In 1880, Chicago

meat-packer Gustavus Swift developed a much more efficient air-cooled freight system and Swift & Co. meat-packing overtook Hammond as the largest meat-packer in the industry. Swift's major competitors, Armour (which bought Hammond in 1901), Morris, Cudhay and, Schwarschild and Sulzberger (later renamed Sulzberger and Sons) quickly adopted the new refrigeration technology and Chicago, St. Louis, Cincinnati and Kansas City became major meat-packing centers in the U.S. for an international cattle meat market. During the 1890s these top five meat-packing companies became known as the "Beef Trust" for their collusion to control prices on the cattle meat market.

In 1873 American farmer Joseph Glidden invented barbed wire, and by the end of the 1880s, thousands of miles of barbed wire fencing tacked up by homesteaders had crisscrossed the great American plains spelling the end of the era of free range cattle drives from Texas. Western cattlemen needed financial backing to establish new fenced in controlled ranges on the plains where the animals could be grazed, watered, and protected from predators and also stocked with Angus and Hereford cattle breeds from Scotland and England. It was at this time that British financiers who fancied American cattle meat began to invest heavily in the American cattle industry. Once the province of hard scrabble American frontiersmen, the cattle industry became a high stakes business venture of fine English gentlemen.

After a steep worldwide economic depression in 1884 and severe winter storms in 1886 and 1887 that decimated cattle herds, only the largest of these cattle companies survived to restock the western plains. Over the next few decades these "cattle barons" undertook the most aggressive land grab in American history. Cattle companies would buy small land holdings from the railroads or make fraudulent small claims under the Homestead Act of 1862, the Timber Culture Act of 1873 and the Desert Lands Act of 1887, and then proceed to fence in thousands of acres of adjacent public lands to which they had no legal claim. This expropriation of public lands for grazing cattle became official U.S. government policy with the Grazing Homestead Act of 1916, and by 1923, 31.4 million acres in all the western states except Texas had been expropriated by cattle companies. The ultimate giveaway of public lands for cattle grazing came with the Taylor Grazing Act of 1934 which, over the next decades, leased tens of millions of acres of public range lands to cattle companies for token fees that didn't even recover the cost of improvements made at government expense for the explicit purpose of raising cattle, such as: stock ponds, seeding with invasive "Cheatgrass", building fences, and predator control (wolf extermination).

In 1935, J.W. Hayward at the University of Wisconsin wrote his PhD dissertation on "*The Effect of the Temperature of Oil Extraction Upon the Nutritive Value of the Protein of Soybean Oil Meal,*" where he showed that heating greatly improves the quality of soybean protein. In 1936 Hayward, et al., demonstrated that cooking soybeans increased the digestibility by about 3% and the biological value or protein quality by about 12%. These discoveries played a major role in expanding the use of defatted soybean meal in animal feed and standardizing the moist heat treatment processing to attain optimum nutritional value. Subsequent research by Hayward found that steaming denatured the soy protein making the amino acids methionine and cystine more available. Hayward went on to work for the major U.S. grain processing corporation, Archer Daniels Midland (ADM), and become a leading authority on the use of soybean meal in animal feed.

The "Ogallala Aquifer" is one of the world's largest aquifers, underlying an area of approximately 174,000 square miles (450,000 square kilometers) in the High Plains region of eight U.S. states: South Dakota, Nebraska, Wyoming, Colorado, Kansas, Oklahoma, New Mexico and Texas. The U.S. Geological Survey has estimated the total water storage capacity of the aquifer at over 3 trillion acre feet. Geologically the aquifer formed between 6 and 2 million years ago when erosion from the Rockie Mountains provided permiable sediments that filled ancient river and stream beds to eventually cover the entire area of the present-day Ogallala Formation. The depth of the aquifer ranges from a few feet to more than 1000 feet (300 meters) and is generally greater in the northern plains. Present-day recharge of the aquifer with fresh water occurs very slowly and much of the water stored in its pourous layers dates back at least to the last Ice Age. Early Anglo settlers of this semi-arid region who had no access to the Ogallala aquifer were plagued by crop failures due to cycles of drought, culminating in the disastrous "Dust Bowl" years of the 1930s. In 1948 an irrigation system called "center-pivot irrigation" was invented by farmer Frank Zybach of Strasburg, Colorado. Center pivot irrigation is a form of overhead sprinkler irrigation consisting of several segments of pipe (usually galvanized steel or aluminum) joined together and supported by trusses, mounted on wheeled towers with sprinklers positioned along its length. The trussed segments move in a circular pattern and are fed with water from the pivot point at the center of the circle. Center-pivot irrigation enables the system to operate in undulating country like the U.S. high plains. Center-pivot irrigation in the High Plains was made feasible by the earlier invention in 1916 of the electric submersible pump (ESP) by the Russian inventor Armais Arutunoff. Arutunoff moved to Bartlesville, Oklahoma, in 1928 at the urging of the Phillips Petroleum Company where he refined his ESP for use in oil wells. In the 1950s the ESP was adapted for use in deep water wells drilled into the Ogallala aquifer and hooked up to central pivot irrigation systems. Substantial water well drilling and ground-water development for irrigation begun in the 1950s transformed the High Plains into one of the most agriculturally productive regions in the world. In 1950, irrigated cropland on the High Plains covered 250,000 acres, but with the development of center-pivot irrigation, by the beginning of the 21st century nearly three million acres of land were being irrigated with water pumped from the Ogallala Aquifer. The High Plains became one of the most productive areas in the U.S. for growing wheat, maize and soybeans mostly to feed livestock. The success of large-scale farming on the semi-arid High Plains depended entirely on groundwater wells for irrigation. Over the course of sixty years this massive irrigation project has drawn down the aquifer by more than 300 feet in some areas. Vast stretches of Texas farmland no longer support irrigation and in west-central Kansas up to one fifth of the irrigated farmland along a 100-mile swath of the aquifer has gone dry. Since 1950, agricultural irrigation has reduced the water volume of the Ogallala Aquifer by an estimated 9% and depletion is accelerating with 2% lost between 2001 and 2009 alone. As of 2013, about 27% of the irrigated land in the U.S. still relies on the Ogallala Aquifer which amounts to about 30% of the ground water used for irrigation in the U.S. Over the decades many advances in center pivot technology have made it an irrigation practice of choice in semi-arid regions around the world including Brazil, Australia, New Zealand, the Sahara and the Middle East.

With the explosion of maize and soybean production that occurred after WWII, along with the concurrent overgrazing of the western plains, the rotation of grazing cattle on the range for 12 to 18 months and then fattening them up on maize and soybean meal for six months before slaughter in massive stockyards called "feedlots" became common practice in the industry. The first large cattle feedlot, what the U.S. Environmental Protection Agency (EPA) calls a CAFO (Concentrated Animal Feeding Operation), to open on the Great Plains was the Lewter Feed Yard near Lubbock, Texas, established by Fred Lewter in 1955. On 125 acres, he built a feed mill, storage tanks and pens for up to 34,000 cattle. Other huge CAFOs began operating in the late 1950s and 1960s with in-house veterinarians and nutritionists and highly automated mechanized feeding systems. CAFO operations are designed to obtain optimal slaughter weight in the minimum time. To this end CAFO operators administer a cocktail of pharmaceuticals to the cattle, including anabolic steroids in the form of time-release pellets implanted in the animals' ears. Cattle are given estradiol, testosterone, and progesterone to increase hormone levels by up to five times which stimulates the animal's cells to synthesize additional protein, add muscle more rapidly and improve weight gain by 5% to 20%, feed efficiency by 5% to 12%, and lean meat growth by 15% to 20%.

Cattle raised in the squalid living conditions inherent to such concentrated confinement are highly susceptible to infectious disease outbreaks, so CAFO operators also began to routinely dose their herds with antibiotics in their feed. As with hormones, antibiotics have the additional effect of speeding up weight gain.

According to the United States Department of Agriculture (USDA), small cattle feedlot operations with less than 1,000 animal capacity compose the vast majority of US CAFOs, but they account for only a relatively small share of fed cattle; feedlots with 1,000 or more animal capacity compose less than 5% of total CAFOs, but they account for 80% to 90% of fed cattle, and CAFOs with 32,000 or more animal capacity account for around 40% of fed cattle. A 2012 USDA report also noted that, *"the industry continues to shift toward a small number of very large specialized feedlots, which are increasingly vertically integrated with the cow-calf and processing sectors..."* While the total number of cattle being fattened in CAFOs goes up or down from year to year, the trend was upward from the mid-1950s to 1975, and then slightly downward ever since. By December 2014 the National Agricultural Statistical Service (NASS) of the USDA reported the number of cattle on U/S. CAFOs with a capacity of 1,000 or more at 10.9 million animals. *(Agricultural Statistics Board, United States Department of Agriculture, Released December 19, 2014, by the National Agricultural Statistics Service.)* USDA Economic Research Service reports indicate that in 1935, 5.1% of the nation's cattle were being fed in CAFOs, in 1963 66%, and in 2012 97%. In 2007 the top five U.S. cattle producing states were Texas, Kansas, Nebraska, Iowa and Colorado.

Before WWII, the maize/soybean fed cattle meat market was limited to wealthy Americans and Europeans, but after the war average middle class Americans began to develop a taste for fatted meat. This change in habit did not occur spontaneously, however, but instead was the result of a cleverly designed marketing ploy by the USDA. Since its inception under President Abraham Lincoln in 1862, the mission of the USDA has always been to promote agricultural production in America. In the early nineteen hundreds the USDA promoted feeding the increasingly bountiful maize harvest from the "Corn Belt" to the cattle grazed on the plains, thus increasing production of both maize and meat. The only problem with this promotional scheme was that the American meat eating public was in the habit of eating lean, range fed meat and had no taste for the grain-fed fatted meat favored by the wealthy. To develop an American market for fatty meat, in 1927 the USDA devised a meat grading system that adopted the English standard of fatted meat as the US standard for high quality. All cuts of meat were graded by meat inspectors based on their fat content from highest to lowest: prime, choice, select, standard, commercial, utility, cutter and canner. Prime, choice and select were to be sold as individual cuts of meat, and the lesser grades were for use in processed meats (hot dogs, sausage, etc.), institutional food services (schools, hospitals, etc.) and pet food. Graded meat was not an instant success with the American public, but after WWII the new regional chain "supermarkets" that took over food retailing in the 1950s and 1960s began using the USDA grading system in their advertising to market marbled meat to American consumers, and fatted cattle meat became all the rage. Today prime cuts are generally served in high end restaurants and sold at specialty meat markets, choice is the most common grade purchased in supermarkets, and select is not widely available.

Most CAFOs are located in sparsely populated rural areas, but their large cattle populations produce as much bodily waste as some of America's largest cities. In 2008, the nongovernmental public interest group, *Union of Concerned Scientists*, issued a briefing on CAFOs entitled, "*The Hidden Cost of CAFOs.*" Below is a summary of their conclusions:

"*CAFOs can appear to operate efficiently because they have been allowed to shift costs onto society as a whole. These "externalized" costs—summarized below—hide CAFOs' true inefficiency.*"

"*CAFOs have been indirectly supported by the federal farm bill, which authorizes huge taxpayer-funded subsidies for grain farmers. Until recently, these subsidies contributed to artificially low prices for corn, soybeans, and other grains, which enabled CAFOs to grow to extraordinary sizes. But some food animals are not well suited to an exclusive diet of feed grains. Cattle, for example, are healthiest when eating their natural diet of grass and forage; eating a grain diet for too long makes these animals sick... indirect grain subsidies to CAFOs between 1997 and 2005 amounted to almost $35 billion, or nearly $4 billion per year, serving to entrench the CAFO system.*"

"Taxpayers pay to clean up CAFO waste—yet most CAFO pollution remains. CAFOs produce some 300 million tons of untreated manure each year (about twice as much as is generated by the entire human population of the United States). The disposal and cleanup cost for all of this manure would hobble CAFOs if they had to pay for it themselves. But another program authorized by the federal farm bill, the Environmental Quality Incentives Program (EQIP), subsidizes the cleanup of some CAFO waste. Extrapolation from the available data suggests that U.S. CAFOs may have benefited from about $125 million in EQIP subsidies in 2007. Nevertheless, the program prevents only a small fraction of CAFO pollution (see below)."

"Even with EQIP subsidies, CAFOs do not effectively manage the enormous amounts of waste they produce. Manure is often handled, stored, and disposed of improperly, resulting in leakage, runoff, and spills of waste into surface and groundwater. CAFO manure has contaminated drinking water in many rural areas, caused fish kills, and contributed to oxygen-depleted "dead zones"(areas devoid of valuable marine life) in the Gulf of Mexico, the Chesapeake Bay, and elsewhere. Ammonia in manure contributes to air pollution that causes respiratory disease and acid rain. Leakage under liquid manure storage "lagoons"pollutes groundwater with harmful nitrogen and pathogens, and some lagoons have even experienced catastrophic failures, sending tens of millions of gallons of untreated waste into streams and estuaries, killing millions of fish. Enforcement of environmental laws against polluting CAFOs has generally proven inadequate."("The Hidden Cost of CAFOs", The Union of Concerned Scientists, Issues Briefing, September 2008)

In 1903 the US Supreme Court issued an injunction to break up the Beef Trust that had formed in the 1890s among the top five meat-packing companies. To get around this injunction, three of the top five – Armour, Swift, and Morris – merged into a giant corporation called the National Packing Co. that operated as a holding company buying up smaller meat companies and other related businesses such as stockyards and slaughterhouses nationwide thus pioneering the business structure known as "vertical integration".

In 1906 investigative journalist Upton Sinclair's horrifying expose of the meat packing industry, *The Jungle,* was published which stoked great public outrage. Sinclair spent seven weeks working undercover in the meat packing plants of Chicago to describe in lurid detail the filthy conditions and the torment of man and beast. In one haunting passage he anguished, *"It was like some horrible crime committed in a dungeon, all unseen and unheeded, buried out of sight and of memory."* In response the US Congress passed the Federal Meat Inspection Act of 1906, but sanitary, working and humane conditions have changed little inside meat packing plants and now over a century later are as horrendous as ever.

In 1912, pressure from federal government regulators forced the dissolution of the National Packing Co., but the big meat-packing companies simply resumed the old Beef Trust with newcomers Sulzberger and Sons and foreign meat-packing companies from Brazil, Argentina and Uruguay that exported cattle meat to Europe and North America. By the end of the decade the new Beef Trust was the most powerful player in the American economy holding interests in livestock companies, railroad terminals, railroads, stockyards, machine supply companies, warehouses, land development companies, banks and many other businesses.

In 1920 the federal government again tried to break up the Beef Trust with a consent decree under the Sherman Anti-Trust Act requiring the Trust to divest of many of its holdings, and in 1921 Congress passed the Packers and Stockyards Act to prohibited packers from engaging in unfair and deceptive practices, but by 1935 Armour and Swift still controlled over 61% of meat sales in the U.S., and by 1957 a Congressional report concluded that concentration in the meat-packing industry was as great as ever.

Then in the 1960s, as the maize/soybean feedlot cattle complex became standard in the industry, new companies using more efficient production methods rose to challenge the old line Beef Trust companies. The first of these was Iowa Beef Processors (IBP) which in 1960 opened a slaughterhouse in rural Denison, Iowa, out of the major meat-packing cities and near to the rural feedlots thereby saving money on transportation expenses and freeing IBP from union labor contracts further saving on wage expenses. In 1967 IBP introduced precut "boxed beef" which they shipped in refrigerated trucks on the country's new interstate highway system to the new chain supermarkets that were growing like mushrooms in the rapidly developing American "suburbs". Precut cattle meat, with the bone and excess fat trimmed away, could be packed much more tightly than whole carcasses resulting in another major savings in transportation costs. IBP built its flagship plant in Dakota City, Nebraska in 1965 and opened massive new plants in Amarillo, Texas in 1974 and Holcomb, Kansas in 1980 by which time they had become the largest beef processor in the world.

Beginning with the merger of Missouri Beef Packers of Plainview, Texas and Kansas Beef Industries of Wichita, Kansas in 1974 to form the MBPXL Corporation which became IBPs top competitor, a merger and acquisition strategy in the cattle meat processing industry over the next 40 years resulted in a new consolidation of the industry even greater than that of the Beef Trust a century before. As of 2013, IBP is owned by Tyson Foods, Inc., which is the largest beef processor in the U.S. The number two beef processor in the U.S. is JBS USA, a Brazilian corporation, which owns Swift & Co. and Smithfield (Including their cattle meat operations in South America, JBS is now the largest beef processor in the world). Number three in U.S. beef processing is Cargill, the number one U.S. grain trader and exporter, which bought MBPXL, changed its name to Excel and then again to Cargill Meat Solutions in 2004. Together these three corporations, Tyson, JBS USA and Cargill control over 70% of the US cattle meat processing industry. These three giant cattle meat processors are also major players in both the chicken and pig meat industries, and also major players in the feed-grains and processed foods industries.

In the century between the late 1880s and the late 1980s, nearly 40% of the continental United States was transformed from a natural prairie ecosystem into a commercial pastureland for cattle, the nations maize and soybean farmers became inextricably dependent upon the cattle feed market and the American people became addicted to eating large amounts of maize/soybean fed fatty cattle meat.

In 1996, the first genetically engineered (GE) seed crops hit the commercial market including four of the world's major field crops – maize, soybeans, rapeseed (Canola) and cotton. By 2007, 12 years after the their commercial introduction, GE crops covered about 250 million acres (101 million hectares), more than half of which were located in the U.S. (136.5 million acres), followed by Argentina (45 million), Brazil (28.8 million), Canada (15.3 million), India (9.5 million), China (8.8 million), Paraguay (5 million), and South Africa (3.5 million). Europe was largely spared this invasion with the exceptions of Spain and Romania.

In the first half of the 20th century, seeds were overwhelmingly bred by farmers and public-sector plant breeders, but in the decades since, agrochemical corporations have used intellectual property laws to highjack the world's seed supply – a business strategy that aims to monopolize control over plant germplasm to maximize corporate profits. Today the GE seed market accounts for a staggering share of the world's commercial seed supply; in less than three decades, a handful of multinational corporations have engineered a heist of the world's staple crop gene bank.

In 1998, the agrochemical giant, Monsanto Corporation entered the seed business in a big way buying Holden's Foundation Seeds, Inc., which at the time controlled 35% of the U.S. maize seed market, and in that same year they also bought DeKalb Genetics Corporation which controlled 11% of the U.S. market and Cargill's international seed products division for access to the global seed market. In 1999 the agrochemical giant, DuPont Corporation, bought Pioneer Hi-Bred which was the world's largest maize seed company. After an agrochemical industry buying binge through the mid 2000s, by 2007 GE seeds accounted for 82% of the global seed market and the top ten seed companies accounted for 67% of that; Monsanto became the world's largest seed company accounting for 23% of the market; the top 3 companies (Monsanto, DuPont, Syngenta) together accounted for 47% of the worldwide GE seed market; these 3 seed companies controlled 65% of the GE maize seed market worldwide, and over half of the GE soybean seed market ("Do biomaterials really mean business," by Emily Waltz, Nature Biotechnol).

The GE giants point to the high adoption rates of GE maize and soybeans by farmers as evidence of strong demand for GE seeds, but the real reason for this demand is that GE seed companies were phasing out their non-GE varieties leaving farmers with little choice but to buy GE seeds. In 2009 University of Illinois entomologist Michael Gray surveyed farmers in five areas of this large maize producing state to ask if they had access to high-yielding, non-GE maize seed; nearly 40% said "no" and in Malta, Ill., 46.6% said they had no access to non-GE maize hybrids. Researcher Angelika Hilbeck, senior scientist at the *Institute of Integrative Biology at the Swiss Federal Institute* of Technology, found the number of non-GE maize seed varieties in the U.S. decreased 67% from 2005 to 2010, while the number of GE maize seed varieties increased 6.7%. Hilbeck and several other researchers found this to be a trend around the world. They analyzed seed catalogs in Spain, Germany and Austria and found that in Spain where GE maize is grown, farmers' seed choices declined overall and increasingly became a choice among GE varieties, whereas in Germany and Austria where GE maize is not grown, farmers have many more seed varieties available to them now than in the 1990s. In Brazil, where it's getting harder for farmers to obtain non-GE soybean seeds, Ricardo Tatesuzi de Sousa, executive director of *ABRANGE* (the Brazilian association for producers of non-GE grains) refers to a commonly used term – the 85/15 rule – which means that distributors will sell 85% GE seeds and just 15% non-GE. A similar situation is occurring in South Africa where the soybean market is dominated by three companies that only offer GE seed ("*The GMO Seed Monopoly: Fewer Choices, Higher Prices*," *The Organic & Non-GMO Report, Food Democracy Now*, October 4, 2013). Cattle meat from these countries is nourished on GE maize and soybeans.

Widespread adoption of GE crops has introduced a whole host of new problems down on the farm. In 2012, Dr. Charles Benbrook, research professor at Washington State University's Center for Sustaining Agriculture and Natural Resources, published a report entitled "*Impacts of genetically engineered crops on pesticide use in the U.S. -- the first sixteen years*," in the September 28, 2012 journal, *Environmental Sciences Europe*. Using U.S. Department of Agriculture (USDA) pesticide use data Dr. Benbrook tracked changes in pesticide use on crops containing GE traits in the US. In the 16 years from the introduction of GE crops in 1996 to 2011, the U.S. went from zero total acres of GE crops to 170 million acres (69 million hectares). This included an estimated 94% of the soybean crop and 72% of the maize crop planted over in herbicide resistant (HR) varieties resistant to the herbicide "glyphosate"(Monsanto trademark *Roundup*®). The GE industry boasts that glyphosate resistant crops reduced the use of glyphosate per acre, but Dr. Benbrook found that in the long run, glyphosate use per acre has actually increased on America's farmland:

> "*Taking into account applications of all pesticides targeted by the traits embedded in the three major GE crops, pesticide use in the U.S. was reduced in each of the first six years of commercial use (1996–2001). But in 2002, herbicide use on HR soybeans increased 8.6 million kgs (19 million pounds), driven by a 0.2 kgs/ha (0.18 pounds/acre), increase in the glyphosate rate per crop year, a 21% increase. Overall in 2002, GE traits increased pesticide use by 6.9 million kgs (15.2 million pounds), or by about 5%. Incrementally greater annual increases in the kilograms/pounds of herbicides applied to HR hectares have continued nearly every year since, leading to progressively larger annual increases in overall pesticide use on GE hectares/acres compared to non-GE hectares/acres. The increase just in 2011 was 35.3 million kgs (77.9 million pounds), a quantity exceeding by a wide margin the cumulative, total 14 million kg (31 million pound) reduction from 1996 through 2002.*
>
> "*Total pesticide use has been driven upward by 183 million kgs (404 million pounds) in the U.S. since 1996 by GE crops, compared to what pesticide use would likely have been in the absence of HR and Bt cultivars. This increase represents, on average, an additional ~0.21 kgs/ha (~0.19 pounds/acre) of pesticide active ingredient for every GE-trait hectare planted. The estimated overall increase of 183 million kgs (404 million pounds) applied over the*

past 16 years represents about a 7% increase in total pesticide use." ("*Impacts of genetically engineered crops on pesticide use in the U.S. -- the first sixteen years*", Charles Benbrook, *Environmental Sciences Europe,* September 28, 2012)

Dr. Benbrook explains the emergence of glyphosate resistant (GR) weeds:

"The emergence and spread of glyphosate-resistant weeds is... by far [the] most important factor driving up herbicide use on land planted to herbicide-resistant varieties.

"Today, the Weed Science Society of America (WSSA) website lists 22 GR weed species in the U.S. [19]. Over two-thirds of the approximate 70 state-GR weed combinations listed by WSSA have been documented since 2005, reflecting the rapidly spreading nature of the GR-weed problem. According to the WSSA, over 5.7 million hectares (14 million acres) are now infested by GR weeds, an estimate that substantially underestimates the actual spread of resistant weeds.

"Why have GR weeds become such a serious problem? Heavy reliance on a single herbicide – glyphosate (Roundup) -- has placed weed populations under progressively intense, and indeed unprecedented, selection pressure [10]. HR crops make it possible to extend the glyphosate application window to most of the growing season, instead of just the pre-plant and post-harvest periods. HR technology allows multiple applications of glyphosate in the same crop year. The common Midwestern rotation of HR corn-HR soybeans, or HR soybeans-HR cotton in the South, exposes weed populations to annual and repetitive glyphosate-selection pressure.

"GR weed phenotypes are forcing farmers to respond by increasing herbicide application rates, making multiple applications of herbicides, applying additional herbicide active ingredients, deep tillage to bury weed seeds, and manual weeding. In recent years the first three of the above responses have been the most common.

"Weed management costs per hectare increase by 50% to 100% or more in fields infested with glyphosate-resistant weeds, as evident in a series of case studies submitted to the USDA by Dow AgroSciences in support of its petition to the USDA seeking deregulation of 2,4-D herbicide-resistant corn [25]."

Dr. Benbrook identifies the environmental impacts of intensive glyphosate use:

"A long list of environmental effects can be triggered, or made worse, by the more intensive herbicide use required to keep pace with weeds in farming systems heavily reliant on herbicide-resistant crops. Glyphosate has been shown to impair soil microbial communities in ways that can increase plant vulnerability to pathogens [36-38], while also reducing availability of certain soil minerals and micronutrients [39]. Landscapes dominated by herbicide-resistant crops support fewer insect and bird species; e.g., a study in the American Midwest reported a 58% decline in milkweed and an 81% drop in monarch butterflies from 1999 to 2010 [40]. Heavy use of glyphosate can reduce earthworm viability [41] and water use efficiency [42]. Several

studies have documented reductions in nitrogen fixation in herbicide-resistant soybean fields sprayed with glyphosate [43,44]. Transgene flow from herbicide-resistant crops can occur via multiple mechanisms and can persist in weedy relatives [45].

"Individually, these environmental impacts appear, for the most part, of the same nature and in the same ballpark as the risks associated with other herbicide-based farming systems, but collectively they raise novel concerns over long-term, possibly serious impacts on biodiversity, soil and plant health, water quality, aquatic ecosystem integrity, and human and animal health." (Ibid)

By 2013, 76% of the U.S. maize crop was planted over in the other major GE crop trait, Bt (*Bacillus thuringiensis*), that produces a natural insecticide within every cell of the plant to kill invasive insect pests including the European corn borer (ECB) and the corn rootworm (CRW). Bt maize is engineered to contain multiple gene expressions of different Bt proteins; this is what the GE industry calls "stacked traits." Stacked Bt maize varieties require considerably less insecticide spray than do their non-Bt equivalents, but if you count the insecticides produced in the Bt plants themselves, then they in fact substantially increase the amount of insecticides actually being applied to the fields. Dr. Benbrook makes this point clear:

"While Bt corn and cotton have reduced insecticide applications by 56 million kgs (123 million pounds), resistance is emerging in key target insects and substantial volumes of Bt Cry endotoxins are produced per hectare planted, generally dwarfing the volumes of insecticides displaced.

"MON 88017 expresses... two Cry proteins... 14-fold more than the insecticides displaced.

"SmartStax GE corn... Total Cry protein production is estimated at... 19 times the average conventional insecticide rate of application in 2010.

"Documenting the full range of impacts on the environment and public health associated with the Bt Cry proteins biosynthesized inside Bt-transgenic plants remains a challenging and largely ignored task, especially given the recent move toward multiple Bt protein, stacked-trait events." (Ibid)

In 2009, the *Union of Concerned Scientists (UCS),* issued a paper entitled, *"Failure to Yield"* in which they presented the most comprehensive evaluation to date of more than two decades of GE research and commercialization aimed at increasing crop yields. Contrary to GE industry claims of significant yield increases for GE commodity crops, the UCS study found that for most crops, GE traits either made no difference or negatively affected yields. The UCS study did find a small increase in yield for Bt maize over non-Bt maize hybrids, but even there, they found it particularly *"significant that the yield increases have been from operational yield—reduction in yield losses—rather than from the intrinsic yield of the crop."* What this means is that unlike conventional High Yielding Variety (HYV) hybrids that actually increased the weight of maize on each stalk, Bt maize only outperformed comparable non-Bt maize varieties that had been hit with corn borer infestations. UCS further noted, *"Moreover, there have been no apparent overall yield increases, operational or intrinsic, from HT [herbicide tolerant] corn and soybeans.*" In other words, GE seeds are not engineered with genes that actually produce higher yielding plants. UCS concludes:

> "*The failure of GE to increase intrinsic yield so far is especially important when considering food sufficiency. Substantial yield increases can be achieved through operational yield, and there is room for achieving huge operational yield increases in much of the developing world. But intrinsic yield sets a ceiling that is proving difficult to surpass. So far, the only technology with a proven record at increasing intrinsic yield is traditional breeding, which now includes genomic methods.*"

As glyphosate resistant weeds and Bt resistant bugs have reduced the effectiveness of these first generation GE crops, the GE industry's response has been to develop second generation of crops with multiple "stacked traits" like the *Genuity® SmartStax® RIB Complete™*, a GE maize by Monsanto that combines Bt and HR (herbicide resistant) traits in the same seed. Stacked herbicide resistant seeds currently in the developmental pipeline include resistance to the highly toxic herbicides *2, 4-D* and *dicamba*, so that even more powerful herbicides can be sprayed on the fields to kill glyphosate resistant weeds. Far from reducing herbicide use, gene stacking has resulted in the ever escalating use of ever more toxic herbicides. In a study conducted by the University of Wisconsin Department of Agricultural and Applied Economics, published in the February, 2013, issue of the journal *Nature Biotechnology*, entitled *"Commercialized transgenic traits, maize productivity and yield risk"* (Nature Biotechnology, February 2013), the authors detected what they called "gene interaction" where genes inserted into crops interact with each other in ways that often reduce crop yields. This study lends credence to the theory of "yield drag" whereby manipulating the genomes of plants causes unintended consequences in their growth habits resulting in less productive crops. This problem of unintended consequences gets to the heart of the problem with GE technology. The interactions of genes within a genome are so immensely complex that contemporary geneticists are just beginning to scratch the surface, so when genetic engineers cram completely foreign genes into a host genome, they really have no idea what the overall impacts their crude experiments will have on the plant, or the cattle, pigs and chickens that eat them, or the people who eat them? Virtually all of the world's GE maize and soybean crop is used to feed cattle, pigs and chickens to produce the meat, milk and eggs that people eat. This public exposure to these novel genes is tantamount to an uncontrolled experiment on an unsuspecting public.

This is the sad state of affairs in world seed technology as of this writing. Based on the above exposé of GE crops, I boldly predict that GE foods will not be the manna from heaven that feeds future multitudes as advertised by the GE industry. Indeed, to the extent that GE crops are contributing to soil infertility on millions of acres of farmland, they are more likely to saddle future generations with poor crop yields and food insecurity.

Central and South America

The history of cattle in Central and South America is as long and notorious as that of North America. First introduced by the Spanish and Portuguese colonists in the early 16th century (see "The Columbian Exchange"), Old World longhorn cattle soon went wild and proliferated by the millions on the great grasslands of Central and South America, particularly the plains of Mexico, the llanos of Venezuela and the pampas of Uruguay and parts of southern Brazil and eastern Argentina. The cattle were so numerous and the population of colonists so small that cattle meat was literally free for the taking; the only commercial value of the animals was for their hides and tallow that were shipped back to European markets. The Spanish and Portuguese crowns granted large land trusts to individual colonial overlords who laid claim to thousands of acres of land where they forced the Indians into servitude. Still today in the early 21st century, a relative few wealthy powerful families own most of the private lands in South America.

The invention of refrigerated freight by George Hammond of the U.S. in the 1870s revolutionized the meat-packing industry by making it possible to ship frozen meat over long distances. At that time South American salted cattle meat jerky was being exported to Europe to satisfy the demand for cattle meat among the growing working class of the Industrial Revolution, but the meat was so hard and dry it was barely edible. In 1878, the *Frigorifique*, became the first refrigerated steamer to cross the Atlantic from Argentina to France with 5,500 frozen cattle carcasses aboard; South America quickly rose to become a major competitor of the U.S. for the European frozen cattle meat market.

Over the course of the 20th century the Brazilian government underwent numerous regime changes and its economic policy vacillated from favoring export oriented markets like coffee, sugar and cattle meat, to favoring internal markets for food and manufactured goods. Despite going through many turbulent years during this period, Brazil developed into one of the world's major food producing regions. From 1950 to 1975, as the population of Brazil doubled from 52 million to 105 million people, cattle ranchers moved north from the grassy pampas region onto the tropical savanna forests of the Cerrado where they burned the trees and planted grass. The poor soils of the Cerrado would only sustain grass for a few years so the ranchers would then move on to burn more forest for range. Brazilian government figures attributed 38% of deforestation from 1966-1975 to large-scale cattle ranching, the rest to subsistence farming and mining.

The Trans-Amazonian Highway was one of Brazil's most ambitious economic development projects. In the 1970s, Brazil planned a 2,000-mile highway to bisect the Amazon and open up the rainforest to settlement by poor farmers from the crowded, drought-plagued north and to developers of timber and mineral resources. Colonists were granted a 250 acre (100 hectare) plots and easy access to agricultural loans in exchange for settling along the highway and converting the surrounding rainforest into agricultural land. The highway was plagued from the start; the geology of the Amazon Basin made paving and drainage impossible, creating a mucky impassable mess during heavy rains, blocking traffic and leaving crops to rot. Crop yields were very poor since the forest soils were quickly depleted, and peasants had to clear new forests annually. Logging was difficult due to the dispersed distribution of commercially valuable trees and rampant erosion, up to 40 tons of soil per acre (100 tons/hectare) occurred after clearing. While a commercial failure, after construction of the Trans-Amazonian Highway, Brazilian deforestation accelerated to levels never before seen and vast swaths of forest were cleared for subsistence farmers and cattle-ranchers.

By 2008 more than 214,000 square miles (554,257 square kilometers) of the Amazon had been turned to agriculture, an area larger than France, and 62% of this deforestation was due to cattle ranching (*"Concerns over deforestation may drive new approaches to cattle ranching in the Amazon", mongabay.com*, September 08, 2009).

The first case of the brain wasting cattle disease "Bovine spongiform encephalopathy" (BSE), more commonly known as Mad Cow Disease, that can be transmitted to humans appeared in the U.S. cattle herd in 2003. As a result, several major markets began to boycott U.S. cattle meat including Mexico, Canada, Egypt, Taiwan, Hong Kong, Japan, South Korea and Russia. While all of these countries eventually reestablished trade in U.S. beef, 2003 marked the first year that Brazil topped the U.S. in cattle meat exports. By 2013, Brazil had far surpassed the U.S. in cattle meat exports with 20.17% of the world market to the U.S. at 12.79% (Foreign Agricultural Service (FAS) of the USDA).

The biggest player in the Brazilian cattle meat industry is the JBS-S.A. corporation, named after the initials of its founder, Jose Batista Sobrinho, who started out as a small town butcher in 1953. In 1956, when Brazil's new capital, Brasilia, was being built 125 miles to the east, he provided meat to its butchers and restaurants. In 1968 he bought a small slaughterhouse bringing his number of cattle slaughtered per day up to 100, and in 1970 a second slaughterhouse boosted his capacity to 500 per day. In the 1990s, Sobrinho's six sons who had taken over management of the company decided to expand first regionally and then nationally by buying several other small meat packing companies in Brazil. In 2005 JBS expanded internationally by buying Swift Armour S.A., Argentina's largest cattle meat producer and exporter, and in 2007 expanded further into the U.S. market buying Swift & Co. and Smithfield Foods. In 2009 JBS continued its acquisition spree merging with another of Brazil's major meat packers, Bertin S.A., and buying a controlling interest in U.S. chicken producer, Pilgrim's Pride. These last two acquisitions made JBS the world's largest cattle meat producer and second-largest chicken meat producer.

Three years after the independent conservation organization, Greenpeace, issued its report *"Eating Up the Amazon"* in 2006 in which they investigated soybean plantations in the Cerrado and Amazon, Greenpeace issued another devastating report in 2009 that investigated cattle ranching in the Amazon entitled *"Slaughtering the Amazon."* Greenpeace's undercover investigation followed the cattle trade from ranches and slaughterhouses in the Amazon to a network of manufacturing hubs and suppliers to some of the world's top corporate global name brands of food, leather and cosmetics products. Their reports exposed the devastating environmental impacts of cattle ranching in the Amazon:

> *"Brazil is the world's fourth largest producer of greenhouse gas (GHG) emissions. The majority of emissions come from the clearance and burning of the Amazon rainforest."*

"Forests play a vital role in stabilising the world's climate by storing large amounts of carbon that would otherwise contribute to climate change. The Amazon is estimated to store 80-120 billion tonnes of carbon. If destroyed, some fifty times the annual GHG emissions of the USA could be emitted. The Brazilian Amazon has the greatest annual average deforestation by area of anywhere in the world."

"The cattle sector is the key driver of deforestation in the Brazilian Amazon. According to the Brazilian government: 'Cattle are responsible for about 80% of all deforestation' in the Amazon region. In recent years, on average one hectare of Amazon rainforest has been lost to cattle ranchers ever y 18 seconds... The largest economic incentive for the expansion of Brazil's cattle sector into the Amazon is lack of governance: contributing factors include corruption, disorganisation, limited capacity and lack of coordination between government departments... Land grabbing in the Amazon is rampant. land titles in the Amazon region are in disarray, with the legal status of roughly half the area uncertain."

"Brazil has the world's largest commercial cattle herd and is the world's largest beef exporter... The Brazilian cattle sector has seen rapid export-oriented growth over the last decade. Exports of beef and veal from Brazil increased almost six-fold in volume between 1998 and 2008. By 2008, nearly one in every three tonnes of beef traded internationally came out of Brazil... To aid Brazil's domination of the global market for agricultural commodities including beef, the Brazilian government is investing in all parts of the supply chain, from farm-level production to the international market... The three processors receiving the lion's share of Brazilian government investment – Bertin, JBS and Marfrig – include one of the world's largest leather traders, the world's largest beef trader (controlling at least 10% of global beef production), and the world's fourth-largest beef trader, respectively... Expansion by these groups is effectively a 'joint venture' with the Brazilian government."

"Greenpeace has tracked the trade in cattle products back from the export-oriented processing facilities of Bertin, JBS and Marfrig in the south of Brazil to three frontiers of deforestation in the Amazon... While the Blue Chip companies behind reputable global brands appear to believe that Amazon sources are excluded from their products, Greenpeace investigations expose for the first time how their blind consumption of raw materials fuels deforestation and climate change... Greenpeace undercover investigations have unpicked the complex global trade in beef products from part-Brazilian-government-owned corporations – Bertin, JBS and Marfrig. Greenpeace has identified hundreds of ranches within the Amazon rainforest supplying cattle to slaughterhouses in the Amazon region belonging to these companies. Where Greenpeace was able to obtain mapped boundaries for ranches, satellite analysis reveals that significant supplies of cattle come from ranches active in recent and illegal deforestation. Trade data also reveal trade with ranches using modern-day slavery. Additionally, one Bertin

slaughterhouse receives supplies of cattle from an illegal ranch occupying Indian lands... These slaughterhouses in the Amazon region then ship beef or hides to company facilities thousands of kilometres away in the south for further processing before export. In a number of cases, additional processing takes place in import countries before the final product reaches the market. In effect, criminal or 'dirty' supplies of cattle are 'laundered' through the supply chain to an unwitting global market... Our evidence links an Amazon-contaminated supply chain to suppliers to many reputable global brands and retailers, including a long list of international Blue Chip companies: Adidas, BMW, Carrefour, Ford, Honda, Gucci, IKEA, Kraft, Nike, Tesco, Toyota, Wal-Mart. The public sector is also exposed; our findings link the chain to suppliers to the UK National Health Service (NHS), and to a supplier in the Middle East whose customers include the British, Dutch, Italian, Spanish and US military forces." ("*Slaughtering the Amazon*" Published by Greenpeace International, Ottho Heldringstraat 5, 1066 AZ Amsterdam, The Netherlands, 2009)

According to Rhett Butler who edits the website http://news.mongabay.com that monitors deforestation in the Amazon:

"Since 2004 the rate of deforestation in the Brazilian Amazon has fallen nearly 80 percent to the lowest levels recorded since annual record keeping began in the late 1980s. Importantly, this decline has occurred at the same time that Brazil's economy has grown roughly 40 percent, suggesting a decoupling of economic growth from deforestation." ("*Deforestation in the Amazon*" By Rhett Butler, http://news.mongabay.com, last updated July 9, 2014)

In the same article Butler reports that while deforestation is down from its peak of 11,220 square miles (29,059 square kilometers) in 1995 to 2,275 square miles (5,891 square kilometers) in 2013, (an area about the size of the US State of Delaware), this still represents a staggering loss of forestland and biodiversity. Under right wing extremist president Jair Bolsonaro who took power in Brazil in 2019, this decline in deforestation was reversed. The November 30, 2020, edition of the Guardian newspaper ran with the headline, *"Amazon deforestation surges to 12-year high under Bolsonaro,"* reporting that, *"Figures released by the Brazilian space institute, Inpe, on Monday showed at least 11,088 sq km of rainforest was razed between August 2019 and July this year – the highest figure since 2008."*

India

Surprisingly, in 2013 the USDA Foreign Agricultural Service ranked India, land of the Hindu and Sikh religions and the Holy Cow, second only to Brazil in world cattle meat exports. How could this be? The history of bovines in India predates that of North and South America by some 6,500 years, going back 7,000 years (5000 BC) to the ancient Indus civilization that domesticated the zebus breed of cattle (*bos indicus*) and the water buffalo. Around 3,750 years ago (1750 BC) Aryan cattle herders from the north invaded the Indus, bringing with them their religious traditions written in Vedic Sanskit that constitute the oldest Hindu texts.

By 2,600 years ago (600 BC), due to population growth and depleted grazing lands, the Brahman ruling class (descendents of the Aryans) could no longer supply cattle meat to the peasant masses and during the next nine centuries, as peasant resentment over the meat heavy Brahman diet grew into violent clashes, the Hindu religion was eventually pressed into adopting a ban on the slaughter of cattle.

Around 1000 AD, India was invaded by Islamic chieftains from Turkey, Persia (modern day Iran), Arabia and Afghanistan where they established an enduring Muslim presence. Muslims did not have cattle in their Middle Eastern homelands since cattle are too water intensive to raise in such arid climates, and it was Muslim religious custom to sacrifice goats, sheep and camels. But once in India where cattle were common place, the Muslims began to sacrifice cattle, particularly on the occasion of *Eid al-Adha*, the "Feast of the Sacrifice." In 1756–57, on his fourth invasion of India, Afghan Chieftain, Ahmad Shāh Durrānī, attacked the Golden Temple in Amritsar and filled its sacred pool with the blood of slaughtered cows; this final act of sacrilege marked the beginning of the long standing bitterness between Indian Sikhs (who expressly forbid consumption of meat from animals killed in sacrificial rituals) and Afghan Muslims.

Major-General Robert Clive was the British army officer credited with securing India for the British East India Company and later the British Raj. As Governor of Bengal in 1760, he built the first cattle slaughterhouse in India in Calcutta. The British built several more slaughterhouses to supply cattle meat to their three main armies in Bengal, Madras (now Chennai) and Bombay (now Mumbai). In 1870, the Sikhs started a cow protection movement known as the Kuka Revolution, in which they revolted against the British and over the 1870s the revolution spread to the Punjab in the Northwest and to the neighboring regions of Oudh (now Awadh) and Rohilkhand. The first *Gaurakshini sabha* (cow protection society) was established in the Punjab in 1882 and the protection society rapidly spread throughout India. The organization rescued wandering cows and cared for them in refuges called *gaushalas*. Charitable networks developed to collect contributions to fund the *gaushalas*. Cow protection sentiment reached its peak in 1893 when large public meetings were held to denounce cattle meat eaters. Riots broke out between Hindus and Muslims in Mau, Azamgarh and Bombay where the Muslim minority called upon British troops to protect their ritual cattle sacrifice. In a letter dated December 8, 1893, England's Queen Victoria wrote to the then Viceroy of India, the 5th Marquess of Lansdowne, about the cow protection movement:

> "*The Queen greatly admired the Viceroy's speech on the Cow-killing agitation. While she quite agrees in the necessity of perfect fairness, she thinks the Muhammadans [Muslims] do require more protection than Hindus, and they are decidedly by far the more loyal. Though the Muhammadan's cow-killing is made the pretext for the agitation, it is, in fact, directed against us, who kill far more cows for our army, &c., than the Muhammadans.*" ("*Report of the National Commission on Cattle*", Report of the National Commission on Cattle, Rashtriya Govansh Ayog, Department of Animal Husbandry & Dairying, Ministry of Agriculture, Government of India, July 2002)

To mobilize public participation in the Indian independence movement in the early 20th century, movement leaders such as Mahatma Gandhi assured the people repeatedly that upon achieving self-rule the first action of the new Indian government would be to ban slaughter of the cow and its progeny by law. In 1947 the Indian independence movement created a Constituent Assembly to draft a new Constitution for an independent India. The Constitution that was passed by the Constituent Assembly made cattle protection a "Directive Principle of State Policy," but it also left the power to legislate the prevention of cattle slaughter up to each of India's 15 (now 28) individual states. Since this Constitution went into effect in 1950, India has had a split personality over the issue of cattle slaughter; while most of the states have enacted laws against cattle slaughter, the national government has consistently promoted the economic advantages of slaughtering older unproductive animals. In 1950, even as the states were taking up legislation on cattle slaughter, the Government of India sent a letter to all State Governments saying: *"Hides from slaughtered cattle are much superior to his from fallen cattle and fetch a higher price. In the absence of slaughter, the best type of hide, which fetches good price in the export market will no longer be available. A total ban on slaughter is thus detrimental to the export trade and work against the tanning industry in the country"* (*"Report of the National Commission on Cattle"*, Report of the National Commission on Cattle, Rashtriya Govansh Ayog, Department of Animal Husbandry & Dairying, Ministry of Agriculture, Government of India, July 2002)

In 1954, the Government of India's Ministry of Food and Agriculture appointed an "Expert Committee on the Prevention of Slaughter of Cattle in India", which issued its report in January 1955. Contrary to the committee's name, the report concluded that there was not enough fodder to maintain more than 40% of India's cattle herd and that 60% should be culled. In the 1970s the Government of India appointed the National Commission on Agriculture which suggested a policy of developing India's buffalo meat industry:

> *"The buffalo should be developed not only for enhancement of milk production but also for making it a source of production of quality meat."*
>
> *"A deliberate and energetic drive should be made to develop for export trade in buffalo meat".*
>
> *"Modernization of slaughter Houses should be undertaken immediately"*
>
> *"Massive programmes for improving the reproductive and productive efficiency of cattle and buffaloes should be undertaken. Low producing stock should b progressively eliminated so that the limited feed and fodder resources are available for proper feeding of high producing animals".*
>
> (*"Report of the National Commission on Cattle"*, Report of the National Commission on Cattle, Rashtriya Govansh Ayog, Department of Animal Husbandry & Dairying, Ministry of Agriculture, Government of India, July 2002)

Over the years since independence, members of the Indian Parliament have introduced legislation to ban cattle slaughter throughout India, but none of these bills has ever passed out of the legislature.

There have also been legal cases on national slaughter bans brought before the Indian Supreme Court where the court has consistently ruled that:

> *"A total ban [on cattle slaughter] was not permissible if, under economic conditions, keeping useless bull or bullock be a burden on the society and therefore not in the public interest."*
> (*"Report of the National Commission on Cattle"*, Report of the National Commission on Cattle, Rashtriya Govansh Ayog, Department of Animal Husbandry & Dairying, Ministry of Agriculture, Government of India, July 2002)

The main players in the Indian beef industry are Muslims who, as of 2014, made up some 13% of the Indian population. But unlike in the U.S. and Brazil where the cattle industry is owned by a handful of large multinational corporations, in India millions of small farmers each own a few dairy cows, oxen or water buffaloes. When the older animals become unproductive, it is an economic burden on these small farmers to feed and care for them, so they become the feed stock for India's beef industry. In India it is illegal to transport cattle over state lines for the purpose of slaughter, but unproductive animals are routinely smuggled illegally into states that have enacted no laws against cattle slaughter. The State of Kerala on the southwest coast has become known as the "Butcher State of India" where cattle are smuggled in from neighboring states with a blind eye cast by the national government authorities. Much of this beef is headed for markets across the Arabian Sea in Muslim Middle Eastern countries. In far northeastern India where several states border on overwhelmingly Muslim Bangladesh, there is a thriving trade in buffalo and cattle meat. And the northern state of Uttar Pradesh, which has a significant Muslim population, is also a leading cattle meat exporter to Southeast Asia and the Middle East. According to the Foreign Agricultural Service of the USDA, in 2013 India exported 1.77 million tons of cattle meat and held a 19.26% share of the global cattle meat export market. The cattle meat export trade has become an important sector of the Indian economy (*"Beef exporter confidence returns in India"*, *The Times of India*, Jul 30, 2014). Though most of India's cattle meat is destined for export, there is a growing internal demand coming from a rapidly expanding urban middle class Hindus.

Indians bred their cattle and water buffalo to be tolerant of India's hot humid climate and to survive on limited food rations which has resulted in animals that yield significantly less milk and meat than western breeds. While the government has developed programs to cross breed Indian cattle with western breeds to improve yields, most of India's herd is still made up of locally bred cattle. The reason India has managed to become the world's second largest cattle meat exporting country despite raising cattle and buffalo that are lower yielding is that India has by far the largest national herd of bovines of any country in the world. In 2014 the Foreign Agricultural Service of the USDA estimated the top five national cattle herds (includes dairy cows, oxen and buffalo) as follows:

Country	# of bovines
India	329,700,000
Brazil	207,960,000
China	104,188,000
US	89,300,000
Argentina	51,095,000

With that many bovines in India, there is a constant large supply of animals entering into their unproductive years to be packed off to the slaughterhouse and sold on foreign markets. India began exporting small amounts of cattle meat in the 1960s, but the industry didn't begin to take off until the early 2000s and in 2007 it kicked into high gear more than doubling by 2012 as India overtook the U.S. and Australia to become the world's second leading beef exporter.

Since the tending of India's cattle and buffalo herds is not done on an industrial scale as in Brazil and the U.S., collecting data on the care and feeding of India's bovine population is a very difficult task. In 2010, researchers from the *Centre of Economic and Social Research,* New Delhi, and the *National Centre for Agricultural Economics and Policy Research,* New Delhi, made the most ambitious attempt at data collection by studying a random sample of livestock-keeping households from all over India *("India's Livestock Feed Demand: Estimates and Projections," Agricultural Economics Research Review,* January-June 2010). Their survey included all of India's 20 agro-ecological zones and 60 sub-zones as mapped by the *Indian National Bureau of Soil Survey and Land Use Planning.* They found that most of India's bovine *"... feed requirement is met from crop residues and byproducts; grasses, weeds and tree leaves gathered from cultivated and uncultivated lands; and grazing on common lands and harvested fields."* They noted that land allocated to cultivate green fodder crops is limited and has hardly ever exceeded 5% of the gross cropped area (GoI, 2009). With such tight limits on green fodder, the authors concluded that *"... the supply of feed has always remained short of normative requirement (GoI, 1976; Singh and Mujumdar, 1992; Ramachandra et al., 2007), restricting realization of the true production potential of livestock."* As India was the world's number one millet and pulse (beans, dried peas, and lentils) producing country, number two rice, wheat and cotton producing country and number four sorghum and maize producing country in 2013, it is largely on crop residues and crop byproducts (husks, bran, oilseeds, oil cakes, meals, and manufactured feeds) that India's massive bovine herd is fed. (Food and Agriculture Organization of the United Nations. FAOSTAT. http://faostat3.fao.org/home/index.html#DOWNLOAD, 2013). Only lactating heifers and working bulls are fed supplemental green fodder crops.

By raising bovines spread out over millions of households across the land, India has managed to avoid the sewerage problems of Concentrated Animal Feed Operations (CAFOs) in the U.S. and deforestation in Brazil, but raising India's vast cattle and buffalo herd has not come without environmental costs. Studies by the Indian Planning Commission concluded that the Thar Desert in the Northwestern Indian states of Rajasthan and Karnataka has been spreading at 50 square miles/year (130 square kilometers/year) for the past 50 years and in that time over-grazing has turned the semi-arid desert into a barren wasteland. According to a team of scientists at the Indian Space Research Organization, 25% of India's land surface is slowly turning into desert. In these areas many of India's cattle are emaciated ("Desertification/Land Degradation Status Mapping of India," *Current Science*, November 25, 2009). In some areas of the Indian central Himalayas, bovine populations exceed the carrying capacity of the land by a factor of 4.5 (*Environment*, <u>29(3)</u> (1987) p. 11). Bovines are also a large source of methane emissions, a greenhouse gas 25 times more powerful than CO_2. In India, although the emission rate per animal is much lower than in developed countries, due to the size of India's national herd the total annual methane emissions from gut fermentation and wastes is about 10,000,000 tons. Cattle and buffalo produce about 20% of India's greenhouse-gas emissions *("Sufferer and cause: Indian livestock and climate change," Climatic Change*, March, 2007).

Hindu farmers' attempts at treating cattle more humanely have had significant unintended environmental impacts. In the 1990s Indian farmers started to administer a drug called *diclofenac* to their cattle as a painkiller, often given to the animals close to death. After the animals die, they were dragged-off to huge communal dumps where vultures would scavenge the carcasses. Since the 1990s vultures have virtually disappeared from rural India and biologists think the vultures were poisoned by the drug that destroys their kidneys and kills them within days. Without the vultures to pick the carcasses clean, packs of wild dogs feed on the rotting carcasses creating a serious health and safety hazard.

Australia

The Foreign Agriculture Service of the USDA ranked Australia as the world's fourth largest cattle meat exporting country in 2013. The first cattle to set hoof in Australia came relatively late compared to the top three cattle meat exporting countries – Brazil, India and the U.S. – not arriving until 1788 with an English fleet of eleven ships containing a cargo of cattle and convicts to establish a penal colony on the far away continent down under. Upon landfall the Englishmen met the aboriginal hunter-gatherer tribesmen who had preceded them on the continent by some 50,000 years. Those first human colonizers happened upon a land located on the Indo-Australian geological plate which is the most stable of all the continents having been the least affected by earthquakes, mountain-building and volcanic forces over the past 400 million years, and it contains some of the world's oldest, shallowest, most weathered and nutrient deficient soils. It is the flattest continent, with an average elevation of 1,082 feet (330 meters) and it is also the driest inhabited continent with over 70% of the land area classed as either semi-arid or arid. The aboriginals proceeded to hunt 90% of Australia's original endemic mega-fauna to extinction and alter the floral landscape by setting fire to vegetative cover.

The Australian continent is divided into three main topographic areas, 1) the eastern highlands, called the Great Dividing Range, which runs north-south from the northern tip of the Cape York

Peninsula down through Queensland, New South Wales and eastern Victoria to the southern island state of Tasmania and includes the Murray–Darling River basin in the southeastern interior which drains around one-seventh of the Australian land mass and is one of Australia's most significant agricultural areas, 2) the central lowlands, which consists of a network of ephemeral rivers that drain into the Gulf of Carpentaria on the north coast and into Lake Eyre in the Great Artesian Basin to the south, and 3) the peneplain, a low plateau spread across the western half of the continent that includes the Great Sandy Desert and the Great Victoria Desert.

After the turn of the early 19th century, the English immigrants began to explore and occupy inland Australia. Early development fanned out to occupy the moist crescent around the semi-arid and arid interior, displacing many aboriginal people and the remaining herbivorous macropods (kangaroos) with sheep and cattle which grazed and multiplied on the vast expanses of native grasslands. The original native grasslands comprised tall warm-season grasses that depended on rainfall and grazing intensity such as kangaroo grass, common tussock-grass, and perennial tussock grass, and also shorter perennial species such as redgrass, bluegrass, windmill grass and the wallaby grasses. In southern Australia, a range of species from around the Mediterranean were introduced inadvertently by the English settlers to become naturalized; these included several cool-season annual grasses such as soft brome (*Bromus, Hordeum*) and hairgrass *(Vulpia* spp.), forbs such as cape weed (*Arctotheca calendula) and* Paterson's curse *(Echium plantagineum*), and annual legumes such as clover (*Trifolium* spp.) and burclover (*Medicago* spp.) During the first century of English colonization, the expanding herds of grazing livestock were sustained by way of a combination of human interventions, such as clearing trees and shrubs, the regular burning of the open woodland-grassland and scrub-grassland communities, the granting of grazing rights and land tenure, fencing, the provision of reliable water supplies, better techniques of animal care and breeding, investment and banking services that followed the discovery of gold in the 1850s, and the building of the Australian railway system from 1855. By 1891, when most of the railway system was in place, more cattle were grazing the Australian landscape than there are today; however, the numbers dropped during the next decade due to a general economic depression and the "Federation drought," which began in the mid 1890s and reached its peak in 1901 and 1902.

The era of scientific agriculture in Australia began late in the 19th century with the establishment of experimental farms, which, during the early 20th century, helped to promote new techniques of dry farming, wheat breeding, superphosphate fertilizer and mechanization. To counteract the depletion of soil organic matter, a technique of ley farming with annual pasture legumes and clover was developed for slightly acidic soils. The person most associated with this period of agricultural development in Australia was Sir Sidney Kidman who was at the time the world's largest individual landholder eventually owning 107,000 square miles (280,000 square kilometers) stocked with about 176,000 cattle and 215,000 sheep. Despite or because of these scientific farming techniques, the severity of soil degradation in the 100 years following 1850 was extreme. Clearing the deep-rooted native vegetation caused loss of ground cover, changes in hydrology, loss of nutrient cycling, erosion and salinization. Overgrazing by livestock and the introduced rabbits caused loss of vegetation cover and type, soil erosion, surface sealing, and nutrient removal. Excessive cultivation caused oxidation of organic matter, surface sealing, compaction, increased wind and water erosion and nutrient losses. Machinery and vehicular traffic caused loss of ground cover and compaction. And fertilizers and chemicals contaminated soil and groundwater.

During the last half of the 20th century, the promotion of sustainable production by research organizations, industry bodies and farmers lowered the rate of soil degradation through understanding the degradation processes and the implementation of more sustainable farming systems and practices including a reduction in stock numbers, the control of rabbits, liming to counteract soil acidity, gypsum treatment for sodic soils, the use of fertilizers and legumes to enhance soil fertility, the adoption of reduced tillage and the increased use of perennial plants for reducing run-off and erosion, and limits on water allocations (pwc.com.au © 2011 PricewaterhouseCoopers).

Australian cattle herds were almost exclusively based on English breeds *(Bos taurus)*, so after WWII, England, which had favorable trade policies with other British Commonwealth countries, signed a "15 year beef agreement" with Australia for the import of Australian cattle meat. This trade marked the beginning of Australia's cattle meat exports. At the end of the trade agreement in 1960 England officially cut its preferential ties with Commonwealth countries and the Australian cattle meat export industry had to scramble to find a new market. At this time, while the U.S. was the world's leading cattle meat exporting country, it was also a large importer of so called "grinder beef" to mix in with hamburger meat, and the U.S. became the prime destination for Australian cattle meat exports. English cattle breeds were well adapted to temperate climates, but were poorly suited for tropical, sub-tropical and semi-arid regions like much of Australia, and parasites, ticks and drought conditions made the animals sickly and less productive. In 1947 pure bred Brahman cattle *(Bos indicus,* aka zebu) imported from the U.S. were introduced in Australia, first as a curiosity, then in substantial numbers in the late 1950s. The Brahman gene pool that originated in tropical India introduced all the characteristics needed to cope with the less favorable Australian environment. From the early 1960s to the late 1980s there was an intense period of breeding activity crossing Brahmans with all the other breeds to produce new stabilized breeds of tropically adapted cattle like the Droughtmaster, Belmont Red, Braford and Santa Gertrudis.

Cattle ranching in Australia is generally divided into the northern and southern regions where farming techniques vary depending on topography and rainfall. Over the second half of the 20th century northern cattle ranchers accounted for 75% of farmed land dedicated to cattle meat, but they accounted for just under 50% of the national herd. Cattle in the northern region typically would forage over sprawling properties, for example the Consolidated Pastoral Company that grazed 360,000 cattle across 5.8 million acres. Cattle meat from these forage fed cattle was considered to be of inferior quality on international markets. Farms in southern Australia are typically intensive feed operations with many more operators running much smaller herds of from 10 to 15 thousand animals. This fed cattle meat is considered "high quality" on the international beef markets. The expanding domestic market for cattle meat in Australia, the grinder cattle meat market in the U.S., and the increasing numbers of Brahman infused cattle all helped to propel Australia's cattle herd to its all time high of 35 million animals in 1974. But then, in 1974 Australia's cattle meat bubble burst; a glut of cattle meat in the US crashed cattle prices and U.S. demand for Australian cattle meat virtually disappeared overnight. By 1978 the Australian herd had been cut in half with many operators going out of business. The U.S. grinder cattle meat market did return thereafter to become the mainstay of Australia's cattle meat export market once again through the 1980s.

In the mid 1980's Australia began to export "quality beef" to Japan. This market was initially opened up by the U.S. as a concession to Japan over the growing trade imbalance between the two countries. Access to the Japanese market was the impetus for the development of the Australian cattle feedlot system and the export of chilled rather than frozen beef. Feedlot operations have grown significantly in Australia since the 1980's, reaching a feeding capacity of over 1 million animals by 2011. The giant U.S. based grain processing corporation, Cargill, has invested in feedlots and packing plants throughout Australia. The Australian meat packing industry is most concentrated in Queensland due to its proximity to the cattle supply. The top five meat packers in Australia account for over 50% of beef production with the four largest are either owned by or in joint ventures with foreign companies including Cargill and Teys (a Cargill joint venture) of the U.S., Swift (now a subsidiary of JBS) of Brazil, and Nippon Meat Packers of Japan.

In the 1990s, other Asian countries, notably Korea and Taiwan, began to import Australian "quality beef" but the most dramatic expansion in the Australian cattle meat market began around 1991 when the South East Asian countries of the Philippines, Thailand, Malaysia and Indonesia began importing live cattle from Australia's northern region. Between 1991 and 1997 this trade in live cattle increased from 70,000 animals annually to 700,000. This rise in Australia's live export market developed at the same time as exports to the U.S. were on the wane. In 1997, Indonesia which accounted for 60% of the live cattle market, suffered a major market crash which again threw the Australian cattle meat industry into a downturn (*"A Brief History Of Australian Beef to 1998," Cattlefacts,* November 1998). When the first case of Bovine spongiform encephalopathy (aka Mad Cow Disease) was detected in the U.S. cattle herd in 2003, Japan banned U.S. cattle meat imports and Australia's share of the Japanese cattle meat market rose by 30% producing a spike in the Australian cattle meat industry. But when Japan lifted its ban in 2006, competition from U.S. producers lowered cattle meat prices and put the financial squeeze on Australian producers. The Australian cattle meat industry has operated under stressed conditions since a run of dry seasons starting in 2001 cut feed crop production and water storage levels in the Murray-Darling Basin to historically low levels due to over-allocation of water rights and competition for irrigation water between agricultural, environmental and community users.

Australia became the world's third leading beef exporting country in 2013 largely by culling its national herd from 28 million in 2011 to down to 26.7 million in 2013 as farmers reduce their stocks. Since the turn of the 21st century the viability of cattle ranching in South Australia has been challenged by the inherent unprofitability of selling "quality beef" in the global marketplace. With under 30 million cattle in 2013, Australia's national herd is small compared to the top cattle meat producing countries (India 329 million animals, Brazil 208 million, China 104 million, U.S. 89 million, Argentina 51 million), but due to low domestic demand from Australia's relatively small human population of 23.5 million people compared to other top beef exporting countries (Brazil 199.32 million people, U.S. 316.37 million and India 1.27 billion), beef exports accounted for 60% of Australia's total production.

Though Australia's national cattle herd is small compared to other cattle meat exporting countries, it is still well beyond the carrying capacity of Australia's impoverished soils and arid climate. In January 2010 the *Australian Bureau of Statistics* issued its 5th edition of a report entitled "*Australia's Environment: Issues and Trends*," in which they drew on a wide range of official statistics to asses the condition of Australia's environment ("*4613.0 – Australia's Environment: Issues and Trends*," *Australian Bureau of Statistics*, Jan 2010). Their analysis paints a stark picture of the environmental impacts of cattle production on the Australian continent:

> "*Grazing accounts for just over half of all land use. Environmental issues associated with sheep and cattle grazing include habitat loss, surface soil loss, salinity, and soil and water quality issues. Drought condition in 2002–03 exacerbated soil loss, leading to the highest dust storm activity since the 1960s (Endnote 1).*"

> "*The impact of grazing varies in different parts of Australia. In the higher rainfall and irrigated areas, livestock grazing has led to the replacement of large areas of native vegetation with more productive introduced pastures and grasses. Grazing also modifies soil structure and leads to soil compaction.*"

> "*In the arid and semi-arid areas of Australia, despite lower stock densities, the impact of grazing on biodiversity can be greater than in high rainfall zones. The low productivity of arid and semi-arid areas limit resources and stock compete with native animals for food and water. The provision of water through bore holes, earth tanks and dams has resulted in grazing occurring in areas previously unsuitable for livestock.*"

> "*More than 80% of farmers reported undertaking activities to prevent or manage pest-related issues. The most common management practices were use of pesticides or insecticides, shooting or trapping, baiting and crutching.*"

> "*The major issues affecting the condition of soil and land on Australian farms in 2006–07 were erosion, soil compaction, soil acidity and surface waterlogging. In that year, farmers spent $649 million to prevent or manage such issues.*"

> "*The agriculture sector provided the second-greatest contribution to Australia's net greenhouse gas emissions in 2007.*"

China

While China is not a major cattle meat exporting country, with over one hundred million bovines (including cattle, water buffalo and yak) it is home to the world's third largest national herd behind only India and Brazil. Biologists and Archaeologists had long thought that humans domesticated cattle independently in two places: the Near East around 10,000 years ago and Southern Asia around 8,000 years ago, but in November 2013 an international team of researchers from the University of York, England and Yunnan Normal University, China, published a study in the journal *Nature Communications*, presenting morphological and genetic evidence for a third independent domestication of cattle in north-eastern China around 10,000 years ago, occurring simultaneously with cattle domestication in the Near East. Water buffaloes *(Bubalus bubalis)* were domesticated in two separate lineages in China: the river buffalo along the Yangtze River basin around 5,000 years ago and the swamp buffalo in southwest China around 4,000 years ago *("Phylogeography and Domestication of Chinese Swamp Buffalo,"* PLOS, February 20, 2013) (*"Wild or domesticated: DNA analysis of ancient water buffalo remains from north China,"* Journal of Archaeological Science, 2008*). Wild yak were first domesticated around 10,000 years ago by the Qiang people in the *Changtang,* an area that covers more than half of Tibet. Yak are acclimated to work at higher elevations between 6,500 and 16,400 feet (2,000 and 5,000 meters) or at lower elevations in more northerly latitudes *("1 ORIGINS, DOMESTICATION AND DISTRIBUTION OF YAK"* FAO corporate Document Repository, Regional Office for Asia and the Pacific).

In ancient China, cattle were ceremoniously slaughtered as a sacrifice to the gods and ancestral spirits, a portion would be set aside as an offering and the rest was eaten by the participants in the ceremony (Schafer, 1963). By the time of the Tang dynasty (618 to 907 AD), bulls had become so valuable as draft animals for cultivating the large staple croplands necessary to sustain China's burgeoning human population, and heifers valuable for milk production that in 831 AD Emperor Wenzong of the Tang dynasty banned the slaughter of cattle on the grounds of his religious convictions to Buddhism (*"China's Golden Age: Everyday Life in the Tang Dynasty,"* Oxford University Press, 2002).

Until the late 20th century, the Chinese people obtained over 90% of their calories from carbohydrates like rice, wheat, millet, beans, and tubers while only consuming meat that was sourced from old unproductive cattle. Draft and milk animals were fed on crop residues, wastes, vegetation, and other biomass (*"China in the Next Decade: Rising Meat Demand and Growing Imports of Feed, USDA Agricultural Projections to 2023,"* Economic Research Service, February 2014). During the Song dynasty (960 AD to 1279 AD), the ethnic Chinese Han people developed an aversion to the milk products that had been introduced by the Mongols back in the 5th and 6th centuries AD (*"The Food of China,"* Yale University Press, 1988). According to eminent French sinologist, Jacques Gernet, this traditional Chinese cuisine sans milk products and cattle meat that was typical of the Chinese diet well into the 20th century, first became popular during the Song Dynasty (*"Daily Life in China on the Eve of the Mongol Invasion,"* Stanford University Press, 1962).

In 1978, China initiated agricultural policy reforms to spur the production of animal foods, especially pigs, chickens, eggs and fish, but also to a lesser extent cattle. Increasing feed grain production was central to this policy and industrialized farming was institutionalized; by 1990 China had over 800,000 tractors in use and by 2008 that number was three million; since the 1970s the area of irrigated farmland has expanded by 32% to 58.5 million hectares in 2010 which amounts to 48% of the total arable land area in China; in 1980 China used 12 million tons of synthetic nitrogen fertilizer, in 2005 48 million tons; China's per hectare pesticide use in grain production more than tripled from 1980 to 2000 and by 1996 China had become the largest pesticide consumer in the world (*"Agricultural machinery - tractors in China,"* TRADING ECONOMICS, 2015) (*"The Fertilizer Situation and Outlook in China,"* China Agriculture University) (*"Ignoring The Labels: An Analysis of Pesticide Use in China,"* Economy and Environment Program for Southeast Asia). While rice and wheat are the major grain crops fed to people, China's largest grain crop is maize which is mostly fed to farm animals. Altogether, China harvested the largest grain crop of any country in history in 2011, a full one third of which went to feed animals. The soybean, which had been a staple of the Chinese diet for millennia, also was turned to animal feed. In 1995 China was self-sufficient in soybean production, but by 2011 it was importing four times more soybeans than it was producing – virtually all from the U.S., Brazil, and Argentina – to feed its multiplying population of livestock. This soybean shortage resulted from the government's policy of grain self-sufficiency which limited the land available for growing soybeans. China alone accounted for 60% of world soybean imports in 2011. Since the agricultural reforms of 1978, China's use of animal feed has shot up more than nine-fold and in 2010, China surpassed the U.S. as the world's number one user of feed (*"Meat Consumption in China Now Double That in the United States"*, Earth Policy Institute, April, 2012).

In 1986 there were around 70 million bovines in China with virtually none slaughtered for meat, by 2012 there were around 103 million with 47 million slaughtered for meat (including milk cows, draft bulls and fed cattle) and cattle meat production had risen from near 0 to 6.51 million tons. Most of this meat came from fattened low-yield milk cows (1.91 million tons) and bull calves (3.68 million tons).

There are four main cattle producing regions in China: 1) the Northeast, 2) Central 3) the Southwest crop farming areas where due to tractor use the population of draft animals is in decline and milk cows on the rise, and 4) the Northwest pastoral grazing region. The Chinese national cattle herd is in transition from mostly draft animals over to milk and meat producers. While cattle meat production is not a priority in China and on average in 2014 the Chinese people ate much less cattle meat per person than Americans (Americans 79 pounds/year, Chinese 8.7 pounds/year), China was still the world's third largest cattle meat producing country ahead of India and Argentina and behind only the U.S. and Brazil. The trend in cattle meat production in China is towards small and large feedlot operations to produce "high quality" fatted meat as cost effectively as possible (*"Inside China's beef and sheep market – agri benchmark,"* Institute of Agricultural Economics and Development, Chinese Academy of Agricultural Sciences, June, 2013).

On October 8th, 1990 the first McDonald's fast food hamburger outlet opened for business in the major city of Shenzhen, located in the southern Guangdong Province just north of Hong Kong. By 2013 McDonald's had over 2,000 outlets throughout China and other American fast food chains like Kentucky Fried Chicken and Pizza Hut were giving it stiff competition for the Americana food experience in China. The proliferation of these American food chains in China played no small part in promoting the transition from a plant-based to an animal-based diet in China.

The environmental impacts of China's move to a more animal based diet by means of industrialized agriculture have been severe. In a 2014 study entitled *"The driving forces of fertilizer use intensity by crops in China: A complete decomposition model,"* *Academic Journals, Scientific Research Essays,* April, 2014), the authors note the water and air pollution caused by high nitrogen fertilizer inputs:

> *"By 2009, the fertilizer use rate in China has reached 504 kg/ha, which was 4 times greater than the global average (Table 1). Such high level of fertilizer use in China has raised concerns about its negative environmental consequences. For example, Zhu and Chen (2002), Ju et al., (2009) and Sun et al. (2012) showed that the high rate of fertilizer use has led to large N [nitrogen] losses and has become the main source of water pollution and air pollution. A nation-wide pollution survey conducted by the Chinese Government identified that fertilizer was a major contributor to water-borne nitrogen, phosphorous pollution, and the increasing frequency of red tides (Zhang et al., 2013). Moreover, it is estimated that fertilizer production has accounted for 30% of agricultural greenhouse gas (GHG) emissions and was the source of about 8% of China's total GHG emissions (Liu and Zhang, 2011;Huang et al., 2012)."*
>
> *("The driving forces of fertilizer use intensity by crops in China: A complete decomposition model." (Dan Pan, Institute of Poyang Lake Eco-Economics, Jiangxi University of Finance and Economics, Nanchang 330013, China, Academic Journals, Scientific Research Essays, Vol. 9(8), pp. 229-237, 30 April, 2014)*

In a 2004 study published in the journal *Agriculture and Biosystems Engineering Publications* by Hongmin Dong et al., of the The Chinese Academy of Agricultural Sciences entitled *"COMPARISON OF ENTERIC [intestinal] METHANE EMISSIONS IN CHINA FOR DIFFERENT IPCC [International Panel on Climate Change] ESTIMATION METHODS AND PRODUCTION SCHEMES,"* the authors note the climate change impacts of methane gas emissions from cattle production:

> *"Enteric fermentation is the third largest source of methane (CH4) emission (ME) in China, following coal mining and rice cultivation. In 1990, China's enteric methane emission (EME) was estimated to account for 25% to 37% of its total ME from agricultural sources (ADB, 1999). The rapid economic development and improvement of living standards in China have led to the steady growth of its livestock production. From 1990 to 2000, livestock inventory in China increased 20.7% for cattle, 38.2% for sheep and goats, and 23.3% for swine, according to the China official government database (China Agriculture Yearbook, 1990–2001; China*

Animal Industry Yearbook, 2001). As a result, EME had been estimated to reach 13,800 Gg in 2000 and 16,900 Gg in 2020, surpassing that from rice cultivation (ADB, 1999). Because of China's large share of livestock production in the world (48% in swine, 8% in cattle, 12.5% in sheep, and 13.7 % in buffalo), accurate and timely determination of EME in China is not only essential to the Chinese national ME inventory, but equally important to the validity of the global greenhouse gas (GHG) inventory."

"The estimated EME for China during the period of 1990 to 1998 are summarized in table 4. The EME for 1996 (peak ME year of the studied period) were estimated to be 8,614; 11,039; 10,533 and 11,469 Gg, respectively, based on Tier 1, Tier 2, the IPCC Good Practices with or without the incorporation of treated straw effect. These EME values were 31%, 28%, 27%, and 20% higher than their respective values for 1990. The increase in ME over this time period was mostly attributed to the population increase in yellow cattle, dairy cattle and goats."

"The magnitude and partitioning of ME by animal species for 1996 are presented in table 5. As can be seen, yellow cattle were the largest contributor to EME in China, accounting for nearly 60% of the total EME. Buffalo and sheep were the second and third largest source, accounting for about 14% and 10% of the total EME, respectively. Emissions by dairy cattle account for less than 3% of the overall EME. However, with the rising demand for dairy products in China, the importance of ME from dairy cattle is expected to increase." ("COMPARISON OF ENTERIC METHANE EMISSIONS IN CHINA FOR DIFFERENT IPCC ESTIMATION METHODS AND PRODUCTION SCHEMES," Agriculture and Biosystems Engineering Publications, American Society of Agricultural Engineers, 2004)

In a 2012 paper entitled *"Pesticide use and farmers' health in China's rice production,"* published in the journal *China Agricultural Economic Review,* of the China Economics and Management Academy, Central University of Finance and Economics, Beijing, China, the authors noted the human health impacts due to the overuse of pesticides:

"China is the world's top consumer of pesticides but almost two thirds of pesticides are wasted, contaminating both land and water, an environment official said last year."

"By 1996, total pesticide supply reached about 340 thousand tons and China is likely to become the biggest pesticide consumer in the world. During the last ten years this has resulted in many health problems with up to 123,000 people poisoned from pesticide use in a year."

"This paper indicates that farmers who spray more pesticides are more likely to have headache, nausea and skin problems. Beside these visible effects, this paper also finds that exposure to pesticides has significant invisible impact on farmers' neurological, liver and kidney systems."

More than 19 percent of soil samples taken from Chinese farmland have been found to contain excessive levels of heavy metals or chemical waste." ("Pesticide use and farmers' health in

China's rice production" Fangbin Qiao et al., (2012) "Pesticide use and farmers' health in China's rice production", China Agricultural Economic Review, Vol. 4 Iss: 4, pp.468 - 484)

In a 2009 study entitled *"Improving crop productivity and resource use efficiency to ensure food security and environmental quality in China"* published in the *Journal of Experimental Botany (September 30, 2011)*, the authors noted the soil degradation caused by monocultures of feed crops:

"Soil degradation, a reduction in soil quality as a result of human activities, is a very serious problem in China. Of the total degraded land area in the world estimated to be 1964 Mha (Oldeman et al., 1991), degraded land in China comprises 145 Mha or 7.4% of the world total (Lal, 2002). The average thickness of topsoil in China over a 50-year period progressively decreased from 22.9 cm in the 1930s to 17.6 cm in the 1980s (Lindert, 2000). Some soils are likely to be even thinner now due to the intensity of erosional and depositional processes." *("Improving crop productivity and resource use efficiency to ensure food security and environmental quality in China," J. Exp. Bot., 2011)*

European Union

In its 2013 ranking of top cattle meat producing and importing countries, the Foreign Agricultural Service (FAS) of the USDA counts the European Union (EU), which includes most of western Europe, as a single economic entity. By this measure the EU was the world's third largest cattle meat producer and sixth largest cattle meat importer. The EU was originally established in 1992 by the 12 signatory states of the Maastricht Treaty, but by 2014 had expanded to include 28 states. In 2004, at a time when the EU had 15 member states, a report by the European Commission Directorate-General for Agriculture found that 3 member states – France, Germany and the UK (England, Scotland, Whales and Northern Ireland) – were the primary cattle meat producers accounting for 55.8% of total EU production (*"The meat sector in the European Union"*, European Commission, 2004).

In Europe during Roman times cattle were bred as draft animals to power plows and carts and these breeds were large boned, lean and slow to mature. In the Middle Ages, after the introduction of the horse collar around 1000AD, horses were used more and more for plowing, and though oxen were still exploited for draft power, their numbers declined throughout Europe (*"Medieval Farming and Technology: The Impact of Agricultural Change in Northwest Europe,"* Brill: Leiden, The Netherlands, 1997) (*"A preliminary description of British cattle from the late twelfth to the early sixteenth century,"* Ark 1980) (*"An Environmental History of the Middle Ages: The Crucible of Nature,"* Taylor and Francis Books: Oxon, UK, 2013).

Cattle were first bred specifically for meat in 15th century England and Scotland where grass was plentiful, the human population was low, and a demand for cattle meat was created by the aristocracy. Development of thickly muscled and fast maturing breeds such as Aberdeen Angus and Hereford began around this time. Cattle meat eating was not common among average European peasants in the Middle Ages as the well sourced treatise, *"Eating Meat: Evolution, Patterns, and Consequences"* (*Population and*

Development Review, December 2002), by Distinguished Professor Emeritus on the Environment at the University of Manitoba, Canada, Vaclav Smil, makes note:

> "[A]nimal foods provided generally less than 15 percent of all dietary protein, and saturated animal fats supplied just around 10 percent of all food energy for preindustrial populations. These conclusions are not in conflict with apparently reliable claims of some relatively high meat intakes among ruling elites, in cities in general and among rich urbanites in particular, or among marching armies—but such high consumption rates were restricted to small segments of populations. Low yields of grain and tuber crops limited the availability of high-quality feeds, and the inherent inefficiency of traditional animal feeding resulted in slow weight gains and low productivities (Smil 1994). These realities, prevalent well into the nineteenth century, had greatly constrained the total amount of available meat in traditional agricultural societies... Perhaps the best way to illustrate the range of reliably documented intakes is to present a few numbers and a few revealing quotations. Even in the richest European countries meat was a rare treat in ordinary households of the late eighteenth century. Antoine Lavoisier (1791) reported in his brochure on the riches of France that large numbers of peasants ate meat only at Easter and when invited to a wedding. The best available data show that at the beginning of the nineteenth century average meat consumption contributed less than 3 percent of all food energy in France (Toutain 1971). Similarly, an English hired hand told Sir Frederick Morton Eden (1797: 227) that in his household they had seldom any butter, but occasionally a little cheese and sometimes meat on Sunday.... Bread, however, is the chief support of the family, but at present they do not have enough, and his children are almost naked and half starved." ("Eating Meat: Evolution, Patterns, and Consequences" by Vaclav Smil, Population and Development Review 28(4):599–639, December 2002)

As the Industrial Revolution swept from England through the rest of Europe over the 18th and 19th centuries, a wealthy merchant class arose that created additional demand for cattle meat. Farmers responded to this demand working to improve their breeds by documenting pedigrees in official "herd books." The oldest known herd book for cattle was initiated in 1775 at the Monastery of Einsiedeln in Switzerland where the grey-brown mountain cattle were bred. The introduction of artificial insemination in 1780 also significantly improved the efficiency of breeding. The first herd books were used primarily in the development of localized breeds in the different regions of Europe, but later into the 19th century the best local breeds were crossbred which further advanced the breeding process. The French Limousin and Charolais meat breeds now popular around the world were developed around this time.

The French Revolution of 1789 and the Napoleonic Wars from 1803 to 1815 profoundly altered the old Middle Ages economic system where feudal lords and church abbots owned the land that was farmed by landless serfs over to a capitalist system where free farmers became peasant proprietors and owner/entrepreneurs. This radical change of land ownership spurred major agricultural innovation throughout much of continental Western Europe over the course of the 19th century. Civil engineering projects drained vast tracts of previously uncultivated marsh lands turning them into productive farmland. Also, by alternating the planting of legumes, turnips, and clover with grains, farmers were able to improve the soil while reducing fallowing from one third to one twelfth of the total cultivated land thereby significantly increasing the number of acres in production. The cultivated land of the continent increased by 38% from 110 million to 151.8 million hectares between 1800 and 1910. Another 3.5 million hectares were irrigated by 1900. Following the publication in 1840 of German biochemist, Justus von Liebig's landmark book on organic chemistry, *"Chemistry and its Application to Agriculture and Physiology,"* the use of nitrogen, phosphate and potash fertilizers (NPK) took off in Europe further improving crop yields. Yields improved by 30% in the first half and another 33% during the next third of the 19th century. These increases in cultivated land and yields produced a surplus of fodder crops that enabled the practice of stall-feeding of cattle over the winter months when pasture was not available. Before the advent of stall-feeding, much of the stock had to be slaughtered as winter came on due to lack of available pasture; this problem proved to be a major impediment to increasing cattle herds. Consequently, after the introduction of stall-feeding, cattle stocks roughly doubled in the second half of the 19th century (*"An Economic History of Nineteenth-Century Europe: Diversity and Industrialization"*, Cambridge University Press, December, 2012).

As the human population in Europe increased rapidly, the system of inheritance split up land holdings into smaller average sizes. By the 1860s, small peasant farms of 1 to 10 hectares made up 28% of the total agricultural lands on the European continent, those of 10 to 40 hectares made up 32%, and larger estates with more than 40 hectares owned roughly 40%. An additional aspect of this agricultural revolution was increasing specialization of production which ended the planting of a great variety of crops on each individual estate or in each regional unit. On the continent even very small farms became specialized and market oriented. The smaller farms tended to be in the lowlands of central Europe where grain production was high and cattle were raised in small scale stall-feeding operations. Larger estates tended to be in the Alpine regions of Switzerland, Austria and Northern Italy as well as in the UK where grains were hard to grow but grass for grazing cattle grew naturally. In the UK, pastureland actually increased from 54% of agricultural land in 1867 to 69% by 1913, but despite this emphasis on cattle meat and milk production, the UK still imported a majority of its meat, butter and cheese over the second half of the 19th century (*"An Economic History of Nineteenth-Century Europe: Diversity and Industrialization"*, Cambridge University Press, December, 2012).

Raising herds of cattle for meat and milk in Western Europe in the 18th and 19th century created conditions ripe for the spread of the fatal ungulate (hoofed animals) disease called "rinderpest" which in German means "cattle-plague." Rinderpest is believed to have originated in Asia over 3,000 years ago, later spreading through the transport of cattle to the Middle East, Europe and Africa. The rinderpest cattle virus is also believed to be the progenitor of the human measles virus sometime around the 11th or 12th centuries. (*"Origin of measles virus: divegence from rinderpest virus between the 11th and 12th centuries,"*

2010). Cattle death rates from rinderpest outbreaks were usually extremely high, approaching 100% in immunologically virgin populations. The virus was mainly transmitted through direct contact or drinking contaminated water, though it could also be transmitted by air. After suffering agonizing symptoms of fever, mouth sores, diarrhea and cellular breakdown, most animals would die in 6 to 12 days after onset. Rinderpest has recurred throughout history, often accompanying wars and military campaigns. Rinderpest hit Europe especially hard in the 18th century, with three long plagues from 1709 to 1720, 1742 to 1760, and 1768 to 1786, leaving millions of dead cattle in its wake. In the mid 19th century (1865-1866), there was a severe outbreak covering the whole of Britain, and in the 1890s there was another major outbreak in the Dutch colony of South Africa. After numerous failed attempts, the first successful vaccine for rinderpest was developed by English veterinary scientist, Dr. Walter Plowright, in 1962. Inoculation programs over the next four decades greatly reduced rinderpest outbreaks and the last confirmed case was reported in Kenya in 2001.

The number of acres under cultivation in western Europe steadily declined over the 20th century from 44.64 million hectares in 1913 to 37.89 million by 1981. World War I (1914 – 1918), the Great Depression (1929 – 1939) and World War II (1939 – 1945) all had devastating impacts on agriculture on the European continent and by the end of WW II grain production was near zero. But grain yields per acre during the inter-war period (1919 – 1938) actually made significant gains largely due to the adoption of the petroleum powered tractor that enabled more intensive cultivation. While fewer cultivated acres with increased yield per acre raised overall grain production to pre-WWI levels by the 1930s, the amount of grain available for cattle feed remained stagnant over the inter-war years (*"A Social and Economic History of Twentieth-century Europe,"* Harvard University Press, November 1989). This limit on silage spurred the development of an alternative feed industry in Europe as a means of increasing meat production. Raw wheat, barley, maize, linseed, cottonseed and fishmeal were imported from abroad as supplemental feed, and feed supplements from domestic sources were mostly derived from by-products of the food industry such as wheat feed left over from flour manufacture; oilseed cakes and meal from the manufacture of margarine and cooking oils; and ominously, meat and bone meal (MBM) from the rendering industry.

The first mention of an early form of MBM as animal feed was published in the book, *"The scientific feeding of animals"* in 1908 by German agricultural scientist, Professor Oscar Johann Kellner, and by the 1920s the use of MBM was well established in the UK (*"The scientific feeding of animals,"* The Macmillan Company, 1913). During WWII the UK set regulations on feed ingredients setting a minimum of 2.5% MBM, which was later increased for young stock to 5%. After the war, with the introduction of synthetic nitrogen fertilizers, the production of grain (especially maize), in western Europe began to skyrocket surpassing its pre-war high of 150 million tons by the mid-1950s to reach 275 million tons by 1981. This increased grain production made more feed available for cattle and as a result the number of cattle in Europe rose commensurately. But even with abundant feed grains, the use of MBM as an ingredient in cattle feed continued to grow after WWII because ruminant nutritionists discovered that cattle digested proteins from MBM more efficiently than proteins from plants. It was also found that MBM provided more absorbable sources of calcium and phosphorus than vegetable protein. In 1980 the Agricultural Research Council of the UK published "*The Nutrient Requirements of Ruminant Livestock*" in which they calculated the optimum amount of MBM to include in cattle feed to maximize milk production to not exceed 5% since inclusion at a higher rate made the feed unpalatable to the cattle. This led to the use of substantial amounts of MBM in place of vegetable proteins which had been the main protein source for milk cows up until then. In 1988 the UK *Ministry of Agriculture, Fisheries and Food* (MAFF) estimated the annual UK production of MBM at 350,000 to 400,000 tons of which about 90% went to pigs and poultry and the rest to ruminant feed.

MBM was considered safe from transmitting infectious diseases since the high temperatures used in processing were thought to kill all known pathogens in the rendered byproducts, but this sense of complacency was shattered in 1986 when the first case of BSE (bovine spongiform encephalopathy – commonly referred to as mad cow disease) was diagnosed in the UK. BSE is a fatal neurodegenerative disease in cattle that causes a spongy degeneration of the brain and spinal cord and loss of motor coordination. American neurologist and biochemist, Dr. Stanley Prusiner M.D., identified a rogue protein called a "prion" as the infectious agent that spreads BSE; unlike infectious bacteria or viruses, prions contain no DNA and are virtually indestructible. Epidemiologists strongly suspect that BSE in cattle originated from MBM sourced from sheep that were infected with the ruminant disease "scrapie" (a disease in sheep and goats similar to BSE in cattle) and the original outbreak was amplified by feeding MBM sourced from BSE-infected cattle (so called downer cows) to calves. Consequent to these findings, the UK introduced a ban on feeding ruminant-derived MBM to cattle in 1988 and the ban was extended to all animal feed in 1990. The entire European Union (EU) prohibited the feeding of mammalian protein to ruminants in 1994 and extended the ban to all other livestock in 2001 (European Union On-Line, 1998) (Brookes, 2001). A 2002 report from the Office International des Epizooties (an intergovernmental organization responsible for improving animal health worldwide) indicated that BSE had been confirmed in 20 countries in the EU with more than 180,000 cases in the UK and another 1,800 elsewhere in the EU including Portugal, France, Switzerland, Germany and Spain (Office International des Epizooties, 2002; United States Food and Drug Administration, 2001). Since the bans went into effect, some MBM is still used as ingredients in petfood but the vast majority is now used as a fossil-fuel replacement in cement kilns, as landfill or is incinerated.

In March 1996, the UK health minister announced that a committee of scientists set up to advise the government on spongiform encephalopathy issues had linked the BSE outbreak in the 1980s to an unusual outbreak of a variant form of human spongiform encephalopathy called Creutzfeldt-Jakob disease (vCJD) that had afflicted 10 people under the age of 42, some in their teens. The first person to develop symptoms of vCJD became ill in 1994 most likely from exposure to prions through the consumption of BSE infected cattle meat products before the ban on MBM feed was instituted in 1988. From October 1996 to March 2011,

175 cases of vCJD were reported in the UK, 25 in France, 5 in Spain, 4 in Ireland, 3 each in the Netherlands and the U.S., 2 each in Canada, Italy and Portugal, and 1 each in Japan, Saudi Arabia and Taiwan. The number of cases of vCJD in the UK peaked in 2000 with 28 deaths declining to about 2 diagnosed cases and 2 deaths per year in 2008 (*Variant Creutzfeldt-Jakob disease*, World Health Organization, Fact sheet N°180, Revised February 2012). As a result of the BSE and vCJD outbreaks, demand for European cattle meat plummeted which led to a significant decline in EU cattle meat production and total cattle herd. Before the BSE outbreak the EU had been a cattle meat exporter, but in 2003, as demand for cattle meat began to rebound, the EU became a net importer due to lack of production capacity.

Back in the early 1960s, several European countries established a predecessor organization to the European Union called the Common Market, and in 1962 the Common Market created a Common Agricultural Policy (CAP) to promote agricultural production among its member states. Though reformed many times, CAP remains the agricultural policy arm of the EU into the 21st century. In order to reestablish the European cattle meat industry after the demand collapse of the late 1980s, strict CAP policies on cattle feeding and rearing practices were put into place in an attempt to regain full consumer confidence that EU cattle meat was BSE free. CAP also established a system of financial subsidies as an incentive for farmers to raised cattle. In the 1990s these subsidies took the form of governments buying surplus production to support the market price paid to farmers; in 1999 the CAP subsidy program was reformed to make direct cash payments to farmers based on their volume of production; and in 2003 the CAP subsidies were reformed again to make the cash payments independent of production volume giving farmers more flexibility to respond to market demand. Without these substantial farm subsidies, raising cattle in the EU would have been unprofitable at world market prices for cattle meat. The cost of replacing the banned high protein MBM feed supplement with imported soy meal from Brazil, Argentina and the U.S. added to the expense of raising cattle in the EU; most of the imported soy meal now fed to European animals comes from genetically engineered (GE) herbicide tolerant RoundUp Ready soybeans and maize developed by the U.S. biotech and seed corporation Monsanto. A second major expense that makes raising cattle in the EU a costly business venture is the heavy dependence on nitrogen and phosphorus fertilizers used on pastures and to grow maize, two-thirds of which is to feed livestock. Spain, Portugal, France, Germany and the Czech Republic are currently growing Monsanto's GE maize for livestock feed.

Another long time scourge of cattle herders has been Foot and Mouth disease (FMD). The first written description of FMD was in 1514 Italy, but it would be until 1897 that German bacteriologist Friedrich Loeffler demonstrated that a filterable agent caused FMD. This was the first demonstration that a disease of animals was caused by a filterable agent and ushered in the era of virology. It was subsequently discovered that the filterable agent was a virus FMDV. The disease affects domestic cloven-hoofed animals, including cattle, swine, sheep, and goats, as well as more than 70 species of wild animals including deer; it is characterized by fever, lameness, and lesions on the tongue, feet, snout, and teats. Although FMD does not result in high mortality in adult animals, the disease has debilitating effects, including weight loss, decrease in milk production and loss of draft power resulting in a loss in productivity for a considerable time. FMD is one of the most highly contagious diseases of livestock, and FMDV rapidly replicates and spreads within the animal and by touch or aerosol to other animals. Outbreaks have occurred in every livestock-containing region of the world with the exception of New Zealand, and the disease is considered endemic to all continents except Australia and North America ("Foot-and-Mouth Disease," *Clinical Microbiology Reviews*, Apr 2004). No effective vaccine has yet been developed against the FMD virus and the strategy to halt outbreaks has been early detection, quarantine of the infected area and destruction of the effected animals. Loses from FMD outbreaks can be considerable as was the case in the UK in the spring and summer of 2001 where around 10 million sheep and cattle were destroyed to halt the spread of the disease (*"Inside Out,"* BBC, Oct. 31, 2007). The 2001 FMD epidemic on the heels of the 1996 BSE/vCJD crisis in the UK shook consumer confidence and sales of British cattle meat went into a severe decline.

Most meat cattle in Europe today come from calves bred to "suckler cows" (females from meat breeds that give all their milk to their calf) under so-called "extensive" systems of production found in the pastoral regions (Ireland, UK and the mountainous areas) where they graze on increasingly fertilized pasture lands. Cattle reared in these regions grow more slowly and produce meat that is less fatty and tougher than maize fed cattle. About 10% of EU cattle meat comes from males born to milk cow breeds that are reared on a liquid diet of a milky gruel for six weeks, then slaughtered for "veal" meat. Milk cows raised in so called "intensive" cereal based systems are more commonly found in the southern and central regions of Europe where grains grow well. Within each of these systems there is a wide range of regional variation involving different breeds of cattle and feed blends. In 2014, the Food and Agriculture Organization of the United Nations ranked the EU as the world's third largest cattle meat producer at 7.58 million metric tons accounting for 12.88% of total world market behind only the U.S. and Brazil, and the EU also ranked as having the world's fourth largest cattle herd (behind only India, Brazil and China) with 88 million animals, up from 59 million in 2000. Some of this increase was due to the expansion of the EU from 15 to 28 member states by 2014.

Up until the beginning of the 19th century, most animal slaughter in Europe took place in private backyard butcher sheds in densely populated urban areas. Beginning in the 18th century, as part of a larger transition from an agrarian to an industrial society, moral reformers argued that "public slaughterhouses" located discreetly out of town would be preferable to private butcher shops in full view of the general public where it reputedly incited violent tendencies. The first public slaughterhouse was built near Paris in 1810 and the French word *abattoir* was introduced to refer to a specific place where animals were brought to be slaughtered for human consumption. In London, public hygiene concerns over cholera outbreaks in the 1840s led to the closure of the city's Smithfield live animal market in 1855 and the subsequent construction of large public slaughterhouses outside the city center. To various extents over the 19th century other Western European countries adopted the public slaughterhouse concept. While termed "public," the real purpose of these new slaughterhouses was to remove animal slaughter from public view (*"A Social History of the Slaughterhouse: From Inception to Contemporary Implications"*, Department of Sociology and Anthropology University of Windsor, Human Ecology Review, 2010). Throughout most of Europe in the 20th century, the methods of processing and marketing animal products developed independently in each country according to long standing customs and traditions; as a result the meat processing industry in Europe is characterized by many small locally based producers rather than a few giant meatpacking firms as in the U.S. While raising and processing chicken and pig meat did concentrate into a few large vertically integrated corporations in the 1980s and 1990s, most cattle raising and processing operations remained in the hands of small farm cooperatives in some regions and small to medium sized private companies in others. Retail "supermarkets" pioneered in the U.S. in the 1930s began to enter the European food market in the 1950s, first in the UK, and then over the next decades on the continent. Large chain supermarkets like Tesco in the UK and Carrefour in France put downward pressure on the supply chain for lower prices forcing producers to consolidate operations into fewer bigger farms. A move towards larger scale cattle operations to satisfy this buyers market is the current trend in the EU.

As in all the major meat and milk producing regions of the world, raising cattle in the EU has outsized environmental impacts. Cattle, no matter where on Earth they are raised, are a significant contributor to the greenhouse gas emissions that are driving global climate change. In a 2010 report by the European Commission Joint Research Centre entitled, *"Evaluation of the livestock sector's contribution to the EU greenhouse gas emissions (GGELS) - Final report -,"* the authors noted:

> *"According to CAPRI-calculations [Common Agricultural Policy Regionalised Impact Modeling System], in the EU-27 384 Mio tons of CO2-eq are, directly and indirectly, emitted by the dairy and cattle sector. 191 Mio tons of those emissions are assigned to the production of beef and 193 Mio tons to the production of milk. This is equivalent to 22.2 kg of CO2-eq per kg of beef and 1.4 kg CO2-eq per kg of raw milk. In case of beef 8.79 kg (39.6%) are emitted in form of methane, 5.77 kg (26%) as N2O and 7.61 kg (34.4%) as CO2, 3.65 kg (16.5%) of CO2 emissions coming from the use of energy and 3.96 kg (17.9%) from land use and land use change (Scenario II)."*

> *"High methane emissions in particular indicate high shares of time animals spend on pastures, or an above average temperature like in Mediterranean countries leading to higher emissions from manure management. N2O emissions increase with the share of solid systems or manure fallen on pastures. Finally, high CO2 emissions indicate a strong dependency on feed imports and, in general, feed crops, and a high use of mineral fertilizers for feed production. In total terms (see Figure 6.4) the largest emitters are France with 45 Mio tons, followed by the United Kingdom, Germany, Spain, Italy and Ireland."*

The much greater use of nitrogen and phosphorus fertilizers in the EU largely to grow more animal feed has led to excessive amounts of nitrates and phosphates in waters and to eutrophication of surface and groundwater throughout Europe, as noted in this *Organisation for Economic Co-operation and Development* report, *"Studies on Water, Water Quality and Agriculture: Meeting the Policy Challenge"*:

> *"Public Opinion across the EU member states has ranked water pollution as one of their major environmental concerns (European Commission 2009). The concern is borne out by the EU Commission's assessment which has identified that 40% of surface water and 30% of groundwater is at risk across the EU of failing to meet the objectives for good chemical and ecological status established under the EU's Water Framework Directive (WFD) (Kanakoudis and Tsitsifli 2010). More detailed analysis at the EU member state level, for example in the United Kingdom, reinforce the EU Commission findings and also points to the importance of diffuse source pollution, mainly from agriculture, as a major cause of pressure on water systems."*

And then there's this notice from the January, 2010 EU Nitrates Directive:

> *"While nitrogen is a vital nutrient that helps plants and crops to grow, high concentrations are harmful to people and nature. The agricultural use of nitrates in organic and chemical fertilisers has been a major source of water pollution in Europe. For the first time mineral fertiliser consumption registered a progressive reduction in the early 1990s and stabilised during the last four years in the EU-15, but across all 27 Member States nitrogen consumption has increased by 6%. Generally, farming remains responsible for over 50% of the total nitrogen discharge into surface waters."*

A report from the European Commission in February, 2010, identifies the worst offending member states:

> *"High nitrate concentrations are found in groundwater in parts of Estonia, south-east Netherlands, Belgium (Flanders), UK (England), several parts of France, northern Italy, north-east Spain, south-east Slovakia, southern Romania, Malta and Cyprus. Particularly high concentrations are found in surface waters in Malta, UK (England), Belgium (Flanders) and France (Brittany)."*

Global Cattle Complex

The statistical service, *Statista,* estimated the worldwide cattle herd in 2012 to be 1.485 billion animals (including meat cattle, milk cows, oxen, water buffalo and yak). In 2013 the Foreign Agricultural Service (FAS) of the USDA reported that the world's total cattle meat production was a staggering 58,856,000 tons. Of that, the top six cattle meat producing countries (counting the European Union as one country) – the U.S., Brazil, EU, China, India and Argentina – accounted for over 70% of world cattle meat production. The top six cattle meat exporting countries – Brazil, India, Australia, U.S., New Zealand and Uruguay – accounted for over 79% of world cattle meat exports, and the top ten cattle meat importing countries (counting the EU as one country) – Russia, U.S., Japan, Hong Kong, China, EU, South Korea, Venezuela, Canada and Chile – accounted for over 71% of cattle meat imports. While these few countries dominate the world's cattle meat markets, the FAS report goes on to list in total 60 cattle meat producing countries, 46 cattle meat exporting countries and 58 cattle meat importing countries. These dizzying statistics on world cattle meat production and consumption can barely convey the massive scope and scale of the worldwide cattle industrial complex.

According to a 2011 FAS report, the top ten cattle meat consuming countries per capita were: Uruguay at 136.9 pounds/person/year, Argentina 123.0, U.S. 85.5, Brazil 83.3, Paraguay 78.5, Australia 77.8, Canada 65.3, New Zealand 64.4, Kazakhstan 59.1 and Hong Kong 52.4. As noted above, there have been few times and places in the history of agrarian societies where cattle meat eating was so commonplace; most notably in 14th and 15th century France and Germany after the Black Death had decimated the human population and cattle were left to forage freely on previously tilled farmlands that had turned to pasture, and in 16th and 17th century South and Central America where the large Indian populations were decimated by European introduced plagues and replaced by a small number of European colonists and multiplying herds of European cattle. In both of these cases, a sudden drop in the human population and simultaneous rise in the cattle population made cattle meat plentiful and cheap. But also in both of these cases, as the human population recovered to prior levels, beef production and consumption once again became uneconomical for the masses of people. Limited cattle meat consumption was the general rule up until the 20th century and the advent of industrialized agriculture. With the introduction of the tractor, massive irrigation systems, synthetic fertilizers and pesticides, hybrid seeds and transportation infrastructure, world production of maize and soybeans began to far outstrip the needs of the rapidly expanding human population with plenty to spare to fatten cattle, pigs, sheep, and chickens for human consumption. In essence, by tapping into a vast pool of energy in the form of underground oil deposits (which in essence is stored ancient solar energy), we humans have managed to rev up the natural cycles of life and plant more acres of faster growing, higher yielding crops. Once again human technologies have managed to forestall the "Malthusian catastrophe." This unprecedented abundance has made cattle meat and other animal products available to large populations of middle class people in amounts unprecedented in human history. With more people than ever before (the UN Population Fund estimated that the world human population exceeded 7 billion on October 31, 2011) eating more cattle meat per person, there is a multiplier effect on world demand for cattle meat, and world cattle meat production has continued on a steady incline.

Of all the animals raised for food, cattle have by far the largest environmental impacts. As we humans go about raising nearly 1.5 billion bovines worldwide for food consumption, we have in effect inverted the natural trophic structure of the world's ecosystems by becoming both the most numerous large mammal on Earth as well as the Earth's top apex predator. Remember: in ecosystems without human intervention, apex predators like wolves and lions embody the least amount of biomass of all the mammals, not the most. This trophic imbalance has so destabilized the flow of energy and the carbon, nitrogen and phosphorus cycles within ecosystems as to have severely compromised their capacity to produce food.

Milk Cows

Human consumption of the milk of other mammals went from zero 8,000 years ago, to become a significant food source for billions of people in modern times. While over that time many different mammals have been exploited for their milk (goats, sheep, camels, reindeer, water buffalo, etc.), cattle have proven to be the most prodigious milk producers and have come to dominate the worldwide milk market. Until modern times when iced dairy products became technically feasible, milk had been consumed in four basic ways: fluid milk, cheese, yogurt and butter. While the history of each of these dairy products goes back thousands of years, it is just in this past century that dairy consumption has become a dietary staple for so many people. Let's take a closer look at how that happened.

Fluid milk

Milk did not enter the diet of adult humans until after the domestication of other mammals. Milk proteins found on ceramic vessels unearthed in modern-day Romania and Hungary provide evidence for dairying as far back as 8,000 years ago (6,000 BC). Most likely these early dairy consuming cultures did not drink fluid milk but instead made milk into cheese to keep it from spoiling.

Back then, humans, like all other mammals, would lose their ability to digest the milk sugar, *lactose*, after being weened from their mother's breast, and drinking raw milk would cause juveniles and adults severe intestinal distress making fresh milk an undesirable food source. Cheese, however, could be tolerated since most of the lactose was removed in the cheese making process. Then, around 7,500 years ago (5,500 BC) some Germanic and Celtic people living in central Europe evolved a genetic mutation that enabled them to continue producing *lactase* (the lactose digesting enzyme) past the age of weening into child and adulthood which enabled people with this *lactase-persistent* (LP) gene to drink raw fluid milk without suffering from indigestion. Due to the survival advantage gained from having this additional fresh food source during the long harsh winter months, dairy farmers carrying the LP gene variant probably underwent a more widespread and rapid population growth than non-dairying groups. The spread of fluid milk drinking from the Balkans across Europe also explains why most Europeans carry the same version of the LP gene; it came in on a wave of population expansion that followed the rapid co-evolution of milk tolerance and dairy farming. There are also four other LP gene variants known to exist in Africa that are thought to have evolved independently in Africa. This genetic diversity is probably the result of the imposition of dairying cultures on a pre-existing farming peoples, rather than the spread of dairy farmers as in Europe. Fluid milk drinking remained restricted to Europe and north Africa until the Europeans spread it around the globe during the age of European colonization. Still, to this day, about 75% of the world's population remains lactose intolerant *(Hertzler SR, Huynh BCL, Savaiano DA. How much lactose is low lactose? J Am Dietetic Asso. 1996)*.

The first cattle bred for milk production was the Holstein around 1 AD in the Netherlands. Farmers bred black cattle of the Batavians with white cows of the Friesians to produce cows that were highly efficient milk producers on limited feed resources. Holsteins are still the most efficient milk producing animal in the world today. As Holsteins and other dairy breeds spread throughout Europe, an increase in milk supply made milk more available to common people.

Raw milk spoils very quickly once it is removed from the cow's udders, and before the 19th century, fluid milk was primarily consumed fresh after milking on farms where most of the population lived and worked. But in the 18th century as the Industrial Revolution caused a mass migration of people away from farms to cities, fresh milk was no longer a dairy option for many urban dwellers since it would spoil before getting to market. In the 19th and 20th centuries, though, significant discoveries and inventions contributed towards making fluid milk a commercially viable product away from the farm.

By the 19th century, the gradual intensification of cattle production had led to a severe problem of bovine tuberculosis (bTB) in cattle herds. Bovine TB is a zoonotic disease that can be transferred from cows to humans through infected milk. In 1882, pioneering German physician and microbiologist, Robert Koch, discovered *"Tubercle bacillus"* as the causative agent of the disease and in 1890 he went on to demonstrate the properties of a tuberculin test for cattle in order to identify those animals with bTB. Finland was the first country in the late 1890s to commence a successful bTB eradication program. It was quickly established that bTB could be eradicated by the use of tuberculin tests. Once test and removal programs were commenced for cattle in other dairying countries, the incidence of clinical cases of bTB rapidly declined in the early 20th century as infected animals were culled from the herds.

A biological discovery of the mid 19th century that later led to improved milk quality was made by French chemist and microbiologist, Louis Pasteur, in 1864, when he found that briefly heating beer and wine would prevent these beverages from turning sour. This process, now called "pasteurization," achieves this effect by eliminating pathogenic microbes and lowering microbial numbers to prolong the quality of the beverage. In the mid-to-late 1800s, milk-born illness like typhoid and tuberculosis created a public health crisis that led to skyrocketing infant mortality rates in the cities. In 1889, a Newark, New Jersey doctor named Henry Coit, urged the creation of a Medical Milk Commission to oversee or "certify" production of milk for cleanliness, finally getting one formed in 1893. In 1895 commercial pasteurization of milk began and the disease rate plummeted.

Through the mid 19th century, cows had always been milked by hand, but this process was slow and laborious and limited the number of cows that could be milked by one person. The first patent for a vacuum milking machine operated by a hand pump was acquired in England in 1851, but the first successful commercial milking machine wasn't introduced until 1891 by a Scottish plumber named William Murchland. Known as the Murchland machine, it was suspended around the cow, attached to the udders with teat cups that would apply continuous vacuum suction to the teats allowing the milk to flow into a pail under the cow that would be emptied into a large vat. Continuous suction proved to be damaging to the cow's teats which spurred the invention of a pulsating vacuum milker called the "Thistle" in 1895 that allowed the teat to recharge before each draw. There have been numerous advances in vacuum milking technology over the course of the 20th century.

The first fluid milk to be transported from farm to city by rail was in the U.S. in the 1840s using 10 gallon tin-plated steel cans loaded onto passenger cars. As volume increased, separate milk cars were developed that were customized with built-in packed ice compartments and insulation to reduce warming during transit. By the late 1800s pre-cooled milk was being loaded onto heavily insulated bulk container tank cars for delivery to creameries in the Eastern cities. Rail transport of milk peaked in 1931 as trucks began to take over the milk transport business and the last milk delivery by train was in 1972. Today, all bulk milk in the U.S. is transported by refrigerated container trucks.

Before milk bottles, milkmen would fill customers' jugs from a vat. In the 1880s several different milk bottles designs with different types of caps were patented. By 1900 the *cap-seat cap* introduced by the Thatcher Manufacturing Company had become standard. Milk bottles were reusable and efficiently refilled at the creamery and delivered to customers or grocery stores by milk trucks. Before mechanization, glass bottles were made by glass blowers blowing molten glass into metal molds. Increasing demand for bottles stimulated many attempts at automated bottle machines in Europe and the U.S. After nine years of refined design work, American, Michael Owens, of Toledo, Ohio, devised the first commercially successful, fully automatic bottle-making machine in 1903. This first automated bottle machine had an average daily production of 50,400 bottles. Since the 1960s in the U.S., glass bottles have almost completely been replaced with either coated paper cartons or plastic containers. These paper and plastic containers are lighter and cheaper than glass to manufacture and ship to consumers.

In 1911, the General Electric Corporation (GE) released a household refrigeration unit that was powered by gas. Home refrigeration extended the time milk and other fresh foods could be kept at home before spoiling. Electric companies that were GE customers did not benefit from this gas-powered refrigerator though, so GE invested in developing an electric model. In 1927, GE released the Monitor Top, the first home refrigerator to run off electricity. In 1930, Frigidaire, one of GE's main competitors, synthesized the synthetic coolant, freon, based on a chlorofluorocarbon (CFC) chemical, that led to the development of smaller, lighter, and cheaper home refrigerators. In the 1970s, CFCs released into the atmosphere were found to be depleting the global atmospheric ozone layer which protects life on Earth from overexposure to solar ultraviolet radiation. The use of CFCs was fazed out worldwide by the international Montreal Protocol treaty of 1987. CFCs have largely been replaced with HFCs (hydrofluorocarbons), which are potent greenhouse gases that are extremely long-lived in the atmosphere.

As the milk supply steadily increased over the first half of the 20th century, the price paid dairy farmers for their milk declined to the point where it became difficult for small operators to make a living producing milk. This led to a movement in the dairy industry toward larger operations with economies of scale that made it possible to earn a profit off milk production. As dairy herds got larger, it became necessary to develop new milking technologies that made it possible for big dairy farms to milk large numbers of animals in a timely fashion. The result of this circumstance was the invention of the "milk parlor" in which several milking machines were connected through pipes to a central collection vat making it possible to milk a number of cows at once and eliminate the time consuming task of emptying individual milk pails. The first milking parlors were designed in the 1930s but it wasn't until the introduction of the "herringbone" milk parlor in New Zealand in the 1950s that milk parlor design became more efficient. In the 1980s, "rotary" milk parlors were introduced which further increased milking efficiency, but these units were very expensive and only affordable by the largest dairy operators. *("Inside the Milk Machine: How Modern Dairy Works," Modern Farmer Media, March 17, 2014)*

The next big development in milking technology was the implementation of electronic milking machines in the 1970s, with "automatic takeoff clusters" and "individual cow identification." It can be harmful for a cow to be over-milked past the point where the udder has stopped releasing milk. Consequently the milking process involves not just hooking up the milking machine to the udders, but also monitoring the process to determine when the animal has been milked out and the milking machine should be removed. While parlor operations allowed a farmer to milk many more animals much more quickly, it also increased the number of animals to be monitored simultaneously by the farmer. The automatic take-off system was developed to remove the milker from the cow when the milk flow reaches a preset level that is customized for each cow using an "individual cow identification" code. These electronic technologies relieve the farmer of the duties of carefully monitoring numerous animals being milked at the same time. An experienced hand milker can milk a herd size of 10 to 20 cows, the number that can be milked in less than an hour. A large automated herringbone milk parlor can milk up to 600 cows with two milkers, and a large automated rotary milk parlor can milk a herd of over 1,000 cows with only one or two milkers.

In 1993, the U.S. Food and Drug Administration (FDA) approved for commercial use the genetically engineered *recombinant Bovine Growth Hormone*, otherwise known as rBGH, rBST, or, by the Monsanto corporate trade name, *"Posilac."* Injecting cows with Posilac has the commercial advantage of increasing milk production per cow. A meta-analysis of studies on *Posilac's* effects on cow health published in the October, 2003, *Canadian Journal of Veterinary Research,* found an average increase in milk output ranging from 11% to 16%. As there has been a milk glut in the U.S. for many decades, the introduction of Monsanto's genetically engineered *Posilac* was a solution in search of a problem. The same study also found that cow's injected with *Posilac* had a nearly 25% increase in the risk of clinical *mastitis* (udder infection), a 40% reduction in fertility, a 55% increased risk of developing clinical signs of lameness, and an overall decrease in the body condition score, even though they had increased feed intake. The milk from *Posilac* injected cows has also been found to contain higher levels of a protein called *"insuline-like growth factor 1"* (IGF-1) which is a known cancer promoter. A 2010, USDA National Agricultural Statistics Service (NASS) survey of Wisconsin dairy farms found that about 18% used *Posilac*. Its use has been banned on health grounds in the European Union, Japan, Australia, New Zealand and Canada.

Besides these technical innovations that have made liquid milk a commercially viable product, the U.S. government has passed numerous laws over the 20th century to increase milk production and consumption:

* 1922, the Capper–Volstead Act exempted milk cooperatives from the Sherman Antitrust Act which had the effect of legalizing farm cooperatives.

* 1937, the Agricultural Marketing Agreement Act of 1937 provided authority for federal milk "marketing orders" which operate like regional cartels to limit competition and keep prices up.

* 1940, the first Federal milk program for public schools and a Federally subsidized milk advertising program under the Works Progress Administration were established.

* 1946, the National School Lunch Act passed which prominently subsidized milk.

* 1949, the Federal Milk Price Support Program began which keeps market prices artificially high by guaranteeing that the government will purchase any amount of cheese, butter, and nonfat dry milk from processors at a set minimum price.

* 1966, the Child Nutrition Act and the Special Milk Program promoted milk consumption for children.

* 1983, the Dairy Production and Stabilization Act created the National Dairy Board for the purpose of dairy product promotion

* 1990, the Fluid Milk Promotion Act was passed to specifically promote the sale of fluid milk.

* 1992, the first USDA Food Pyramid was released which recommended 2 to 3 servings of dairy per day to American food consumers. (The original food pyramid was updated in 2005 and 2011 and is now called "My Plate" with no specific recommended dairy intake, instead graphically depicting dairy as a side dish.)

Despite the U.S. government's continued effort to increase consumption of fluid milk by American consumers, milk consumption peaked in the 1970s at 20.7 gallons/person/year, and by 2010, had fallen to fewer than 5.7 gallons/person/year. This large decline in per capita fluid milk consumption in the U.S. was largely due to the introduction of dozens of alternative drinks on the market especially for the 2 to 19 year old age group. At 5.7 gallons/person/year, Americans rank far down on the list of nations for per capita milk consumption which is dominated by Scandinavians and Europeans. Here is a list of the top ten cow's milk consuming people in the world in 2010:

Nationality	gallons/year
Finns	48.6
Swedes	38.4
Irish	34.3
Dutch	32.5
Spanish	31.5
Norwegians	30.8
Swiss	29.7
English	29.4
Australians	28.1
Canadians	25.0

2011 MooMilk.com

Cheese

The first dairying cultures of central Europe likely used milk to make cheese. It is hypothesized that the process of cheese making was discovered accidentally by storing milk in a pouch made from the stomach of a ruminant animal, resulting in the milk being turned into curds (milk solids) and whey (milk liquid) by the rennet (stomach enzymes) that remained in the animal's stomach. This observation that curdling milk in an animal's stomach gave better-textured curds may have led to the deliberate addition of rennet to further enhance the process. The process of making cheese removes a lot of the lactose as it is drained off with the whey, thus overcoming the problem of lactose intolerance.

There is written evidence of cheese making in ancient Sumerian cuneiform texts and depictions of cheese making in Egyptian tombs dating back to around 2000 BC (4,000 years ago). Late Bronze Age Minoan tablets record the inventorying of cheese on the island of Crete around 1,500 BC (3,500 years ago). The earliest cheeses were likely sour, hard and salty. By Roman times, cheese was a common food and cheese making a more refined process. The English word "cheese," as well as the Spanish "queso" and German "kaese" and some other words for cheese can all be traced back to the Latin word for cheese, *caseus*. The Romans primarily used goat and sheep milk to make cheese. In 65 AD Lucius Columella, who wrote the most comprehensive, systematic and detailed treatise on Roman agriculture ever written entitled, *De Re Rustica* (On Agriculture), described a cheese making process involving rennet coagulation, pressing of the curd, salting, and aging. Cheeses produced in Europe where climates are cooler than in the Middle East required less salt for preservation making the curd a better host for the microbes and molds that give aged cheeses their distinctive flavors. In Pliny the Elder's famous work, *Natural History* (77 AD), he devotes two chapters to describing the diversity of cheeses eaten by early Romans. As Rome expanded into new territories that had their own cheese making traditions, cheeses in Europe diversified further and various locales developed their own distinctive cheeses.

In the Middle Ages after the fall of Rome, cheese lost its luster among the noble class and was considered peasant fare unfit for royal consumption. During the Middle Ages cheese was made and improved by monks in the monasteries of Europe. The Po Valley in Italy became the cheese making center of Europe in the 10th century.

Cheese was virtually unheard of in Asian cultures, in the pre-Columbian Americas, and in most of Africa before European colonization spread its use worldwide. Cheese is still rarely considered part of local ethnic cuisines outside of Europe, the Middle East, and the Americas.

Up until the mid 19th century AD, the great majority of people in Europe and North America lived in rural agricultural areas and milk and milk products were primarily made for home or local consumption. Due to the physical demands of twice daily milkings, individual farmers could only tend small herds and dairy farms were limited in size. However, with the population movement from farms to cities that occurred during the Industrial Revolution, the demand for cheese also moved from local rural areas to densely populated urban areas. To supply these distant markets with cheese, it became necessary to make major changes in how cheese was made and distributed.

In 1851, dairy farmer Jesse Williams of Rome, New York, opened up the first successful cheese factory where he took in milk from his neighbors to a centralized cheese making facility where the cheese was made on an assembly line to create a uniform standardized product. The Williams Cheese Factory was the seminal inspiration for our modern industrialized food system. Soon Williams' was utilizing the milk of 300 to 400 cows and in his first season of operation, produced 100,000 pounds of cheese – more than five times the amount produced on the typical farmstead. By the end of the Civil War in 1865, there were 500 such cheese factories in New York State alone.

In 1845, a band of Swiss immigrants settled in Green County, Wisconsin and started making European cheeses in America. Over the next decades Swiss immigrants turned Wisconsin into the largest cheese producing state in America. The wholesale cheese industry underwent phenomenal growth during the latter half of the 1800s.

The first Holstein cow was imported from Holland to the U.S. in 1852 by a Massachusetts man named Winthrop Chenery. Chenery was so impressed with his Holstein's milk production that he imported more in 1857, 1859 and 1861, and soon many other dairy farmers followed suit to establish lines of Holstein in the U.S. By 1885 there were enough dairy farmers interested in the breed to start the *Holstein-Friesian Association of America* to maintain herdbooks and record pedigrees of Holstein cows in the U.S. (In 1994, the association changed its name to *Holstein Association USA, Inc.*)

The 1860s saw the beginnings of mass-produced rennet, and by the turn of the 20th century scientists were producing pure microbial cultures. Before then, bacteria in cheese making had come from the environment or inoculation from a prior batch of whey which made for an inconsistent product. These pure laboratory cultures meant a more consistent product could be manufactured for mass markets.

By 1880 there were 3,923 dairy factories nationwide which were reported to have made 216 million pounds of cheese representing almost 90% of that year's total cheese production. By the turn of the 20th century, farm production of cheese had become insignificant; the 1904 government census only reported factory output, which weighed in at over 317 million pounds.

As mass production made cheese more available to urban consumers, simple cost-effective storage solutions for cheese gained popularity. Ceramic cheese dishes became one of the most common ways to prolong the life of cheese in the home, and remained the most popular until the introduction of the home refrigerator in 1911.

The first processed cheese was developed by Walter Gerber and Fritz Stettler in Switzerland in 1911. In this process, natural cheese was heated with sodium citrate to produce a homogeneous product which firmed-up upon cooling. The intent of this process was to improve shelf-life of cheese shipped to warmer climates. In 1916, American, James Kraft, who was working independently on blending and heating natural cheeses in the U.S., took out the first patent on processed cheese.

Prior to the mid 19th century, most people considered cheese a specialty food produced in small batches and eaten sparingly. Advances in dairying and factory production in the century between 1850 and 1950 made cheese a more affordable condiment for average working people in the U.S. and Europe, but it wasn't until further advances in factory production after World War II that cheese consumption per capita shot up to the amounts people eat today in the early 21st century. Based on 2009 statistics by Eurostat, the Canadian Dairy Information Centre and the Wisconsin Milk Marketing Board, Americans ranked 11th in the world, consuming 31 pounds of cheese per person in 2009, up from 12 pounds per person in 1950 (*"The Human-animal Relationship: Forever and a Day", edited by Francien Henriëtte de Jonge, Ruud van den Bos, pg 252, 2005).* The top eleven cheese consuming people are:

Country	pounds/person/year
Greeks	68
French	53
Maltese	48
Germans	46
Dutch	46
Romanians	46
Italians	44
Finns	44
Poles	41
Swedes	40
Americans	31

In the U.S., in 1955, 13% of milk was made into cheese. By 1984 this percentage had grown to 31%, and currently over one-third of U.S. annual milk production is devoted to making cheese. Total natural cheese production in the U.S. grew from 418 million pounds in 1920 to 10.6 billion pounds in 2011. Processed cheese also experienced a surge in consumer demand with annual production exceeding 4 billion pounds a year by 2011. In 2011 the U.S. was the world's top cheese producer at 5,163,564 metric tonnes. The top 10 cheese producers were:

Country	Metric Tonnes
U.S.	5,163,564
Germany	2,047,453
France	1,942,375
Italy	1,133,756
Netherlands	746,263
Poland	651,316
Egypt	644,564
Russia	604,753
Argentina	580,375
Canada	408,825

According to the U.S. Department of Agriculture Foreign Agricultural Service (FAS), U.S. cheese exports were 224,306 metric tons in 2011 and the top buyers were Mexico, South Korea and Japan. U.S. imports of cheese were 142,146 metric tons and the top sources were Italy and France.

Yogurt

Yogurt dates back to around 3,000 BC (5,000 years ago) when goatherds in Anatolia (modern day Turkey) first fermented goat's milk in a goatskin pouch to conserve it. Like cheese, yogurt was probably discovered accidentally when a goatherd stored some sun dried milk in a goatskin pouch and it spontaneously fermented when it came into contact with the natural bacteria contained in the goatskin. The result, a thick tart paste that preserved well, was called "yogurt", a word derived from a Turkish verb that means "*to be curdled or coagulated; to thicken.*"

The fermentation of the milk sugar, lactose, by these bacteria produces lactic acid which acts on milk protein (casein) to give yogurt its characteristic creamy texture and tart flavor. Fermentation breaks down the lactose thus overcoming the problem of lactose intolerance. Milk from goats, sheep, water buffalo, yaks, camels and horses is still used in some parts of the world to produce yogurt, but worldwide, cow's milk is now the most common source.

Making yogurt became widespread in ancient civilizations. In ancient India, the combination of yogurt and honey was called *"the food of the gods."* Persian traditions hold that Abraham, father of Judaism, Christianity and Islam, owed his fertility and longevity to regular ingestion of yogurt. The cuisine of ancient Greece included a dairy product known as oxygala which is believed to have been a form of yogurt. The prominent Greek physician, surgeon and philosopher, Galen, (129 AD – 200 AD) mentioned that oxygala was consumed with honey, similar to the way thickened Greek yogurt is eaten today. The oldest writings mentioning Turkish yogurt are those of the Roman, Pliny the Elder, in the 1st century AD, who wrote about ancient barbarous nations that knew how *"… to thicken the milk into a substance with an agreeable acidity."* The Turkish books written in the 11th century use the word "yogurt" and describe its use by nomadic Turks. Yogurt wasn't introduced into central Europe until 1542 when King François I of France was suffering from severe diarrhea and his royal doctors could offer no cure. The Sultan of the Ottoman Empire and political ally of France, Suleiman the Magnificent, sent a Turkish doctor who cured the king with yogurt. So impressed was François that he became a leading advocate in Europe for the health benefits of yogurt. By the 19th century the use of yogurt had spread to the Balkans, the Russian Empire (especially Central Asia and the Caucasus) and into Western Asia.

In 1905 a Bulgarian student of medicine in Geneva, Switzerland, named Stamen Grigorov, first examined the microflora of Bulgarian yogurt. He described it as consisting of a spherical and a rod-like lactic acid bacteria. In 1907, this rod-like bacterium was named *Bacillus bulgaricus*. The Russian biologist, Ilya Ilyich Mechnikov, of the Institut Pasteur in Paris, was influenced by Grigorov's work and hypothesized that regular consumption of yogurt was responsible for the unusually long lifespans of Bulgarian peasants and he worked to popularize yogurt as a foodstuff throughout Europe.

In 1919, Isaac Carasso, from Ottoman Salonika, started the first industrialized production of yogurt in a small shop in Barcelona, Spain. He named his business Danone, or "little Daniel", after his son. The brand later expanded to the United States under the name Dannon. In 1933 yogurt with added fruit jam was patented in Prague, present day Czech Republic, by the Radlická Mlékárna dairy.

Americans first began to take notice of yogurt in the first decade of the 20th century after the Russian zoologist Ilyich Mechnikov, published his book *The Prolongation of Life; Optimistic Studies* (1908), in which he recommended daily ingestion of lactic-acid bacillus from yogurt to increase life span. Yogurt was further popularized in America by Dr. John Harvey Kellogg, M.D., at his Battle Creek Michigan Sanitarium, where it was used both orally and in enemas. Like Mechnikov, Kellogg believed that most disease is alleviated by a change in intestinal flora, that a poor diet favors harmful bacteria that can then infect other tissues in the body, and that intestinal flora is improved by eating a well-balanced vegetarian diet favoring low-protein, laxative, and high-fiber foods. Kellogg recommended that this natural change in flora could be sped by enemas seeded with the favorable bacteria in yogurt. In the 1950s and 1960s, the dairy industry began promoting yogurt as a health food in the U.S. and by the late 20th century, it had become a common American food item.

According to the leading independent market research firm, *Euromonitor International, AC Nielsen,* the top ten per capita yogurt consuming nations as well as the U.S. and India, in 2013 were:

Country	pounds/person/year	kilograms/person/year
Netherlands	78.8	35
Turkey	77.7	35
France	77.3	35
Germany	76.5	34
Saudi Arabia	61.2	27
Spain	55.8	25
Austria	52.4	23
Czech Republic	37.5	17
Poland	36.0	16
Russia	33.8	15
U.S.	17.0	7
India	5.0	2

Though the U.S. lags far behind much of the yogurt consuming world in per capita consumption, yogurt sales have grown exponentially since the early 1990s. In 1993, Americans consumed three times as much fluid milk as they did yogurt, but by 2004 yogurt had surpassed milk in average annual consumption. Even with approximately $7.6 billion in sales in 2012, America is still considered an emerging market by the yogurt industry *(The Yogurt Wars, Scott Goodson, Forbes, Apr 13, 2013)*. The people of India actually consume much more yogurt (called dahi) than is indicated in the above statistics, but the researchers only counted commercially produced product, while most of the yogurt consumed in India is home made. China has a very low yogurt consumption per capita, but China has embarked on a very active dairy program in the 21st century and is expected to be a major growth market in the future.

In 2014 there was a $2.5 billion worldwide export market in yogurt which represented a 21.4% gain from 2010, but most yogurt is still consumed in the country of origin *(Top Yogurt Exporters, Daniel Workman, Forbes, August 6, 2015)*.

Over the decade between 2002 and 2012, the commercial yogurt industry underwent a consolidation where a few large international corporations such as Danone, Yoplait, Ehrmann, Chobani and Fage bought up many smaller producers who already had ongoing operations and a retail presence. Today, there are so few yogurt producers that the market is practically monopolized *("The Yogurt Wars", Scott Goodson, Contributor, Forbes, Apr 13, 2013)*.

Mass marketing campaigns have been tremendously influential in directing consumer trends towards yogurt consumption. The rising interest in Greek yogurt in America coincided with a marketing blitz by the major yogurt producers, and now, Greek yogurt is virtually synonymous with yogurt in America (*"The Yogurt Wars", Scott Goodson, Contributor, Forbes, Apr 13, 2013*). Yogurt was primarily marketed as a health food and this is largely how it is perceived by most consumers today. But in 2008, Dannon was taken to the U.S. District Court for the Northern District of Ohio in a class-action lawsuit alleging that they had lied when marketing their Activia and DanActive yogurts by trumpeting health benefits that didn't exist. Product labels said the yogurt has *"... a positive effect on your digestive tract's immune system."* Rather than have the actual nutritional science on yogurt's health effects exposed in an open courtroom, Dannon settled the case agreeing to pay duped consumers $35 million in reimbursement for products bought under false pretense, and to change the wording on the label to say yogurt will *"... interact with your digestive tract's immune system."*

Butter

The origin of butter goes back about 8,000 years when it was first made from sheep and goat milk, as cattle had not yet been domesticated. The first butter is believed to have been made by filling a goat skin with half milk and half air, the skin would be hung with ropes from a tripod of sticks and rocked until the agitation led to the formation of butter. Butter is produced by agitating the cream in milk which damages the membranes that separate the fat globules allowing the milk fats to conjoin and separate out from the other parts of the milk.

The oldest written reference to butter was found on a 4,500 year old (2,500 BC) limestone tablet in Mesopotamia illustrating how butter was made. It is generally believed the word butter originates from the Greek *bou-tyron* meaning "cow cheese", but it may have been derived from the ancient Scythian language spoken by nomadic Eurasian cattle-herders. The ancient Greeks and Romans seemed to have considered butter a food fit more for the northern barbarians. The Greek poet, Anaxandrides, refers to the Indo-European Thracians as *"butter-eaters",* and in *"Natural History,"* Pliny the Elder calls butter *"... the most delicate of food among barbarous nations."* In the first century AD, the Greek physician Galen described butter as a medicinal agent. Modern historian and linguist, Andrew Dalby, says most references to butter in ancient Near Eastern texts should more accurately be translated as *ghee*. Ghee is a clarified butter that is prepared by simmering butter and removing the liquid residue. This process flavors the ghee, and also produces antioxidants that help protect it from rancidity. Because of this, ghee can be stored from six to eight months in warmer climates. Ghee is mentioned in Roman shipping manifests as a typical trade article around the Red Sea and Arabian Sea in the first century AD, and the Roman geographer, Strabo, describes it as a commodity of Arabia and Sudan. In India, ghee has been a symbol of purity and an offering to the gods, especially the Hindu god of fire, Agni, for more than 3,000 years. References to the sacred nature of ghee appear numerous times in the ancient Hindu text, the *Rigveda*. Since prehistory in India, ghee has been both a staple food and used for ceremonial purposes such as fueling holy lamps and funeral pyres.

After the fall of Rome and throughout much of the Middle Ages, butter was a common food across most of Europe, but like cheese, it had a low reputation and was consumed mostly by peasants. In the cooler climates of northern Europe, people could store butter longer before it spoiled; Scandinavia has the oldest tradition in Europe of a butter export trade, dating back at least to the 12th century. Butter slowly became more accepted by the upper class in Europe after the Roman Catholic Church allowed its consumption during the Lent fasting period in the 12th century. Bread and butter became regular fare among commoners, especially in England which gained a reputation for the liberal use of melted butter as a sauce on meat and vegetables. France became well known for its butter, particularly in Normandy and Brittany.

By the 1860s, butter had become so in demand in France that Emperor Napoleon III offered prize money for an inexpensive substitute to supplement France's inadequate butter supplies. A French chemist named Hippolyte Mège-Mouriès won the prize with the invention of margarine in 1869. The first margarine was cattle meat tallow (fat) flavored with milk and worked like butter; vegetable margarine followed after the development of hydrogenated vegetable oils by the French chemist, Paul Sabatier, in 1897.

Until the 19th century, the vast majority of butter was churned by hand on farms. The first butter factories appeared in the U.S. in the early 1860s, after the successful introduction of cheese factories a decade earlier. The centrifugal cream separator was marketed successfully by Swedish engineer, Gustaf de Laval, in the late 1870s. This machine dramatically sped up the butter-making process by eliminating the slow step of letting cream rise to the top of milk naturally. Initially, whole milk was shipped to the butter factories, and the cream separation took place there. Cream-separation technology quickly became small and inexpensive enough to do the separating on the farm, and the cream alone shipped to the factory. By 1900, more than half the butter produced in the U.S. was factory made; Europe soon followed suit. In 1920, Otto Hunziker authored *The Butter Industry, Prepared for Factory, School and Laboratory*, a well-known text in the butter industry. As part of the efforts of the *American Dairy Science Association*, Professor Hunziker and others published articles on butter-making that helped standardized industry practices around the world.

Per capita butter consumption declined in most western nations during the 20th century, in large part due to the rising popularity of margarine, which is less expensive and, as a result of mass marketing, perceived as healthier than butter. In the U.S., consumption of margarine overtook butter during the 1950s, and more margarine than butter is eaten in the U.S. and in the European Union still today.

According to the Canadian government's Canadian Dairy Information Center, the top ten per capita butter consuming countries as well as India and the U.S., in 2013 were:

Country	pounds/person/year	kilograms/person/year
France	17.44	7.9
Germany	13.69	6.2
Switzerland	12.13	5.5
Australia	11.69	5.3
Iceland	11.44	5.2
Austria	11.00	5.0
Czech Republic	10.81	4.9
New Zealand	10.81	4.9
Poland	9.00	4.1
Pakistan	8.38	3.8
India	8.19	3.7
U.S.	5.50	2.5

According to the USDA FAS, in 2010 the top ten butter consuming countries (counting the EU as one country) were:

Country	1,000 metric tonnes/year
India	5,025
EU-27	2,170
U.S.	854
Russia	368
Mexico	227
Ukraine	111
Canada	96
Australia	91
Brazil	90
Japan	72

And in 2010, the top ten butter producing countries (counting the EU as one country) were:

Country	1,000 metric tonnes/year
India	5,035
EU-27	2,275
U.S.	900
New Zealand	580
Russia	240
Mexico	195
Australia	115
Ukraine	110
Brazil	95
Canada	90

Global Dairy Complex

To produce the four major dairy products – fluid milk, cheese, yogurt and butter – as well as the many other dairy products on the market such as dried powdered milk, whey protein, buttermilk, kefir, cream, sour cream, ice cream, frozen yogurt, etc., an enormous amount of milk is required. An analysis by the Food and Agriculture Organization (FAO) of the United Nations for 2013 notes:

"World cow's milk production in 2013 stood at 636 million tonnes, with the top ten producing countries accounting for 56.1% of production. The USA is the largest cow's milk producer in the world accounting for 14.4% of world production, producing 91 million tonnes in 2013, an increase of 0.4% when compared to 2012.

"India is the second largest cow's milk producer, accounting for 9.5% of world production and producing nearly 61 million tonnes in 2013.

"Of the top ten largest milk producing countries, Turkey and Brazil have shown the largest percentage growth from 2012 to 2013 at 4.2% and 6.0%, respectively."

According to the FAO report, the top ten milk producing nations in 2013 were:

Country	million tonnes
U.S.	91
India	61
China	36
Brazil	34
Germany	31
Russia	30
France	24
New Zealand	19
Turkey	17
UK	14

To produce these quantities of milk worldwide requires an enormous global herd of milk cows. In 2012, the FAO reports over 264 million milk cows worldwide. According to the FAO report, the top ten national milk cow herds were:

Country	million cows
India	44
Brazil	23
Sudan	15
China	13
Pakistan	10
Kenya	9
U.S.	9
Russia	9
Tanzania	7
Ethiopia	7

In the 27 European Union countries there were 23 million milk cows producing 136 million tonnes of milk making the EU the top milk producing region in the world with 42% of world production. The Americas are the second largest producing region at 29% of world production and Asia is third at 21%. A careful examination of these statistics indicates that the EU and former British colonies (U.S., New Zealand and Australia) produce a lot more milk with far fewer cows than in Asia and Africa. There are three main reasons for this: 1) in countries with a European tradition of farming, dairy farms mostly breed Holstein cows rather than Asian and African breeds that are less productive, 2) milk cows in these countries get considerably more high nutrient feed, and 3) milk cow operations in these countries are highly mechanized and automated.

By the 1980s, the typical Western style dairy operation was dominated by corn-soy-alfalfa fed Holstein cows. Holsteins make up over 90% of the U.S. dairy herd. The modern Holstein is a product of human engineering, as people have altered its genome through selective breeding by 22% since the 1970s. Bred to tolerate a high-nutrient, grain and legume diet as opposed to the cow's natural diet of grass, the average Holstein produces around 23,000 pounds of milk, or 2,674 gallons of milk each lactation cycle which usually lasts about 305 days; that comes out to 75 pounds, or almost 9 gallons of milk/cow/day. Today's average milk cow produces six to seven times as much milk as she did a century ago.

Milk cows spend their lives being fed in an indoor stall or a crowded feedlot. They are artificially inseminated to keep them constantly impregnated in order to produce more milk. Newborn calves are separated from their mothers within days and the grieving mothers are visibly in emotional distress moaning with big sad eyes for days. The economic reality is that if calves were allowed to suckle on their mothers for a few months, as nature intended, the farmers would lose their slim profit margin; a high percent of milk production comes during these first few months after birth. The female calves are raised to be milkers and the males are sold for "veal" meat after 18 to 20 weeks or raised to full adult weight in 18 to 24 months and slaughtered for cattle meat.

In the U.S., antibiotics and hormones are routinely administered to milk cows to reduce infections and increase milk production. Milk cows are pushed hard, and after three or four years when their production slackens, they are sold off for hamburger meat.

According to the USDA Economic Research Service, the trend in U.S. dairy farming since the 1970s is towards fewer larger operators:

"Between 1970 and 2006, the number of farms with dairy cows fell steadily and sharply, from 648,000 operations in 1970 to 75,000 in 2006, or 88 percent (fig. 1). Total dairy cows fell from 12 million in 1970 to 9.1 million in 2006, so the average herd size rose from just 19 cows per farm in 1970 to 120 cows in 2006. Moreover, because milk production per cow doubled between 1970 and 2006 (from 9,751 to 19,951 pounds per year), total milk production rose, and average milk production per farm increased twelvefold. These changes reflect a trend toward greater specialization as well as greater size. However, like much of agriculture, dairy

farms come in a wide range of sizes. The largest U.S. dairy farms have over 15,000 cows, though farms with 1,000–5,000 cows are more common. Large dairy farms account for most inventory and production in Western States, and a growing share of production elsewhere." ("Profits, Costs, and the Changing Structure of Dairy Farming" / ERR-47 *Economic Research Service/USDA)*

In assessing the environmental costs of cattle production, governmental and non-governmental organizations statistically combine meat and milk cattle to measure the total impact of the species. As noted above in the section on meat cattle, there are approximately 1.5 billion cattle in the world today including both meat and milk cattle, and, of all domesticated animals, raising cattle causes the greatest environmental impacts including emissions of greenhouse gasses into the atmosphere, pollution of fresh water with nitrates, and overdraft of fresh water aquifers. In California, the leading milk producing state in the U.S., alfalfa to feed milk cows is the #1 water intensive crop in the state using 5.2 million acre feet/year (1 acre foot = 325,851 US gallons) in 2009, while sucking down the Central Valley aquifer. An increasing percentage of California grown alfalfa is being exported to China to feed its expanding dairy industry, even as California was suffering through a mega four year drought in the 2010s. Soybeans and maize from Brazil are exported to Europe and China to feed meat and milk cows as the Amazon rainforest is sacrificed at the alter of human gods. The human addiction to cattle meat and milk is the single most environmentally destructive anthropogenic activity on Earth.

It is interesting to note here that the words "cattle" and "capital" have shared origins, both trace back to the early 13th century French word "chattel," which refers to personal property or wealth; in turn, chattel traces back to the medieval Latin "capitale" and to an earlier Latin "capitalis" both of which trace to "caput" which means "head." What this etymology suggests is that back in the Middle Ages capital as represented by head of cattle was considered the measure of a man's wealth and status. In effect, cattle owners were the world's first capitalists and the origins of capitalism go back much farther than the industrial revolution and Adam Smith's capialist opus, *The Wealth of Nations (1776).*

17

CHICKENS

The modern day bird we call the "chicken" (from Old English *cicen* meaning "young fowl") was originally domesticate from a wild red junglefowl native to Southeast Asia called *Gallus gallus.* From these obscure beginnings 8,000 years ago, the chicken has become the most populous bird species on Earth and a major source of food for humans around the world. Let's take a closer look at how that happened.

While chickens were first domesticated in Southeast Asia (South China, Burma, Thailand, Laos, Cambodia, Vietnam) for the purpose of cock fighting, around 8,000 years ago, many geneticists now think a chicken that was domesticated independently by the Harappan civilization of the Indus River valley (present day Pakistan and Northwest India) around 4,500 to 4,100 years ago (2500 to 2100 BC) is the genetic progenitor of the egg and meat bearing birds common throughout the world today.

Although inconclusive, evidence suggests that the Harappan civilization carried on a brisk trade with the Middle East more than 4,000 years ago (2000 BC). Archaeologists have recovered ancient chicken bones from Lothal, a once thriving Harappan sea port on the Northwest coast of India, raising the possibility that chickens could have been transported west across the Arabian Sea to the Arabian Peninsula as cargo or provisions. Cuneiform tablets from Mesopotamia around 2000 BC refer to "the royal bird of Meluhha," which Professor Piotr Steinkeller, a specialist in ancient Near Eastern texts at Harvard University, believes most likely refers to the chicken.

Richard Redding, professor of anthropology at the University of Michigan, and an expert on animal bones in archaeological contexts, notes in his article, "*The Pig and the Chicken in the Middle East: Modeling Human Subsistence Behavior in the Archeological Record Using Historical and Animal Husbandry Data*" (*Journal of Archaeological Research, Dec 2015*), that as pig meat consumption declined in the Near East, chicken consumption sharply increased. Adam Thake of the *New Historian* online magazine points out there is a logical reason why ancient Mesopotamians chose chickens over pigs:

> "*Chickens have several advantages over pigs. First, they are a more efficient source of protein than pigs; chickens require 3,500 litres of water to produce one kilo of meat, pigs require 6,000. Secondly, chickens produce eggs, an important secondary product which pigs do not offer. Third, chickens are much smaller and can thus be consumed within 24 hours; this eliminates the problem of preserving large quantities of meat in a hot climate. Finally, chickens could be used by nomads. While neither chickens nor pigs can be herded in the same way as cattle, chickens are small enough to be transported.*" ("*People Ate Pork in the Middle East Until 1,000 B.C.—What Changed? A new study investigates the historical factors leading up to the emergence of pork prohibition,*" New Historian, 2015)

Chickens arrived in Egypt some 250 years later, where depictions of chickens as fighting birds and additions to exotic menageries adorned royal tombs. It would be another 1,000 years, during Ptolemaic times, before the chicken would become a popular commodity among ordinary Egyptians. By then the Egyptians had mastered the technique of artificial incubation, which freed hens from brooding (egg sitting) to devote themselves to laying more eggs. Chicken eggs naturally hatch in three weeks, but only if the brood hen keeps the temperature constant at around 99 to 105 degrees Fahrenheit and the relative humidity close to 55%. The hen must also turn the eggs three to five times a day, to avoid physical deformities developing in the embryo. The Egyptians constructed extensive incubation complexes made up of hundreds of "ovens." Each oven was a large chamber connected to a series of corridors and vents that allowed attendants to regulate the heat from fires fueled by straw and camel dung. The Egyptian egg attendants kept their methods secret from outsiders for centuries.

The chicken also spread south and east from Asia to many Pacific island chains, but since these island cultures had no written language, there is no documentary evidence of the chicken's origins there. DNA evidence, however, indicates that the chicken began to spread across the Pacific around 3,000 years ago (1000 BC). A study entitled, *"Using ancient DNA to study the origins and dispersal of ancestral Polynesian chickens across the Pacific"* published in the *Proceedings of the National Academy of Sciences (PNAS,* February 2014), indicates the human migration into the South Pacific took place in two phases, the first of which began around 1000 BC. Professor Alan Cooper of the University of Adelaide's *Australian Centre for Ancient DNA* and co-author of the PNAS study notes, *"We can show [from chicken DNA] that the trail heads back into the Philippines. We're currently working on tracing it farther northward from there."* From the Philippines the chicken spread south to the Malaysian and Papua New Guinea archipelagos and from there highly skilled seafarers known as the "Lapita" set off east into the great unknown of the Pacific to colonize hundreds of tropical islands including Vanuatu, Fiji, Tonga, Samoa and New Caledonia. They sailed as colonists, not explorers, bringing with them everything they might need to settle on the lands they hoped to find, like flints for tool making, pottery, and foodstuffs – including chickens. A second much later phase of human migration beginning around the year 800 AD (1,200 years ago), saw the Lapita and their chickens extend even further east into the vast expanse of the eastern Pacific to inhabit Tahiti, Bora Bora, the Marquesas, Easter Island, and Hawaii.

As in the Pacific, the chicken was also first introduced into Western Europe around 1000 BC when Phoenician traders spread chickens along the Mediterranean coast as far as Iberia (modern day Spain). The first pictures of chickens in Europe are found on Corinthian pottery of the 7th century BC. In the mid-5th century BC Greek poet, Cratinus, called the chicken "the Persian alarm" and in Aristophanes's Greek comedy *The Birds* (414 BC) he called a chicken "the Median bird", suggesting an eastern origin. In ancient Greece, chickens were still rare and considered a prestigious food for elite men at the symposia. The Greek island of Delos seems to have been a center of chicken breeding *(Columella, De Re Rustica 8.3.4).*

Chickens were a delicacy among the Romans, whose culinary innovations included the omelet and the practice of stuffing birds for cooking. In 162 BC, a Roman law called the "Lex Faunia" forbade fattening hens as a means to conserve grain rations *("A History of Food By Maguelonne Toussaint-Samat," John Wiley & Sons, March, 2009).* To get around this law, Romans discovered that castrated roosters, called capons, would double in size on the same rations. The Romans also used chickens for oracles. According to 1st century BC Roman philosopher, statesman and orator, Cicero, special attendants called "pullarius", would open the chickens' cages and offer them pulses or a special kind of soft cake when a divination was needed; if the chickens stayed in their cage, made noises, beat their wings or flew away, the omen was bad, if they ate greedily, the omen was good *(Cic. de Div. ii.34).* The aforementioned 1st century AD Roman author, Columella, gave detailed advice on chicken breeding and raising in the eighth book of his 12 book treatise on Roman agriculture, *De Re Rustica*. In the "Apicius", a collection of Roman cookery recipes thought to have been compiled in the late 4th or early 5th century AD, there are 17 recipes for chicken, mainly boiled with a sauce. All parts of the animal were used including the stomach, liver, testicles and tail.

The chicken's status as a food source in Europe appears to have diminished with the collapse of Rome. According to Dr. Kevin MacDonald, professor of archaeology at University College in London, *"In the post-Roman period, the size of chickens returned to what it was during the Iron Age,"* more than 1,000 years earlier. MacDonald speculates that the big, organized farms of Roman times which were well suited to raise large flocks of chickens and protect them from predators simply disappeared. As the centuries went by, the chicken was replaced on the medieval menu with other naturally adapted native fowl species like geese and partridge. At the same time, the chicken's status as a religious icon gained currency: in the 6th century AD, Pope Gregory I declared the rooster the emblem of Christianity and in the 9th century AD Pope Nicholas I ordered the figure of the rooster placed on every church steeple.

Introduction of the chicken into the Western Hemisphere is still a matter of dispute among archaeologists with some claiming a pre-Columbian origin on the Pacific coast of South America by prehistoric Polynesian seafarers, but the most current and exhaustive DNA analysis strongly suggests that it occurred with the European colonization of the Americas in the 16th century AD *(PNAS, February, 2014)*. English settlers landing at Jamestown, Virginia in 1607 brought a flock of chickens that helped them survive their first harsh winters and chickens were also brought by the Pilgrim's to Plymouth Rock, Massachusetts in 2020. But the popularity of the Old World fowl soon faded, as turkey, goose, pigeon, duck and other hardier native birds were plentiful. In 1692, the Virginia General Assembly made it illegal for African slaves to own horses, cattle or pigs, but not chickens, which were considered not worth mentioning. This loophole offered an opportunity for slaves from West Africa, where raising chickens had a long history, to emerge as the chicken merchants of the North American colonies. One of the West African specialties that caught on among the English was chicken pieces fried in oil – the fried chicken that is now considered a quintessential American dish.

Slaves laid the foundation for the American taste for chicken, but it was the forced opening of China by the West in the 1840s that brought specimens of Asian chickens never seen before in America. Breeders crossed the large and colorful Chinese birds with the smaller but hardier Western breed to produce a bird that could lay more eggs and provide more meat. The results of this breeding are the famous varieties Plymouth Rock and Rhode Island Red. Still, up to the end of the 19th century, chicken rearing in the United States remained a small-scale family business mostly to produce eggs which were considered somewhat of a luxury.

This began to change with the arrival of millions of Eastern European Jewish immigrants in the 1890s who used chickens primarily as a meat source. By 1900, 1,500 kosher butcher shops were operating in New York City alone that were being supplied with live chickens that arrived in train box cars from farms in the Midwest where rural women ran much of the chicken business. The market for inexpensive chicken meat soon extended beyond immigrant Jews to include millions of people who were leaving their Midwestern and Southern farms for factory jobs in the Northeastern cities. World War I gave chickens another boost, when cattle and pig meat stocks were diverted to the troops. While the market for chicken meat expanded, chicken farming remained in the hands of many small farmers since large flocks could not be kept over the cold dark North American winters. A chicken farmer in the early 20th century would keep a dozen hens and a rooster over winter, and allowed the hens to hatch a brood of chicks each in the spring, bringing the flock to around 85 birds. The old rooster would be slaughtered after the chicks had hatched. The old hens and most of the young chickens would be sold in the fall, and one rooster and twelve hens would be kept over the next winter. Chickens were kept on diversified farms, so they mostly fed themselves with bugs, grubs and seeds, and spilled feed from other barnyard animals. The chickens generally had free rein of the barnyard where they would peck apart manure from horses and cows, and some farmers would let the hens into the vegetable garden for an hour or so of monitored bug control. By having 85 chickens during the plentiful summer months and only 13 over the lean winter months, farmers did not need to supplement the chickens feed with grain. This feeding regimen kept the chickens fed, but it did not produce a lot of eggs with the average hen laying only 83 eggs per year in 1900.

In 1923 a housewife named Celia Steele from Oceanview, Delaware, ordered 50 chicks from a hatchery and was sent 500 by mistake. She decided to keep all the birds, and by dosing them with the newly discovered vitamin A and D supplements, she was able to keep them crowded into large sheds throughout the winter. With such a strong chicken meat market in New York City, by 1926 Steele was raising 10,000 birds a year and by 1935 250,000. Celia Steele had invented the first factory farm.

The rise of chicken farming continued through the Great Depression, when raising chickens supplemented a small farmer's income. Henry Wallace, President Franklin Roosevelt's agriculture secretary (and later Vice President) from Iowa, argued that the chicken was the savior of poverty-stricken rural Americans. In 1936, Wallace and his business associates established Hy-Line International which was the first modern genetics company to incorporate hybridization into its breeding program for chickens to produce egg laying hens on a commercial scale. Hy-Line is still one of the major hybrid chicken breeding companies in the world. By the 1930s Arthur Perdue and John Tyson, had begun their own factory farmed chicken operations and they invested heavily in revolutionizing the chicken industry. Using cheap government subsidized hybrid maize for feed, Perdue and Tyson introduced automated chain-driven feeders and debeaking to prevent the birds from pecking at each other in close quarters. Electric fans made even greater densities possible and automated lights allowed for the manipulation of growing and egg laying cycles. By the 1940s sulpha drugs and antibiotics were being added to chicken feed to stimulate growth and hold down infectious diseases prevalent under conditions of intense confinement. Perdue and Tyson are still two of the largest chicken producing companies in the world.

By the 1950s chicken breeders had developed two distinct varieties of chickens: "layers" for egg production and "broilers" for meat production. The genetics and life-cycles of modern day chickens have been so altered by humans that they bear little resemblance to their ancestral jungle fowl. Broilers are so grotesquely overweight and contorted out of physical proportion that they can barely stand up. A wild chicken's natural life span is 15 years, but factory farmed broilers are slaughtered after only 42 days when they have reached market weight which is three times faster than in the 1950s. A project led by Michael Zody of Sweden's Uppsala University, researched the genetic differences between the wild red junglefowl and its modern day descendants. The researchers found important mutations from selective breeding in a thyroid-stimulating hormone receptor gene. In wild chickens this gene coordinates reproduction with day length, confining breeding to specific seasons. The mutation disabled this gene enabling chickens to breed and lay eggs all year long. By 2000 the average hen produced well over 300 eggs per year, more than three times the production in 1900. In the U.S., laying hens are usually slaughtered for "soup meat" after one to two years when their egg production starts to decline.

With such a fast turnover of millions of layers and broilers, maintaining a steady supply of new birds constantly running through the system became a major industry. The breeding process is a multi-staged operation. To maintain pure bred lines, "primary breeder flocks" are raised in hatcheries to produce true breeds that are delivered to "parent stock breeders." On parent stock breeding farms, chicks are raised to 20 weeks of age where they receive no more than 10 hours of light per day so they don't start laying eggs prematurely. After 20 weeks the chicks are transported to a "breeder farm" where they are raised in open floor houses with automatic watering, feeding, and egg collection systems. Roosters and hens are allowed to mate naturally. Hens begin producing eggs around 24 weeks of age and lay efficiently for 40 weeks per cycle. An average breeder hen will lay 150 to 180 eggs per year. The eggs are automatically collected daily, transported to the hatchery, and stored at 55-65° F and 70% humidity. The eggs are held at the hatchery for three to ten days prior to being placed in an incubator. Incubators hold thousands of eggs in a very controlled environment. The eggs are then transferred into hatching baskets where they hatch after 21 days. Within 12 hours of hatching the chicks are sexed, vaccinated, counted and placed in baskets for delivery to a "grow-out" farm. Rooster chicks of the laying breeds can't lay eggs and are unsuitable for meat production, so they are destroyed soon after sexing by breaking their necks, suffocation with carbon dioxide, or thrown live into a high speed grinder. After about a year of production, spent breeder chickens are slaughtered for "soup meat."

Harland Sanders (better known as "Colonel Sanders") made a major contribution to the popularization of chicken in the latter half of the 20th century. Sanders identified the potential of franchising restaurants by opening his first "Kentucky Fried Chicken" (KFC) outlet in Utah in 1952. By 2013, KFC was the world's second largest franchise restaurant chain (as measured by sales) in the world after McDonald's with 18,875 outlets in 118 countries and territories around the world. Though Sanders sold the franchise in 1964, his iconic image is still synonymous with KFC the world over.

In the 1960s, doctors made the link between cattle meat consumption and heart disease and chicken meat was widely recommended as a healthier, lower fat, lower cholesterol alternative. By 1992 chicken meat consumption had surpassed cattle meat consumption in the U.S. and has remained on top ever since.

Statistics on worldwide chicken meat consumption by the FAO lump chicken in with other "poultry" which includes turkey, quail, pigeon, duck and geese, but chicken accounts for the largest portion of the world's total poultry consumption *("FAOSTAT: ProdSTAT: Livestock Primary," 2007).* According to a 2012 FAO report, the world's top 15 poultry meat consuming countries per capita were:

Country	pounds/person/yr	kilograms/person/yr
1. Kuwait	166.9	75.7
2. Israel	149.7	67.9
3. U.S.	114.2	51.8
4. Bahamas	104.1	47.2
5. French Polynesia	102.5	46.5
6. Luxembourg	87.7	39.8
7. Australia	86.6	39.3
8. Canada	82.5	37.4
9. UK	64.4	29.2
10. Spain	60.2	27.3
11. Argentina	59.1	26.8
12. Iceland	57.3	26.0
13. Portugal	56.0	25.4
14. Czech Republic	52.2	24.6
15. France	46.7	21.2

According to the FAO, the top 15 chicken meat consuming countries by tonnage on average between 2010-2012 (counting the EU as one country) were:

Country	million tonnes
1. U.S.	19.2
2. China	17.1
3. Brazil	13.1
4. EU	12.4
5. Russia	3.2

6.	India	2.9
7.	Mexico	2.8
8.	Argentina	1.8
9.	Indonesia	1.7
10.	Iran	1.7
11.	Turkey	1.6
12.	Malaysia	1.5
13.	South Africa	1.5
14.	Japan	1.4
15.	Canada	1.2

According to the *US Poultry and Egg Association*, yearly egg consumption in the U.S. topped out at 258.1/person/year in 2007 and stood at 247.9/person/year in 2010. According to the International Egg Commission, the top 15 egg consuming countries per capita in 1999 were:

Country	eggs/person/yr
1. Japan	320
2. Czech Republic	297
3. Mexico	295
4. Hungary	268
5. France	264
6. US	255
7. Belgium	242
8. Denmark	239
9. Austria	235
10. Russia	227
11. Germany	224
12. Italy	224
13. Spain	221
14. Cyprus	218
15. China	206

According to the FAO, the top 10 egg producing countries in the world in 2011 were:

Country	egg production (X 1,000)
1. China	477,940,000
2. US	91,855,000
3. India	63,500,000
4. Japan	41,377,000
5. Mexico	47,622,740
6. Russia	40,778,280
7. Brazil	40,730,688
8. Indonesia	24,911,000
9. Ukraine	18,428,100
10. France	14,087,635

In 2009, an estimated 62.1 million metric tons of eggs were produced worldwide from a total laying flock of approximately 6.4 billion hens. *(WATT Ag Net – Watt Publishing Co)* and more than 50 billion chickens were reared annually as a source of both meat and eggs. According to the FAO, the world's average chicken population on any given day is almost 19 billion, nearly three times the human population. To produce this massive quantity of eggs and meat, over 99% of layers and broilers raised in America today are factory farmed and factory farming is now a common practice around the world. According to the Worldwatch Institute, 74% of the world's poultry meat and 68% of eggs are produced on factory farms *("Towards Happier Meals In A Globalized World", World Watch Institute).*

Factory farmed broilers and layers are housed inside large sheds containing up to 20,000 birds living under artificial light their whole lives. In the U.S., chickens are routinely dosed with anti-biotics in their feed to reduce the prevalence of infectious diseases that can spread quickly through flocks under such crowded conditions. This wide scale indiscriminate use of anti-biotics has led to the evolution of anti-biotic resistant bacteria that are increasingly making anti-biotics ineffective to control bacterial infections in humans. Broiler chickens live in open floor space until they reach six weeks old when "chicken catchers" come into the shed, grab them violently by the legs and throw them into crates for transport to the slaughterhouse. Most layers are raised in battery cage systems, so called because the rows and columns of the identical wire cages the hens live in share common divider walls resembling the cells of a battery. In these wire cages where about 95% of laying hens spend their entire one to two year lives; each hen is given about 76 square inches of space (a standard 8 1/2" by 11" sheet of paper measures 93.5 square inches) and the floor of the cage is also wire mesh so their feces drops down to the floor for convenient removal. The chickens live constantly breathing in the overwhelming stench of ammonia. After 12 months of laying, commercial hens' egg-laying capacity starts to decline to the point where they are uneconomical so many flocks are "force-molted", to reinvigorate egg-laying. This involves complete withdrawal of food for 7 to 14 days to cause body weight loss of 25 to 35% which forces the hen to lose her feathers, but also reinvigorates egg-production. In 2003, more than 75% of all flocks in the U.S. were force-moulted.

More than one million chickens are slaughtered every hour in the U.S. alone. To slaughter this many chickens every hour of every day requires slaughterhouses that are highly mechanized assembly line operations. At the slaughterhouse, the chickens sit jammed in crates on delivery trucks without food or water for up to 9 hours waiting to be killed. They are then dumped out of the crates where workers again violently grab them and force their legs into shackles so that they are hanging upside-down on a movable conveyor belt. The birds' heads and upper bodies are then dragged through an electrified water trough called a "stunner." This electric shock does not actually render the birds unconscious, its purpose is to immobilize them to keep them from thrashing on the slaughter line and to paralyze the muscles of their feather follicles so that their feathers will come out easily after they are killed. The birds are intentionally kept alive during the slaughter process so that their hearts will continue to pump blood during the "bleedout" process. Following the "stun" bath, the paralyzed but fully conscious birds' throats are cut by a rotating machine blade and/or a manual neck cutter. Although both carotid arteries should be severed quickly to ensure a relatively rapid death, these arteries are often missed, and many birds enter the "bleedout tunnel" still alive. They hang upside down for 90 seconds in the bleedout tunnel where they are supposed to die from blood loss, but millions of birds do not die and are plunged into the scalding-hot water of the "defeathering" tanks still conscious. According to one former slaughterhouse worker, when chickens are scalded alive, they *"... flop, scream, kick, and their eyeballs pop out of their heads. They often come out of the other end with broken bones and disfigured and missing body parts because they've struggled so much in the tank."* ("Poultry Slaughter The Need for Legislation", United Poultry Concerns, Machipongo, Virginia 23405 US, 2007).

In 2007, over 9 billion chickens were slaughtered in the U.S., 640 million in Canada, 7 billion in Europe, and 850 million in Great Britain. Worldwide, approximately 52 billion poultry were reported slaughtered in 2007, more than 50 billion of them chickens, including egg-laying hens *(WATT Executive Guide To World Poultry Trends 2009/10).*

Avian influenza (commonly known as bird flu) is a disease that infects birds with Type A influenza viruses. These viruses occur naturally among wild aquatic birds worldwide and can infect domestic poultry and other bird and animal species. Symptoms include: sudden death without any signs; lack of coordination; purple discoloration of the wattles, combs, and legs; soft-shelled or misshapen eggs; lack of energy and appetite; diarrhea; swelling of the head, eyelids, comb, wattles and hocks; nasal discharge; decreased egg production; coughing, sneezing. Bird flu was first recorded in Italy in 1878. Originally known as Fowl Plague, there were several outbreaks in poultry flocks in the early 20th century, including two in the U.S. in 1924 and 1929. In 1955, it was discovered that the Fowl Plague was caused by the influenza virus. It wasn't until 1997, however, when a highly pathogenic bird flu strain identified as H5N1 was discovered to have infected humans in Hong Kong, that the avian influenza virus had mutated into a zoonotic disease (a disease that can be passed between animals and humans). The 1997 outbreak of H5N1 bird flu in poultry flocks spread to numerous other countries in Asia, Africa, the Middle East and Europe, and by 2011, 573 people had become infected of whom 336 died. In modern factory farmed poultry operations where thousands of genetically similar birds live in dark, moist, crowded conditions that act as incubators for disease, bird flu outbreaks spread like wildfire. When a flock is infected the only remedy for the chicken farmer is to destroy the entire flock. In June 2015, a major avian influenza outbreak hit poultry flocks in the Midwestern U.S. and according to the U.S. Department of Agriculture led to the death of more than 48 million birds in a dozen states. Iowa was the hardest hit, euthanizing more than 31 million birds, including approximately 40% of the state's 60 million laying hens. Euthanizing and disposing of millions of infected carcasses presents major logistical problems. For laying hens, most of which are housed in battery cages, euthanasia by carbon-dioxide gas is the preferred method and for broiler chickens which are floor-reared, the use of water-based foam similar to that used by firefighters is used to suffocate large flock in a short period of time. Depending on local conditions, the dead birds are composted on-site, composted off-site, buried, moved to landfills or incinerated. Composting, in which dead birds are laid in rows, mixed with a bulking agent such as wood chips or saw dust, is the preferred method of disposal because the virus is killed by the heat produced as the birds decompose. Buried in landfills the virus can survive and contaminate the soil or groundwater. Although H5N1 hasn't yet evolved into a virus that can spread easily among people, scientists have found a few small differences in newer strains. Some of the H5N1 strains that are circulating now are becoming better at spreading disease among animals. Since viruses are masters of mutation, some scientists worry that its only a matter of time before a highly pathogenic avian influenza mutates into a form that can spread readily from human to human.

Over the course of the 20th century, as commercial chicken farming grew from small scale production for local consumption to large scale production of a staple food for billions of people, the structure of the industry underwent a complete makeover. Like the cattle industry, the chicken industry is now vertically integrated to where large corporations like Tyson and Perdue own and control multiple stages of production including the breeder flocks, hatchery, slaughterhouse, processing plant, feed mill, transportation, and marketing. According to the chicken industry trade group, WATT Global Media, of the thousands of vertically integrated poultry corporations they analyzed worldwide in 2014, the top 9 were:

Corporation	Country	Chickens slaughtered annually, in millions
1. JBS S.A.	Brazil	3,380
2. Tyson Foods, Inc.	U.S.	2,310
3. CP Group	Thailand	939
4. Industrias Bachoco	Mexico	702
5. New Hope Group	China	700
6. Perdue Farms	US	654
7. Koch Foods Inc.	US	624
8. Uifrango Agroindustrial	Brazil	520
9. Arab Company for Livestock Development	Saudi Arabia	500

These vertically integrated poultry corporations own every step of the process from top to bottom, except one – the farming. The integrated corporation provides all the chicks and the feed to "independent" farmers, who contract to house and feed them. The farmer grows the birds to market size and when the poultry corporation picks them up for slaughter, the farmer gets paid. The size of the payment depends on how efficiently the farmer converted feed to meat. The corporations grade on a curve; the farmers that grow the biggest chickens get a bonus and the farmers with relatively smaller birds get penalized. Scott Marlow, Director of the nonprofit *Rural Advancement Foundation International – USA* (RAFI), a farmer advocacy group, notes that under this contract system:

> "No matter what happens, some of the farmers are always going to win and lose, but the company always wins. Farmers have to consistently compete, but the company's average payment is always the same. Most poultry farmers take out very expensive loans for their facilities. A million plus is an average loan. In most cases the farmer's home, land, and assets are tied to those big loans. If a person gets dropped in their ranking, then they are unable to start paying back these loans, so it forces farmers to chase after upgrades in the hope they can make more money. At first farmers who invests their nest egg into a big loan from the bank do well, but as time passes, other farmers surpass them, and they start making less and less. Finally, they go bankrupt, and sell the farm to the next round."

Under this contract system of chicken farming, the economic fate of independent chicken farmers is totally in the hands of the vertically integrated poultry corporations.

To raise this enormous worldwide flock of chickens requires huge amounts of chicken feed and chicken feed has become a significant segment of the livestock feed industry. Cereal use for poultry production differs across countries, with maize dominating in Brazil, China and the U.S., and wheat in the EU. Maize is the predominant grain used in commercial poultry feed because it has a high energy content and is easy for the chickens to digest. The amino acid profile of the protein in maize complements the amino acid profile of the other ingredients typically used in feed. Other grains are evaluated in relation to maize. Sorghum, barley, wheat and rapeseed are also commonly used in chicken feed. Fats and oils added to the feed provide a concentrated source of energy. Sources of fat include tallow (cow fat), lard (pig fat), poultry fat and reprocessed restaurant grease and cooking oil. Additional protein sources include fish meal, meat and bone meal, field peas, soybeans and cereal byproducts. Cereal byproducts are the by-products from the production of flour such as grain hulls, bran, germ, gluten meal, tailings, chaff, weed seeds and broken grains. Commercial feed producers also supplement feed with vitamins and minerals. U.S. feed suppliers supplement with the mineral arsenic to promote faster growth and increased feed efficiency, that is, fatter chickens on less feed. Arsenic is a cancer causing mineral that gets into the chicken meat that people eat. Most of the producers of animal feed are part of the vertically integrated corporations that control the chicken industry. According to the WATT Global Media group cited above, the top 10 livestock feed (which includes poultry, cattle and pig feed) corporations worldwide in 2014 were:

Corporation	Country	annual production (x1000 metric tons)
1. Cargill	US	19,500
2. New Hope Liuhe	China	15,710
3. Purina Animal Nutrition	US	12,700
4. CPP	China	12,400
5. Wen's Food Group	China	12,000
6. BRF	Brazil	10,360
7. Tyson Foods	US	10,000
8. East Hope Group	China	7,600
9. Jah Zen-Noh	Japan	7,200
10. Shuangbaotal Group	China	6,600

Providing this much chicken meat and eggs to billions of people worldwide is having major environmental impacts on a local and global scale. A 2007 paper published by the *Animal Production and Health Division of the FAO* entitle, *"Poultry production and the environment – a review,"* identifies these local impacts:

> *"Poultry facilities are a source of odour and attract flies, rodents and other pests that create local nuisances and carry disease. Odour emissions from poultry farms adversely affect the life of people living in the vicinity. Odour associated with poultry operations comes from fresh and decomposing waste products such as manure, carcasses, feathers and bedding/*

litter (Kolominskas et al., 2002; Ferket et al., 2002). On-farm odour is mainly emitted from poultry buildings, and manure and storage facilities... Flies are an additional concern for residents living near poultry facilities. Research conducted by the Ohio Department of Health indicated that residences that were located in close proximity to poultry facilities (within half a mile) had 83 times the average number of flies... Pesticides used to control pests (e.g. parasites and disease vectors) and predators have been reported to cause pollution when they enter groundwater and surface water. Active molecules or their degradation products enter ecosystems in solution, in emulsion or bound to soil particles, and may, in some instances, impair the uses of surface waters and ground water (World Bank, 2007)... Improper disposal of poultry carcasses can contribute to water-quality problems especially in areas prone to flooding or where there is a shallow water table. Methods for the disposal of poultry carcasses include burial, incineration, composting and rendering. In the case of recent highly pathogenic avian influenza (HPAI) outbreaks, the disposal of large numbers of infected birds has presented new and complex problems associated with environmental contamination. Large volumes of carcasses can generate excessive amounts of leachate and other pollutants, increasing the potential for environmental contamination... Poultry slaughterhouses release large amounts of waste into the environment, polluting land and surface waters as well as posing a serious human-health risk. The discharge of biodegradable organic compounds may cause a strong reduction of the amount of dissolved oxygen in surface waters, which in turn may lead to reduced levels of activity or even death of aquatic life. Macronutrients (nitrogen, phosphorus) may cause eutrophication of the affected water bodies. Excessive algal growth and subsequent dying off and mineralization of these algae may lead to the death of aquatic life because of oxygen depletion (Verheijen, et al., 1996).

Slaughterhouses are usually located in urban or peri-urban locations, where transport costs to markets are minimized and where there is abundant labour supply. This situation increases the risk of environmental impacts: first, because slaughterhouses often lack the land required to set up waste-management facilities; second, because the pollutants that are emitted add to those emitted by other human activities; and third, because neighbouring communities are directly affected by surface-water and groundwater contamination... The rapid growth of intensive poultry production in many parts of the world has created regional and local phosphorus imbalances (Gerber et al., 2005). The application of manure has resulted in more phosphorus being applied than crops require, and increased potential for phosphorus losses in surface runoff. Too much phosphorus input into a body of water leads to plant overgrowth, shifts in plant varieties, discolouration, shifts in pH, and depletion of oxygen as a result of plant decomposition. A drop in the level of dissolved oxygen in surface water has deleterious effects on fish populations (Ferket et al., 2002). Thus, increased out puts of phosphorus to *fresh water can accelerate eutrophication, which impairs water use and can lead to fish kills and toxic algal blooms. In general, 80 percent of the phosphorus contained in animal feed is subsequently excreted (Burton and Turner, 2003)... With increasing use of metals not only as growth promoters, but also as feed additives to combat diseases in intensive poultry production, manure application has emerged as an important source of environmental contamination with some of these metals. Metals such as arsenic, cobalt, copper, iron, manganese, selenium and zinc are added to feeds as a means to prevent disease, improve weight gain and feed conversion, and increase egg production (Bolan et al., 2004; Jackson et al., 2003)... The excretion of hormones from poultry has been cited as a possible cause of endocrine disruption in wildlife. Endocrine disruptors are a class of compounds (either synthesized or naturally occurring), which are suspected to have adverse effects in animals. They affect organisms primarily by binding to hormone receptors and disrupting the endocrine system. Endocrine disrupting chemicals (EDCs) include pesticides, herbicides and other chemicals that interact with endocrine systems (University of Maryland, 2006)... Atmospheric ammonia (NH_3) is increasingly being recognized as a major air pollutant because of its role in regional-scale tropospheric chemistry and its effects when deposited into ecosystems. Ammonia is a soluble and reactive gas. This means that it dissolves, for example in water, and that it will react with other chemicals to form ammonia-containing compounds... The concentrations of ammonia in the air are greatest in areas where there is intensive livestock farming... Impacts of ammonia deposition include; soil and water acidification, eutrophication caused by nitrogen enrichment with consequent species loss, vegetation damage, and increases in emissions of the greenhouse gases such as nitrous oxide."*

The FAO report cites the following global impacts of the poultry industry:

"The extraordinary performance of the poultry sector over the past three decades has partially been achieved through soaring use of concentrate feed, particularly cereals and soybean meal (FAO, 2006a). We estimate that in 2004 the poultry sector utilized a total of 294 million tonnes of feed, of which approximately 190 million tonnes were cereals, 103 million tonnes soybean meal and 1.6 million tonnes fishmeal... Estimates put the global use of cereals for feed (all species included) at 666 million tonnes, or about 35 percent of total world cereal use (FAO, 2006a). This implies that in 2004 cereal utilization as feed by the poultry sector represented about 28 percent of the cereal and 75 percent of soybean meal used by the livestock sector... Demand for feed by the livestock sector has been a trigger for three major global trends: the intensification of feed production, agricultural expansion and erosion of biodiversity. The production of feed has an impact on the environment at various stages of crop production. In terms of the environment, these three trends have had a number of global impacts, which include land and water pollution, air pollution, greenhouse gas emissions, land-use change

through deforestation and habitat change, and overexploitation of non-renewable resources... Intensification of feed production affects land and water resources through pollution caused by the intensive use of mineral fertilizer, pesticides and herbicides to maintain high crop yields. It is estimated that only 30–50 percent of applied nitrogen fertilizer (Smil, 1999) and approximately 45 percent of phosphorus fertilizer (Smil, 2000) is taken up by crops. Steinfeld et al. (2006) estimated that about 20 million tonnes of nitrogen fertilizer were used in feed production for the livestock sector. Based on the estimation that the poultry sector utilizes 36 percent of feed concentrates (cereals and soybean), we can attribute about 7.2 million tonnes of nitrogen fertilizer use to feed production for the sector... The application of nitrogen fertilizer to cropland is a major source of air pollution through the volatilization of ammonia. Assuming an average mineral fertilizer ammonia volatilization loss rate of 14 percent, it has been estimated that global livestock production can be considered responsible for a global ammonia volatilization from mineral fertilizer of 3.1 million tonnes of NH3-N (nitrogen in ammonia form) per year (Steinfeld et al., in FAO, 2006b). Based on these same assumptions, the poultry sector can be considered responsible for about 1.1 million tonnes of ammonia volatilization from mineral fertilizer per year... Increases in feed production, have to some extent been related to the expansion of cropland dedicated to feed... For example, the land area for soybean production in Brazil increased from 1 million hectares in 1970 to 24 million hectares in 2004 – half of this growth came after 1996, most of it in the Cerrado, with the remainder in the Amazon Basin (Brown, 2005)... Changes in land use can have profound impacts on carbon fluxes, leading to increased carbon release and fuelling climate change. In addition to changes in carbon fluxes, deforestation also has an impact on water cycles and increases runoff and consequently soil erosion. WWF (2003) estimates that a soy field in the Cerrado loses approximately 8 tonnes of soil per hectare per year... Feed production is also driving biodiversity erosion through the conversion of natural habitats and the overexploitation of non-renewable resources for feed production. Intensive feed production contributes to biodiversity loss through land use and land-use change, and modification of natural ecosystems and habitats. The demand for feed has triggered increased production and exports from countries such as Brazil... The production of fishmeal for the poultry sector is an important factor contributing to the overexploitation of fisheries... Current estimates are that around 40 percent of global fishmeal production is used for the livestock sector of which 13 percent is used by the poultry sector (Figure 2) (Jackson, 2007)... The relatively high energy input in intensive livestock systems has given rise to concerns regarding greenhouse gas emissions and climate change. The energy consumption of industrially produced poultry is relevant because of the production of carbon dioxide (CO2) along the production chain. Carbon dioxide emissions are produced by the burning of fossil fuels during animal production and slaughter, and transport of processed and refrigerated products, but importantly also through land use and land-use change, and the use of inputs for the production of feed... On-farm energy consumption includes direct and indirect energy input – direct energy refers to fossil energy used for the production process (e.g. energy input for poultry housing systems), and indirect energy to that used as an integral part of the production process (e.g. feed processing)... The energy used for heating, ventilation and air conditioning systems typically accounts for the largest quantity of energy used in intensive poultry operations... Other sources of carbon dioxide emissions include energy used for feed preparation, on-farm transport and burning of waste (EU, 2003). Generally, on layer farms, artificial heating of housing is not commonly applied, due to the low temperature needs of birds and the high stocking density. The activities that require energy are ventilation, feed distribution, lighting, and egg collection, sorting and preservation. On broiler farms, the main energy consumption is related to local heating, feed distribution and housing ventilation... it is estimated that about 52 million tonnes of carbon dioxide are emitted per year... In poultry abattoirs, fossil fuel is mainly used for process heat, while electricity is used for the operation of machinery and for refrigeration, ventilation, lighting and the production of compressed air. Ramírez et al. (2004) in an analysis of energy consumption in the EU meat industry found poultry slaughtering to be more energy intensive (3096 MJ/tonne dress carcass weight) than other meat sectors (1390 MJ/tonne dress carcass weight for beef and 2097 MJ/tonne dress carcass weight for pork)... Using the Ramírez et al. (2004) estimates of energy consumption values for poultry, we estimate that carbon dioxide emissions from poultry slaughtering facilities amount to 18 million tonnes... International trade in poultry meat contributes significant carbon dioxide emissions – induced by fossil fuel use for the shipping of poultry meat. Steinfeld et al. (in FAO, 2006b) estimated carbon dioxide emissions by combining traded volumes with respective distances, vessel capacities and speeds, fuel use of main and auxiliary power generators for refrigeration, and their respective emission factors. Based on this analysis, trade in poultry meat was found to contribute an estimated 256 000 tonnes of carbon dioxide (representing about 51 percent of the total carbon dioxide emissions induced by meat-trade ocean transport)... Emissions of greenhouse gases such as carbon dioxide and nitrous oxide are influenced in an indirect way by intensification of feed production, which requires energy input for the production of mineral fertilizer and the subsequent use of this fertilizer in the feed production process... [Carbon dioxide] gas is produced by the burning of fossil fuels during the manufacture of fertilizer... [Poultry production] results in an estimated annual carbon dioxide emission of 18 million tonnes – about 44 percent of that ascribed to the livestock sector... Poultry production is indirectly associated with the greenhouse gas nitrous oxide because of the sector's high concentrate-feed requirements and the related emissions from arable land due to the use of nitrogen fertilizer. FAO–IFA (2001) reported a 1 percent N2O-N (nitrogen in nitrous oxide) loss rate from nitrogen mineral fertilizer applied to arable land. By applying this loss rate to the total nitrogen fertilizer attributed to the poultry sector, we estimate that nitrous oxide emissions from poultry feed related fertilizer to be 0.07 million tonnes of N2O-N per year – about 35 percent of the global nitrous oxide emissions attributed to the livestock sector from mineral fertilizer application. Overall, intensive poultry production (indirectly and directly) contributes an estimated 3 percent of the total anthropogenic greenhouse gas and is responsible for about 2 percent of the total greenhouse gas emissions from the livestock sector. This estimate however does not include emissions from land use and land-use change associated with feed production or emissions related to transport of feed."

While chickens are far more efficient at converting feed grains into animal protein than are cattle, it is simply not possible to produce chicken meat and eggs as staple foods for billions of people worldwide without causing severe environmental impacts on both a local and global scale. To raise and process billions of chickens every year is simply an unsustainable agricultural practice. As we humans increasingly place ourselves atop the trophic pyramid, so we preside over the ecological decline of our planet.

18
FISH

According to FishBase, the world's largest fish database: as of April, 2015, over 33,000 species of fish had been described taxonomically with about 250 new species discovered every year. That is more than the total number of species of mammals, amphibians, reptiles and birds combined. Unlike mammals, amphibians, reptiles and birds that are each thought to have evolved from one common ancestor, fish are thought to have evolved from multiple ancestors that include jawless, cartilaginous and vertebrate types.

Fish species are divided between salt water (oceans and seas) and fresh water (rivers and lakes) ecosystems. There is 10,000 times more salt water in the oceans and seas than there is fresh water in all the Earth's rivers and lakes, yet only 58% of fish species are salt water as compared to 41% fresh water, with the remaining 1% being anadromous or catadromous fish that inhabit both salt and fresh water at different times in their life cycles. This disproportionate diversity of fresh water species is due to their inhabiting tens of thousands of distinct lake ecosystems which promotes greater diversity through isolation and speciation. Whether by species count or abundance, most fish species live in warmer environments with relatively stable temperatures.

Coral reefs in the Indian and Pacific Oceans are the most diverse sites for salt water species of fish, and the Amazon, Congo and Mekong River basins are the most diverse sites for fresh water species.

Exceptionally rich fresh water sites such as Cantão State Park in the Amazon River basin, can contain more fresh water fish species than occur in all of Europe.

Fish are also categorized as "demersal" (those that live on or near the bottom of oceans or lakes) or "pelagic" (those that live up from the bottom). Pelagic fish are further categorized as "epipelagic" (inhabiting sunlit waters down to 650 feet), "mesopelagic" (inhabiting deeper twilight waters down to 3,300 feet), or "bathypelagic" (inhabiting the cold pitch black depths below 3,300 feet). Seventy-eight percent of salt water pelagic species live near the shoreline in the relatively shallow waters of the continental shelf, while only 13% live out in the open ocean.

Ninety-six percent of all fish species are vertebrates known as "teleosts" (Greek: *teleios*, "complete" + *osteon*, "bone"). The main difference between teleosts and the other 4% of vertebrate fish species is in their jaw bones; teleosts have a movable bone in their upper jaw that allows them to protrude their jaws outwards from the mouth. Teleosts range from the giant oarfish that can measure 25 feet (7.6 meters) long to the ocean sunfish that can weigh over 2 tons, to the tiny anglerfish just 1/4 inch (6.2 millimeters) short that barely tips the scale. Teleosts take a great variety of shapes including torpedo-shaped, elongated cylinders, flat bodied either vertically or horizontally, and even segmented with bony armor, upright posture and a curled tail like the seahorse. Teleosts ply the waters of the Earth from pole to pole inhabiting the ocean depths, estuaries, rivers, lakes and even swamps.

Of the over 33,000 identified fish species, the relatively few species consumed by humans are nearly all teleosts; the more common of these species include: anchovy, bass, carp, catfish, cod, flounder, grouper, haddock, halibut, herring, mackerel, perch, pike, pollock, rockfish, salmon, sardine, smelt, snapper, sole, sturgeon, swordfish, tilapia, trout, tuna and whitefish. While evidence suggest that our early *homo erectus* ancestors likely hunted fish as long as 500,000 years ago, fish predation did not become a wide spread practice by H. sapiens until neolithic times around 11,500 years ago. From these primitive beginnings, fish consumption has become a major source of animal protein for billions of people around the world in modern times, especially those living in coastal areas and near inland rivers and lakes. Let's take a closer look into the history of human fish predation and consumption.

The earliest permanent human settlement known to have depended on fish as a staple food source was discovered at an archaeological site called Lepenski Vir, located in modern day Serbia. Radiocarbon dated bones from this site on the banks of the Danube River indicate that a fish hunting culture flourished there during Neolithic times from 11,500 to 8,000 years ago (9500 to 6000 BC). The settlement at Lepenski Vir sits on a narrow plateau squeezed between cliffs on the river banks, ideal for hunting fish but offering little in the way of terrestrial food resources. Fish hunting communities of this type were common in the wider Danube valley region during the early stages of this period. Genomes of 235 ancient inhabitants of Lepenski Vir were mapped, indicating that around 9,500 years ago (7500 BC), Neolithic agriculturalists from Asia Minor (modern day Turkey), began to mix with the indigenous population of Lepenski Vir and they introduced a completely new way of life. With them came farming of the first grain crops and tending of the first domesticated herd animals. Lepenski Vir is the rare archaeological site that provides evidence of the transition from the hunter gatherer way of life in Upper Paleolithic times (50,000 to 10,000 years ago) to the agricultural food economy of Neolithic times (12,000 to 6,500 years ago).

Archaeological sites as far flung as Europe, Japan and India indicate that hunting fish with barbed tipped harpoons became widespread in the Upper Paleolithic period. The famed Cosquer cave drawings in Southern France dating back over 16,000 years depict harpoons being used to hunt seals. But most of the fish hunting technologies that are in use today, such as hook and line, weirs, and nets, were first invented by Neolithic agriculturalists as they emigrated around the globe between 8,000 and 4,000 years ago.

The Hook and Line

While archaeological remains of the first fish hooks (called "gorges") that were made of bone date back ~7,000 years, the first evidence of humans using line to hunt fish are depictions in Egyptian art from around 4,000 years ago. Archaeologists assume that vines were used as the first line long before the Egyptian civilization, but since line was made of organic materials that quickly decomposed, there is no trace of them left in the archaeological record. The first account of silk fishing line dates back to between 4,400 and 4,300 years ago (2400 BC and 2300 BC) Chinese text that describes fish hunting with a silk line, a bamboo pole, and a hook made from bone and baited with cooked rice. In 15th century AD England (500 years ago), fish hunters braided horse hair into line, and 16th century English diarist, Samuel Pepys, wrote of line made with catgut. As Christian Crusaders brought silk production back to Western Europe from the Middle East, particularly Italy and France, manufacture of stronger more durable silk line became the standard. Around this same time, long linen lines woven from flax were used to hunt large ocean fish.

The first direct antecedent of the modern fish hook was a device archaeologists call a "gorge". A gorge was a piece of bone or wood that was notched in the center so a line could be tied to it. The gorge was baited and when the fish swallowed it, the line was yanked so the gorge would set cross-wise inside the fish and catch so the fish could be hauled in. One of the earliest types of gorge was unearthed from a peat bed 22 feet below the surface in Somme, France, estimated to be about 7,000 years old. There is also evidence of Native Americans on the coast of present day California hunting fish with gorges around 7,000 years ago.

The earliest known examples of bent barbless hooks are from the 1st Egyptian Dynasty approximately 5,000 years ago (~ 3000 BC), and the first metal barbed fish hooks appeared during the 12th dynasty between 4,000 and 3,800 years ago (2000 BC and 1800 BC). Egyptians using hook and line to hunt Nile perch, catfish and eels from small reed boats is depicted on the walls of tombs and on surviving papyrus scrolls. In the early Egyptian civilization, fishing with hook and line was depicted as a subsistence means of obtaining food for commoners, but depictions in the later 18th and 19th Egyptian dynasties show upper class Egyptian officials and their wives hunting fish with hook and line as a form of leisure.

Fish hooks were developed independently by many different cultures around this time, but perhaps the best chronology of the progressive development of the fish hook is seen in artifacts left by the cultures that lived in the Swiss Lakes country. Once they began to work with bronze, they designed a metal gorge that was a wire straight on either side, but with a little hump in the middle where the line was attached. The next change was to give a slight curve to the wire arms of the gorge that were later bent further into the shape of a hook. Then some ancient artisan twisted the wire so an eyelet was formed in the center. Fish hunting cultures from Europe, Middle East, Asia, and Africa likely developed fish hooks in a similar fashion.

In ancient Greece, fish was a common food of coast dwellers. As early as 800 BC (2,800 years ago), the Greek writer, Homer, in his famous "Iliad" describes baited hook and line. While fish was a subsistence food for coast dwellers in ancient Greece, fish hunting was considered of low status and not generally the subject of art. There is a rare scene, however, on a wine cup dating back to 500 BC (2,500 years ago) of a boy crouched on a rock with a fishing pole in his hand and a fish trap in the water below. Later, during the heyday of ancient Greek culture in the 4th and 5th centuries BC, Greek philosophers Herodotus, Plato and Aristotle wrote of hunting fish with hook and line. In a 2nd century BC account from the 40 volume tome, "*Histories*," by the Greek historian, Polybius, is a description of hunting swordfish using a harpoon with a barbed and detachable head. And in his "*Comparative biographies*" of famous Greeks and Romans written in the 1st century AD as Rome was ascendant, Greek writer, Plutarch, gave tips on fish hunting with hook and line.

There are also references to hunting fish with hook and line found in ancient Chinese, Assyrian and Hebrew texts.

Between 177 and 180 AD, Greco-Roman poet, Oppian of Corycus, composed a series of didactic poems in Greek hexameter: one on hunting land animals (*Kynēgetiká*), one on hunting birds (*Ixeutiká*), and one on hunting fish (*Halieutiká*). His poem on hunting fish is dedicated to Emperor Marcus Aurelius, who historically has come to symbolize the Golden Age of the Roman Empire. In the 3rd century AD (between 1,800 and 1,700 years ago), Roman rhetorician, Claudius Aelian, wrote about hunting Macedonian trout using artificial flies as lures. In the 6th century AD, after the Roman Empire had moved its center of government to Constantinople (present day Istanbul, Turkey), the enlightened Emperor, Justinian I, convened a council of legal scholars to conduct a uniform rewriting of Roman law that produced the "*Corpus Juris Civilis*," ("*Body of Civil Law*") which is still the basis of civil common law in many modern countries. Known as the Justinian Code, it was in this document that the right of common people to access fish bearing waters for subsistence fish hunting was first established. This legal concept is the forerunner of the modern day "Public Trust Doctrine" that sets aside natural resources as a public good:

> *"By the law of nature these things are common to mankind – the air, running water, the sea,*
> *and consequently the shores of the sea. No one, therefore, is forbidden to approach the seashore,*

provided that he respects habitations, monuments, and buildings which are not, like the sea, subject only to the law of nations."

"The seashore extends as far as the greatest winter flood runs up. The public use of the seashore, too, is part of the law of nations, as is that of the sea itself; and, therefore, any person is at liberty to place on it a cottage, to which he may retreat, or to dry his nets there, and haul them from the sea; for the shores may be said to be the property of no man, but are subject to the same law as the sea itself, and the sand or ground beneath it."

Modern versions of the public trust doctrine generally allow for governments to regulate the private take of public trust assets like fish and wildlife.

Modern day "sport fishing" had its origins in 15th century England; the first mention of sport fishing comes from the essay *"Treatyse of Fysshynge wyth an Angle"* (*"Treatise of Fishing with an Angle"*) in 1496 by Dame Juliana Berners, the prioress of the Benedictine Sopwell Nunnery on the River Ver in southeastern England. Her treatise describes the construction of hooks and rods for the new sport of "angling." For about 150 years it was the basis of sports fishing knowledge in England. In 1653, English angler Isaac Walton published *"The Complete Angler"*, or the *"Contemplative Man's Recreation"*, considered by some historians to be the most influential book ever published on sport fishing. In it Walton describes the art of constructing tackle, the science of basic aquatic biology, and the philosophy of recreational anglers. Around this same time unknown anglers invented the reel to take up and hold long lines, and attached a wire loop at the tip end of the rod which allowed a running line, useful for casting and "playing" a hooked fish. Sport fishing was initially reserved for the wealthy classes, but in the 18th century as technological advances meant better equipment could be manufactured relatively cheaply, it gradually became more accessible to the less affluent. When the first motorboats appeared in the 19th century, big-game fishing started to become popular. Marine biologist Charles Frederick Holder is generally considered the father of this branch of fishing. Hand braided horsehair was used as line from the time angling first became a sport in the 15th century, until it was later replaced with superior braided silk line. Silk fiber is much stronger and longer than horsehair which meant it could be braided by machines instead of by hand, making it readily available to the growing numbers of sports fishermen. Linen line made from flax also appeared around this time and was used for big-game fishing. While silk and linen were superior to horsehair for fishing line, as organic materials they did not solve the problem of bacterial decay or damage from ultraviolet light. One spin-off from World War II was the invention of synthetic materials that were later applied to making fishing line. The first synthetic fishing line in the 1950s was made of polyester (marketed as Dacron by Du Pont). Dacron is still known for its strength and durability. With Du Pont's later invention of nylon, came the monofilament line made from a single, high-strength strand which is still in use today. Depending on the application, there are now specialty fishing lines made of various synthetic materials that are exceptionally strong and durable.

In modern times, fishing with hook and line whether for subsistence or sport accounts for only a tiny fraction of the worldwide fish catch.

The Weir

The English word "weir" comes from the Anglo-Saxon *wer*, meaning a device to trap fish. Weirs were probably in use predating the emergence of modern humans and have been used by people around the globe ever since. They were usually constructed of wood or stone and placed in tidal waters or in the flow of a river in such a configuration as to direct the passage of fish into a trap where they could be easily extracted from the water. Weirs were used very effectively to hunt marine fish in the inter-tidal zone, and to hunt anadromous fish such as salmon as they migrate up river to spawn, or catadromous fish such as eels as they migrate down river to spawn in the ocean.

Regional differences in weir construction techniques, materials used and species caught, depended on the resources available on site. Weirs can vary in size from small temporary brush frameworks to extensive complexes of stone walls and channels. Weirs on rivers or streams can be circular, wedge-shaped, or ovoid rings of posts or reeds, with an upstream opening. As the fish swim in they are trapped within the circle upstream of the current and cannot escape. Tidal fish traps are typically solid low walls of boulders or nets stretched across tidal basins. The fish swim over the top of the barrier at high tides, and as the water recedes with the tide, they are trapped behind.

In September, 2014, researchers from the University of Victoria, British Columbia, using a remote-controlled underwater vehicle turned up evidence of a sophisticated coastal community that existed around the time humans were first migrating to the New World. This underwater archaeological discovery was made near the Haida Gwaii archipelago 30 to 40 miles (45–60 kilometers) off the north Pacific coast of Canada. The area under investigation is now submerged under the Hectate Strait, but thousands of years ago it was lush, rolling landscape above sea level that provided a migration corridor for both animals, and the first humans to cross the Bering land bridge from Asia to North America. Archaeological digs on Haida Gwaii put humans on the islands 12,700 years ago, but researchers suspected the shallow waters in the Hectate Strait contained evidence of human habitation as far back as 17,000 years ago. With their remote-controlled underwater vehicle, they discovered a line of rocks that appears to be a fish weir, which at over 13,700 years old, makes it the oldest weir discovered thus far anywhere in the world.

Fish weirs are difficult to date, in part because while they may have been in continuous use for decades or even centuries, they were necessarily dismantled and rebuilt many times in the same locations, so the archaeological remains are often not from the original structure. Fish bone assemblages from adjacent middens are used by scholars as a proxy for dating fish weirs, as well as sediments containing pollen or charcoal at the bottom of the weirs. Another proxy used to date weirs is to identify local environmental changes such as changing sea level or the formation of sandbars that would impact the weir's use. Archaeological evidence of fish weirs built by hunter-gatherer peoples have been found all around the world dating to the Mesolithic period in Europe (12,000 to 7,000 years ago), the Archaic period in North America (10,000 to 4,000 years ago), and the Jomon period in Asia (16,000 to 3,000 years ago).

The earliest known fish weirs in Europe are in marine and freshwater locations in the Netherlands, Denmark and Ireland dated to between 8,000 and 7,000 years ago. Two weir sites in Zamostje, Russia near Moscow, are dated to more than 7,500 years old, and wooden structures at Wooton-Quarr on the Isle of Wight and along the shores of the Severn estuary in Wales have been dated to over 6,500 years old.

Muldoon's Trap Complex is a stone-walled weir at Lake Condah in western Victoria, Australia, constructed around 6,600 years ago by aboriginals who removed basalt bedrock to create a bifurcated channel to trap eel. Muldoon's is one of many weirs located near Lake Condah.

Fish bone assemblages from marine sites in southern Africa suggest stone-walled weirs (called visvywers) dating back to 6,000 years ago.

The aforementioned Haida Gwaii weir off the north coast of British Columbia, is the oldest known weir in the world, but prehistoric weirs have also been discovered in many other locations across North America. A stake from the Sebasticook Fish Weir in central Maine, returned a radiocarbon date of 5,770 years old. A weir at Glenrose Cannery on the mouth of the Fraser River in British Columbia, dates from 5,280 to 4,500 years old. In the Back Bay area of Boston, Massachusetts, wooden stake remains of the Boylston Street Fishweir discovered while excavating subway tunnels and building foundations was determined to be a series of weirs built near the tidal shoreline between 5,200 and 3,700 years ago.

In South America stone weirs were in use on Chiloé Island off the coast of Chile 6,000 years ago, and a large series of weirs in the Baures region of Bolivia appears to have supported a dense human population around 5,000 years ago.

The earliest weirs in Japan are associated with the end of the Jomon period from 4,000 to 3,000 years ago.

Through much of the Middle Ages (500 AD to 1500 AD) in Western Europe, kings owned the rivers and lakes, and fish hunting for everyone else was strictly regulated. By the 13th century, human population expansion in England had placed heavy demands on rivers as sources of food and commerce, and the king's weirs on rivers around the country had diminished fish stocks and created barriers to commercial shipping. In 1215 AD this conflict came to a head, and King John was forced by rebel barons to sign the Magna Carta which, among other demands, required the king to remove his weirs, "... *throughout the whole of England, except on the sea coast*." Enforcement of the Magna Carta was a continuing source of conflict between the crown and the local gentry over the next five centuries. In 1535, a regulation enacted under King Henry VIII (1491-1547), apparently at the instigation of his chief minister and leading proponent of the "English Reformation," Thomas Cromwell, appointed commissioners in each county to oversee the *"putting-down"* of weirs. A collection of correspondences between courtiers, royal officials, friends and relatives of Henry VIII known as *"The Lisle Papers"* is considered by historians an important contemporary source of information on domestic life in the Tudor age. In this correspondence there is a detailed account of the struggle of the owners of the weir at Umberleigh in Devon to be exempted from this

1535 regulation. Successive "Salmon Fisheries Acts" in the 17th, 18th and 19th centuries placed heavy fines and prison sentences on anyone found guilty of obstructing salmon passage to their spawning grounds.

English settlers in North America quickly adopted the indigenous people's age old practice of building weirs which eventually became the source of conflict with other river stakeholders. In 1768, the Maryland General Assembly ordered all weirs on the Potomac River destroyed, and for the next six decades a concerted effort was made to destroy weirs that were considered an obstruction to navigation and a detriment to sport fishing. In the southeastern region of North America, now encompassing the States of Tennessee, Alabama, Georgia, South Carolina and North Carolina, the Cherokee Indian tribe had used weirs continuously for millennia before Europeans arrived. While much of the evidence of Cherokee life was destroyed during the forced removals conducted by the U.S. government throughout the 1800s, in 1775 an early Irish trader in the region named James Adair recorded this description of Cherokee weirs:

> *"The Indians have the art of catching fish in long crails, made with canes and hiccory splinters tapering to a point. They lay these at a fall of water, where stones are placed in two sloping lines from each bank, till they meet together in the middle of the rapid stream, where the intangled fish are soon drowned."*

Over the course of the next century, however, colonial settlers who poured into the region began to outlaw weirs as obstructions to commercial waterways, and by the 1870s most of the traditional Cherokee weirs had been abandoned.

As human populations continued to grow around the world, the ancient use of weirs on waterways to catch fish became increasingly at odds with exploitation of these valuable resources by commercial fishing and shipping interests. As of this writing in the early 21st century, weirs account for only a tiny fraction of the worldwide fish catch, and their use is primarily confined to indigenous peoples living in sparsely populated areas such as the far northern reaches of Canada.

Nets

Twine braided from grass, flax, tree fibers, or cotton knotted into a mesh to make netting has been used by humans to hunt fish since at least Neolithic times (12,000 to 6,500 years ago); the oldest archaeological remains of fish netting dating back to 11,540 years ago was found among other fishing equipment in the Karelian town of Antrea on the border between present day Russia and Finland. While ditching a swamp meadow in 1913, a local farmer dug up several objects that Finnish archaeologist, Sakari Pälsi, later identified as 18 floats, 31 weights and parts of a net. All the items were found in a relatively small area preserved in the bottom clay layer of what was then an ancient lake, suggesting the artifacts had come to rest all at one time as if a fisherman's boat had capsized. The net was made from willow and is 90 feet (27 meters) long by 4 feet (1.3 meters) wide, with a 2.4 inch (6 centimeters) mesh. This mesh size is suitable for fishing salmon and common bream. The net is laced with a knot called Ryssänsolmu which was used for thousands of years in the Baltic Sea region.

By Neolithic times, using nets to catch fish was widely practiced worldwide. Two cultures separated by thousands of miles of Pacific Ocean that developed highly sophisticated netting systems to catch fish, exemplify this diversity: the Chinookan of North America and the Maori of New Zealand.

Teaming salmon runs on the Columbia River and its tributaries in the Pacific Northwest of North America provided the indigenous people with a seemingly endless supply of fish to eat. The Chinookan peoples who inhabited these areas used purse seine nets to catch migrating salmon. The purse seine is a net drawn in a circle with floats at the top and weights at the bottom that is dropped to the river bed around a school of fish. The bottom of the net has a purse-string line that was drawn tight to capture the fish which were then hauled in to shore. Chinookan purse seine nets were made from wild grasses or fiber from spruce roots, the top line was floated with cedar sticks and the bottom line was weighted with stones.

Archaeological sites on the southwestern Pacific islands of New Zealand predating by thousands of years the arrival of the Englishman, Captain Cook, in 1769, reveal a trove of intricately carved hooks and lures made from shells by the indigenous Maori people. But other indicators of Maori fishing prowess suggest that they caught most of their fish with nets made of vegetable fibers that did not survive in the archaeological record. When Cook mapped the coastline of New Zealand, he noted vast arrays of wooden stakes used to support nets all along the shallower shores. Cook described nets of up to 33 feet (10 meters) deep and over 33 hundred feet (1 kilometer) long. This size of netting amounts to industrial-scale fishing, and indeed, fish bones and scales in coastal middens show a decrease in fish size over time, indicating a decline in fish numbers of netted species such as snapper, spotted shark, mackerel, maomao and mullet. The Maori also used hand scoop nets and large hoop nets lowered to the bottom, then raised up around a school of fish. The Maori were so technically proficient at catching fish, that Cook commented none of his men were a match for them as fishermen.

Tomb paintings depicting ancient Egyptians using nets to catch fish are dated to 3000 BC, and Japanese records from the Edo period (1603–1867 AD) trace gill net fishing there to 1000 BC. Roman poet Ovid, who wrote *Metamorphoses* in the 1st century AD, and the aforementioned Greco-Roman poet, Oppian, who wrote the *Halieutica* in the 2nd century AD, describe different kinds of fish nets. With the exception of now being made of modern synthetic materials, these ancient fish net designs have changed little to the present day:

- **Cast net** – relatively small round net (from 1.5 to 4 meters) with weights at its edge which is cast by hand to catch small fish when the net is hauled back in.
- **Lift net** – placed horizontally into the water with its opening facing upwards, it is then lifted by hand or mechanical device to capture and haul in fish.
- **Push net** – net with a large "belly" placed in a rigid frame that is pushed along the bottom in shallow waters in order to catch shrimps and small fishes that live at the bottom.
- **Purse seine net** – used to surround schools of fish, then a line is pulled which closes the bottom of the net trapping the fish and a whole net is hauled into a ship.

- **Gill net** – vertical net with floats at the top and weights at the bottom that ensnares fish behind the gill when they try to pass through the mesh.
- **Tangle net** – a variant of the gillnet but with smaller mesh size that ensnares fish not by their gills, but by their teeth or fins.

Gill nets are composed of vertical panels of netting that hang from a line with regularly spaced floaters at the top line and weights along the bottom line that are adjusted to hold the net vertically in the water at the desired depth. Gill nets work by allowing fish to passes only part way through the mesh, and as it struggles to free itself, the twine slips behind its gill-cover thus preventing escape. Archaeological evidence from the Middle East and Japan indicates that gillnets were in use by these civilizations in ancient times. Pre-Columbian Indians of northwest North America used gillnets made with nettles or the inner bark of cedar, floated with wood and weighted with stones. Gill nets were suspended by hand in shallow water close to shore or from canoes as drift nets out in the open ocean.

Commercial Fishing

Norwegian fishermen have a long cultural history of using gill nets to catch herring and cod. While fisher people the world over had sold their surplus catch at local fish markets for millennia, it was in the 10th century AD (~1,000 to 1,100 years ago) on the Lofoten Archipelago, in northern Norway where the Norse Vikings developed the first large scale commercial fishery. In this region, the regular seasonal spawning of Atlantic cod coincided with climatic conditions ideal for the freeze drying and long-term preservation of cod (aka "stockfish" or "klippfisk" in Norwegian) without the use of expensive salt. These unique conditions produced a high protein food source with a long shelf life that could be transported by Viking longship over great distances to markets in the burgeoning cities along the northern coast of Europe during the Middle Ages.

In 13th, 14th and 15th century Europe, as the continent was being carved-up into the rough outlines of the nation states we know today, much political, economic, and military power was vested in the larger cities which had developed as centers of increasingly inter-regional commerce. During this period in what is now northern Germany, dozens of cities joined together in a loose alliance called the Hanseatic League, with the port city of Lübeck on the Baltic Sea at its center. Initially the alliance was made for the purpose of providing mutual protection against raids from marauding pirates and bandits. In 1241, Lübeck, which had access to the Baltic Sea herring and cod fishing grounds, formed an alliance with Hamburg which had access to the North Sea fishing grounds and which controlled the salt-trade routes to the inland city of Lüneburg. These allied cities came to dominate the salt-fish trade by gaining control over the Scania Market in what is now southern Sweden. The Scania Market was then the world's largest fish market which took place annually and was one of the most important events for trade around the Baltic Sea. Scania served as a distribution hub for western European goods bound for eastern Scandinavia. The Scania Market continued to be a vital trade center for 250 years and was a cornerstone of the Hanseatic League's wealth. Over this time the League expanded by making treaties with cities on the rim of the North Sea in Germany, Belgium, England and Norway, and cities on the rim of the Baltic Sea in Poland, Latvia and finally, in 1436, Russia, putting an end to Scandinavian control over Baltic Sea trade-routes. The economic leverage that League merchants secured in the countries that needed their goods, was the mainstay of Hanseatic power. The bargain was German manufactured goods such as woolen and linen fabrics, carved and turned wood, engraved metals and armor, in exchange for natural resources such as copper, iron, timber, furs, and of course, salt cod and herring that was traded throughout Germany.

Dogger Bank

Scandinavian shipbuilding technology failed to advance beyond that of the Viking days, and while traditional Viking longships performed well in the relatively tranquil summer waters of the Medieval Warming Period (950 to 1250 AD), the stormy seas of the late 13th century rendered these vessels dangerous to the point of obsolescence. In the early 14th century, craftsmen along the Atlantic seaboard of western Europe developed new boats capable of withstanding the choppy seas and gales that became common in the North Sea even in the summer months. A Dutch design called the "dogger" became the primary fishing vessel in the North Sea, and for which the fertile fishing ground off the east coast of England called the Dogger Bank was named. Doggers were designed to fish for cod in shallow waters with hook and line. They were slow single-masted boats, but sturdy and capable of withstanding the rough conditions of the North Sea. They were wide-beamed and barrel shaped, about 50 feet (15 meters) long, and weighing in at about 13 tons. Doggers could carry a ton of bait, three tons of salt, half a ton each of food and firewood for the crew, and return with six tons of fish. Decked areas forward and aft provided sleeping, storage and cooking areas. An anchor allowed extended periods fishing in the same spot in waters up to 60 feet (18 meters) deep. Later, in the 15th century, the Dutch introduced another new type of fishing boat called the "Herring Buss," that became the workhorse of their North Sea fishing fleet. The two or three masted Herring Buss was a larger vessel at about 65 feet (20 meters) long and weighing up to 100 tons. At night, crews of 18 to 30 men would set out long drifting gill nets, and in daylight they would retrieve the nets and set about salting and barreling the catch on the broad deck. They sailed in fleets of 400 to 500 ships to the prime herring and cod fisheries of the Dogger Bank. The Dutch buss fleets would stay at sea for weeks at a time and the catch was transported back to their home port cities in special boats called *ventjagers*. In the 17th century, the English developed a two masted dogger that was an early prototype for a "sailing trawler." Dogger Bank fishing ground was contested between the English and the Dutch, and both sides accompanied their fishing fleets with naval escorts leading to periodic skirmishes. The first modern sailing trawler was developed in the 19th century at the English fishing port of Brixham on the English Channel. By the early 19th century, Brixham fishermen needed to expand their fishing area further out to sea due to depletion of stocks in the over-fished waters of southern England. The Brixham trawler they developed was of sleek design with a tall central mast and large sails both fore and aft that gave it sufficient power and speed to make long distance trips to fishing grounds out in the open ocean, and to tow long trawl lines in deep water. This revolutionary design made large scale trawling in the open ocean possible for the first time, which resulted in a massive migration of the English fishing industry from ports in the south, to villages on England's northeastern seaboard such as Scarborough, Hull, Harwich, Yarmouth and Grimsby. The small village of Grimsby grew to become the largest fishing port in the world by the mid 19th century. The docks at Grimsby incorporated many innovations for the time such as dock gates and cranes that were operated by hydraulic power with a 300 foot (91 meter) tall water tower built to provide sufficient water pressure. The port was served by a rail link to London's Billingsgate Fish Market which gave Grimsby fishers direct access to their largest customer base. By the end of the 19th century there were over 3,000 Brixham trawlers operating out of England, with almost 1,000 out of Grimsby alone. Brixham trawlers were sold to fishermen around Europe, and the design influenced ship builders around the world.

Grand Banks

In 1497, around 500 years after the Vikings' failed attempt to establish a colony on the island of Newfoundland off the northeast coast of North America, and only 5 years after Italian explorer Christopher Columbus' first voyage across the Atlantic Ocean to the Caribbean islands, Italian explorer, John Cabot, sailed west from England to the east coast of present day Canada. Unlike other European explorers of the day, Cabot kept very poor logs of his voyage, but upon his return to England, the Italian ambassador to England reported hearing Cabot assert that the sea was "*... swarming with fish, which can be taken not only with the net, but in baskets let down with a stone.*" While the exact site of Cabot's expedition is unknown, historians believe that he was referring to the fishery off the coast of present day Newfoundland now called the Grand Banks.

The continental shelf off the southeast coast of Newfoundland is divided into a series of underwater plateaus called "banks" that are relatively shallow ranging in depth from 50 to 300 feet (15 to 91 meters). These underwater shallows are also located at a juncture where the cold "Labrador Current" mixes with the warm "Gulf Stream" current, which causes an up-welling of plankton (a diverse collection of tiny animal and plant organisms that inhabit the pelagic zone of water bodies that provides the nutritional foundation for the aquatic food web), creating the ecological conditions for one of the richest fisheries in the world. Fish species include capelin, cod, haddock, halibut, herring, mackerel and swordfish; shellfish include scallop and lobster.

While Cabot claimed all of Canada for his sponsor England, the European countries of France, Portugal and Spain also sent fishing fleets to the Grand Banks. By 1576, there were 250 French vessels and 200 vessels from other European nations fishing the Grand Banks. But apart from temporary drying stations on shore, the Europeans made no attempts to establish permanent on-shore settlements as this was a period in Europe when royal families were preoccupied with fighting religious wars of succession between Catholic and Protestant heirs. In 1585, these religiously inspired wars in Europe spilled over to the Grand Banks fishery; Protestant England allied with Protestant Netherlands against Catholic Spain for control of the North Atlantic. To this end, Queen Elizabeth I of England commissioned privateers to raid and capture Spanish and Portuguese fishing fleets on the Grand Banks. Queen Elizabeth's aggressive military adventurism paid off, and in conjunction with the English defeat of the Spanish Armada just three years later in 1588, effectively ended all Spanish and Portuguese commercial ambitions in North America.

Throughout the 17th and 18th centuries, the fisheries of Newfoundland, Labrador and the Saint Lawrence River estuary were hotly contested between the English and the French. The English used small, flat-bottomed, pointy tipped row boats called "dories" to fish with hook and line in the shallow bays close to shore. They practiced the "dry fishery" technique, which involved building temporary outposts on shore for drying cod placed on open air racks, before shipping the cured jerky back to Europe. Alternatively, the French practiced "green fishery," which involved processing the catch with salt aboard ship before shipment back to Europe. By the early 19th century, as the Napoleonic Wars (1803 – 1815) raged across Europe, and as England was preoccupied in the War of 1812 against the fledgling United States of America, significant change came to the bay fisheries of Newfoundland and Labrador. Fisheries in France and New England had declined due to the wars, and Newfoundland and Labrador cod became more valuable on the international market which lured many English and Irish fishermen to permanently relocate to North America rather than make the arduous trans-Atlantic crossing each summer to catch fish. In the decade from 1805 to 1815, the settler population of Newfoundland and Labrador nearly doubled from 21,975 to 40,568. With this influx of permanent residents, the bay fisheries became family operated businesses. Fishers, usually men, rowed or sailed out on the bay in their dories where they fished for cod using hook and line. When they returned home with the catch, the entire family helped clean and cure the fish. They would then trade their prize to merchants to pay for gear and supplies they had previously obtained on credit. Throughout the 1800s, as more bay fishermen caught larger volumes of fish, cod stocks in Conception, Trinity, and Bonavista Bays, where fishers had been fishing the longest, became depleted. To compensate, fishers adopted more efficient fishing gear including purse seine nets, gill nets, trawl lines with hundreds of baited hooks, and cod traps. Some fishers also relocated from fishing grounds on the inner bay, to areas on the outer headlands. Fishing the outer headlands required larger vessels that were very costly to build, and were only available to fisherman who could afford to invest in a "schooner" weighing up to 20 tons.

In the 18th and 19th centuries, sleek shaped schooners had become popular vessels in North America for coastal trade as they were fast and versatile, and required a smaller crew for their size than ocean crossing square rigged ships. Larger three-masted schooners were introduced around 1800. As more efficient nets and boats became widespread in the mid-1800s, fishermen caught much larger volumes of fish in less time than the traditional hook and line method, which put even more intense pressure on bay cod stocks. Bay fishers protested against this severe stock depletion, but in the end, they either invested in new fishing gear themselves, or they went to work aboard a schooner owned by someone who did. Schooners would anchor in favorable locations and launch a number of dories into the water. From these small boats two or three men fished for cod using hand lines or trawl lines. At daybreak, they would row to a fishing spot and return to the mothership several times throughout the day to unload their catch. At night, back on board the mothership, they would clean and salt the cod.

As the bay fisheries of Newfoundland and Labrador continued to decline throughout the 1800s, the provincial government of Canada encouraged fishers to move out to the Grand Banks by offering subsidies, and by the mid-1870s, fishers started arriving in the first steam powered fishing trawlers. These were large steel hulled vessels 80 to 90 feet (24 to 27 meters) long weighing up to 50 tons that could travel up to 11 knots (13 miles per hour) even on windless days. Steam power allowed fishers to go farther and fish deeper than ever before, and cod fishing remained profitable in Newfoundland and Labrador throughout the 1880s, peaking in 1889 with 4,401 fishers hauling in more than 13,200 tons of cod. But from the 1890s on, the catch steadily declined, and by 1920 many fishing communities had ceased operations.

The first steel hulled diesel powered "motor trawler" was built in Grimsby, England, in 1920, and in 1931, the first side mounted motorized "power drum" was deployed that enabled the use of larger nets and to draw them in much faster, thereby revolutionizing the fishing industry. But it wasn't until after World War II in the fisheries of northeastern North America where motor trawlers were first deployed in force. After the war, diesel powered trawlers that were used as minesweepers were refitted as fishing trawlers, which allowed fishermen to trawl larger areas, at greater depths and for longer periods than ever before. In 1947, a ship builder based in Leith, Scotland, refitted the surplus minesweeper, HMS *Felicity*, with refrigeration equipment and a stern ramp, to produce the first combined "freezer/stern" factory trawler. The first purpose built freezer/stern factory trawler was *Fairtry* built in 1953 in Aberdeen, Scotland. At 280 feet long and grossing 2,600 tons, this ship was much larger than any other trawlers then in operation, and it inaugurated the era of the "super trawler." As these factory ships pulled their motorized nets in over the stern, they could lift and process up to 60 tons of fish at a time. The *Lord Nelson* followed in 1961, installed with more advanced vertical plate freezers and equipped with radar, electronic navigation systems and sonar that allowed fishers to target the cod with unerring accuracy. These investor-owned super-trawlers served as prototypes for expanding corporate fishing fleets around the world in the following decades. Nylon gillnets introduced in the 1960s were another boon to commercial fishing: they were larger, cheaper, easier to handle, lasted longer, and required less maintenance than natural fibers, and were virtually invisible in the water, which helped to increase the catch considerably. The tonnage of cod caught by these super-trawlers on the outer Grand Banks increased each year until 1968 when it peaked at 810,000 tons, after which it declined precipitously, and by 1974 was down to 34,000 tons. Part of the problem was that these enormous nylon gill nets not only hauled in huge numbers of fish, when nets were lost at sea they would still entangle fish by the gills and then sink to the bottom where the fish would die, and after scavenger fish cleaned the nets of those dead fish, these so called "ghost nets" would float up to snare even more fish; this cycle would repeat for decades until the nets would finally break down into small pieces. Ghost-nets now make up about 10% of all marine litter. Fishers also developed massive bag-like drag nets that could sweep up all the fish in their path. A "rock-hopper" dredge was another type of net attached to large wheels that allowed it to trawl near the ocean bottom without snagging on rocks or other obstructions.

For centuries the unofficial "Law of the Sea" adhered to by most maritime nations was that national sovereignty extended 3 miles out from the seashore, and beyond that, the "high seas" were open to exploitation by ships from any nation. By the 1970s, with super trawlers vacuuming up fish stocks just beyond the 3 mile limit, Canada, with the longest coastline in the world, played a leading role in shaping the *United Nations Convention on the Law of the Sea* (UNCLOS) that took place between 1973 and 1982, that extended national sovereignty out to 200 miles from shore, an area referred to as an Exclusive Economic Zone (EEZ). The idea was that if individual countries could manage territorial fish stocks, they would enact sustainable limits on the fish take. Canadian fisheries experts advised that for Grand Banks cod stocks to recover, the Total Allowable Catch (TAC) should be limited to 16% of the cod population. In 1989, due to an over estimation of the cod population, the *Canadian Department of Fisheries and Oceans* over estimated the TAC for cod that year to be 125,000 tons, but under pressure from the fishing industry, the *Canadian Minister of Fisheries* arbitrarily raised that limit to 235,000 tons, which turned out to be an estimated 60% of the cod population. As a result of this extreme over fishing, by 1992 the Northern cod stock on the Grand Banks, once the largest in the world, collapsed down to 1% of its pre-industrial fishing level, and despite the government completely closing down the fishery, 30 years later the cod had not returned. In effect, overfishing on the Grand Banks dramatically altered the ecology of the entire aquatic food chain. Besides cod, the super trawlers caught as "by-catch" enormous volumes of other fish species including mackerel, herring and capelin. In the natural ecosystem, herring feed on cod eggs, and mackerel feed on herring which kept their population in check, and capelin were the main food source for the cod. As all these species were swept up in massive trawl nets, the entire natural food chain was destroyed. Rock-hopper dredges were particularly devastating to the cod as they fished the ocean bottom that had previously been a refuge for young cod. The waters of the Grand Banks now appear to be dominated by crab and shrimp rather than fish.

Australia

While the closure of the Grand Banks due to over-fishing is the most spectacular fishery collapse in history, over-fishing has led to the collapse of many other fish stocks around the world. The English colonization of Australia tells a similar cautionary tale. English settlers in the late 1700s were amazed at the quantity and size of the fish in the waters of Australia, but by the mid 1800s, fisheries at Port Jackson and Botany Bay located near the rapidly-growing city of Sydney in New South Wales (NSW) were already showing signs of over-fishing. Practices such as "stalling" netted off entire tidal flats with fine mesh nets that trapped everything behind them as the tide receded; fishers picked out the larger fish such as bream, whiting and flathead for market, and simply left piles of small fish to rot. Alexander Oliver, who in 1880 was appointed to a special commission to study the declining fisheries in NSW, noted that while the *"… net of the fishermen gradually increased in length, meshes decreased in width, so that nothing escaped, and bushels upon bushels of small fry—the young of the very best fishes—were left on the beaches."* That same commission also reported that fish *"... are followed up every creek and cranny by their relentless human enemies,"* and *"... perpetually harassed and hunted."* In the late 1920s, less than a decade after the introduction of ocean trawl fishing, stocks of flathead south of Sydney completely collapsed. In 1919, 2.3 million tons of flathead were fished from the Botany Bay fishery; in 1928, flathead stocks crashed, and by 1937 only 0.2 million tons were hauled up by the trawling fleet. Ninety years later, flathead stocks had only recovered to 40% of pre-1915 levels, suggesting that complex aquatic ecosystems, once over-fished beyond a certain point, may never fully recover to their previous state.

South China Sea

The South China Sea encompasses an area of 1.4 million square miles (3.63 million square kilometers) that is one of the most biodiverse marine ecosystems on Earth. In 2015, 10 million tons of fish were caught in the South China Sea accounting for 12% of the global fish catch, and more than half of the fishing vessels in the world were estimated to operate there. Six countries with coastlines on the South China Sea – Brunei, China, Malaysia, the Philippines, Taiwan, and Vietnam – have competing claims on this fishery. China, by far the dominant military power in the region, claims an exclusive historical right to fish almost the entire sea and has demarcated a broad U-shaped area called the "9 dash line" that includes international waters and also encroaches on the 200 mile Exclusive Economic Zones (EEZs) of all the other countries under the *1994 United Nations Convention on the Law of the Sea*. As a result of over-fishing since the 1950s, total fish stocks in the South China Sea have declined by 70-95%, and since 1995, catch rates have declined by 66-75%.

The marine food web in the South China Sea concentrates around coral reefs, but due to destructive fishing practices by fishers over the past 70 years, these reefs have been declining at a rate of 16% per decade. A common practice by small artisanal fishers has been "blast-fishing," using dynamite or grenades to indiscriminately kill fish by rupturing their internal organs, which also causes collateral damage to nearby reefs. Bottom trawling with rock-hopper trawl nets by large Chinese factory trawlers has further caused extensive reef damage. And in the 2010s, China dredged and built artificial islands for military installations which destroyed 62 square miles (160 square kilometers) of reefs. All of these destructive practices taken together have severely damaged more than half of Southeast Asia's coral reefs. Further exacerbating the decline in fish stocks are thousands of miles of ghost nets lost at sea by industrial trawlers that haunt the South China Sea, killing countless fish, dolphins, whales, turtles, and other marine animals. Another destructive fishing practice commonly employed by small artisanal fishers is "poison-fishing" using sodium cyanide to stun fish making them easier to catch. Poison-fishing, blast-fishing and bottom trawling are all illegal in most Southeast Asian countries, but these methods continue to be widely used due to lack of enforcement.

All of these threats to the South China Sea fishery are particularly acute around the Spratly Island archipelago that contains over 600 coral reefs, where disputed claims to marine resource compound the problem of unregulated fishing. Much of the over-fishing in the South China Sea is attributable to IUU, which stands for Illegal, Unreported, and Unregulated fishing. IUU fishing is common practice region-wide, with violators ranging from small-scale local artisanal fishermen to large-scale industrial trawler fleets operated by China. In recent years, there have been numerous incidents of Chinese military vessels and industrial trawlers triggering violent clashes with small fishing boats from other countries on the high seas. As competition for diminishing fish stocks becomes more intense, marine biologists warn that the entire South China Sea fishery is rushing head-long into an irreversible collapse.

Deep Sea Fisheries

Most marine fisheries are located in the Exclusive Economic Zones (EEZ) of countries within 200 miles from shore in the shallow waters of the continental shelf, since that is where most of the fish live. But there are a number of commercially fished species that live out in the "deep sea" mostly near "sea mounts" which are large geologic land-forms that rise-up from the ocean floor but do not break the surface. Typically formed from extinct volcanoes, sea mount peaks usually remain many hundreds to thousands of feet below the ocean's surface. Oceanographers have mapped more than 14,500 sea mounts under the Earth's oceans covering a total area of 3,396,210 square miles (8,796,150 square kilometers). Underwater currents as well as the elevated position of sea mounts attracts plankton and deep sea corals that form the foundation of the food web upon which large pelagic deep sea fish such as mackerel, marlin, ocean cod, sharks, swordfish and tuna, depend for survival.

Japan was the first country to foray into commercial tuna fishing in the 1920s, investing in longline operations around islands in the Western Pacific Ocean. In the early 1950s, tuna fishing was largely confined to islands in the Western Pacific and to the west coasts of North and Central America in the Eastern Pacific, but as advanced fishing and freezer technologies became widely dispersed after World War II, exploitation of deep sea tuna fisheries expanded rapidly, and by the 1980s, deep sea tuna fisheries had become active in equatorial and temperate waters in the Pacific as well as the Atlantic and Indian Oceans, resulting in an exponential growth of the global tuna catch. Pacific tuna catches increased from around 310,000 tons in 1950 to over 4.1 million tons in 2016; Atlantic tuna catches increased from 38,000 tons in 1950 to around 840,000 tons/year by the mid-1990s, declining gradually thereafter to just over 600,000 tons in 2016; Indian Ocean tuna catches increased from around 330,000 tons/year in the mid-1980s, to a peak of slightly over 990,000 tons/year in the mid-2000s, declining gradually thereafter to 700,000 tons in 2016.

In the Pacific, Japan had been the dominant fisher country since the 1950s, peaking at 900,000 tons in 1986 accounting for 40% of the total catch, before declining more recently to around 350,000 tons/ year accounting for 10% of the total Pacific catch. The U.S. was also a major fisher in the Pacific peaking in 1987 at 540,000 tons accounting for 27% of the total Atlantic catch, after which it declined to around 400,000 tons/year by the mid-2010s. Since the 1990s, other Asian countries have contributed significantly to the catch in the Pacific, including Taiwan, Indonesia, South Korea and the Philippines. These four Asian countries together caught nearly1.5 million tons of large pelagic fish in 2016.

In the Atlantic Ocean, during the 1960s, Japan had also been the dominant fisher with a peak catch of over 160,000 tons in 1965 accounting for well over 40% of the total catch, but by 2016, Japan's catch of 38,000 tons had fallen off to 8% of the total Atlantic catch. Spain took over as the dominant fisher in the Atlantic in the 1980s, peaking at over 210,000 tons in 1991, declining gradually thereafter to around 106,000 tons/year by the mid-2010s, accounting for around 17% of the total. France, became the second highest fisher in the 1980s, peaking in the early 1990s at 130,000 tons/year, and declining ever since. In the mid-1990s, Ghana saw its catch rise to around 79,000 tons/per year, accounting for 13% of the total Atlantic catch in the mid-2010s; this statistic is deceptive, however, since the industrial tuna fleet flying under the Ghanaian flag was in fact majority-owned by Japanese and Korean investors under joint venture arrangements with Ghana.

Catches of large pelagic fish in the Indian Ocean had also been dominated by Japan until the late-1960s, but by 2016, Japan accounted for only 2% of the total Indian Ocean catch. Massive increases in Indian Ocean catches in the 1980s and 1990s were driven largely by Taiwan, Spain, France and Indonesia, which together caught around 320,000 tons in 2016 accounting for 44% of the total.

There are six varieties of commercially fished tuna: Albacore, Atlantic Bluefin, Bigeye, Skipjack, Southern Bluefin and Yellowfin. Their prevalence varies depending on the ocean they inhabit, which is reflected in the worldwide catch data. In the Pacific, through the mid-2010s Skipjack and Yellowfin were the main varieties caught averaging around 3.0 million tons/year accounting for 76% of the total Pacific catch of large-pelagic fish. While tuna was the main target species of fishers in the Pacific, the fifth most caught large-pelagic fish was the non-target, Blue Shark, with 82,000 tons caught as "by-catch" in 2016. The most widespread fishing gear used by tuna fleets in the Pacific was purse seine nets accounting for 69% of the 2016 catch, followed by longlines at 17%.

In the Atlantic in the 1950s, the tuna catch was mainly comprised of Atlantic Bluefin and Albacore, while Skipjack and Yellowfin rapidly increased after 1960. More recently, catches have been dominated by Skipjack at around 230,000 tons/year accounting for 39% of the total Atlantic catch, followed by Yellowfin at about 100,000 tons/year accounting for 16%, and Bigeye at 75,000 tons/year accounting for 13%. The fishing gear primarily used by Atlantic fishers was longline and purse seine nets, with a recent strong movement to purse seine nets.

In the Indian Ocean, Southern Buefin contributed on average 36% of the total catch in the 1960s but now accounts for less than 1%. Yellowfin and Skipjack were caught in roughly equal amounts, each accounting for 18% of the total Indian Ocean catch, though in the 2010s, the catch of Skipjack was trending higher at about 23%. Longlines were used almost exclusively in the Indian Ocean up to the late 1960s, but subsequently, purse seine and to a lesser extent gillnets, became popular and now account for 55% of the total catch.

All of the above catch numbers of large pelagic fish in deep sea areas came from a report titled *"Using harmonized historical catch data to infer the expansion of global tuna fisheries"* (*Fisheries Research*, Volume 221, January 2020) that summarized catch data provided by six *"Regional Fisheries Management Organizations"* (RFMOs) that are international bodies of stakeholder countries with an interest in managing and conserving tuna stocks in ocean areas beyond the 200 mile EEZs of individual nations. Stakeholder countries include coastal states whose EEZs are part-time homes to migrating deep sea tuna stocks, and "distant water fishing nations" (DWFN), whose fleets travel to international deep sea areas where tuna stocks also congregate.

RFMOs were established by international agreements or treaties and each has different reporting requirements for by-catch of non-tuna large pelagic fish, which has made determining the total by-catch in the world's deep sea fisheries difficult. By extrapolating from available data, marine biologists have calculated the bycatch of large pelagic species from 1950 to 2016 in the Pacific, Atlantic and Indian Oceans. Sharks account for the largest tonnage of large pelagic fish bycatch, sometimes rivaling in weight the tuna catch. A catch of over 6 million tons of shark was reported by the RFMOs since 1950, and researchers estimate another 5.7 million tons went unreported across the same time period. Of the shark catch reported by the RFMOs, 66% was blue shark which is now listed by the International Union for Conservation of Nature (IUCN) as a "near threatened" species. Research biologist estimates of the total unreported by-catch for all fish species by the world's industrial tuna fleets increased from around 450,000 tons in 1950 to approximately 5.6 million tons in 2016.

In September, 2015, the *World Wide Fund for Nature* and the *Zoological Society of London*, issued a joint report titled the *"Living Blue Planet Report,"* which assessed the state of the world's marine fisheries from 1970 through 2010. According to this report:

> *"Of the marine [ocean] fish in the LPI [Living Planet Index] (930 species), 1,463 populations (492 species) are recorded as utilized, whether for local subsistence or commercial use. The index for all utilized fish species indicates a 50 per cent reduction in population numbers globally between 1970 and 2010 (Figure 2). Of the utilized fish populations, data sources for 459 contain information on threats. Exploitation is identified as the main threat in the vast majority of cases; other threats listed include habitat degradation/loss and climate change impacts.*

> *"For fish species of importance for regional economies, livelihoods and food, the decline may be even more dramatic. This can be seen in the case of Scrombidae, the family of mackerels, tunas and bonitos. An index for Scrombidae, based on data from 58 populations of 17 species, shows a decline of 74 per cent between 1970 and 2010 (Figure 3). While the most rapid decline is between 1976 and 1990, there is currently no sign of overall recovery at a global level."*

The report goes on to note:

"More fish are being caught at greater depths than ever before (Figure 18). Around 40 per cent of the world's fishing grounds are now in waters deeper than 200m and many deep-water species are likely to be overexploited (Roberts, 2002). Only a few decades ago it was virtually impossible to fish deeper than 500m: now, with technological improvements in vessels, gear and fish-finding equipment, bottom trawling is occurring at depths of up to 2,000m (UNEP, 2006, Ramirez-Llodra et al., 2011). Most deep-sea fisheries considered unsustainable (Norse et al., 2012) have started to target fish populations that are low in productivity, with long lifespans, slow growth and late maturity (Morato et al., 2006). This leads to rapid declines in the population (Devine et al., 2006) and even slower recovery once the stock has collapsed (Baker et al., 2009).

"As a result of this growing pressure, the number of fish stocks that are overfished and fully fished has increased, while less than 10 per cent of fisheries have any capacity for expansion (Figure 20). Yet this huge increase in fishing effort does not mean we are catching more fish: the total weight of fish landed in marine capture fisheries in 2012 was 79.7 million tonnes, compared to 80.7 million tonnes in 2007 (FAO, 2014b). For some species, the increased fishing pressure has had an adverse effect, as seen in the overall decline in the utilized fish species index presented in Chapter 1, and the even steeper 74 per cent decline in the Scrombridae group.

"Small-scale fisheries are not immune to overcapacity, overfishing or destructive fishing practices. In some cases, the activities of the small-scale fleets themselves have been a root cause of depletion and environmental degradation. In many other cases, the difficulties faced by small-scale fleets have been compounded (or even initially caused) by the arrival of industrial-scale fleets in their traditional waters. These factors are not exclusive to small-scale fisheries. In many developing countries, fisheries continue to have open access with no effective controls on the quantities of fish harvested or the techniques used. Lack of political will, data deficiencies and inadequate financial and human resources are often blamed for weak governance and management (CSR, 2006; FAO and OECD, 2015).

"The fisheries sector is often a buffer for populations marginalized by conflicts, climate events, poverty or unemployment which makes it politically difficult to restrain access to resources, placing vulnerable populations in even more precarious situations. At a global scale, IUU [Illegal, Unregulated and Unreported] fishing has escalated over the last two decades. IUU fishing is estimated to take 11-26 million tonnes of fish each year, adding to the pressures on stocks (Agnew et al., 2009). This represents 12-28.5 per cent of global capture fisheries production (FAO 2014b).

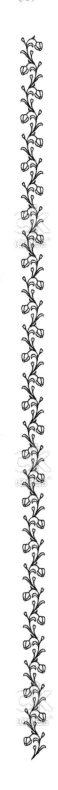

On global bycatch, the report gives this dire assessment:

"Overfishing is also closely tied to bycatch, which causes the needless loss of billions of fish, along with marine turtles, whales and dolphins, seabirds and other species. Global bycatch levels (excluding IUU fishing) are estimated at 7.3 million tonnes (Kelleher, 2005)."

"Globally, catches of sharks, rays and related species such as skates rose more than threefold from the 1950s to a high in 2003 and have been falling since (Dulvy et al., 2014). This decrease is not so much a result of improved management, but of the decline in populations (Davidson et al., 2015). As most catches of sharks and rays are unregulated, total catch could be three to four times greater than reported (Clarke et al., 2006; Worm et al., 2013).

Around one in four species of sharks, rays and skates is now threatened with extinction, due primarily to overfishing (Dulvy et al., 2014). Sharks and their relatives include some of the latest maturing and slowest reproducing of all vertebrates (Cortés, 2000): these species are especially vulnerable to overexploitation.

Many shark species are apex predators; others are filter feeders or carnivores of a lower trophic level. While the effects of falling shark numbers are still being studied, there is widespread concern about the damage to ecosystem health. Research has shown that the loss of apex predators nearly always results in further marine ecosystem degradation (Estes et al., 2011)."

The report identifies the causes of deep sea fisheries depletion:

"A growing world demand for fish, overcapacity – partly driven by fishing subsidies estimated at up to US$35 billion per year, equivalent to around a fifth of the industry's overall revenue (Sumaila et al., 2013) – and the lack of new or alternative opportunities are all contributing to a 'race to fish.' This is depleting many coastal fisheries and causing fishing fleets to look further and fish deeper into international waters. New species and areas are being targeted as traditional stocks become exhausted. Figure 19 shows the huge expansion in heavily fished areas: only the deepest and most inaccessible parts of the ocean are yet to feel pressure from fisheries."

On January 5, 2019, *The New York Times* reported that a 613 pound (278 kilogram) bluefin tuna sold for a record $3.1 million (¥333.6 million) at the *Tsukiji* fish market in Tokyo, Japan. The fish was purchased by Kiyoshi Kimura, the self-styled *"King of Tuna,"* who runs the *Sushi Zanmai* chain of sushi restaurants. Near the end of the *Times* story, almost as a footnote, the reporter got to the meat of the matter:

"Fishermen, driven by the high value, have begun using advanced techniques to catch the prized fish, leaving the population on the verge of collapse. An estimated 80 percent of the world's catch of bluefin tuna goes to Japan for use in sushi and sashimi, and the country has opted out of global conservation efforts in the past."

As long as there are wealthy people eager to pay any price to eat an endangered species, extinction can not be far behind.

Anchoveta

As noted in *The Living Blue Planet Report* cited above, large deep sea apex predator species such as shark and tuna that are slow to mature are particularly vulnerable to depletion by over-fishing, but as a consequence of the major advances in fishing technology since the 1950s, even massive fish stocks of small, fast breeding, prey species such as anchovies and sardines are now at risk of population decline due to over-fishing.

For untold millennia, vast schools of Peruvian anchovy, known as anchoveta, have inhabited the Pacific coastal waters of South America offshore from northern Chile, Peru, and in some years, extending further north to Ecuador. Anchoveta can live up to 3 years, reach a length of 8 inches (20 centimeters), and females can first reproduce at about 1 year of age. Anchoveta eat mostly phytoplankton and zooplankton such as krill and small crustaceans that thrive in the waters of the "Humboldt Current" where cold water off the coast of southern Chile flows north into warm tropical water off the coast of northern Peru, causing an upwelling of nutrients that provides the trophic foundation for the most productive marine ecosystem on Earth.

The anchoveta were first exploited by humans over 5,000 years ago (3000 BC) when the earliest coastal dwellers figured out how to make fishing nets with a species of wild cotton that enabled them to catch anchoveta offshore. During the historical period from 1950 to 2001, modern day fishers using purse seine nets caught over 274 million tons of fish off the Peruvian coast, 209 million tons of which were anchoveta, leading the *International Union for Conservation of Nature* (IUCN) to list the Peruvian anchoveta as *"... the most heavily exploited fish in world history."*

In conjunction *with the Humboldt Current, a* second naturally occurring environmental phenomenon that has a major impact on the anchoveta population is the irregular variation in winds and sea surface temperatures that periodically appears in the southeastern Pacific Ocean known as El Niño. El Niño events cause warm water to drift over the cold Humboldt Current and lower the depth of the upwelling of nutrients which leads to a drop-off in plankton and a corresponding crash in the anchoveta population. Typically, the population of fast reproducing anchoveta bounced back quickly from El Niño induced crashes, but after the El Niño of 1972 – 1973, combined with the record anchoveta catch of 13.1 million tons in the prior year of 1971, there was an unprecedented crash in the anchoveta population that did not fully recover until the 1990s. By 1994, the anchoveta catch had crept back up to 11 million tons, and the 1997–1998 El Niño event, the strongest on record, caused another devastating crash from which the anchoveta catch has yet to fully recover. From 2008 to 2012, the annual anchoveta catch varied between 4.2 and 8.3 million tons, which was still more than any other wild caught fish species in the world.

The *Marine Research Institute of Peru* (IMARPE) is the scientific institution responsible for monitoring fish stocks and recommending catch limits in Peru's anchoveta fishery, and the *Ministry of Production* (PRODUCE) is the government agency that regulates Peru's fishing industry, but their effectiveness at managing the anchoveta fishery has been called into question by the fish buyers industry group, *FishSource. FishSource* is an online database created by major world fish buyers to collect all the publicly available scientific and technical data on the status of world fisheries and fish stocks so they can make informed buying decisions. In *FishSource's* 2019 report, they were critical of the Peruvian authorities for their weak management of the anchoveta fishery:

> *"Since 2015 both IMARPE and PRODUCE are gradually improving transparency regarding the management of this fishery. IMARPE publishes daily landing records from both industrial and artisanal/small-scale fleets (IMARPE 2017f). However, the decision making process is not made publicly available; there is no explicit harvest control rule that anticipates reducing fishing effort if spawning stock biomass drops to the limit level (4 million tonnes) nor mechanisms explaining how catch levels are defined among the alternative scenarios presented by IMARPE before a fishing season is opened."*

PRODUCE established a catch limit for juveniles of 10% of the total catch to protect the recovery capacity of the anchoveta fishery, but according to the non-governmental ocean protection organization, *Oceana*, the actual percentage of juveniles caught in 2015 was far higher. In their February, 2016, report entitled, *"Overfishing and El Niño Push the World's Biggest Single-Species Fishery to a Critical Point,"* Oceana contextualized the El Niño event of 2015 – 2016:

> *"Last October [2015], fishermen and scientists argued that a total halt to the second anchoveta (Engraulis ringens) season would be necessary to protect fish stocks from the combined effects of El Niño and overfishing. Strong El Niño years, such as 2015-16 and 1997-98, can tip anchoveta populations into collapse unless fishing pressure is reduced, says Patricia Majluf, Oceana's vice president for Peru.*

> *"The warning signs were evident in the first anchoveta season of 2015, which ran from March through June in the north of Peru. There are usually two anchoveta fishing seasons in one year, with separate management and seasons for the southern anchoveta fishery. Though the government assured the public that catches would increase dramatically from 2014, fishermen hauled in low numbers of fish, and those that they did catch were small, skinny and sexually immature.*

> *"The Peruvian Marine Research Institute (IMARPE) conducted a routine survey of anchoveta populations in October and found that the northern stocks had sunk to a low of 3.38 million metric tons. Of this, only 2 million metric tons were reproductive-age fish, well below the 5 million metric tons required by law to open the fishery. The fishing industry, which used a different methodology, estimated that stocks hovered at a healthier 6.8 million metric tons. Despite the discrepancy in these two numbers, the Ministry of Production [PRODUCE] allowed the opening of the northern anchoveta fishery's second season on November 17. The ministry set a catch quota of 1.1 million metric tons — half of the 2 million metric tons taken during the first season.*

"'The real stock assessment resulted in a volume [of anchoveta] that should not have allowed fishers,' says Majluf, referring to the estimate from IMARPE.

"Sexually immature fish made up 50 percent of the second opening's catch, with some commercial boats' haul going as high as 90 percent. National fishing regulations mandate that juveniles make up no more than 10 percent — by numbers, not by volume — of allowable landings."

"As stocks of Peruvian anchovies struggle, government-imposed catch limits for 2015 and 2016 have failed to keep pace. While fishermen report low landings and high numbers of immature and pregnant fish, scientists fear for the long-term viability of what the United Nations calls 'the most heavily exploited fish in world history.'"

PRODUCE also set a limit on bycatch at 5% of total catch, but according to FishSource, "Data on protected and non-target species is scarce, and compliance on the percentage bycatch limit is not reported." PRODUCE further claims to manage the anchoveta fishery by applying an "adaptive system to account for high ecosystem variability and consequent uncertainty and rapid fluctuations in biomass, typical of this resource and the Humbolt ecosystem" (EUR-OCEANS, 2008), but FishSource begged to differ:

"The main threat posed by this fishery consists of reduction of food availability to protected predator species (Gislason, 2003), as anchovy is a forage species. An inverse relationship was found between the anchoveta fishing mortality and populations of seabirds and pinnipeds [seals and sea lions]. Also, a negative trend was observed for anchoveta landings from 1990 to 2012, what was also seen for other commercial species, which rely on anchoveta directly or indirectly through the trophic chain, underpinning the key role of anchoveta in Peruvian marine ecosystem (IMARPE, 2014a)."

"Several authors and most recently, (Hervás and Medley 2016) have raised concerns about the justification of the thresholds used by IMARPE in relation to the impact on predators and the need to analyze if these reference points are sufficient, taken also into account the role of anchoveta in the ecosystem. Recommendations have been included in a fishery improvement project (SNP and CeDePesca 2017)."

PRODUCE mandated that artisanal fishers operate exclusively between 3 and 10 nautical miles from shore and their catch be used exclusively for human consumption. Ostensibly these policies were to protect sensitive breeding grounds from overfishing, but in practice it has limited effect since catch records indicate that only 2% of the anchoveta catch actually goes to feed people directly, the remaining 98% is fished by industrial trawler fleets using massive purse seine nets fishing 10 to 70 nautical miles from shore and the catch goes to producing fish-meal and fish-oil that is then sold to Chile, the United States and China as high protein feed for factory farmed pigs and salmon. It can require several pounds of wild fish to produce one pound of farmed salmon; so what this means is that the largest marine fishery in the world is also one of the most inefficient food production systems in the world.

Artisanal fishers have been predicting for years that industrial fishing would be the end of the anchoveta fishery. In a 1996 interview broadcast on the syndicated radio show, *Living on Earth*, reporter Jyl Hoyt engaged artisanal fisher David Bravo in this dialogue:

> *"HOYT: A larger fleet equipped with the latest technology means Peruvians can capture more and more fish. That same high tech advancement shows up in seaports around the world, pushing fish stocks to or past their limit. Seagulls and pelicans swoop over fishermen as they unload mounds of anchovies from their grimy, brightly painted boats. Most of the catch will be ground into fish meal, then exported and used as animal feed. Peru's fish meal industry is now the second most important economy in the country. Peruvian fishermen caught 11 million tons of anchovies in 1994. The government and the private sector have invested heavily in Peru's fishery, so much so that now the fleet can bring in 4 times as much fish as the government recommends. There is strong pressure to make good on these investments, and that worries fisherman David Bravo.*
>
> *BRAVO: (Speaks in Spanish)*
>
> *TRANSLATOR: They're building all these new plants, all these new ships. That means now they have a lot of financial obligations to pay off all their new investments. It's obvious. In the future they'll have beautiful plants, marvelous boats, and not one single fish left."*

It takes a simple fisherman to state the obvious: commercial fishing is not about fish, it is about money.

The Great Lakes

Most of the fish biomass caught by the world's commercial fishers is made up of salt water species, since most of the world's fish live in the seas and oceans. But over the course of the 19th and 20th centuries there have also been some relatively large commercial fisheries operating on many of the world's largest fresh water lakes. The Great Lakes on the border between the United States and Canada sustained just such a fresh water fishery from the 1850s to the late 1950s.

Historically, of the five Great Lakes – Superior , Michigan, Huron, Erie and Ontario – Lake Erie contained the most abundant fish populations largely due to its very shallow average depth of only 63 feet as compared to the second shallowest Lake Huron averaging 195 feet, and the deepest Lake Superior averaging 483 feet. Such shallow water makes Lake Erie the warmest of the Great Lakes which promotes algal and plankton growth that provides the trophic foundation for the aquatic food pyramid. While Lake Erie holds the least volume of water of the five Great Lakes, it is estimated to contain 50% of all the Great

Lake's fish, including the commonly fished native species of cisco (lake herring), lake trout, northern pike, smallmouth bass, turbot, walleye, whitefish and yellow perch.

For millennia before European settlers colonized its shores, Indian nations vied for access to Lake Erie's coveted fishing grounds, including the Erie, Attawandaron, Iroquois and Anishinaabe. European settlers began to establish commercial fisheries on the lake in the pre-Civil War years, as railways encircled the lake by1852 and it had become a major thoroughfare for commercial shipping traffic. In the 1860s, the huge, slow maturing, lake sturgeon, was so abundant it was considered bycatch and either dumped back into the lake, fed to pigs, used as fertilizer, or even dried to burn as fuel. Once its food value was established, fishers began to target the bottom dwelling sturgeons with trapnets, poundnets and gillnets, one year hauling in over 5 million pounds from Lake Erie alone. The sturgeon fishery collapsed entirely by 1900, and despite its designation as a protected species, lake sturgeon still remain exceedingly rare in the lakes over a century later.

Lake Erie and parts of downstream Lake Ontario provided a unique food niche for a fish first identified as a blue pike, but after definitive mitochondrial DNA analysis performed years later, was reclassified as a blue walleye, a subspecies of the more common yellow walleye. Through the mid-1900s blue walleye were so abundant there were no catch limits for commercial fishers, and in many years they accounted for over 50% of the total commercial catch. But suddenly, in the 1950s, the blue walleye population began to show signs of instability: between 1950 and 1957, catches in the U.S. and Canada fluctuated between 2 million and 26 million pounds (910,000 and 12 million kilograms) per year. Then in 1959, the catch plummeted to 79 thousand pounds (36,000 kilograms), and in 1964 dwindled to 200 pounds (91 kilograms). In 1967 the U.S. declared the blue walleye an endangered species, and in 1983, extinct. The main cause of the blue walleye's demise was the insatiable appetite for fish by the millions of people who were flooding into the rapidly industrializing cities that ring the perimeter of Lake Erie, including Buffalo New York, Cleveland and Toledo Ohio, Erie Pennsylvania, Detroit Michigan and Windsor Ontario. For nearly a century, blue walleye was a staple on the menu in millions of homes and restaurants proximate to the lake.

Even as the blue walleye was being fished to extinction, the catch of other commercial species such as northern pike, yellow walleye and whitefish were also in decline due to billions of gallons of pollution pouring into the lake from industry, farms and housing developments. As the industrial mid-western cities grew up around the Great Lakes in the 1900s, they used the lakes as giant open-pit cesspools for disposal of untreated industrial wastes, silt eroded from deforested land cleared for agriculture, farm fertilizer run-off, and human sewerage. Lake Erie, with the least volume of water to dilute the pollutants, became the most polluted of the five Great Lakes, causing massive die offs of fish that would wash-up on shore and rot. In 1969, the oily sludge floating on the surface of the Cuyahoga River that flows into Lake Erie at Cleveland actually burst into flames, turning the lake's pollution problem into an international embarrassment. In December 1970, the U.S. Justice Department along with the newly established Environmental Protection

Agency (EPA) filed lawsuits against 12 corporations in north eastern Ohio that were dumping cyanide directly into the Cuyahoga River in violation of the 1899 Rivers and Harbors Act. Also in 1970, the city of Cleveland passed a $100 million bond initiative to replace the city's sewer lines and upgrade their sewerage treatment plant. In 1972 the U.S. Congress passed into law the Clean Water Act, and the U.S. and Canada joined in an International Water Quality Agreement to establish water pollution limits on the Great Lakes. This joint U.S. – Canada effort forced hundreds of major industrial polluters to upgrade their waste treatment facilities and municipalities to upgrade their sewerage treatment plants to meet the new clean water standards. Also at this time, the U.S. Congress mandated that the U.S. Army Corps of Engineers design and develop a program for the *"rehabilitation and environmental repair of Lake Erie"*. The Army Corps commissioned the Lake Erie Wastewater Management Study (LEWMS) which identified phosphorus from agricultural runoff as the nutrient most affecting the eutrophication (oxygen depletion) of Lake Erie, and called for implementation of conservation tillage, and in some cases, no-till farming on the U.S. side of the lake to achieve phosphorus reduction targets.

Lake Erie's lower water volume than the other four Great Lakes made it more susceptible to becoming over-burdened with pollution, but on the plus side, the lake's small size worked to its advantage in accelerating the clean-up. Due to its small size, the water in Lake Erie completely turns-over every 2.6 years, much faster than the other four Great Lakes. As the sources of new pollutants flowing into the lake were systematically shut off, the fast turn-over of Lake Erie's water quickly turned it clear again, and the fish responded favorably; sport fishers caught 112,000 yellow walleyes in 1975, by 1985 that catch was up to 4.1 million out of a total estimated population of around 33 million. The numbers were improving, but still, all was not well in the fishery; some of the industrial chemicals spewed into the lake such as PCBs (Polychlorinated biphenyls), methylmercury, DDT (Dichlorodiphenyltrichloroethane – thank goodness for acronyms), and Dioxins, are resistant to breaking down in the environment and have persisted as toxins in the sediments at the bottom of the Great Lakes for decades despite the massive clean-up efforts. At the bottom of the food chain are tiny mollusks that eat by filtering water for organic particulates. As they filter water, they also filter out these persistent toxic chemicals which are then stored in their bodily tissues. As small fish eat the mollusks by the thousands, and bigger fish eat the smaller fish by the thousands, these toxic chemicals work their way up the trophic pyramid to become highly concentrated in the tissues of the fish species at the top that people like to eat.

As it became clear to medical science that these toxic chemicals were a serious public health risk, in 1974 the U.S. Environmental Protection Agency (EPA) was obliged to publish a "National Listing of Fish Advisories" notifying the fish eating public that:

"Advisories may be issued for the general public or for specific groups of people at risk, such as:

- *People who eat a lot of fish*
- *Elderly men and women*
- *Pregnant women*

- *Nursing mothers*
- *Children*

An advisory for a specific waterbody or type of waterbody may address more than one affected fish or shellfish species or contaminant. Advisories can be issued by federal, state, territorial or tribal agencies."

Based on the levels of PCBs and methylmercury contamination found in the fish, every state and locality in the U.S. with a fishery now issues advisories to sports fishers on "safe" limits of fish to eat, ranging from no limit, to ½ pound per week, to ½ pound per month, to Do Not Eat! Such advisories on fish consumption negatively affected consumer demand for Great Lakes fish, and by the 1990s the only commercial fishery left on Lake Erie was on the Canadian side and restricted to catching yellow perch. On the U.S. side, despite concerted protests from commercial fishers, sports fishers have laid claim to the Lake Erie fishing industry.

Back in the 1960s and early 1970s, massive blooms of blue-green algae resulting from unchecked agricultural runoff had become a yearly phenomenon on Lake Erie, but through the mid 1970s and 1980s, as agricultural run-off was significantly curtailed, the blooms disappeared. The improved farming practices of the 1970s that resulted in this improvement were only voluntary, however, and by the 1990s agricultural run-off was once again pouring into the lake which, in 1993, resulted in a return of the blue-green algae bloom. Blue-green algae is actually not an algae at all, but a type of cyanobacteria (bacteria capable of photosynthesis) that can grow rapidly in the warm calm waters of ponds and lakes when phosphates and nitrogen are present in large amounts. Blue-green algal blooms are a triple threat to the Lake Erie fishery. Typically, they arrive late each summer and form large surface mats 10 inches thick that deprive other phytoplankton of sunlight, which collapses the entire trophic pyramid over large areas of the lake. Blue-green algae can also produce both nerve and liver toxins (microcystins) that can kill fish directly, not to mention unsuspecting dogs and people who ingest it. And third, after the blue-green algae die, bacterial degradation of their biomass requires oxygen consumption, which depletes the water of oxygen creating large "dead zones" where fish cannot survive. A U.S. EPA study reported the dead zone in 2003 as a 10-foot-thick layer of cooler water at the bottom of the lake that stretched 100 miles across the center and lasted the entire month of August, up from two weeks back in 1993, the year the algal blooms returned. In 2014, the city of Toledo, Ohio's, water supply was contaminated with the toxic microcystins and residents had to resort to bottled water for cooking and bathing. The U.S. National Oceanic and Atmospheric Administration (NOAA) now measures the bloom using satellite imagery. According to NOAA, the largest Lake Erie algal bloom to date occurred in 2015, and the second largest was in 2011. University of Windsor professor of biology, Dr. Robert McKay, is the director of the *Great Lakes Institute for Environmental Research* (GLIER), and is the preeminent researcher studying the algal blooms on the Great Lakes. GLIER researchers confirmed satellite images that show the 2019 algal bloom stretching up to 500 square miles (1,300 square kilometers) in Lake Erie's western basin with its epicenter near Toledo.

In early August, 2019, GLIER researchers collected 60 samples of the algal bloom from pre-selected sites on the Canadian side of the lake. In an article about his work published in the August 7, 2019, *University of Windsor Daily News*, Dr. McKay reflected:

> *"Field work is important to understanding the bloom, [McKay] said. 'What satellites do not tell us is what's going on inside the bloom itself.'*
>
> *"Water samples will allow researchers to measure toxin levels, develop toxin profiles, and measure the nutrient levels feeding them.*
>
> *"Lake Erie's western basin is the perfect breeding ground for algal blooms, McKay said. The water is shallow, allowing it to be warmed faster than other parts of the lake. Nutrients flow into the lake from the high population density and agricultural lands that surround it.*
>
> *"McKay said Ohio residents can see evidence of the algal bloom on their beaches. On this side of the border, the bloom is further offshore, making Wednesday's water sampling important.*
>
> *"'Without this, in Ontario, it's out of sight, out of mind.'"*

Since the early 1900s, the Lake Erie fishery has been under constant threat from non-native invasive species, some introduced intentionally, others not. In 1912, eggs of the anadromous rainbow smelt taken from the landlocked Green Lake in Maine, were intentionally introduced into the Crystal Lake in Michigan, in the hope of increasing the forage available for larger predatory fish, and also to create a springtime fishery when the anadromous smelt swim up-stream on the lake's tributaries to spawn. Crystal Lake drains into Lake Michigan which is connected to all the other Great Lakes through natural waterways, and before long all the Great Lakes were infested with non-native rainbow smelt. Rainbow smelt are sensitive to temperature and light, so in shallow Lake Erie they kept to the cooler, darker, mid-waters of the lake, which was the natural habitat of the native blue walleye. Although adult rainbow smelt grow to only 6 inches long and did serve as forage for the much larger blue walleye, the smelt were also predators of the tiny blue walleye fry (baby fish), and are believed to have contributed to the eventual extinction of the blue walleye. Rainbow smelt thrived in Lake Erie, and the commercial catch peaked in 1941 at 4.8 million pounds, after which the smelt population showed large fluctuations until the so called "smeltdown" of 1993 from which they have yet to recover. The *Great Lakes Science Center* does annual prey fish surveys in the lakes, trawling the lake bottom and counting what they find; they found that their 2013 count of smelt was only 6% of the long-term average count. In a report on Lake Michigan prey fish populations, scientists from the *Science Center* wrote, *"Rainbow smelt biomass in Lake Michigan during 1992-1996 was roughly four times higher than rainbow smelt biomass during 2001-2013."* Rainbow smelt had become the primary forage species in each of the five Great Lakes for predatory species in the lakes, so the crash in the smelt population rippled through the entire trophic structure of the Great Lakes.

The return of the algal bloom in 1993, and the 1988 arrival of another non-native invasive species in the Great Lakes called the zebra mussel are thought to be responsible for the smelt's final undoing. The zebra mussel is a fingernail sized clam with a striped shell that is native to the Black and Caspian Seas where Eastern Europe meets Western Asia, but has been dispersed around the world encrusted on ocean going cargo ships. Six to seven weeks after a female zebra mussel attaches herself to a surface, she begins to generate eggs: one female can bear up to 40,000 eggs at a time, up to 1 million in a year, and up to 5 million over the course of her four to five year lifetime. With a proliferation capacity like this entering a nutrient dense ecosystem like the Great Lakes with no natural predators, hundreds of billions of zebra mussels quickly overran the entire Great Lakes system and completely altered the trophic structure of the lakes once again. Zebra mussels are filter feeders that filter out plankton from the water that was a main source of food for the rainbow smelt. Some researchers suspect the zebra mussels are to blame for the smeltdown.

Another non-native species introduced to the Great Lakes, this one unintentionally, was the highly invasive and extremely destructive sea lamprey, which looks like an eel, but in fact is a scaleless, jawless, cartilaginous, anadromous fish that can grow up to 40 inches (100 centimeters) long that is native to the Atlantic Ocean. Outflows from Lake Ontario form the headwaters of the Saint Lawrence River which drains into the Atlantic Ocean at the Gulf of Saint Lawrence near the present day city of Quebec, Canada. The first recorded sighting of the sea lamprey in the Great Lakes was in Lake Ontario in 1835, but the Niagara Falls served as a natural barrier preventing them from moving farther upstream to Lake Erie and from there on to the rest of the Great Lakes. In the late 1800s and early 1900s, however, improvements were made to the Welland Canal that bypassed Niagara Falls to provide a shipping channel between Lake Ontario and Lake Erie, which allowed sea lampreys to circumvent the falls and spread throughout the Great Lakes system, to Lake Erie by 1921, Lake Huron by 1936, Lake Michigan by 1937, and Lake Superior by 1938. Sea lampreys were able to thrive once they invaded the Great Lakes because of the availability of excellent spawning and larval habitat in lake tributaries, an abundance of host fish, a lack of predators, and their high reproductive rate – a single female can produce as many as 100,000 eggs. Sea lampreys are parasitic fish that attach to other fish with their suction cup mouth then dig their teeth into its flesh for grip; once securely attached, they rasp through the fish's scales and skin with their sharp tongue and feed on the fish's bodily fluids by secreting an enzyme that prevents blood from clotting. In their native Atlantic Ocean habitat, due to co-evolution with ocean fish, sea lampreys rarely are fatal to their hosts, but in the Great Lakes where no such co-evolutionary link existed, each adult sea lamprey can typically kill up to 40 pounds (more than 20 kilograms) of fish over their 12-18 month feeding period. The sea lamprey invasion had an enormous impact on the trophic structure of the Great Lakes; in 1920, before the sea lamprey invaded the upper Great Lakes, Canada and the U.S. caught about 15 million pounds of lake trout alone, but by the early 1960s, after decades of predation by the sea lamprey, the total combined catch of lake trout, whitefish, and cisco – the backbone of the Great Lakes' commercial fishery – had plummeted to around 300,000 pounds. Meanwhile, as the sea lamprey decimated the population of lake trout and whitefish that preyed upon the non-native smelt, the smelt population also exploded. In Lake Michigan the commercial catch of rainbow smelt went from 86,000 pounds in 1931, to 4.8 million pounds in 1941, in Lake Superior it went from 21,000 pounds in 1953, to over 4 million pounds in 1976. As the rainbow smelt population thrived, the native cisco population dived as cisco eggs and larvae were a favorite food of the smelt. By the 1950s, native ciscoes had virtually disappeared from much of the Great Lakes basin; in effect, the rainbow smelt had replaced the cisco as the main forage for the Great Lakes' dwindling populations of native predatory fish species.

By the 1950s, the Great Lakes fishery was in such bad shape that in 1954 the U.S. and Canada co-created the *Great Lakes Fishery Commission* to deal with the multiple hazards facing the fish that were destroying the fishery, including the sea lamprey, habitat destruction, poor water quality, and overfishing. Fishery biologists from major universities on both sides of the lakes were tasked by the Commission with finding a solution to the seemingly intractable sea lamprey problem. According to a post in the 10/2/2017 bulletin, *Fish Tales from Ohio,* published by the *Ohio State University College of Food, Agriculture and Environmental Sciences*:

> "*When trying to combat the sea lamprey, wildlife managers tried using barriers to prevent the sea lampreys from breeding in streams. Physical barriers such as dams were designed prevent lampreys from passing through, while still allowing other 'good' fish to pass. Electrical barriers were put in place to prevent lampreys from entering rivers to lay their eggs. While these barriers were somewhat effective and are still in place today, they were not able eliminate the problem of the sea lamprey (Great Lakes Fishery Commission 2000; Smith and Tibbles 1980). In 1958, managers started using a chemical called 3-trifluromethyl-4-nitrophenol, commonly abbreviated as TFM, to control lamprey populations. TFM is a lampricide, a chemical designed to kill lamprey in their breeding streams when they are still young. This prevents them from growing up and doing damage to fish populations. The lampricide proved to be effective, greatly reducing population sizes of the sea lamprey (Smith and Tibbles 1980). This has allowed some fish populations decimated by the lamprey to increase, but it will take more time for the fisheries to fully recover (USGS NAS 2016). However, treatments with TFM are ongoing to prevent the sea lampreys from ever reaching their 1950s numbers. Researchers are continuing to search for other treatments that reduce sea lamprey numbers to reduce dependence on TFM, which could have negative effects on other fish living in areas where lampricide has been used (Birceanu et al. 2014; USGS NAS 2016). Researchers at the Hammond Bay Biological Station, a partner of Michigan State University, are examining how pheromones (chemicals that animals release into the environment) can be used to alter movements of sea lamprey and to lure them into areas where they can be easily captured or killed (USGS Great Lakes Science Center 2016).*"

Notably, this strategy of using barriers and poisons, while not without its own environmental consequences, did prove effective at greatly reducing the population of sea lamprey, and by 2016, had allowed some native fish populations in the lakes to increase, but will still require eternal vigilance for the fisheries to fully recover.

Yet another invasive species unintentionally introduced to the Great Lakes that has played havoc with the lakes' trophic structure was the alewife. Alewife are an anadromous planktivore (eat plankton), adults grow 10 to 12 inches (25 to 30 centimeters) long, and are native to the Atlantic Ocean. In the ocean alewife are preyed upon by Atlantic salmon. Atlantic salmon long ago colonized Lake Ontario via their spawning route up the Saint Lawrence River, but as with the sea lamprey, Niagara Falls acted as a barrier preventing them from colonizing the other Great Lakes. The Atlantic salmon population of Lake Ontario acted as gate keepers preventing the alewife from becoming established in the lake, but in the mid 1900s, the Atlantic salmon were so widely over-fished that in 1873, for the first time, an alewife was spotted in Lake Ontario. With no natural predator to check its population growth, the alewife quickly colonized Lake Ontario, and then followed the same route as the sea lamprey to colonize the other four Great Lakes, through the Wellen Canal bypassing Niagara Falls; alewife were first detected in Lake Erie in 1931, Lake Huron in 1933, Lake Michigan in 1949, and Lake Superior in 1954. By the late 1960s, the population of alewife, each female of whom could produce 7,500 offspring, spiked in the polluted waters of Lake Michigan, feeding on small crustaceans that are now nearly extinct. Alewife were so prolific that they would often overshoot their own food source, and mass die-offs became common in the 1960s and 1970s with piles of dead fish stretching for miles along beaches around the Great Lakes. In 1967, contemporaneous news reports tell of a massive die-off near Chicago, Illinois and Gary, Indiana, where one billion pounds of dead fish were hauled away to two dumps in Indiana devoted exclusively to disposing of decomposing fish. The drinking water on the North Side of Chicago became so contaminated that the city issued an order for all residents to boil their tap water before use. Alewife are very resilient fish, however, and their populations always managed to bounce back quickly in regular feast-or-famine cycles. By the mid-1960s, alewife had overtaken rainbow smelt as the primary forage fish species in the lakes, so when they had these periodic die-offs, it caused starvation among the lakes predator species and contributed to the already steep population declines in lake trout, turbot, walleye and whitefish. In 1964, the Michigan Department of Natural Resources (DNR) hired a fish biologist named Howard Tanner to figure out how to deal with the alewife problem in Lake Michigan, encouraging him to, *"Make it spectacular."* Tanner considered the alewife simply as a forage fish for predator species, and since the native predators had largely been extirpated from the lakes, he settled on restocking with a non-native predator species from the Pacific Northwest – the Pacific Chinook salmon. Tanner's "spectacular" vision was to turn the Great Lakes into the world's premier sports salmon fishery, and in 1966, the DNR released the first Pacific Chinook salmon into the Great Lakes ecosystem. Tanner's vision turned out to be a spectacular success, the newly introduced salmon consumed alewife, reducing their numbers such that die-offs no longer occurred, and by the mid-1980s, the biomass of alewife in Lake Michigan was less than 20% of the historic high. At the same time, salmon grew rapidly and became the backbone of a recreational charter boat industry on the lakes estimated at the time to generate $7 billion annually. But all was not well in the Great Lakes sports fishery, and by the late 1980s, the Chinook salmon boom turned to bust. The following post excerpted from the May 25, 2020, *Great Lakes Fisheries Commission's* online newsletter, *eForum*, untangles this complex ecological web:

"Management agencies continued to stock Pacific salmon in increasing numbers, with more than 25 million fingerlings being stocked in the Great Lakes basin during the early 1980s. Initially, managers were quite pleased with results, because harvest increased linearly with stocking increases. Yet, during the late 1980s, alewife populations were declining and, as a result, so was the size of salmon. In response to pressure from recreational fishers, management agencies eliminated commercial fisheries for alewife by 1991 because the commercial fisheries competed with salmon for alewife. Agencies also reduced the number of stocked salmon in an attempt to balance predator (salmon) abundance with lower levels of prey (alewives) to maintain a highly valuable, but much smaller recreational fishery for Pacific salmon.

"As a management philosophy, balancing predator (Pacific salmon) with available prey (alewives) prevails. Although alewives serve as a key source of food for Pacific salmon, they also have a down side. The species exerts strong, negative impacts on many fish: they consume the pelagic early life stages of native species such as yellow perch and lake trout and compete with coregonines for zooplankton. Further, alewives contribute to Thiamine Deficiency Complex which impairs early development of salmonines, thereby threatening the rehabilitation of native species as well as the viability of stocked fingerlings.

"New invasive species - such as zebra and quagga mussels - are also exerting adverse impacts on the ecosystem. Since 2002, cladocerans, a type of zooplankton, have declined by 90% in Lake Huron thereby reducing the food available for early life stages of pelagic fishes. Alewife populations collapsed after 2003 resulting in fewer resources to sustain the salmon fishery. Compounding the pressure on alewives, Chinook salmon are now naturally reproducing in lakes Michigan, Huron and Ontario resulting in a higher demand, yet fewer resources to sustain alewife and hence Chinook salmon.

"Since 2004, the Lake Huron system has changed from one dominated by alewife and Chinook salmon to one where alewife have been nearly eliminated and Chinook salmon biomass has been reduced to a fraction of their recent (pre-2003) biomass. As a result, angler effort has declined by about 90% and recruitment of native fishes, including lake trout, walleye, cisco, bloater, and emerald shiners, is increasing. Thus, the introduction of some unwanted aquatic invasive species is changing the ecosystem from the state desired by anglers (strong Pacific salmon fishery) to an alternative state where native species are becoming dominant.

"Fishery managers must now make the difficult decision of whether to manage for short-term economic success by attempting to maintain a balance between the demand for Pacific salmon fisheries and the declining alewife populations that support these fisheries, or to embrace ecosystem change and manage primarily for rehabilitation of native fishes that appear to be *better suited to the ongoing ecosystem changes. The case can be made for managers to direct fewer resources toward active management of Pacific salmon in favor of efforts to restore native species in a changing food web. Conversely, the popular and economically important recreational fishery for Pacific salmon creates an environment in which managers are pressured to maintain the Pacific salmon fishery at least at current levels, despite a reduced capacity in the ecosystem to provide for the very characteristics desired by the anglers: high catch rates and large size. Although this decision choice may become moot following fundamental ecosystem shifts, this remains a significant paradox for fishery managers."*

The five Great Lakes of North America are the largest group of freshwater lakes on Earth by total area, and a close second to Lake Baikal, Russia, in total volume, containing 21% of the world's surface fresh water. The lakes began to form at the end of the last glacial period around 14,000 years ago, as retreating ice sheets carved out and exposed the basins which then filled with meltwater. Over several millennia, a highly complex ecosystem with a wide diversity of species and a well defined trophic structure (food pyramid) colonized the lakes. The first humans arrived around 10,000 years ago, and estimates of their pre-Columbian population range between 60,000 and 120,000 people. On the grand scale of the Great Lakes ecosystem, there is no evidence that this relatively small number of people fishing with archaic gear had any significant impacts on the dynamic equilibrium of the lakes as established over millennia through natural selection. European settlers began to fish the Great Lakes commercially in the 1840s, and to their great detriment, the lakes have been exploited commercially ever since. In that time, dozens of industrial cities grew up on the shores of the lakes creating an enormous demand for fish that resulted in overfishing, enormous amounts of industrial pollutants, farm chemicals and residential sewerage pouring into the lakes, and a parade of non-native invasive species colonizing the lakes, that turned the Great Lakes fishery into an out of balance and severely dysfunctional ecosystem. The fishery biologists cited above from the *Great Lakes Fisheries Commission* are right: fisheries managers around the Great Lakes are faced with a decision whether to bend to commercial sports fishing interests and continue restocking the lakes with non-native Pacific Chinook salmon in a desperate attempt to breathe life into a gasping sports fishing industry, or to manage the lakes for the long term recovery of native species. In 2020, the U.S. Environmental Protection Agency (EPA) estimated the human population of the Great Lakes basin at 30 million people. If sports fishing in a market of this size continues to drive fishery policy for much longer, then there is little hope the troubled waters of the Great Lakes fishery will ever again return to a state of ecological balance. The sad story of the Great Lakes fishery is a cautionary tale for every freshwater fishery on Earth.

Wild Salmon

About 1% of all fish species are anadromous or catadromous, that is fish that inhabit both salt and fresh water at different times in their life cycles. This remarkable genetic trait traces back an estimated 65 – 95 million years ago, when, as a result of an "autotetraploid event," fishes of the Salmonidae family inherited twice the number of chromosomes and twice the DNA content of other closely related ray-finned fishes which enabled them to survive in both fresh and salt water. While living this double life must have been an adaptive advantage for Salmonidae over the millions of years of their evolution, the threats to their survival in the current Anthropocene Epoch may be their final undoing. The Salmonidae fish family includes trout, char, grayling, whitefish, and of course, the most prized of all – salmon.

The earliest salmon were part of a broad divergence of ocean fishes that adapted over eons to the cold, northern waters of the upper Northern Hemisphere around the Arctic Circle. Both the fossil record and molecular data indicate that the Atlantic salmon (*Salmo – Latin "to leap"*) along with brown trout, and their relatives, had diverged from Pacific salmon (*Onchorhynchus*), steelhead trout and their relatives, by the early Miocene Epoch (15 – 20 million years ago), perhaps following the cooling of the Arctic Ocean. Atlantic salmon spread to the rivers and streams of northeastern North American, Greenland, Iceland, Ireland, Britain, northern Europe south to Spain and Portugal, the Baltic region, Scandinavia and northwestern Russia. Pacific salmon spread to the rivers and streams of far northeastern Russia, Alaska, Canada and Northwest U.S. Approximately 6 million years ago, Pacific salmon further diverged into five distinct species – Chinook, chum, coho, pink and sockeye. David Montgomery, Professor of Geomorphology at the University of Washington, in his paper, *"Coevolution of the Pacific salmon and Pacific Rim topography"* (*Geology*, Dec. 2000), has postulated that speciation of Pacific salmon was driven by the active Miocene geologic history of Northwestern North America over the past 70 million years in contrast to the relatively stable Atlantic drainages. Along the Pacific coast, tectonic uplift created the mountain ranges that characterize the region today, as well as a diverse and changing array of habitats that promoted isolation, specialization, and speciation. Over the last 2.58 million years, an alternating series of glacial and interglacial periods known as the Pleistocene glaciation further contributed to this constantly changing array of habitats. During glacial periods as glaciers expand, more water is bound up in ice causing sea level to fall, and during interglacial periods as glaciers melt, sea level rises. As sea level rose and fell over the course of the Pleistocene Epoch, the shorelines of the continents constantly changed and coastal estuaries where fresh river water mixes with salty ocean water were continuously in flux. Free to navigate the seas and inland rivers of this ever changing habitat, Pacific salmon thrived and speciated. Over the last 5,000 years, dominant habitat features in the Pacific Northwest have held relatively stable, and the five species of Pacific salmon we know today are thus the product of recent evolution overlaid on top of historical lineages evolved over the last 2.58 million years during the recurrent glacial episodes of the Pleistocene glaciation.

The life cycle of salmon is complex: they spend one to five years (depending on the species) growing to adults out in the open ocean preying on forage fish, before swimming upriver against the current and leaping over rapids to the freshwater tributary of their birth to spawn the next generation. Salmon can make epic journeys, for example: Chinook and sockeye salmon of central Idaho travel over 900 miles (1,400 kilometers) and climb nearly 7,000 feet (2,100 meters) from the Pacific Ocean as they return home to spawn. Once the adults reach their destination, the females use their tails to excavate a shallow depression in the gravely stream bed called a redd, where they deposit up to 5,000 yellow to orange eggs (roe). One or more males approach the female in her redd, depositing milt (semen) over the roe; the female then covers the eggs by disturbing the gravel at the upstream edge of the redd with her tail before moving on to excavate another redd; females may make several redds before their egg supply is exhausted. In all five species of Pacific salmon, the adults die within a few days or weeks of spawning, but between 2% and 4% of female Atlantic salmon survive to spawn again. The salmon eggs hatch into tiny "alevin" still feeding on their egg yokes, quickly grow into spotted "fry" on a diet of zooplankton, then develop into vertically stripped "parr" on a diet of aquatic insects. The parr stay in their natal stream for six months to three years developing into bright silvery "smolts"; typically, only about 10% of all salmon eggs survive to this stage. The freshwater smolts then migrate downstream to its estuary where their body chemistry changes allowing them to survive in the salt water ocean where they feed on krill and other tiny shellfish to amass body weight and mature into adults. When, according to their internal biological clock, it comes time for the adult salmon to spawn, they use the Earth's magnetic fields to guide them back to the estuary where they first entered the ocean and then rely on their sense of taste and smell to guide them back to their ancestral tributary. Consistently, the salmon home in on their place of birth, not only to pass down the best evolutionary genetic lines, but also the unique adaptive differences of their clan, which allowed them to detect, recall and locate that singular place of their birth.

Over millennia, innumerable salmon clans eventually colonized every available food niche within the species' broad geographical distribution. That salmon begin and end their lives in rivers and tributaries makes them particularly vulnerable to human predation, and the first aboriginal people to inhabit these far northern watersheds of salmon habitat thousands of years ago quickly adopted them as a staple food source. Early aboriginal subsistence salmon fishers also developed a brisk trade in dried salmon with inland tribes, but for thousands of years this relatively minor level of human exploitation had little impact on the swarming salmon runs, and the fish returned in abundance year after year to spawn in their natal streams.

It wasn't until the 1800s that overfishing began to take its toll on salmon populations, when the industrial process of canning made it practical to preserve and transport fish to far away markets without spoilage. By 1810, Frenchman, Nicolas Appert, had perfected preservation of food in sealed glass jars by placing the jars in boiling water, and in that same year Englishman, Peter Durant, patented his own method of preservation, packing food in tin cans. Tin cans were first used to preserve salmon in Scotland in the 1830s, and by the 1840s, salmon canning had reached across the Atlantic to Maine and New Brunswick in North America. But it wasn't until 1864, in the spirit of early stage capitalism, that the four Hume brothers brought industrial scale canneries to the west coast salmon fisheries. The Humes' built the first industrial scale cannery on a barge in the Sacramento River that runs through central California and empties into the Pacific Ocean at the estuary on San Francisco Bay. Only two years later, in1866, the brothers decided that their fortunes would be better made further north on the less crowded, salmon rich, Columbia River on the border between Oregon and Washington. The Columbia River has its headwaters in Canada and is over 1,250 miles long. Its main tributary, the Snake River, is over 1,000 miles long, and the total length of the Columbia and all its tributaries is about 14,000 miles. The entire Columbia River Basin is larger than the country of France. This watershed that carries a quarter-million cubic feet of fresh water per second to the Pacific Ocean is second only to the Mississippi as the largest navigational transportation system in the U.S. The Hume brothers set up shop 50 miles upstream from the mouth of the Columbia at a site near present day Astoria, Oregon. In the years that followed, the salmon industry on the Columbia grew by leaps and bounds from 2 commercial fishing boats in 1866, to 100 by 1872, 250 by 1874, 500 in 1878 and 1,200 in 1881. In addition to gillnets, fishers also used purse seine nets pulled by horses, fish traps, and the ruthlessly efficient "fish wheel" that was positioned in the river so that their steel mesh buckets, driven by the current, would scoop fish from the water and drop them into a chute that was directly connected to a cannery. By 1883 the Northern Pacific Railroad had punched inland to The Dalles, Oregon, and with access to the railroad the canneries thrived; the commercial catch of wild salmon on the Columbia reached its brief peak yield in 1883 and 1884 with totals of over 42 million pounds, and the total number of canneries peaked at 39 between 1883 and 1887. Through the mid-1880s, canneries did not set catch limits and commercial salmon fishers often caught more than the canneries could process, so the excess, as many as 500 dead salmon a day, were simply dumped back into the river. By the late 1880s the salmon catch and cannery operations were already in steep decline, and by 1890 the total catch was down to 29.6 million pounds and the total number of canneries down to 21.

Another factor contributing to this decline in salmon populations in the late 1880s and 1890s was the environmental impacts to upstream spawning areas of human land use practices such as farming, road building, and logging. Salmon require gravely stream beds to lay their eggs and cold water for their young to survive; their greatest nemesis: silted up stream beds and loss of shade cover caused by human land development. A third major obstacle to the salmon of the Columbia River Basin in their epic struggle to survive was the era of hydroelectric dam building to supply electricity to the ever growing human populations of the Pacific Northwest. A report from the 1976 *Pacific Northwest Regional Commission* listed 23 dams that were built on salmon producing tributaries in the Columbia River Basin between 1889 and 1920. A 1933 report by the *Fish Commission of Oregon* estimated that about half of the salmon spawning habitat in Columbia River tributaries had been wiped out by irrigation and hydroelectric dams. Major hydroelectric dam construction continued apace well into the 1980s, and there are now 136 hydroelectric power dams along the 1,250 mile long Columbia, and only 44 miles of river that still runs free. These dams effectively blocked passage to vast drainages where salmon had spawned for thousands of generations.

Declining Chinook runs in the Columbia's tributaries was observed as early as 1875, when Spencer Baird, the U.S. Fish Commissioner, advised the commercial fishing industry that the problems of overfishing, habitat loss and dams could all be overcome through artificial propagation of fish, that is, raising sufficient numbers of fish in hatcheries to stock tributaries below the dams where fish passage would not be obstructed on their way to the ocean as juveniles or back from the ocean as spawning adults, and where upstream habitat destruction would not matter. Baird saw artificial production as a better means of protecting the commercial salmon fishery than attempting to protect naturally spawning fish by limiting the catch or regulating upstream land uses, and this approach to salmon preservation prevailed for more than a century, even in the face of declining salmon populations. Early attempts at establishing hatcheries from 1877 through the 1890s were poorly financed and ill conceived, and failed to stem the decline in salmon runs. In 1898, Washington State Fish Commissioner, A.C. Little, alarmed by the declining Chinook runs in the upper Columbia tributaries called for more aggressive artificial production to rebuild and save them, writing, *"[The salmon catch has reached] the highest point attainable unless radical measures are taken towards keeping up the supply. In no way can this be done successfully but by artificial propagation."* In effect, Little argued that the only way to reverse the salmon decline was to ignore its obvious causes and simply produce more hatchery fish. This was the predominant thinking among fishery biologists of the day, despite clear evidence to the contrary. In 1909, the state of Oregon constructed the Central Hatchery, (later renamed the Bonneville Hatchery), on the lower Columbia River just upstream from the present-day Bonneville Dam. The Central Hatchery served as a place to incubate salmon eggs brought in from other hatcheries, with the resulting fry shipped to streams all over the Northwest. The theory was that the Central Hatchery could serve as a nursery to assist in rebuilding salmon runs in streams where they were depleted by transferring salmon stock from other parts of the basin where they were still plentiful. These so called "stock transfers" involved taking eggs from one part of the basin to a hatchery, where they were incubated and hatched, and then transferred to another part of the basin for release. Scientists of the time believed they could rebuild the depleted Columbia salmon runs with fish from other rivers, but in actual effect, these stock transfers produced a biological disaster. It wasn't until the late 20th century that fish biologists began to understand the impacts that hatchery fish had on fish that spawn in the wild. Through careful observation, scientists learned that fish raised in the hatchery environment become acclimated to artificial conditions, and when released into the wild they carry this learning into the natural environment. Hatchery fish raised by the hundreds of thousands in open concrete tanks called raceways were fed pellets at regular intervals. The fish learned to dash for the pellets when they appeared, and to be fearless of predators. When released into natural streams, hatchery fish behaved in the same way. Alternatively, wild fish spawned in natural streams learn to conserve energy, avoid predators, eat when food is available and disperse to places in the aquatic environment where food, shelter and appropriate water temperatures are available. When hatchery salmon released into the natural environment competed with the native wild salmon, the hatchery salmon out-competed the wild salmon for food, but also were easy targets for natural predators. This comingling of hatchery and native fish had negative impacts on both: it starved native salmon which severely reduced their survival rate, and it increased predation on hatchery salmon which limited the adult fish available for commercial fishers. In

1908, when the annual release of hatchery salmon fry into the Columbia River reached 34 million, the Oregon Fish Commission expressed alarm at the continuing decline of the spring Chinook runs, but for decades thereafter, fisheries managers assumed that hatcheries could compensate for lost spawning and rearing habitat by simply outproducing nature, even as it was becoming evident that hatchery fish were contributing to the decline of wild fish by introducing fish that looked the same as their wild counterparts but behaved much differently.

Hatchery fish faced many of the same obstacles to survival as fish spawned in the wild – water pollution, degraded stream habitat, high water temperatures, the effects of predators and overfishing – but one problem unique to hatchery fish was "genetic erosion" caused by stock transfers. Scientists at Oregon State University published a study in the journal, *Nature Communications (February, 2016)*, titled, *"DNA evidence shows that salmon hatcheries cause substantial, rapid genetic changes."* This research has verified that Pacific hatchery stock salmon differ genetically from wild salmon and the differences accrue from the first generation of breeding. Researchers measured *"differential gene expression"* in the offspring of wild and of first-generation hatchery fish reared in a common hatchery environment. Surprisingly, they found that there were *"723 genes differentially expressed between the two groups of offspring."* Further analysis using *"gene-enrichment analyses"* revealed that genetic adaptation to the hatchery environment involved responses in wound healing, immunity and metabolism, suggesting to researchers that the earliest stages of domestication may involve genetic adaptations to highly crowded hatchery conditions. Through this process of genetic erosion, most Pacific salmon in the Columbia River Basin are no longer wild fish, but instead genetic impostors.

In the early 20th century, troll fishing for hatchery salmon began on the lower Columbia and steadily increased in both number of boats and in gasoline-powered boats that could range farther than the traditional sail-powered boats, even venturing out into the ocean. Trollers dragged multiple lines from booms that extended from either side of their boats. By 1915 there were 500 boats trolling in the lower Columbia, and by 1919 a thousand. 1915 also was the year that the number of gillnet boats peaked on the lower Columbia at 2,856. In 1914, the total catch jumped to 38.5 million pounds and in 1915 to 42.7 million pounds. It stayed above 40 million pounds per year through 1919 but then, despite continued mass stocking of hatchery fish, began to steadily decline, reaching above 40 million pounds one last time in 1925. In the 1930s, when the states would periodically close the river to allow more fish to escape capture, many fishers simply took to trolling out in the Pacific near the mouth of the Columbia, and in the mid 1930s, as the catch of albacore tuna began to increase farther out to sea, salmon fishers realized they could take both salmon and tuna if they fished farther off shore. Ocean trolling for salmon near the mouth of the Columbia and beyond, continued at high levels into the early 1980s. The commercial catch of hatchery salmon continued to decline decade upon decade in the 20th century, to 18.8 million pounds in 1938, dropping below 10 million pounds for the first time in 1953 only to rise above one more time thereafter through 1969.

On the Snake River, the longest tributary of the Columbia that wends its way through the states of Wyoming, Idaho, Oregon and Washington, cannery and catch records suggests that in the 1800s about 1.5 million salmon and steelhead returned to the Snake River each year to spawn; a more recent count from the U.S. National Marine Fisheries Service (NMFS), estimated annual returns of Snake River spring/summer Chinook in the 1960s at just 125,000 fish, and by 1979 at just 12,000 despite increased hatchery production after 1966. The U.S. Endangered Species Act (ESA) was signed into law by President Richard Nixon in 1973, and in 1980, in an attempt to avoid listing Columbia River Basin salmon as threatened or endangered species which would have require extensive costly mitigations by fishers, irrigators, electric dam operators and industrial electric power users, the U.S. Congress passed the Northwest Power Act, which authorized the four Northwest states that share the bulk of the Columbia River Basin to form the *Northwest Power Planning Council* (changed to *Northwest Power and Conservation Council* in 2003), and directed the Council to write a program to mitigate the impacts of hydropower dams on fish in the river basin. The Council adopted its first version of this program in 1982 that included recovery measures for salmon such as spawning habitat improvements, increased production of hatchery fish, improved fish bypass systems at the dams and, particularly on the Snake, transporting smolts around the dams on barges. These measures appeared to be working in the mid-1980s as counts of adult fish at the dams increased compared to the 1970s, but runs began to decline again in the late 1980s; in 1983, the commercial salmon and steelhead catch in the Columbia River totaled 1.25 million pounds, but by 1995, for the first time since 1866, dropped below 1 million pounds. Some populations, particularly Snake River sockeye, which spawn in mountain lakes at the headwaters of the Salmon River in central Idaho, the Snake's largest tributary, declined from several thousand fish in the 1950s to several hundred in the 1960s to just one in the years 1988, 1989, 1992 and 1994. In 1990, the number of naturally spawning Snake River fall Chinook, as opposed to hatchery fish, was estimated at just 78 fish, and in 1994, the number of naturally spawning Snake River spring/summer Chinook was estimated at just 1,822 fish. As the runs continued to diminish through 1990s, the states, much to the anger of commercial fishers, were forced to set shorter and shorter commercial fishing seasons. Even when the total catch of hatchery fish rebounded to nearly 5 million pounds per year in the early 2000s, it had become clear to commercial fishers that they could no longer earn a living off salmon fishing on the Columbia River, and most either retired or moved to Alaska where salmon fishing was still profitable. Since the early 2000s, even as wild salmon faced extinction, the Oregon and Washington Departments of Fish and Wildlife still opened fishing seasons and sold fishing licenses for both river and ocean salmon.

In April, 1990, the Shoshone-Bannock Indian Tribe, whose reservation is in southeastern Idaho and whose members historically fished the headwaters of the Salmon River, petitioned NMFS to list the Snake River sockeye as an endangered species under the ESA. Two months later, petitions to list Snake River spring/summer and fall Chinook as threatened species were filed by a coalition that included *Oregon Trout*, the *Oregon Natural Resources Council*, the *Northwest Environmental Defense Center*, *American*

Rivers, and the *American Fisheries Society*. Over the course of the 1990s, as population sizes continued to dwindle, 12 populations of Columbia River Basin salmon and steelhead were eventually listed as threatened or endangered:

- Snake River sockeye, 1991
- Snake River spring/summer run Chinook, 1992
- Snake River fall run Chinook, 1992
- Snake River steelhead, 1997
- Upper Columbia River steelhead, 1997
- Upper Columbia River Chinook, 1999
- Lower Columbia River Chinook, 1999
- Columbia River chum, 1999
- Middle Columbia River steelhead, 1999
- Lower Columbia River steelhead, 1999
- Upper Willamette River steelhead, 1999
- Upper Willamette River Chinook, 1999

In 1992, NMFS, which is the federal agency that implements the ESA for salmon and steelhead, appointed the *Snake River Salmon Recovery Team* to make specific recommendations for the recovery of the fish and they released their first set of recommendations in 1993 which included improving fish ladders to increase survival of adult salmon swimming upstream, installing screens on dam turbine intakes to prevent smolts swimming downstream from being sucked in, transporting smolts around the dams in specially designed barges and trucks, and building several new hatcheries on the Snake to release millions more smolts into the river each year. In other words, no significant changes from the recommendations made more than a decade earlier by the *Northwest Power Planning Council* that had failed to recover the fish. The most controversial recommendation that was left off the table by the *Snake River Salmon Recovery Team* due to powerful political opposition from the electric utilities industry, industrial scale electricity users, and navigable river shipping interests, was to breach the four Snake River hydroelectric dams in central Washington and allow the river to run free to give the salmon free passage up and down stream. While all 250 dams on the Columbia River Basin have played a role in the salmon's decline, the 4 dams on the lower Snake River are prime targets for removal because they have become a financial liability to the Bonneville Power Administration, and their removal would inordinately benefit salmon; the Snake River watershed constitutes 70% of the habitat available for Chinook in the entire Columbia River Basin, no other dam removals would open up as much habitat. Even though the dam operators spent billions of ratepayer dollars on fish ladders and other fish passage mechanisms, the dams have made salmon passage to and from the sea so difficult that all but a few ever make it back home to spawn in their ancestral streams. The salmon recovery effort has cost Bonneville Power ratepayers more than $16 billion since 1980, much of it spent on the basin's 178 salmon hatcheries that not only haven't helped wild salmon recover, but have actually diminished their chances of survival. While the hydroelectric dams have been an unmitigated disaster for the salmon, they have also been disastrous for the other 137 species that are part of the trophic pyramid including apex predator orcas (killer whales) living off the Pacific coast of Washington that are dying of starvation due to the near-absence of Chinook salmon which are the foundation of their diet. By 2019, the three local orca pods were down to 73 animals, and marine biologists feared their population had dropped below sustainable levels.

As ESA listings of distinct salmon and steelhead populations continued throughout the 1990s (see listings above), the failure of status quo measures to recover the fish was once again confirmed. In 2007, a team of NMFS researchers published a study, *"Pacific Salmon Extinctions: Quantifying Lost and Remaining Diversity,"* in the journal, *Conservation Biology*, where they systematically enumerated extinct Pacific salmon populations and characterized lost genetic diversity and ecological life history in the northwestern U.S. In this study, researchers pieced together historical salmon ranges from archaeological reports and historical accounts left by explorers, surveyors and early settlers. This evidence indicated that before Europeans arrived, 1,383 distinct Pacific salmon populations thrived in the river systems from central California to the Canadian border that drain into the Pacific Ocean; each population a geographically cohesive group of fish that did not spawn with any others, rendering it genetically isolated and distinct from all other salmon that had adapted to a particular stream. Since the arrival of Europeans in the late 18th century, a total of 406, or 29% of these genetically-distinct populations have become extinct, and as of the early 21st century, more than one-third of the remaining 977 populations have been listed as threatened or endangered under the ESA. Geographically, extinctions are proportionally fewer in coastal drainages, compared with interior watersheds mainly due to dams and other human alterations to the salmon's stream habitat. On the Columbia River Basin the researchers found 26 populations of sockeye, Chinook and steelhead to be completely extirpated from the Columbia River headwaters in British Columbia, Canada. The mid and upper sections of the Columbia River and its tributaries have lost over 50% of salmon populations, including all coho populations. The upper Snake River watershed is also now devoid of salmon, having lost all 51 of its Chinook, sockeye and steelhead populations. The study determined that at the beginning of the 21st century on the Columbia River and its tributaries: 54% of chinook, 47% of sockeye, 21% of chum, and 18% of pink salmon populations had become extinct.

When federal agencies such as NMFS propose actions that affect an endangered species, the U.S. National Oceanic and Atmospheric Administration (NOAA) is required to produce a biological opinion call a "BiOp" that directs further action on species recovery. The first NOAA BiOp for Snake River salmon and steelhead recovery was produced in 1993/1995, which was followed by BIOps in 2000, 2004, 2008/10 and 2014, each of which was challenged in federal court by coalitions of tribal nations, environmental NGOs, and state governments, for failing to comply with the ESA. Since the court's first ruling in 2000, federal judges have sided with plaintiffs in every case finding that NOAA's plans do not go far enough to recover the endangered fish, and are merely a perpetuation of the status quo. In 2016, Federal District Court Judge Michael Simon admonished NOAA to produce a BiOp that includes an analysis of new alternatives such as removal of the 4 Snake River dams which he suggested *"… may elucidate an approach that will finally move the listed species out of peril [and] break through any bureaucratic logjam that maintains the status quo."* As of 2020, the dams still stand, and the salmon be damned.

(Full disclosure: I live on the north coast of California in the Eel River Basin that was once premier salmon habitat before European immigrants like my ancestors arrived. The Eel River and its tributaries form the third largest watershed entirely in California, draining an area of 3,684 square miles (9,540 square kilometers) flowing north that empties into the Pacific Ocean 10 miles south of the Humboldt Bay. The story of the Eel River exactly mirrors that of the Columbia River. Salmon canneries flourished on the lower Eel from the 1870s to the 1920s, and declined thereafter due to decreasing runs caused by overfishing, intensive logging, road building, farming, and construction of two hydroelectric dams built between 1900 and 1908 that cut off 100 miles (160 kilometers) of prime salmon spawning habitat in the Eel River's upper headwaters. These dams added ecological insult to environmental injury by diverting water from the Eel River Basin into the Russian River Basin that flows south and empties into the Pacific Ocean 60 miles north of the San Francisco Bay. Even as these antiquated dams have become a financial albatross to their owner, Pacific Gas & Electric Co., powerful economic and political interests to the south that control the water behind the dams have prevented their removal to the detriment of the salmon. Artificial propagation of salmon in hatcheries was first deployed on the Eel River in 1857, well before it was on the Columbia, and the Eel was routinely stocked with millions of fry hatched from chinook eggs taken from the Sacramento, Noyo, and Russian Rivers, resulting in the "genetic erosion" of native Eel River salmon. When European settlers first arrived in the latter 1800s, historical evidence suggests that in wet years with good ocean conditions the Eel River Basin supported salmon and steelhead runs of well over a million fish, with about half that number in unfavorable years. But since the 1960s, the total salmon and steelhead run has averaged around 3,500 fish (+/- 1,000 Chinook, 500 coho, and 2,000 steelhead), which represents a greater than 99% decline in numbers. By the early 2000s, the commercial fishery for salmon at the mouth of the Eel was closed. Eel River Chinook were federally listed under the ESA as threatened in 1999, steelhead in 2000, and Coho listed as endangered in 2002. Despite these listings, as of July 29, 2020, the California Department of Fish and Wildlife is still issuing sports fishing licenses to catch salmon and steelhead in the ocean and on the Eel River (confirmed by phone call to CDFW, Eureka office, 7/29/2020). A report issued in 2010 by the *University of California Center for Watershed Sciences* concluded *"… coho salmon, Chinook salmon, and steelhead are all on a trajectory towards extinction in the Eel River basin, with only winter steelhead being widely enough distributed and abundant enough to persist beyond the next 50 years."*)

As dire as the situation is for Pacific salmon, it is even worse for Atlantic salmon. In March, 2016, highly respected scientist, scholar and writer, Kathleen McKeoghain, who specializes in genetics, agriculture, biodiversity and conservation, published a widely disseminated article on the internet, *"Atlantic Salmon Is Basically Extinct: You're Eating a Genetically Eroded Version,"* where she exposed the tragic plight of the Atlantic salmon:

"Today, 99.5 percent of all native Atlantic salmon has disappeared from the wild. In Europe, Scandinavia and around the Baltic Sea, native indigenous salmon has vanished from the Russian rivers Neva and Narva, the LuleÃ¤lven and UmeÃ¤lven of Sweden, from the Odra and Wisla in Poland, and the Vilia of Belarus. In fact, only 10 of the many rivers which empty into the Baltic arm of the northern Atlantic Ocean sustain wild salmon populations any longer, and the wild Baltic salmon genome is the only one with natural resistance to the destructive Gyrodactulus salaris parasite.

"Around the British Isles, in Ireland and across the pond to North America, wild salmon populations are extinct or endangered or threatened. The Kola Peninsula of Russia is known to be a current refuge for wild type Atlantic salmon, yet is also known to harbor military and radioactive waste at ecologically harmful levels. The grand TorneÃ¤lven of Sweden, called Tornionjoki where it traverses Finland, is one of the last rivers to host wild Atlantic salmon in the world. (For more on the status of Atlantic salmon, see the International Union for Conservation of Nature Red List <u>map</u>. *Researchers at the Swedish Agency for Marine and Water Management have produced a* <u>report</u> *on the Baltic extinctions. Anna Tonteri, a conservation geneticist at the University of Turku in Finland has written an excellent doctoral* <u>thesis</u> *about the population genetics of north European Atlantic salmon.)*

"The Baltic salmon extinctions were largely enabled by human destruction of migration routes for spawning, upon the building and operation of hydroelectric dams. Further molecular DNA studies of the hatchery stock salmon from this exemplary sea have demonstrated a genetic "homogenization." Stock salmon populations constitute more of a weak puree than a chunky soup, in terms of "population genetic structure," another statistical measure of diversity. This is why — although the map above may demonstrate a wide range and lesser areas of extinction — the actual number of wild salmon living within the extant areas is quite small at around 0.5 percent. In other words, the orange areas showing extant salmon are overall 99.5 percent inhabited by farmed stock salmon.

"We have learned to overlay DNA diversity upon geography and geologic history, in a relatively new field called landscape genomics. The important data is not just in the map or the numbers of fish, but in the genetic quality and the relationships of the individual salmon that comprise the families, clans and populations. An apparent abundance by numbers does not mean a population is healthy, self-sustaining and diverse.

"In Ireland, the release of farmed salmon has not only caused genetic erosion, but has disrupted the capacity of wild populations to adapt to warmer waters. This is a problem for salmon across its geographical range for the obvious reason of climate change. Strong and well founded recommendations for saving the remaining wild salmon include cessation of stock salmon releases and re-establishment of native spawning grounds. The future effects of warming waters, however, are unknown and not hopeful."

"Stock salmon cannot survive without human intervention. The overcrowded hatchery conditions in which it grows cause numerous fish body abnormalities and require nutritional supplementation to cover for shortfalls in bone development and other physiological problems."

"Moreover, the pollution and operation of inland fish tanks is costly. At this point in the Anthropocene, conservation interests may want to rise up another step against the introduction of industrialized, non-native food species (call them what you will) into the only biosphere we have in which to live, until we are able to halt any further species genetic erosion. Salmon has been swimming upstream against the depleting force of "genetic erosion" for at least a century, a force that has claimed its wild genome, its clans and its tribes, its genetic diversity, and which has nearly eliminated a once self-sustaining, powerful ocean species. Now, salmon cannot live without us.

"Atlantic salmon is essentially extinct because we have demanded too much of this natural resource through over-consumption and environmental exploitation. The wild gene forest that once lived, the old trees, the towering antiquarians of genetic variation, are gone, lost in the fire of a rapid, wholesale, industrial Homo sapiens sapiens taking, consumed in an anthropocentric fire we could even see burning, when one looks at the timeline of scientific data."

In researching this segment on salmon, I collected information from a broad range of sources including independent scientists, government agencies, tribal nations, environmental organizations, commercial fishing interests, sports fishing interests and hydroelectric dam operators, and there was one thing they all had in common: their stated goal is to recover wild salmon stocks to sustainable levels so that we can continue to exploit them as a food source as we have always done. With the lone exception of Kathleen McKeoghain above, the realization that it is commercial exploitation that has driven this iconic species to the brink of extinction never seems to dawn on them. Many scientists expressed optimism that salmon are genetically well equipped to survive the rapidly changing environments of the Anthropocene Epoch since the species has proven so resilient over the last 2.58 million years adapting to the constantly changing habitats of the Pleistocene glaciation. What these optimists fail to take into account is that the diverse genetics of wild salmon have been so eroded by hatchery fish, that they can no longer survive in the wild without human intervention.

Farmed Fish

Of the 1,500 fish stocks around the world that are known to be commercially fished, comprehensive estimations of abundance currently exist for only around 500. In most cases these are fish stocks which have been commercially fished for many decades and accurate records have been kept of species and tonnages caught, including the age and size of the fish. Very little is known about the other 1,000 fish stocks, particularly those in the Exclusive Economic Zones (EEZs) of many developing countries. Some developing countries provide catch data alone, without any scientific assessment, and others provide no catch data at all. Due to the dearth of reliable data from these fisheries, the UN Food and Agriculture Organization (FAO) makes limited use of such information which in effect means that FAO statistics do not reflect the conditions of a large proportion of the world's fish stocks. To fill in this major gap in the FAO data base, an independent joint American-German research group of scientists called the *World Ocean Review* (WOR), developed their own mathematical model to estimate the status of all fisheries by using catch reports alone.

The WOR researchers diligently requested information from the authorities of the countries responsible for regions with no catch data at all. According to the WOR model, a fish stock is depleted when the catch decreases conspicuously within a few years. Based on their findings, which takes into account 1,500 commercially exploited fish stocks and another approximately 500 fish stocks exploited by small scale artisanal and subsistence fishers – world fisheries are in even worse shape than assumed by the FAO. By 2008, 56.4% of fish stocks were over exploited or depleted, not 29.9% as claimed by the FAO. Despite the uncertainties of counting fish, WOR scientists and the FAO have both agreed on one thing: over the years the situation has continued to worsen. According to the *2010 State of World Fisheries and Aquaculture* (SOFIA) report of the FAO Fisheries and Aquaculture Department, after temporary fluctuations, the percentage of "fully exploited" stocks increased from 51% in 1974 to 57% in 2009, the percentage of "over exploited" or "depleted" fish stocks increased from 10% to 29.9%, and the percentage of "non-fully exploited" stocks declined from near 40% to only 12.7%. A clear trend was emerging: as far as overfishing and the intensive exploitation of the oceans is concerned, the situation is not improving – it is steadily growing worse.

Critics of this dire assessment of world fisheries cite the fact that the total annual world catch of wild fish remained relatively stable from its peak years in the 1990s of between 50 and 60 million tons (not including mollusks, crustaceans and seaweed) into the next decade from 2000 to 2010, as evidence that wild fish stocks were not being depleted. But by relying on the total world catch figures as their only metric, such critics completely missed the boat. The reason overall fish catches remained relatively stable into the first decade of the 21st century was not because of healthy wild fish stocks, but because as coastal fisheries became fished out, the fishers expanded from their traditional fishing grounds of the North Atlantic and North Pacific, further and further south. They also expanded into ever deeper waters; only a few decades ago it was virtually impossible in technical terms to drop nets deeper than 1,600 feet (~500 meters), today the fisheries are operating at depths of up to 6,500 feet (~2000 meters). Moreover, once the stocks of traditional species were exhausted, fishers turned to other species; some fish were given new appealing names in an effort to make them more marketable, for example: the "slimehead" became the "orange roughy", and the "Patagonian toothfish" became the "Chilean seabass". With modern technologies in the early 2000s, it was possible to remove virtually the same amount of fish from the sea as in the peak years of the 1990s, but below the water's surface, the composition of global fish stocks was undergoing profound changes – consistent catches are not an indicator of sustainable fisheries or stable ecosystems.

In a study published in the journal *Science* in 1998, (*Science* 06 Feb 1998), titled *"Fishing Down Marine Food Webs,"* researchers found that from 1950 to 1994 there was a decline in the trophic level of the species groups caught as reported in FAO global fisheries statistics. According to the researchers this decline:

> *"… reflects a gradual transition in landings from long-lived, high trophic level, piscivorous [fish that feed on other fish] bottom fish toward short-lived, low trophic level invertebrates and planktivorous [fish that feed on plankton] pelagic fish. This effect, also found to be occurring in inland fisheries, is most pronounced in the Northern Hemisphere. Fishing down food webs (that is, at lower trophic levels) leads at first to increasing catches, then to a phase transition associated with stagnating or declining catches. These results indicate that present exploitation patterns are unsustainable."*

Over the seven decades spanning 1950 to 2020, as new fishing technologies enabled commercial fishers to penetrate farther and deeper into the fishes natural habitat, the world's human population was spiraling upward. In 1950, the world's total human population was estimated at 2.584 billion people, by 2020 that number had more than tripled to 7.794 billion. In absolute terms, this amounts to 5.21 billion more mouths to feed in 2020 than in 1950. Another factor contributing to the ever increasing demand for fish was a steady increase in the average per capita fish consumption of people around the world from 21.8 pounds (9.9 kilograms)/person/year in the 1960s, to 36.3 pounds (16.4 kg)/person/year in 2005. With more people eating more fish, world demand for fish exploded over these seven decades.

Into the early1970s, over 94% of all fish consumed by people around the world came from wild caught species living in natural aquatic ecosystems, but by 1980, the practice of fish farming had begun to take off, and in the decades since, farmed fish has supplied an ever increasing percentage of the world's demand for fish and other aquatic species. From 1970 to 2008 the production of fish farms (including fish, mollusks, crustaceans and seaweed) grew at a rate of 8.3% per year, compared to less than a 2% increase for wild caught fish, and 2.9% increase for terrestrial livestock. In 1970, farmed fish supplied 5.2% of world fish demand, by1980 that percentage had nearly doubled to 9.7%, increasing again to 16.4% by 1990, 30.6% by 2000, 46.8% by 2010, and in 2013, farmed fish overtook wild fish, supplying 51.4% of the world's demand. In the 1990s, as the wild fisheries catch plateaued at over 90 million tons/year (including mollusks, crustaceans and seaweed), fish farming continued to expand at an accelerating rate, increasing by 24.87 million tons/year in the 1990s, to 36.30 million tons/year in the 2000s. The 2010 FAO report noted that the world's population increased by 6.3% from 2004 to 2009, whereas fish farm production increased by 31.5% over those same five years.

Fish farming, otherwise known as "aquaculture", is nothing new to the human Neolithic experience. In 2003, Dr. Heather Builth, an honorary research associate with Monash University in Melbourne, Australia, provided convincing evidence of the world's oldest know fish farm built by the aboriginal Gunditjmara people of Lake Condah about 220 miles (~350 kilometers) west of what is today Melbourne. Although the land was drained in the late 19th century by European settlers, Dr. Builth measured every hill and valley in the landscape and used a computerized geography simulation program to "re-flood" the land. Dr. Builth's simulated flood revealed an artificial system of ponds connected by canals, covering more than 30 square miles (~75 square kilometers). Dr. Builth told *ABC Science Online*, "*The community excavated channels to get direct access to baby eels that were migrating from the sea, and to bring them into prepared wetlands. It was a gigantic aquaculture system.*" Supporting evidence for Dr. Builth's theory was found in the sediments underneath trees and in the remaining swamps near Lake Condah. Dr. Barry Sankhauser of the Australian National University in Canberra used mass spectrometry and gas chromatography to find evidence of eel lipids (fats) in the sediments beneath hollowed-out trees which were likely used by the Gunditjmara people as smokehouses and cooking hearths. Dr. Peter Kershaw, a Monash University palynologist (expert in ancient pollen) studied the pollen record in the swamp sediments and found evidence of a sudden change in vegetation consistent with an artificial pond system; radiocarbon dating of the soil samples indicated the ponds were created up to 8,000 years ago. Dr. Builth, who argues that the community was smoking eels to preserve and trade them, asserts that the "*Guditjmara weren't just catching eels; their whole society was based around eels. And that to me was the proof.*" The second oldest record of fish farming goes back to 3500 BC (5,500 years ago) in China, and the oldest textbook on fish farming dates back to 475 BC (2,475 years ago) when a Chinese government official and self-taught fish farmer named Fan-Li wrote a book covering pond construction, brood stock selection and pond maintenance. Ancient Chinese fish farmers fed silkworm feces and nymphs to carp raised in ponds on silkworm farms. Around 2000 BC (4,000 years ago), ancient Egyptians developed an elaborate irrigation system used to desalinate land for agriculture in which they fish farmed tilapia. In 600 BC (2,600 years ago), wealthy Romans built "Assyrian vivariums" in their homes, which were a kind of artificial pond where fish and crustaceans caught in lagoons were kept alive until shortly before they were eaten. Wealthy Romans also cultivated fish such as mullet and trout in ponds called "stews." The European Middle Ages (5th to the 15th century AD) saw the stew pond concept further developed, particularly by monks at monasteries, at least in part to augment declining wild fish stocks in rivers. Sound familiar? As far back as the 4th century AD, the Mayan civilization of Central America practiced a form of aquaculture; they created fertile plots of land in swampy areas by digging canals and placing the excavated mud on mats made of woven reeds two feet above the water level. Fish, turtles and other aquatic species that entered the canals were caught for food. In the 10th century AD, native Hawaiians farmed a wide range of salt-tolerant and freshwater fish such as mullet, silver perch and Hawaiian gobies, in highly productive "taro fishponds" that were fed by runoff from irrigation streams as well as hand-made estuaries connected to the ocean tides.

While fish farming goes back millennia, never before in human history has it been the worldwide economic juggernaut it has become in modern times. Modern fish farming can trace its roots back to the early 1950s, when John Hanson, an employee of the New Mexico Game and Fish Department, began experimenting with the dietary regimen of hatchery trout using formulations for dried fish pellets. Until the end of World War II, most fish hatcheries relied on raw meat (mostly horse meat) as a dietary staple, but Hanson's formulation included other ingredients such as fish meal and fish oil made from fisher "by-catch" (non-commercial fish species caught by commercial fishers), vegetable proteins, cereal grains, vitamins and minerals, that he dried and formed into easily digestible pellets. Throughout the 1950s, Hansen experimented with the recipe for fish feed pellets at the Red River Hatchery near Taos, New Mexico, to improve on the conversion ratio of food intake to fish growth. When Hanson's fish feed pellets were applied to aquaculture, what had been a marginal business enterprise became a profitable business model. Then, in the 1970s, the introduction of new, lighter, more durable and relatively inexpensive construction materials such as plastic tubing and nylon netting, enabled the cost effective manufacture of large fish cages that could float in the open ocean rather than having to construct expensive artificial saltwater ponds on land made of glass, steel and concrete. These new materials and methods enabled the rapid expansion of marine (salt water) aquaculture that took place from the 1970s into the first decades of the 21st century. While over 220 species of fish and shellfish species are commercially farmed, Atlantic salmon, carp and tilapia are the most commonly farmed fish species around the world; shrimp are also farmed on an industrial scale in modern day aquaculture.

Atlantic salmon were first successfully farmed in Norway in the 1960s in on-shore tanks. A technological breakthrough came around 1970 when the first fish cage was constructed allowing salmon to be farmed off-shore out in the open ocean. Salmon eggs were hatched and reared to juveniles in on-shore hatcheries, then transferred to the off-shore cages to grow to adult slaughter weight. This cage system has changed little since those early days, basically, a closed net hangs down in the water from a floating, square, hexagonal or circular ring made of steel or plastic tubing that is moored to the sea bottom. Cage surface areas range from 4,300 square feet to 11,800 square feet (~400 square meters to 1,100 square meters), volumes range from 106,000 cubic feet to 1.4 million cubic feet (~3 000 cubic meters to 40,000 cubic meters), and depths range from 33 feet to 130 feet (~10 meters to 40 meters). The salmon are fed a formulation of dry feed. These open net fish cages allow sea water to flow through, thus eliminating the need for expensive pumping and filtration systems required to operate on-shore fish tanks. This innovation turned salmon farming into a highly profitable business enterprise.

By packing hundreds of thousands of fish into these massive enclosures similar to feedlots (Concentrated Animal Feeding Operations – CAFOs) on land where cattle are grown to slaughter weight, these salmon factories churn out adult fish like clockwork in 14 to 30 month cycles, producing from

800 to 4,000 tons/cage/cycle. The long and sheltered coastline of Norway, with its thousands of fjords and islands as well as its cold and stable ocean temperature, provided the perfect setting for this kind of intensive fish farming. Norwegian salmonid farming companies have come to dominate the world's farmed salmon industry: in 2016, 11 of the top 20 producers were from Norway. Since the year 2000, the Norwegian company "Marine Harvest" has held the top spot as the world's largest salmonid farming enterprise, slaughtering almost as much fish annually as the next three largest producers combined. Their salmon farming operations extend well beyond the coast of Norway to Ireland, Scotland, the Faeroe Islands, Canada, U.S. and Chile.

As in overcrowded feedlots on land, disease runs rampant in overcrowded salmon cages. Salmon anemia is one of the most pernicious viral diseases of farmed salmon. This highly contagious disease was first described in Norway in 1984, and it continues to be a problem there despite control measures. Since the late 1990s, outbreaks have also been reported in Chile, the Cobscook Bay in Maine, U.S., the Bay of Fundy in New Brunswick, Canada, the Faroe Islands and Scotland. With an initially low mortality rate, the cumulative mortality can sometimes exceed 90% if the disease remains unchecked. While the farmed salmon industry has spent tens of millions of dollars to eradicate the disease, it has killed millions of fish and left the flesh of survivors riddled with lesions. In November, 2019, the *Sea Shepherd Conservation Society* documented a mass salmon die-off event at salmon farms within Clayoquot Sound, a UNESCO listed World Biosphere Reserve. The video footage reveals the presence of hundreds of thousands of dead and decomposing salmon being loaded onto barges at salmon farming sites while clean-up crews operated around the clock to clean up the mess. Alexandra Morton, an independent biologist, confirmed the presence of "Piscine Orthoreovirus", a virus from Norway that appears to cause jaundice in farmed salmon, stating *"neither farmed or wild salmon are surviving this cheap and dirty way of farming."* Sea *Shepherd* founder and CEO, Paul Watson, sees salmon farming as such a serious threat to wild salmon that he has initiated a major campaign against salmon farms stating overtly, *"Our objective is to shut them down."*

Sea lice are a natural parasite that co-evolved with wild salmon over millions of years, but with the exponential growth of salmon farming over the late 20th century, unprecedented sea lice infestations are now threatening wild salmon populations in their native northern hemisphere. In the study, *"Declining Wild Salmon Populations in Relation to Parasites from Farm Salmon,"* published in the October, 2006, *Proceedings of the National Academy of Sciences (PNAS)*, researchers studied sea lice transmission and pathogenicity to estimate the impact of salmon farms on the survival of wild juvenile pink and chum salmon migrating through the Broughton Archipelago off the coast of western Canada. Usually considered benign on adult salmon, sea lice are a severe pathogen of wild juvenile pink salmon; survival with one or two sea lice is poor, and with more than two is fatal. In the wild, juvenile salmon do not cohabitate with adults (and their parasites) for the first several months of their marine life. However, salmon farms located on juvenile salmon migration routes undermine this natural spatial divide with juveniles swimming near to the overcrowded salmon farm cages where sea lice proliferate. This change in the timing and magnitude of parasite transmission undermines the functional role of migration in protecting juvenile salmon from parasites associated with adult fish. The researchers concluded that salmon farm induced sea lice infestations have depressed wild pink salmon populations and may lead to their local extinction. By 2016, sea lice had infested nearly half of Scotland's salmon farms, killing thousands of tons of farmed fish and causing skin lesions and secondary infections in millions more. Scotland has some of the worst sea lice infestations in the world, but the problem is growing worldwide. In 2016 for the first time, total production in Norway fell by 60,000 tons due to sea lice, and all salmon farms in the northern hemisphere where sea lice are endemic sustained significant losses. The salmon farming industry is estimated to spend more than $1.3 billion/year on pesticides and antibiotics in their effort to eradicate the sea lice and the diseases they bring. The pesticide "ivermectin" is commonly administered through feed to treat salmon for sea lice infestations. A high proportion of the chemical is excreted unchanged by the salmon, and accumulates in marine sediments below and in the vicinity of the fish farm. Studies have shown ivermectin in existing concentrations to be very toxic to many species that live in these sediments. Ivermectin is particularly lethal to a class of marine worms called polychaetes that are a crucial part of the marine food chain. They are key to the decomposition of accumulated organic matter such as fish feces and uneaten feed that accumulates under salmon farms. The worms constantly turn over the marine sediment allowing oxygenated water to reach aerobic decomposing bacteria. Without them, the marine sediment can become depleted of oxygen and aerobic decomposition cannot occur. Two other pesticides, "cypermethrin" and "azamethiphos," used on salmon farms have been shown to have toxic effects on lobster larvae and azamethiphos can also kill shrimp and adult lobster at low doses. To date there are few studies on the effects these pesticides have had on actual marine ecosystems.

As on land based factory farms where disease also runs rampant, a variety of antibiotics are administered to the fish through their feed in an attempt to control disease outbreaks. The most common antibiotics used are "oxytetracycline" and "fluorfenicol" both of which are also known to persist in marine sediments. Researchers have shown that antibiotics can significantly alter the microbial community found in marine sediment, not only reducing the total amount of bacteria but also the relative abundance among the different bacteria species. Sediment-dwelling bacteria provide a number of important ecosystem services by cycling key nutrients such as nitrogen, phosphorous and sulfur. Measurements reveal that antibiotics found in marine sediment near salmon farms lower the conversion rates for sulphates and nitrates. Studies also reveal that antibiotics result in an increase in antibiotic-resistant bacteria in farmed salmon which has led to a steady increased in antibiotic use and a concurrent increase in environmental risk. Here again, to date there are few studies on the effects these antibiotics have had on actual marine ecosystems.

Another threat to wild salmon posed by farmed salmon is when escaped farm salmon breed with native wild salmon, thereby changing their DNA. Escapes due to storm damage, predator damage and equipment malfunction are common on salmon farms, with reported escapes in Norway alone of approximately 200,000 fish/year. All farmed salmon breeding stocks were selected from wild Atlantic salmon taken from a few rivers in Norway and bred for specific genetic traits such as fast growth and high feed to growth ratios, neither of which predisposes them to survive in the wild, whereas wild salmon have evolved over millennia to survive local conditions of temperature, flow rate and pH levels. The resulting interbreeding between escaped farmed salmon and wild salmon has an irreversible effect on the genetic integrity of wild stocks, weakening them and reducing their production and survival rates. Researchers have found that over 71% of Norwegian rivers have been affected by interbreeding and in 29% of rivers the genetic contamination is at a critical level, such that the genetic integrity of wild fish is changing to that of farmed fish. One of the largest escapes of farmed salmon in Newfoundland happened in 2013, when more than 20,000 salmon got away from a farm in Hermitage Bay. That incident led scientists from the Canadian Department of Fisheries and Oceans to study the DNA of salmon in rivers on Newfoundland's south coast the next year, where they found hybrid salmon in 18 of the 19 rivers studied. In total, 1,700 fish we sampled and about 27% showed some farmed salmon genes. Even more alarming, some of the salmon tested were "feral" meaning both parents were of direct farm descent. The effects of escaped farm salmon on already depleted wild salmon stocks has been little studied.

Proponents of aquaculture claim that one of the benefits of fish farming is that it reduces demand for wild caught fish, but with respect to farmed salmon the exact opposite is true. Salmon are carnivorous and small wild caught forage fish such as anchovy and sardine are a major ingredient in the fish pellets that are fed to farmed salmon. In fact, 4 of the top 5 wild caught forage fish species are used in fishmeal and fish oil production for aquaculture as well as for pig and chicken feed. Salmon require 2.5 to 5 times as much forage fish biomass in their feed as the salmon biomass produced for human consumption. The proportion of fishmeal used in salmon farming feed rose from 10% in 1988 to 17% in 1994 to 33% in 1997. From 1988 to 1997, fish biomass used for feed rose from 10 million tons to 29 million tons. In effect, feeding wild caught forage fish to farmed salmon significantly increases demand for wild caught fish. It also significantly reduces the overall supply of wild fish that could potentially be consumed directly by people. As noted above in the section on the world's largest fishery in Peru, 98% of the Peruvian anchoveta catch is exported to produce fishmeal while in 2002, over 25% of indigenous Peruvian children under age 5 suffered from chronic malnutrition. All Atlantic salmon sold to consumers in North American and Europe comes from farmed salmon.

As we have seen, farmed salmon live under very different conditions than wild salmon and as a result the constituent of their tissues differs considerably from wild salmon. Wild salmon swim freely in the ocean eating a diet of krill and shrimp while farmed salmon are confined in densely populated cages where they are fed a diet of formulated pellets consisting of fish oil and fish meal made from ground-up herring and anchovies, maize gluten, ground-up feathers, soybeans, chicken fat, genetically engineered yeast, and the additive "astaxanthin" which is a caratenoid pigment found in krill and shrimp that gives wild salmon flesh its distinctive reddish-orange color. Some of the astaxanthin pigment used by fish farmers is made from algae or pulverized crustaceans, but most comes from the pharmaceutical corporation Hoffman-LaRoche that patented a cheaper synthetic version made with petrochemicals to reduce costs which still amounts to 20% of the price of feed pellets. The synthetic astaxanthin produced from petrochemicals possess a significantly different chemical structure than the natural chemical found in krill and shrimp. Natural astaxanthin is a very potent carotene-class antioxidant which serves a vitamin-like role in wild salmon and is essential to their health and survival, whereas one study on the synthetic petrochemical-sourced astaxanthin showed that fish consuming it grew more slowly than fish consuming the same amount of natural astaxanthin, indicating that synthetic astaxanthin is not functionally identical to natural astaxanthin in salmon metabolism. The main reason salmon farmers use this expensive chemical additive in their feed is not for the health of the fish, but because without it, the salmon flesh would be an unappetizing gray color making it unsalable. Thanks to a lawsuit in 2003 brought by consumers against three giant U.S. supermarket chains (Albertsons, Safeway and Kroger), in the U.S. farmed salmon must now be labeled as containing artificial chemicals for coloring.

Farmed salmon are fed diets far richer in fish oils than the natural diet of wild salmon so that they grow faster and reach market size sooner, but this fatty diet completely changes the fat profile of farmed salmon relative to its wild counterpart. Farmed salmon contain over twice as much total fat/gram as wild salmon, more than three times as much saturated fat/gram, and nearly six times as much Omega-6 fatty acids/gram. This fat profile is extremely unhealthy for the salmon and for the people who consume them. Also, the fat soluble persistent organic pollutants (POPs) – dioxins, furans, and PCBs (polychlorinated biphenyls) – are concentrated in fish oil fed to farmed salmon, and as a result farmed salmon contain about ten times more of these extremely toxic carcinogenic synthetic chemicals than wild salmon.

As noted above, due to the high density of fish in salmon cages, farmed salmon are more susceptible to infections and disease than wild fish, so to counter this problem antibiotics are frequently added to fish feed. Antibiotics in farmed salmon have been shown to promote antibiotic resistance in fish bacteria which, through gene transfer, increases the risk of antibiotic resistance in human gut bacteria. In effect, farmed salmon have been so manipulated by human intervention that they barely resemble the wild species fishmongers claim them to be.

(Note to readers: As I write, the Norwegian fish farming corporation, *Nordic Aquafarms*, is applying for a permit to raise Atlantic salmon in an onshore fish farming facility located on the Pacific coast of California in Humboldt County just 100 miles north of where I live. A coalition of local and national environmental organizations have filed a "joint comment" to the "draft environmental impact report" (DEIR) for the project making note of its significant environmental impacts:

> *"At full build out, [the fish farm] would use 21% of the county's electricity— as much as the cities of Eureka and Fortuna combined. And yet the DEIR concludes there would be no significant impacts from greenhouse gas emissions, truck traffic, bay intakes that*

will draw 10,000,000 gallons and an ocean discharge of 12,000,000 gallons of treated wastewater a day."

"Although its wastewater would have a lower nitrogen concentration than the effluent from antiquated municipal wastewater treatment plants around the bay, it would add to the existing nutrient load. It would also discharge warmer water with lower pH and salinity than the receiving waters. This combination has the potential to exacerbate the toxic algae blooms that have devastated the crab and clam fisheries in recent years."

Despite these significant environmental impacts on an already degraded ecosystem, *Nordic Aquafarms'* **permit will very likely be approved.)**

Genetically Modified (GM) Salmon

The final indignity suffered upon this iconic species by humans was the genetic engineering of its genome to extract every last pound of flesh humanly possibly from this marvel of evolutionary biology. After years of research, in 1989 two Canadian genetic engineers working at the Memorial University of Newfoundland succeeded in patenting a transgene created with a growth hormone gene taken from the fast growing Pacific Chinook salmon and a gene promoter sequence taken from the eel like fish, ocean pout. The growth gene and gene promoter sequence, which acts like an "on" switch, enabled the genetically modified (GM) salmon to grow year-round instead of seasonally like wild or farmed salmon. By 1992, with the aid of an $8.2 million federal grant for which the Canadian government negotiated a 10% royalty for itself on GM salmon sales, the researchers had successfully inserted this transgene into the DNA of the Atlantic salmon.

AquaBounty Technologies Inc., (a subsidiary of Intrexon, a biotech firm owned by U.S. billionaire Randal J. Kirk), headquartered in Waltham, Massachusetts, obtained the patent rights to the genetically engineered salmon. According to AquaBounty, the advantage of their innocuously named AquAdvantage® GM salmon is that it grows to adult size in half the time of wild or traditionally farmed salmon (about 16 to 18 months vs. 32 to 36 months) on 25% less feed. As the first GM animal ever considered for commercial sales, the AquAdvantage® GM salmon languished in regulatory limbo for over two decades until 2013 when AquaBounty announced that Environment Canada had approved the commercial production of GM Atlantic salmon eggs on Prince Edward Island off the east coast of Canada. This approval was given despite neither Canadian nor U.S. regulatory agencies having done any safety testing of their own, instead relying solely on studies conducted by AquaBounty that proved to be woefully deficient.

The AquAdvantage® GM salmon grows faster than wild fish because the transgene inserted into its genome causes the fish to continuously produce the growth hormone IGF all the time instead of just seasonally like wild or farmed salmon. Higher levels of IGF is known to lead to higher levels of cancer, yet AquaBounty conducted no long term health studies of AquAdvantage® GM salmon to test for carcinogenicity. The AquAdvantage® GM salmon was also found to contain less of the desirable Omega-3 fatty acids than either wild or farmed salmon suggesting that the transgene that makes GM fish grow faster changes the fishes metabolism in ways that are unknown. AquaBounty tested the AquAdvantage® GM salmon for allergic reactions on a tiny sample of just six fertile and six infertile fish. They found that the fertile AquAdvantage® GM salmon were 40% more allergenic than non-GM salmon, while the infertile group was 19% more allergenic than non-GM. AquaBounty claimed that the infertile allergenicity level wasn't statistically significant, and even if it was significant, it didn't matter because only infertile fish would be sold. Margaret Mellon, senior scientist with the non-government organization *Union of Concerned Scientists*, voiced strong disagreement with AquaBounty arguing there is good reason to be concerned about the potential allergenicity of all GM foods:

> *"You have this technology that allows you to essentially move proteins around from food to food. You can move a highly allergenic protein into a new food, and no one will know to avoid the new food."*

Michael Hansen, senior scientist with non-governmental organization *Consumers Union* also found fault with Aquabounty's allergenicity testing protocols noting that their test wasn't double blind meaning the researchers knew which fish were part of which test group, the sample size of just six infertile fish was woefully insufficient, and although AquaBounty is going to try to turn all its market-bound fish into sterile females, the process isn't perfect, and some 5% can be expected to end up as the more allergenic fertile females. This is particularly problematic when you consider that if a fertile female escapes into the wild, it could interbreed with wild fish. Canadian researchers had already found that AquAdvantage® GM salmon readily breed with wild brown trout, a closely related species common to areas surrounding AquaBounty Prince Edward Island facilities, posing serious risks to wild populations that are already under stress. Canada's approval of AquAdvantage® GM salmon egg production despite its inadequate testing was the first time any government had given the go-ahead to commercial scale production involving a GM food animal. The salmon eggs produced on Prince Edward Island were then shipped to laxly regulated Panama to be raised to adult slaughter weight in onshore grow-out tanks for export back to the U.S. and Canada.

In 2016, Canada became the first country to allow human consumption of AquAdvantage® GM salmon. The first shipments totaling 4.5 tons were flown into Montreal from Panama in June 2017 under cover of strict secrecy that was later exposed by the food watchdog group out of Quebec, *Vigilance OGM*, that obtained the import documents. Import-export data indicated that a Panama-based company called *Soterion Development* delivered the GM salmon to Canadian fish importers *Montreal Fish Co.* and *Sea Delight Canada*. According to the documentation, the refrigerated GM salmon fillets were then sold to unidentified supermarket chains, food-service distributors, restaurant chains and fish traders. When questioned about these retail outlets, Dave Conley, AquaBounty's director of corporate communications, said, *"It is our policy not to discuss our buyers, for obvious reasons."* Since Canada has no rules requiring labeling of GM products, Canadian fish consumers have in effect been denied their right to make informed choices about whether to consume GM foods or not.

The reason AquaBounty, a U.S. headquartered corporation, built their production facilities in Canada and Panama is that they did not yet have final approval from the U.S. Food and Drug Administration (FDA) that the AquAdvantage® GM salmon was safe for human consumption, approval they needed before locating production facilities in the U.S. The FDA did give Aquabounty preliminary approval, however, which allowed them go ahead with production outside the U.S., arguing that the *"[U.S. National Environmental Policy Act (NEPA)] does not require an analysis of environmental effects in foreign sovereign countries."* Documents AquaBounty submitted to the Securities and Exchange Commission (SEC) as part of it's bid to join the NASDAQ Stock Market, indicated that in 2013 AquaBounty handed over management of its Panamanian facility – including regulatory compliance, security of the facility, and other day-to-day operations – to an independent contractor about whom the FDA knew little. Subsequently, at the Panamanian facility there were disease outbreaks, security lapses that led to "lost" salmon, and a $9,500 fine from the GM friendly Panamanian regulators who found the company had repeatedly violated Panamanian environmental laws. Wenonah Hauter, Executive Director of the non-governmental organization *Food & Water Watch,* remarked:

> *"The horrendous environmental record of AquaBounty, which includes a security lapse that*
> *lead to 'lost' salmon in Panama and regulatory violations related to environmental safety, are*
> *a predictable consequence of the company's cavalier approach to raising this risky fish."*

The FDA is supposed to protect public safety, yet their environmental review of AquAdvantage® GM salmon was done in the form of an environmental assessment (EA) instead of the more thorough environmental impact statement (EIS) that would have fully considered the threat this GM fish could pose to wild fish populations and ecosystems. Another red flag on the U.S. approval process for AquAdvantage® GM salmon was that the FDA didn't even have an established protocol for reviewing the health risks of GM animals, so instead they arbitrarily decided to assess the GM fish using the same protocols they use for reviewing new animal drugs.

Despite AquaBounty's clear disregard for public safety, and despite a storm of public protest, and despite the FDA's inadequate approval process, in November, 2015, the AquAdvantage® GM salmon became the first genetically modified animal approved as safe for human consumption by the U.S. FDA. Just a few weeks later, however, the FDA banned the import and sale in the U.S. of AquaBounty AquAdvantage® GM salmon eggs from Canada and adult fish from Panama pending approval of consumer labeling guidelines for GM foods that were at the time under development by the U.S. Department of Agriculture (USDA). In the years following 2015, Senator Lisa Murkowski of Alaska (where virtually all wild salmon come from) inserted an amendment into FDA appropriations bills that required the FDA to issue mandatory labeling guidelines for GE salmon, using clear, on-package labeling stating that these fish are genetically engineered. In March of 2019, in defiance of Murkowski's amendment, the FDA lifted its import ban on GM salmon eggs bound for AquaBounty's new production facility constructed in the U.S. state of Indiana, based on the new guidelines issued by the USDA which did not explicitly require labeling of GM salmon as "genetically engineered." Instead the new FDA guidelines allowed GM food producers to force consumers to scan a "QR code" on their smart phone or call 1-800 numbers to find out if a product was genetically modified or not. Upon the FDA's lifting of the import ban on GM salmon, George Kimbrell, Legal Director at the *Center for Food Safety* (CFS), remarked:

> "USDA's new guidelines don't require adequate mandatory labeling, don't require calling the fish "genetically engineered" and don't help consumers know what kind of fish they are buying. These guidelines don't require mandatory labeling of GE [genetically engineered] salmon, and instead allow producers to use QR codes or 1-800 numbers for more information. That clearly is not what the Murkowski amendment requires."

Besides defying the Murkowski amendment, the FDA's lifting of the import ban on GM salmon eggs also came amidst a pending lawsuit against the FDA challenging its legal authority to even approve this genetically engineered fish as a "new animal drug". In March, 2017, CFS in coalition with environmental groups and commercial fishing trade associations sued the FDA for its approval of the AquAdvantage® GM salmon, objecting to the regulation of genetically engineered animals as though they were veterinary drugs, an obviously inappropriate testing protocol pointed out by Senior Policy Analyst at CFS, Jaydee Hanson:

> "This isn't what was meant by an animal drug. It's actually a whole new animal, the animal itself becomes the drug."

The plaintiffs further argued that with at least 35 other species of GM fish as well as GM cows, chickens, and pigs in the development pipeline, the FDA's approval of the AquAdvantage® GM salmon as a drug sets a bad precedent for the approval process for GM food animals in the future. CFS Legal Director Kimbrell added:

> "AquaBounty has not been able to follow the law because it lacks the capacity, sophistication, will, or all of the above. The FDA is dangerously out of touch, advancing AquaBounty's application based on its promises, not reality."

This is a polite way of saying that the U.S. regulatory system for genetically modified foods is corrupt to the core and dictated by the corporate titans of the genetic engineering industry.

In advance of AquaBounty's planned first-ever slaughter of GM salmon at its facility in Indiana for sales in the U.S. planned for the fall of 2020, consumer groups pressured over 80 grocery retailers, fish wholesalers, food service corporations and restaurant chains with more than 18,000 locations nationwide to issue public statements they will not sell GM salmon, including supermarket giants Albertsons, Costco, Kroger, Sprouts, Target, Trader Joe's, Walmart and Whole Foods, as well as the national restaurant chain Red Lobster.

In August, 2020, at a U.S District Court hearing on the CFS et al lawsuit against the FDA, District Judge Vincent Chhabria, unimpressed with the environmental assessment (EA) the FDA used to approve the AquAdvantage® GM salmon, said he was concerned that AquaBounty might use the FDA's finding of "no significant impact" to expand the program without realizing its full impact on local ecology. While Judge Chhabria did not issue a formal ruling at the hearing, he did say he was inclined to reject the EA and order the FDA to take a closer look at the project's potential hazards. As of this writing in September, 2020, U.S. salmon consumers are in the dark about the genetic heritage of the fish they are buying and eating.

In the debate over the efficacy of genetically modified food animals that has raged since the AquaBounty AquAdvantage® GM salmon became a reality in the early 1990s, genetic engineering proponents mounted a furious public relations campaign designed to denigrate and discredit critics of genetic engineering as anti-science and ignorant of the science of genetics. The reason the genetic engineering industry found it necessary to frantically attack their critics was because they knew that trusted public interest groups like *Center for Food Safety* and *Food & Water Watch* had been extremely effective at informing the general public that genetically engineered foods offered them no benefits while likely putting their personal health and the larger environment at risk. Of course, the truth is that independent molecular scientists who are not employed by the genetic engineering industry are highly skeptical of the safety claims made by the industry. In 2008, a group of distinguished French and Canadian scientists, published a review in the peer reviewed journal *Environmental Science & Policy* to specifically address the state of the science on the AquAdvantage® GM salmon, titled, *"Factors to consider before production and commercialization of aquatic genetically modified organisms: the case of transgenic salmon."* Their review contains detailed assessments on many problematic issues such as, *"Threat to wild salmon population," "Genetic risk," "Health risk," "Allergy," "Toxicity," "Environmental risk," "Biodiversity considerations"* and *"Socio-economic risk,"* replete with 179 supporting footnotes referencing leading peer reviewed studies on genetic modification taken from the scientific literature. But what I found most compelling was the authors' critique of the very process of genetic engineering itself which is inherently fraught with unknown risks:

> *"Transgenesis [genetic modification] is not simply a technological extension of [selective breeding], but represents a revolution in that it makes it possible to modify a given part of the genome even somewhere where natural scission would not occur. This allows crossing the barriers of species or even of realms, a phenomenon that is still very little understood and surely generates novel physiological and metabolic conditions."*

> *"Genetic engineering succeeds in overcoming natural limits in transplanting nuclei, manipulating the number of sets of chromosomes, or transferring DNA sequences. Aquatic GMO [genetically modified organism] engineering may be considered as another step in this biology which circumvents natural cells and nuclear barriers by microinjection (Chourrout*

et al., 1986), electroporation (Inoue et al., 1990), sperm transfer (Muller et al., 1992), gold microparticule bombardment (Kolenikov et al., 1990), retroviral infection (Kurita et al., 2004), muscular injection (Tseng et al., 1995) or transposition (Raz et al., 1997), in order to introduce one foreign DNA fragment into the genome of a germinal cell. All these techniques represent an insertion by chance of one or several very precise genetic sequences in an unknown genome.

"Thus, the novel trait of an aquatic GMO represents a qualitative change because most of the time it does not occur in natural populations of the parental species, or a quantitative one when the quantity of a natural substance is changed compared to the wild species. These changes affect a wide range of endpoints such as metabolic rates or endocrine controls, influencing a variety of functions such as reproduction, immune defence, nutrition, development and growth. In practice the most frequently observed phenotypic contribution derived from these changes is growth enhancement, and may also affect resistance or tolerance to threats such as disease, parasites or other adverse environmental conditions (see Section 2.5)."

"Despite rapid advances in molecular biology since two decades, scientists do not have the capacity to control nor really understand the genome of living organisms. In particular, the risks of transgenesis arise from the lack of control over the number of sequences and sites of insertion, the rate of expression of the transgene, the complexity of interactions between the gene networks, the multiplicity of gene functions, epigenetics [the study of heritable changes in gene function that do not involve changes in DNA sequence] and the interactions with environment.

"Different families established from separate GH[growth hormone]-transgenic salmons yield lines with unique growth characteristics suggesting important site-of-integration effects on transgene expression (Devlin et al., 2004a). The disadvantage of transgenesis is that, at present, the control of the transgene is unpredictable despite the known artificial promoter. It can thus not be expressed, or it may modify another gene by blocking it, by slowing it down, by stimulating it or by changing its function. Thus, the transgene could make other genes function in an aberrant way.

"If some handbooks of biochemistry or molecular biology still retain and restate the axiom "one gene, one protein, one function," reality seems now to be much more complex, agreeing more with the theory of polygenic characters (Mather, 1979). In fact, the number of genes is smaller than the number of functions signifying that one gene plays several roles. Furthermore, interactions between genes are multiple and complex and generate novel functions; for example, most of the time a multitude of factors act synergetically to control one gene expression and this varies according to physiological and environmental conditions

(Shrimpton and Robertson, 1988). Moreover, one gene can naturally exist in the form of several copies that "work" differently in different tissues or during different development stages (Se´ ralini, 2004). In the rainbow trout, for example, it has been clearly demonstrated that the pituitary adenylate cyclase-activating polypeptide and growth hormone-releasing gene change their expression during development, notably through alternative splicing and variation in the gene copy number (Krueckl and Sherwood, 2001). Increasingly there is a debate around the very concept of the gene. Philipp A Sharp noted in his Nobel lecture (1993): "what exactly the gene is has become somewhat unclear" (Sapp, 2003). Indeed, our knowledge about hereditary mechanisms continues to evolve, including the fact that "the transfer of genes across the phylogenetic spectrum is now known to occur naturally" (Sapp, 2003). Today, genetically based knowledge is in a process of flux due to observations of an unanticipated "mind-boggling complexity" involving, for instance, overlapping genes, genes within genes, transcription (including overlapping transcripts, fused transcripts) converting many segments of genome (from either of the DNA strands) into multiple RNA ribbons of differing lengths and epigenetic inheritance (Pearson, 2006)."

"Health risks may arise if the transgenic organism produces a new substance or an anticipated substance at higher concentration, compared to the non-transgenic equivalent species; this could therefore result in allergenic or toxic characteristics (Berkowitz, 1993). The GMO may also tolerate a new toxic compound or be sensitive to a pathogen (Se´ ralini, 2000, 2004). Furthermore, in particular in the case of a hormonal substance, a complete change in many metabolic pathways could arise, rendering the aquatic GMO markedly different in chemical composition and thus contributing to unexpected risks which would need to be assessed (Malarkey, 2003).

"It remains a problem that in some countries like USA and Canada, in contrast to the European Union and most countries that have signed and applied the Carthagena protocol [an international agreement on biosafety that seeks to protect biological diversity from the potential risks posed by genetically modified organisms resulting from modern biotechnology], it is supposed in regulation that the whole GMO is equivalent to the corresponding wild species, necessitating no labelling nor mid- or long-term toxicity tests. This approach presumes that if only one new trait has been added, this will result in the production of only one new substance that does not change significantly the composition. For example the transgenic growth hormone salmon could be considered as a banal salmon that has only the particularity of producing more GH or a normal level of GH but all year round. This approach called "substantial equivalence" is risky because it is based on an oversimplified understanding of the complexities entailed in transgenic modification."

"Because of the random insertion and the genome complexity described previously, transgenesis can modify some biochemical pathways and/or physiological regulations in an aquatic GMO, which may then become, for example, a larger bio-accumulator of a pollutant that it tolerates (Kapuscinski and Hallerman, 1994). For instance polybrominated diphenyl ethers used as flame-retardants in several products of daily life, are now sometimes measured at levels averaging 1.46 ng/g wet weight in farmed Atlantic salmon in Chile (Montory and Barred, 2006). It was also often measured in human blood. Nothing guarantees that this rate could not increase in GH salmon that grows faster and have less time to eliminate this kind of toxic chemical.

"Salmon dietary qualities are of interest in human nutrition and are associated with a positive image. Notably, proteins, polyunsaturated fatty acids (including the omega-3 group) (Sidhu, 2003), vitamin A and carotenoids (Rajasingh et al., 2006) content are high, especially in wild salmon. Evaluation should verify that these characteristics persist, especially in an animal that grows faster. Growth-enhanced transgenic salmon, compared to control fish, exhibited a 10% improvement in gross feed conversion efficiency, but body protein, dry matter, ash, lipid and energy were significantly lower relative to controls while moisture content was significantly higher (Cook et al., 2000)."

"In particular, environmental impacts should be studied in depth, as the release of genetically modified animals would, as for genetically modified plants, be irreversible. The introduction of new species in a given environment could be considered as similar to the introduction of a cocktail of new substances into a body: interactions and impacts are very complex and thus not subject to systematic predictability. Thus, as for toxicity, tests, and notably long-term tests, are necessary (Se´ralini, 2003; Se´ralini et al., 2007). These are conditions to maintain food quality for a high level of human health. Respect for protection against serious or irreparable harm is called for in Article 15 of the Declaration of Rio, even in the absence of scientific certitude."

Simply put, genetic engineers have no idea of the consequences of their actions. Genetic engineering proponents are not the keepers of the sanctity of science as they claim, but rather the manipulative anti-science soothsayers they disingenuously project onto their critics.

Proponents of the AquAdvantage® GM salmon make the claim that their primary motivation in genetically modifying Atlantic salmon to grow faster is purely altruistic: to expand the world's food supply at a time when the planet's human population is expanding at a rate of over 80 million people per year. Here, the authors of the review expose this claim for the sophistry that it truly is:

"Protein is of course, for a carnivorous fish such as salmon, an important part of the diet. This could make transgenic salmon a contestable choice in regard to the lack of food

supply within the world. Lipid requirements are higher than for other marine species, around 25% of feed weight in adult food and even more in young stages. Although the conversion rate of this food into salmon flesh is high, sometimes attaining a figure near 1.5 kg food to obtain 1 kg salmon flesh (the rate depends on food quality, temperature, fish age, etc.) (Chamberlain, 1993), yet it should be recalled that millions of tons of small fish and crustaceans are transformed and through flour and oil enter the composition of food pellets destined to aquaculture. Most of the time, for each kilogram of flesh, salmon farmers use between 1.2 and 1.4 kg dry pellets, that is to say 4 or 5 kg of fresh fish and shellfish (Naylor et al., 2000).

"In any case, there are increasing doubts regarding the longterm sustainability of farming systems based entirely upon these fishery resources (Naylor et al., 2000), in particular concerning the efficiency and ethics of feeding potentially food-grade fishery resources back to animals rather than feeding them directly to humans (Best, 1996; Hansen, 1996; Pimentel et al., 1996; Rees, 1997). It should be noted also that herring and sardines, important nutritional sources in salmon farming feed, are themselves excellent protein sources including sources of omega-3. This then poses a double set of socio-economic and ethical issues: the loss of food-grade fishery resources, and the transfer of these resources from the South (Africa and South America) towards the North (principal commercial outlet for salmon farming products)."

In other words, farming GM salmon faster on less feed than conventionally farmed salmon was never about expanding the world's food supply, it was always just a devious   scheme to transfer food resources from the impoverished global south to the wealthy global north. AquAdvantage® GM salmon offers no advantages to food consumers, only unknown risks from an unproven product. The only true advantage of AquAdvantage® GM salmon accrues to the factory farming AquaBounty corporation: it is within its own corporate self-interest to increase profits by speeding up the production line. The unrelenting pursuit of profit is the implacable logic of global corporate capitalism.

Global Industrial Fish Complex

In 2000, 90% of the world's total aquaculture production was in southeast Asia, and of that over 70% was produced in China alone (2002 FAO report). China dominates world aquaculture; while global aquaculture production increased by 0.4-0.7 million tons per year until 1992, productivity in China increased by about 2.6 million tons per year. This tremendous growth in production was largely due to increased emphasis on the freshwater species carp and tilapia, with pond farming producing about 67% of the total yield. In China, silver and bighead carp make up 60-80% of stocked fish. While I could find no studies on the environmental impacts of carp farming in China, studies from other countries where this non-native species is farmed suggest impacts may be substantial. The following fact sheet put out by *Feral Cleaning Australia* sums it up well:

> "*Carp cause their main environmental impacts through their feeding habits. As adults, they usually feed on the bottom of rivers and ponds. They feed by sucking soft sediment into their mouths, where food items are separated and retained and the sediments are ejected back into the water. This habit (known as roiling) leads to a suspension of sediment in the water. When carp are present in high densities, the resultant suspended sediment can result in a number of problems, including: • direct deterioration of water quality due to sediment and increased nutrient levels • reduced light penetration, resulting in reduced plant growth • smothering of plants, invertebrates and fish eggs • clogging of gills of other fish species • inhibited visual feeding by other fish species. The process of feeding can also result in fewer aquatic plants: carp will graze on plants directly and uproot plants during feeding. Carp are also effective grazers of surface films on plants and rocks. Their direct impact on plants can also have a number of related impacts, including: • reduced populations of invertebrates that are dependent on the plants • reduced stability of bottom sediments through loss of aquatic vegetation.*"

> "*Juvenile carp in particular also feed directly on zooplankton in the water. If zooplankton numbers are reduced, algal growth might increase, as the zooplankton normally feed on algae. There are also records of carp feeding on fish eggs and on small fish. The introduction and/or spread of disease by introduced species are often cited as a likely impact threatening native fauna... Some parasites such as the external parasitic anchor worm Lernaea cyprinacea and the tapeworm Bothriocephalus acheilognathi might have been introduced with carp and they are now found on or in native species. The impact of these parasites is unknown. Carp can potentially impact Australian native fauna through a variety of mechanisms: • indirectly, through habitat disturbance and alteration • directly, through competitive exclusion, predation and possible pathogens. The end result of one or a combination of these impacts will be reduced water quality and/or reduced abundance and diversity of native species... Despite limitations in the methods used in trying to determine the impacts of carp, it is impossible to conclude that our inland ecosystems would not be better off without them. Carp are certainly consuming resources that could otherwise be available to native species.*"

Tilapia is a tropical freshwater fish native to Africa and the Middle East that is a member of the Cichlid family. China, Indonesia and Egypt are the three leading aquaculture producers of tilapia, but because this species can tolerate varying concentrations of salt, high concentration of pesticides, medication residues, and fertilizers, they are farmed in over 135 tropical countries and on every continent in the world except Antarctica. The U.S. Food and Drug Administration (FDA) tests imported fish for chemicals banned in the U.S.: in 2014, 82% of tilapia coming from China were rejected due to contamination as were two thirds of tilapia from South America that contained the antimicrobial "malachite green" and the antiseptic "gentian violet," both of which are known carcinogens; all samples of tilapia tested positive for at least one heavy metal such as mercury, cadmium, arsenic, or lead. Tilapia feed mostly on algae and plankton, although they can eat nearly anything including maize and soy. Most tilapia worldwide are farmed without the use of modern compound feeds, however, modern intensive farming systems rely heavily on added feeds because fish are stocked at high densities that cannot be supported by natural food sources. As with carp, I could find no studies on the environmental impacts of tilapia farming in China, but studies from other countries where this non-native species is farmed suggest impacts may be substantial. One study out of the University of Arizona found that introduced tilapia can negatively impact native fish species:

> *"A series of dams and diversion of most of the [Colorado River] caused massive environmental changes. The dams stopped the normal flooding cycle, altered the algal community and increased salinity. Introduction of tilapia for aquatic weed control in the irrigation canals allowed them to eventually migrate into the Colorado River mainstream. Tilapia, along with, many other exotics introduced as sport fish, completely changed the fish community. In some areas of the river, tilapia now represent 90% of the fish biomass and virtually all of the native species are endangered."*

The same study found that effluent from tilapia farms has negative environmental impacts:
> *"There are several environmental impacts associated with the discharge of waste waters from tilapia farms. The most obvious of these are the nutrients that are released from fecal wastes and uneaten food. Nitrogen, phosphorus and other macro and micro nutrients contribute to algae and plant growth in receiving bodies of water. Biochemical oxygen demand, lower levels of dissolved oxygen and higher levels of total suspended solids in fish effluents also contribute to eutrophication. This problem is common to all forms of tilapia culture. Pond effluents impact receiving streams, cage culture impact the surrounding lake or pond, salt water culture impacts nearby reefs or other marine systems, and recirculating systems in an urban setting can impact the municipal sewage system."*

According to a press release published by the FAO Representation in the Islamic Republic of Iran, outbreaks of Tilapia Lake Virus have become a major international problem on tilapia farms:
> *"Tilapia Lake Virus (TiLV) has now been confirmed in Colombia, Ecuador, Egypt, and Thailand. While the pathogen poses no public health concern, it can decimate infected populations. In 2015, world tilapia production, from both aquaculture and capture, amounted*

to 6.4 million tonnes, with an estimated value of USD 9.8 billion, and worldwide trade was valued at USD1.8 billion.

"It is not currently known whether the disease can be transmitted via frozen tilapia products, but 'it is likely that TiLV may have a wider distribution than is known today and its threat to tilapia farming at the global level is significant,' GIEWS said in its alert.

"The disease shows highly variable mortality, with outbreaks in Thailand triggering the deaths of up to 90 percent of stocks. Infected fish often show loss of appetite, slow movements, dermal lesions and ulcers, ocular abnormalities, and opacity of lens."

In many tropical countries with long coastlines, natural mangrove forests thrive in the brackish marshes at the shores' edge. Mangrove forests are key to these coastal zone ecosystems providing the main source of organic matter, as well as habitat for countless aquatic and avian species. Mangrove forests further provide other ecosystem services acting to buffer against coastal erosion and storm damage, filter pollutants and sequester carbon. Unfortunately, mangrove forests are also located on prime real estate for shrimp farming.

Shrimp ponds are conveniently situated on the coast as it allows the tides to create a natural flow of water through the ponds that is necessary for shrimp survival. Researchers have documented that from 1975 to 1993, construction of shrimp ponds has devastated millions of acres of mangrove forest: 521,000 acres (~211,000 hectares) of mangrove forest were razed to build shrimp ponds in Indonesia, 508,000 acres (~205,500 hectares) in the Philippines, 356,000 acres (~144,017 hectares) in Thailand, 252,000 acres (~102,000 hectares) in Vietnam, 161,000 acres (~65,000 hectares) in Bangladesh, and 53,000 acres (~21,600 hectares) in Ecuador. Worldwide, mangrove forest cover has declined from 48.9 million acres (~19.8 million hectares) in 1980 to less than 37.1 million acres (~15 million hectares) in 2000. Although the rate of deforestation slowed from 1.7% in the 1980s, to 1.0% in the 1990s, mangrove deforestation continues into the 21st century.

Intensive shrimp farms are essentially a grid pattern of individual ponds. Shrimp larvae are raised in small nursery ponds and then transferred to large grow-out ponds, where they are raised to adult size. Each pond is connected on one side to a supply canal and on the other side to a drain canal. The supply canal carries water from the ocean into the pond and the drain canal returns the water to the ocean. It has been estimated that, for each million shrimp farmed, four to seven million other organisms are killed by trapping in the nets of the pond's inlet. The natural nutrients in the circulated ocean water is not enough to feed the shrimp living under such unnatural high density conditions so to meet their nutritional requirements they are fed large amounts of feed in the form of pellets containing wheat flour, soybean meal, and fishmeal. Because shrimp nibble rather than eat the pellets whole, up to 40% of the added feed is left to break down into dissolved nitrogen (N) and phosphorus (P). Also, of the feed eaten by the shrimp 77% of the nitrogen and 89% of the phosphorus is not absorbed but excreted which further adds to the pond's N and P load. This pond water with extremely high concentrations of N and P is then released untreated back into the ocean where it causes red tides (algae blooms) and hypoxia (oxygen depletion) leading to massive dead zones where animals and plants cannot survive. One study (Biao and Kaijin, 2007) found that in China, 43 billion tons of wastewater from shrimp farms is released back into Chinese coastal waters every year.

Whether farming salmon, carp, tilapia or shrimp, aquaculture over the past 70 years has caused vast devastation to the world's natural ecosystems.   In the dozens of articles and studies I read to research this segment on fish farming, virtually every one emphasized the increasingly elaborate technical fixes that have been taken or are proposed to be taken to mitigate these severe environmental impacts, yet, as aquaculture continues on its exponential growth trajectory, so far the destruction has only been compounded.

The 2018 FAO report estimated total world production of fish (including fish, mollusks, crustaceans, cephalopods, etc.,) by weight to be 194,821,743 tons which broke down to 93,736,944 tons from capture fisheries (wild caught) and 101,084,799 tons from aquaculture (farmed). The top 15 producers were as follows:

Country	Total	Captured	Aquaculture
1) China	81,500,000	17,800,000	63,700,000
2) Indonesia	23,184,419	6,584,419	16,600,000
3) India	10,785,334	5,082,332	5,703,002
4) Vietnam	6,420,471	2,785,940	3,634,531
5) U.S.A	5,375,386	4,931,017	444,369
6) Russia	4,931,017	4,773,413	173,840
7) Japan	4,343,257	3,275,263	1,067,994
8) Philippines	4,228,906	2,027,992	2,200,914
9) Peru	3,911,989	3,811,802	100,187
10) Bangladesh	3,878,324	1,674,770	2,203,554
11) Norway	3,529,576	2,203,602	1,326,216
12) South Korea	3,255,171	1,395,951	1,859,220
13) Myanmar	3,090,034	2,072,390	1,017,644
14) Chile	2,879,355	1,829,338	1,050,117
15) Thailand	2,493,154	1,530,583	962,571

As can be seen, China dwarfs the rest of the world in both capture fisheries and aquaculture production with Indonesia a distant second and India a further distant third, while the next 12 of the top 15 countries all totaled well over 2 million tons. The following 11 countries in order of production – Mexico, Egypt, Morocco, Brazil, Spain, Ecuador, Iceland, Iran, Canada and Nigeria – all produced between 1 and 2 million tons, and the following 54 countries in the FAO report all produced between 100 thousand and 900 thousand tons. All told, 202 countries and territories were listed with Mongolia at the bottom producing 15 tons.

In 2018, fish and fish products were the most traded food items in the world with 67 million tons traded internationally representing almost 38% of all fish caught or farmed worldwide. The 2018 FAO report described the export trade in fish and fish products as follows:

"In addition to being by far the major fish producer, China has also been the main exporter of fish and fish products since 2002, and since 2011 the third major importing country in terms of value. China's imports have increased in recent years partly as a result of the outsourcing of processing from other countries, but also reflecting China's growing domestic consumption of species not produced locally. According to the latest available estimates for 2019, China's exports declined by 7 percent compared with 2018 (USD 20 billion versus USD 21.6 billion), possibly impacted by trade disputes between China and the United States of America.

"Since 2004, Norway has been the second major exporter, now followed by Viet Nam, which has become the third major exporter since 2014. Catches by the Norwegian fleet comprise large volumes of small pelagics and groundfish species such as cod, while Norway's aquaculture sector for salmonids (salmon, trout, etc.) is the largest in the world. High cod and salmon prices worldwide saw Norway's seafood export industry achieve record export revenues in recent years, peaking at USD 12 billion in 2018 before slightly declining (–0.1 percent) in 2019. Meanwhile, Viet Nam has successfully maintained steady growth in recent years, thanks mainly to strong trading connections with a fast-growing Chinese market, an expanding Pangas catfish (Pangasius spp.) aquaculture sector in the Mekong Delta, and a booming processing and re-export industry.

"Since 2017, India has become the fourth major exporter, boosted by a steep increase in farmed shrimp production. However, after peaking at USD 7.2 billion in 2017, the value of India's exports declined by 3 percent in 2018 and by a further 1 percent in 2019 (USD 6.8 billion), driven primarily by a decline in shrimp prices. In Chile, aquaculture production of Atlantic salmon, coho salmon and rainbow trout has grown into a modern multibillion dollar industry, second only to Norway in global aquaculture production. Chile has been has seen sustained export revenue growth on the back of strong global demand for salmonids throughout the Americas, Europe and Asia and increase in prices.

In 2018, Chile became the fifth major exporter of fish and fish products, but in 2019 their value declined by 3 percent to USD 6.6 billion. Thailand, the sixth major exporter, has experienced a significant decline in exports since 2012, mainly as a result of its reduced shrimp production due to disease outbreaks that have eroded its competitiveness at the global level.

"The steady increase in developing countries' share of international trade flows, with faster rates of growth compared with developed countries (Figure 30), has been a defining feature of global fish market development. From 1976 to 2018, exports from developing countries increased by an average of 8.4 percent per year in value terms, compared with 6.8 percent for developed countries. In the period 1976 – 2018, the share of developing countries of trade in fish and fish products increased from 38 percent of global export value to 54 percent, and from 39 percent to 60 percent of total quantity (in live weight equivalent), supported by strong aquaculture production growth and heavy investment in export market development. China, the rest of developing East Asia, Southeast Asia and South America made the most substantial gains in this period. In 2018, fish exports of developing countries were valued at USD 88 billion, and their net fish export revenues (exports minus imports) reached USD 38 billion, higher than those of other agricultural commodities (such as meat, tobacco, rice and sugar) combined."

The 2018 FAO report described the import trade in fish and fish products as follows:

"For many decades, three major markets have accounted for a large proportion of total imports – the European Union, the United States of America and Japan – all heavily dependent on imports to meet consumer demand, often of relatively more expensive species than those consumed in other countries. In 1976, the value of imports by the European Union, the United States of America and Japan represented 33 percent, 22 percent and 21 percent, respectively, of the global total. In 2018, while the share of the European Union was largely unchanged (34 percent), the shares of the United States of America and Japan had fallen to 14 percent and 9 percent, respectively. According to the latest available estimates, these trends continued in 2019. Their declining shares are rather the result of much faster demand growth in many emerging economies, particularly in East and Southeast Asia.

"While developed markets still dominate fish imports, the importance of developing countries as consumers as well as producers of fish and fish products has been steadily increasing. Urbanization, improved disposable income and expansion of the seafood-consuming middle class, have been fueling demand growth in emerging markets that is far outpacing that observed in their developed counterparts. In 2018, fish imports by developing countries represented 31 percent of the global total value and 49 percent by quantity (live weight), compared with 12 percent and 19 percent, respectively, in 1976. As *consumer purchasing power increases and preferences evolve, an increasing proportion of production that would previously have been exported to developed markets is now being directed to meet the demand of regional and domestic consumers. Countries such as Brazil and China are now large consumers of high-value species such as shrimp and salmon. For LIFDCs [Low-Income Food-Deficit Countries], the value of imports has been increasing at an average annual growth rate of about 6 percent in the period 1976–2018, but in most cases these values remain at very low levels relative to the rest of the world."*

"Interregional trade flows (Figure 31) continue to be significant, although this trade is often not adequately reflected in official statistics, in particular for Africa and selected countries in Asia and Oceania. Oceania, the developing countries of Asia and the Latin America and the Caribbean region remain solid net fish exporters. Interregional trade flows (Figure 31) continue to be significant, although this trade is often not adequately reflected in official statistics, in particular for Africa and selected countries in Asia and Oceania. Latin American exports, comprising primarily shrimp, tuna, salmon and fishmeal from Ecuador, Chile and Peru, were boosted in 2018. Europe and North America are characterized by a fish trade deficit (Figure 32). Africa is a net importer in volume terms but a net exporter in terms of value, reflecting the higher unit value of exports, which are destined primarily for developed country markets, particularly Europe. Africa imports consist largely of cheaper pelagic species such as mackerel or tilapia…

"The growing importance of regional trade flows has been facilitated by a steady increase in the number of regional trade agreements since the 1990s. These agreements are reciprocal trade agreements establishing preferential terms of trade among trading partners in the same geographical region. They currently apply to a large proportion of global trade in fish and fish products and are expected to continue to play a prominent role in the structure and dynamics of international trade."

With the spectacular growth in trade of fish and fish products around the world, fish consumption by people the world over also saw dramatic increases. The 2012 FAO report described the per capita consumption of fish and fish products by country as follows:

"Notwithstanding the strong increase in the availability of fish to most consumers, the growth in fish consumption differs considerably among countries and within countries and regions in terms of quantity and variety consumed per head. For example, per capita fish consumption has remained static or decreased in some countries in sub-Saharan Africa (e.g. the Congo, South Africa, Gabon, Malawi and Liberia) and in Japan in the last two decades, while the most substantial increases in annual per capita fish consumption have occurred in East Asia (from 10.6 kg in 1961 to 34.5 kg in 2009), Southeast Asia (from 12.8 kg in 1961 to 32.0 kg in 2009)

and North Africa (from 2.8 kg in 1961 to 10.6 kg in 2009). China has been responsible for most of the increase in world per capita fish consumption, owing to the substantial increase in its fish production, in particular from aquaculture. China's share in world fish production grew from 7 percent in 1961 to 34 percent in 2009. Per capita fish consumption in China has also increased dramatically, reaching about 31.9 kg in 2009, with an average annual growth rate of 4.3 percent in the period 1961 2009 and of 6.0 percent in the period 1990 2009. In the last few years, fuelled by growing domestic income and wealth, consumers in China have experienced a diversification of the types of fish available owing to a diversion of some fishery exports towards the domestic market as well as an increase in fishery imports. If China is excluded, annual per capita fish supply to the rest of the world was about 15.4 kg in 2009, higher than the average values of the 1960s (11.5 kg), 1970s (13.5 kg), 1980s (14.1 kg) and 1990s (13.5 kg). It should be noted that during the 1990s, world per capita fish supply, excluding China, was relatively stable at 13.113.5 kg and lower than in the 1980s as population grew more rapidly than food fish supply (at annual rates of 1.6 and 0.9 percent, respectively). Since the early 2000s, there has been an inversion of this trend, with food fish supply growth outpacing population growth (at annual rates of 2.6 percent and 1.6 percent, respectively)."

"Differences in fish consumption exist between the more-developed and the less developed countries… The actual values may be higher than indicated by official statistics in view of the under-recorded contribution of subsistence fisheries and some small-scale fisheries. In 2009, apparent per capita fish consumption in industrialized countries was 28.7 kg, while for all developed countries it was estimated at 24.2 kg. A sizable share of fish consumed in developed countries consists of imports, and owing to steady demand and declining domestic fishery production (down 10 percent in the period 2000 2010), their dependence on imports, in particular from developing countries, is projected to grow. In developing countries, fish consumption tends to be based on locally and seasonally available products, and the fish chain is driven by supply rather than demand. However, in emerging economies, imports of fishery products not available locally have recently been growing."

By every measure – captured fish, farmed fish, import/export of fish and fish products, and per capita fish consumption – human exploitation of the Earth's endowment of fish and other aquatic animals for food is at an all time high and growing at an alarming rate. As we have seen in the discourses presented above on the world's major capture fisheries and the fish farming industry, virtually every major aquatic ecosystem in every corner of the globe is in severe decline due to human predation. In the Anthropocene Epoch, H. sapiens that evolved as herbivores in terrestrial ecosystems, have become apex predators in aquatic ecosystems around the world. There is no place on Earth safe from the human apetite.

Effects of Plastics and Climate Change on Aquatic Ecosystems

Besides predation, fish and other aquatic life are also under assault by other anthropogenic activities, most notably plastic waste accumulating in the oceans and climate disruption.

A study published in the on-line open sourced peer reviewed journal *Plos One* in 2014, attempted to determine the global abundance and weight of floating plastics in the world's oceans. To conduct this unprecedented study, researchers made 24 expeditions between 2007 and 2013 across all five sub-tropical gyres (large systems of rotating ocean currents) in the North Pacific, North Atlantic, South Pacific, South Atlantic and Indian Ocean, as well as to the Bay of Bengal, the Mediterranean Sea and the coast of Australia. Using an oceanographic model of floating debris dispersal and correcting for wind-driven vertical mixing, they conservatively estimated a minimum of 5.25 trillion plastic particles weighing 268,940 tons floating in the oceans. The data broke down the plastic particles into four size classes: macroplastics (8 inches in diameter, 200 millimeters), mesoplastics (2 inches in diameter, 50 millimeters), and two sizes of microplastics (0.015 – 0.047 inches, 0.33 – 1.00 millimeters and 0.048 – 0.187 inches, 1.01 – 4.75 millimeter). By weight, 233,400 tons consisted of macro and meso plastics and 35,540 tons consisted of microplastics. When the researchers compared between the four size classes, a tremendous loss of microplastics was observed from the sea surface compared to expected rates of fragmentation of macro and meso plastics, suggesting there are mechanisms at play that remove microplastic particles from the ocean surface. These include UV degradation, biodegradation, decreased buoyancy due to fouling organisms, suspension in the water column, beaching, and ingestion by organisms. It is through ingestion by small organisms at the bottom of marine food chain that microplastics work their way up through trophic levels to concentrate in the tissues of top predators, ultimately including humans.

In May, 2020, *Science of the Total Environment*, published a study on the effects of ingested plastics with the rather lengthy descriptive title, *"Microplastics in wild fish from North East Atlantic Ocean and its potential for causing neurotoxic effects, lipid oxidative damage, and human health risks associated with ingestion exposure."* The researchers studied a total of 150 specimens of European seabass, Atlantic horse mackerel and Atlantic chub mackerel fished with trawls in Northwest Portuguese coastal waters in March and April of 2018. Microplastics were found in 73 of the 150 examined fish, 52 fish had microplastics in the gastrointestinal tract, 54 fish had microplastics in the gills and 48 fish had microplastics in the dorsal muscle. Microplastics were found in all three species. The fish with microplastics had more "lipid peroxidation" (damaged fats) in gills, muscle and brain tissue than fish without microplastics. Lipid oxidative damage can lead to a wide range of adverse effects: gill lipid peroxidation damage has been shown in other studies to compromise respiration; muscle lipid peroxidation to disrupt neuromuscular functions resulting in problems of movement coordination and decreased swimming performance; brain lipid peroxidation damage to cause the disruption of membranes of pre-synaptic vesicles containing neurotransmitters resulting in negative effects such as discoordination, confusion and visual impairment. Based on the total mean of microplastics found in fish muscle and on the consumption of fish per capita in selected countries, the researchers estimated human intake of microplastics through fish consumption ranged from 518 microplastic items/year/capita in Brazil to 3,078 microplastic items/year/capita in Portugal.

In another study presented at a meeting of the *American Chemical Society* (ACS) in August, 2020, researchers found microplastics in all 47 out of 47 human liver tissues sampled. Researcher Varun Kelkar, who presented the study at the ACS meeting, calmly intoned:

> *"We never want to be alarmist, but it is concerning that these non-biodegradable materials that are present everywhere can enter and accumulate in human tissues, and we don't know the possible health effects. Once we get a better idea of what's in the tissues, we can conduct epidemiological studies to assess human health outcomes. That way, we can start to understand the potential health risks, if any."*

If any? Lol. In other words, by 2020, the effects of this ubiquitous pollutant on human health had yet to be studied.

According to a report by the *Ellen MacArthur Foundation* released at the World Economic Forum in 2016, if current trends continue, and so far there is no indication otherwise, world plastics production is expected to double by 2036 and nearly quadruple by 2050. If plastics production is not drastically curtailed and effectively prevented from entering the oceans, they predict the oceans will contain one ton of plastic for every three tons of fish by 2025, and by 2050 plastics in the ocean will outweigh fish. In this pitch battle for ocean supremacy between fish and plastic, plastic is winning.

The United Nations International Panel on Climate Change (IPCC), the world's preeminent scientific body studying the phenomenon of anthropogenic caused climate disruption, has concluded that due to an increase in the atmospheric concentration of greenhouse gases (GHGs) resulting from human gas and oil combustion, deforestation and intensive agriculture, the Earth's average surface temperature has increased by more than 0.8 °C since the middle of the 19th century, and is now warming at a rate of more than 0.1 °C every decade. The ocean has absorbed more than 90% of this additional heat energy generated between 1971 and 2010 and absorbed 30% of emitted anthropogenic generated carbon dioxide (CO_2). Ocean temperature trends have risen over most of the globe, though the rise has been most pronounced in the Northern Hemisphere, especially the North Atlantic.

In 2018, a comprehensive analysis of dissolved oxygen in the oceans published in the journal *Science* (*"Declining oxygen in the global ocean and coastal waters"*, Science 05 Jan 2018), indicated on average a 2% decline in dissolved oxygen in the oceans during the 50-year period since 1960 with the greatest losses occurring near the equator. As atmospheric global warming warms the oceans from the surface down, the surface layer becomes more buoyant since warmer water is lighter than colder water, making it harder for fresh oxygen from the air to mix down into the deeper layers where the oxygen-poor zones are located. This forces pelagic fish species that normally ply these deeper waters such as tuna, herring, shad, mackerel, cod, marlin, swordfish and sharks, into ever-smaller bands of oxygen-rich water near the surface. Concentrating all these species near the surface makes them easier prey for surface predators, including humans. For some pelagic species, low oxygen waters can impair reproduction, impair immune systems, increase disease, shorten lifespans and even affect future generations by altering gene expression.

As atmospheric CO_2 concentrations increase, the oceans absorb more CO_2 which decreases the water's pH causing ocean acidification. Since the beginning of the industrial era in the mid 1800s, ocean pH of surface water has decreased by an average pH of 0.1 corresponding to a 26% increase in acidity. Observed trends in global ocean pH already exceed the range in natural seasonal variability over most of the oceans and are expected to exceed it further in coming years. Ocean acidification is known to negatively affect calcification rates of marine invertebrates such as shell fish (mollusks and crustaceans), zooplankton that forms the base of the marine food chain, coral reefs that provide habitat for many tropical fish species, as well as the development of marine vertebrates (fish) in their egg and larval stages.

Between 1900 and 2016, sea level rose by 6.3 – 8.3 inches (16 – 21 centimeters) due to global warming. Data gathered by NOAA from satellite measurements in 2017 reveal an accelerated rise of 3.0 inches (7.5 centimeters) between 1993 and 2017, mostly from global warming caused thermal expansion of seawater and the melting of land-based ice sheets and glaciers on Greenland and Antarctica. Scientists expect the rate to further accelerate during the 21st century with NOAA projecting a worst case scenario global mean sea level (GMSL) rise of 6.6 feet to 8.9 feet (2.0 meters to 2.70 meters) by the end of the 21st century. Sea level rise has been shown to alter coastal ocean currents and change the salinity of estuaries adversely effecting the rich diversity of aquatic species that inhabit these coastal zones.

In a study published in the journal *Science* titled, *"Impacts of historical warming on marine fisheries production"* (Mar 2019), researchers used temperature-dependent population models to measure the effects of ocean temperature on the global catch of 235 fish and invertebrate populations including 124 species in 38 ecoregions, representing approximately 33% of the reported global catch, to estimate past temperature-driven changes in maximum sustainable yield (MSY) from 1930 to 2010. They concluded that from the 1930s to the 2010s, the combined MSY from the 235 populations studied decreased by 4.1%, from 35.2 million metric tons to 33.8 million metric tons. The greatest losses in catch occurred in the Sea of Japan, North Sea, Iberian Coastal, Kuroshio Current, and Celtic-Biscay Shelf ecoregions with the East Asian ecoregions experiencing some of the largest warming-driven declines from 8% to 34%.

In the FAO's *Fisheries and Aquaculture Technical Paper 627*, *"Impacts of climate change on fisheries and aquaculture,"* presented at the Rome meeting of the FAO in 2018, researchers projected the effects of anthropogenic climate disruption to the end of the 21st century. Using two different models, the projected catch was estimated under the lowest and highest greenhouse gas (GHG) emission scenarios. Application of these two models resulted in projections that the total maximum catch potential in the world's exclusive economic zones (EEZs) is likely to decrease 2.8% to 5.3% by 2050 (relative to 2000) under the lowest emissions scenario, and 7.0% to 12.1% under the highest scenario. Extending the projections out to 2095, under the lowest emissions scenario the projected total maximum catch changed little from the 2050 projection, but under the highest emission scenario the decrease in catch more than doubled to 16.2% to 25.2%. These projected decreases in catch varied substantially across regions and the impacts could be much greater in the EEZs of countries in the tropics, most notably in the South Pacific regions. The catch potential in the temperate Northeast Atlantic was also projected to decrease between 2000 and 2050. The FAO paper noted that their projections are highly speculative and depend on decisions made by fisheries managers on establishing and enforcing MSY catch limits. This is wishful thinking by the FAO; considering that unlimited growth is central to corporate capitalism which is the world's predominant economic system, the worst case scenario for human predation of world fisheries is virtually inevitable.

In a study published in the journal *Science* titled, *"Impacts of Biodiversity Loss on Ocean Ecosystem Services," (Science* Nov 2006), researchers gave a more dire projection for the world's fisheries:

> *"Our data highlight the societal consequences of an ongoing erosion of diversity that appears to be accelerating on a global scale (Fig. 3A). This trend is of serious concern because it projects the global collapse of all taxa currently fished by the mid–21st century (based on the extrapolation of regression in Fig. 3A to 100% in the year 2048). Our findings further suggest that the elimination of locally adapted populations and species not only impairs the ability of marine ecosystems to feed a growing human population but also sabotages their stability and recovery potential in a rapidly changing marine environment."*

(Note to readers: Throughout history, human predation of fish and other aquatic animals has been mythologized in the classic literature of every culture to glorify the epic struggle of man against beast. This heroic narrative has become so drilled into the human psyche that in all the scores of articles, papers, reports and studies that I read to research this chapter on fish, whether authored by fisher interests, government agencies, environmental organizations or independent scientists, expressed the implicit bias that extracting aquatic animals from the world's water bodies for food is essential for human well-being. For the purposes of this book, however, which is to lay out the facts of how our species came to dominate the animal kingdom, I have deliberately weeded out any and all such allusions to this implicit bias with the intention of letting the pertinent facts speak for themselves. Also in the interest of a fact based presentation, I have striven to excise the implicit biases that I hold against the human exploitation of other animal species.)

Fish and Food Security

The Food and Agriculture Organization (FAO) of the United Nations was established in 1945 as the world's preeminent international agency to achieve food security for all people on Earth. In this capacity, the FAO has emerged as the world's leading promoter for exploitation of world fisheries to feed the hundreds of millions of hungry people living in impoverished nations around the world. The FAO justifies their position based on these four assertions: 1) eating fish is a healthy source of good nutrition;

2) catching and processing fish provides employment for millions of otherwise marginalized people; 3) trading in fish products is an indispensable sector of the global economy; 4) providing fish to people on a global scale can be done sustainably. While these rationals may at first appear legitimate, even a shallow dive into the disciplines of nutritional science, economics and ecology exposes them as false promises.

The FAO's report, *"State of World Fisheries and Aquaculture 2012"* states:

"Fisheries and aquaculture make crucial contributions to the world's well-being and prosperity. In the last five decades, world fish food supply has outpaced global population growth, and today fish constitutes an important source of nutritious food and animal protein for much of the world's population."

With this statement the FAO, a world authority on food and nutrition, perpetuates the commonly held assumption that animal protein is a good source of nutrition for people despite the fact that modern nutritional science has clearly demonstrated that animal protein contributes to many of the intractable diseases that plague the human race. Dr. Michael Greger, M.D., is an internationally recognized speaker on nutrition, food safety, and public health issues, a licensed general practitioner specializing in clinical nutrition, and a founding member and Fellow of the American College of Lifestyle Medicine. Dr. Greger is also publisher of the website Nutritionfacts.org where he shares with the lay public state of the art studies on nutritional science. In the excerpt below from one of his many posts on the adverse health effects of animal protein, Dr. Greger warns:

"The adverse effects associated with long-term, high protein-high meat diets may include disorders of bone and calcium balance, increased cancer risk, disorders of the liver, and worsening of coronary artery disease.

"What about our kidneys? Harvard University researchers followed thousands of healthy women for more than a decade to look for the presence of excess protein in their urine, a sign that kidneys may be starting to fail. The researchers found three dietary components associated with this sign of declining kidney function: animal protein, animal fat, and cholesterol. Each is found in only one place: animal products. No association was found between kidney function decline and intake of plant protein or fat.

"High animal protein intake may induce hyperfiltration, a dramatic increase in the kidney's workload. Within hours of consuming meat, whether beef, chicken, or fish, our kidneys may rev up into hyperfiltration mode, whereas an equivalent amount of plant protein causes virtually no such stress on the kidneys.

"Animal protein consumption also appears to trigger the release of insulin-like growth factor 1 (IGF - 1), a cancer-promoting growth hormone. IGF-1 levels rise during childhood to power our development and diminish when we reach adulthood. Should the levels remain too high, however, our cells will constantly receive a message to grow, divide, and keep going and growing. Not surprisingly then, the more IGF-1 in our bloodstream, the higher our risk for developing

some cancers. Animal protein appears to stimulate IGF-1 production whether it's the muscle proteins in meat, the egg-white protein in eggs, or the milk proteins in dairy. After just 11 days of cutting back on animal protein, however, our IGF-1 levels may drop by 20 percent.

"Watching our animal-to-plant protein ratio may be useful for cancer prevention. The largest diet and bladder cancer study found that a 3 percent increase in animal protein consumption was associated with a 15 percent increased risk of bladder cancer, while a 2 percent increase in plant protein intake was associated with a 23 percent decreased cancer risk."

By promoting consumption of animal proteins, the FAO is putting millions of people at addition risk for disease. Alternatively, the FAO should be promoting the consumption of healthy plant proteins which are in plentiful supply on the world food market.

While it is of course true that presently millions of poverty stricken people worldwide earn a living by fishing, their employment is anything but secure as it depends on fish stocks that are in steady decline largely due to overfishing, pollution, climate disruption and sea level rise, especially in southeast Asia where most subsistence fishing occurs. For the FAO to advocate fishing as a means to effect world food security when it is human activity that is pushing aquatic ecosystems to the brink of collapse, is a short sighted solution to hunger that will inevitably lead to even greater food insecurity for increasing numbers of people over the course of the 21st century.

The FAO's contention that the fish trade is indispensable to the global economy relies entirely on citing the dollar value of fish products traded on world food markets, while completely ignoring the market value of substitute food products that could readily replace fish. Ironically, this glaring omission is exposed in another FAO report that documents the enormous volume of food waste inherent to the world's inefficient food marketing system. In their 2013 report, *"Food Wastage Footprint"*, the FAO estimated that annually around 1.3 billion tons of food produced for human consumption in the world (about 1/3 of total food production) is lost or wasted which includes 45% of all fruits and vegetables and 30% of all cereal grains, (it does not include the 70% to 75% of world soybean production or the 40% of world grain production fed to livestock that could be diverted to human consumption). In shear tonnage, this weight of food waste dwarfs the FAO's estimated 179 million tons of fish produced in 2018. I submit that the reason the FAO does not even consider the redistribution of surplus fruits, vegetables and grains as a replacement for fish on world food markets is at least in part due to their aforementioned implicit bias toward fishers. Another reveal of the FAO report is the enormous disparity in food waste between wealthy countries of the global north and poor countries of the global south: decadent consumers in Europe and North America throw away around 209 – 254 lbs/person/year (95 – 115 kg/person/year), while frugal consumers in sub-Saharan Africa and South/South-East Asia waste around 13 – 24 lbs/person/year (6 – 11 kg/person/year), largely due to lack of infrastructure and refrigeration equipment. What the FAO report never considers is how the world's food economy incentivizes overfishing of wild fish stocks in the global south while at the same time incentivizes inefficient fish farming in the global north. The prevailing world economic system of corporate capitalism is driven by the singular motive of profit, and there is no profit to be made selling surplus plant foods to large populations of poor people in the global south. This disparity in food security forces people in the global south to be dependent upon intensive artisanal and subsistence fishing to survive. Conversely, it is highly profitable for corporate fishers to buy cheap forage fish such as anchoveta and sardines from impoverished countries in the global south to make fish meal that is fed to farmed salmon which are then sold at high prices to affluent consumers in the global north. As long as the logic of corporate capitalism is what drives the world's food economy, rich people will be profligate, poor people will be desperate, and ecosystems will be destroyed.

In support of its contention that fishing can be practiced sustainably on a global scale, the FAO points to examples of local fisheries where the catch has increased year over year, but as we have seen in the preceding discourse on major world fisheries, reported catch numbers are not an accurate reflection of ecosystem health or sustainability. The FAO attributes increased catches to local fisheries management policies that set maximum sustainable yields (MSY), but the lessons of history tell use that fishery management is an inexact science that is systematically corrupted by the political demands of corporate capitalism. The sad tale of the North Sea cod fishery is illustrative of this capitalist logic playing out in real time as told by investigative journalist Eveline Vouillemin in her article, *"North Sea cod on brink of collapse"*:

> *"In the 1970s, the North Sea cod population peaked at 270,000 tons. In the decades following there was a long period of decline and then in 2006 cod stocks collapsed dramatically to just 44,000 tons. After a decade of recovery efforts, numbers gradually began to recover and in 2017 it received a 'blue tick' from the Marine Stewardship Council (MSC). However, continual fishing of North Sea cod at levels above the 'Maximum Sustainable Yield' (the largest average catch that can be captured from a stock under existing environmental conditions), because of ministers frequently setting the total allowable catches above scientific advice, has now [in 2019] led to another dramatic fall in stock levels and has left North Sea cod fishery in a precarious situation."* (*Geographical*, July 2019)

In 2017, the United Nations Department of Economic and Social Affairs estimated the current world population at 7.6 billion people and projected the population to reach 8.6 billion by 2030, 9.8 billion by 2050 and 11.2 billion by 2100. As this plague of human beings proceeds to indulge its voracious appetite for fish and other aquatic animals, there will be constant pressure on fishery managers to push fish stocks beyond their natural limits. As we humans continue our relentless pursuit of aquatic animals, and as we continue to defile our planet's hydrosphere, the Anthropocene Epoch is rapidly collapsing the trophic structure of the Earth's aquatic ecosystems. Even by its own data, the FAO concedes the long term prognosis for global fish populations is steadily downward.

19

THE GLOBAL ANIMAL BIOMASS EXCHANGE

Before humans began to domesticate sheep, pigs, cattle and chickens (as well as many other animals) starting around 10,000 years ago, 100% of the biomass (the weight of all living animal species) was contained in wild animal species. Today, the biomass contained in humans and our associated livestock far exceeds that of all the world's remaining wild terrestrial mammal and bird species combined. What I have termed "The Global Animal Biomass Exchange" is the legacy of the global animal industrial complex. This startling reality is reflected in the report, "*The biomass distribution on Earth,*" (*Proceedings of the National Academy of Sciences*, 2018), by environmental scientist Yinon Bar-On et al,

The authors were able to make use of several recent major technological and scientific advances such as next generation genetic sequencing, better remote sensing tools, and global sampling that added more definition to continent-specific details, to make an improved quantitative estimate of the Earth's total biomass. With these tools, they were able to separate biomass into the seven existing taxa (in descending order) – plants, bacteria, fungi, archaea, protists, animals, and viruses – and they were also able to separate animal biomass into distinct components including humans, domesticated animals and wild animals.

The authors report biomass in gigatons of carbon (Gt C), as a measure that is independent of water content and has been used extensively in the literature. According to their estimate, only 2 Gt C accounting for 0.0036% of the Earth's total biomass of 550 Gt C is contained in animal species, and of that, only 0.06 Gt C accounting for 0.03% of animal biomass is contained in humans. For a species that contains such a tiny fraction of the Earth's biomass, we humans have had an out-sized impact on the biomass distribution of life on Earth over the past 10,000 years. Here the authors give their quantitative estimates of the human impact on the Earth's biomass distribution:

> "*Over the relatively short span of human history, major innovations, such as the domestication of livestock, adoption of an agricultural lifestyle, and the Industrial Revolution, have increased the human population dramatically and have had radical ecological effects. Today, the biomass of humans (≈0.06 Gt C; SI Appendix,* Table S9*) and the biomass of livestock (≈0.1 Gt C, dominated by cattle and pigs; SI Appendix,* Table S10*) far surpass that of wild mammals, which has a mass of ≈0.007 Gt C (SI Appendix,* Table S11*). This is also true for wild and domesticated birds, for which the biomass of domesticated poultry (≈0.005 Gt C, dominated by chickens) is about threefold higher than that of wild birds (≈0.002 Gt C; SI Appendix,* Table S12*). In fact, humans and livestock outweigh all vertebrates combined, with the exception of fish. Even though humans and livestock dominate mammalian biomass, they are a small fraction of the ≈2 Gt C of animal biomass, which primarily comprises arthropods (≈1 Gt C; SI Appendix,* Tables S13 and S14*), followed by fish (≈0.7 Gt C; SI Appendix,* Table S15*).*

Here the authors compare their current estimate of the Earth's biomass distribution to their estimate of the biomass distribution that existed before humans arrived on the scene:

"*Comparison of current global biomass with prehuman values (which are very difficult to estimate accurately) demonstrates the impact of humans on the biosphere. Human activity contributed to the Quaternary Megafauna Extinction between ≈50,000 and ≈3,000 y ago, which claimed around half of the large (>40 kg) land mammal species (30). The biomass of wild land mammals before this period of extinction was estimated by Barnosky (30) at ≈0.02 Gt C. The present-day biomass of wild land mammals is approximately sevenfold lower, at ≈0.003 Gt C (SI Appendix, Pre-human Biomass and Chordates and Table S11). Intense whaling and exploitation of other marine mammals have resulted in an approximately fivefold decrease in marine mammal global biomass [from ≈0.02 Gt C to ≈0.004 Gt C (31)]. While the total biomass of wild mammals (both marine and terrestrial) decreased by a factor of ≈6, the total mass of mammals increased approximately fourfold from ≈0.04 Gt C to ≈0.17 Gt C due to the vast increase of the biomass of humanity and its associated livestock. Human activity has also impacted global vertebrate stocks, with a decrease of ≈0.1 Gt C in total fish biomass, an amount similar to the remaining total biomass in fisheries and to the gain in the total mammalian biomass due to livestock husbandry (SI Appendix, Pre-human Biomass). The impact of human civilization on global biomass has not been limited to mammals but has also profoundly reshaped the total quantity of carbon sequestered by plants. A worldwide census of the total number of trees (32), as well as a comparison of actual and potential plant biomass (17), has suggested that the total plant biomass (and, by proxy, the total biomass on Earth) has declined approximately twofold relative to its value before the start of human civilization. The total biomass of crops cultivated by humans is estimated at ≈10 Gt C, which accounts for only ≈2% of the extant total plant biomass (17).*"

These estimates are nothing short of breathtaking. The total biomass of wild terrestrial animals before human domestication was estimated at ≈0.02 Gt C; today, the biomass contained in wild terrestrial animals has plummeted down to ≈0.003 Gt C, an absolute decline of 85%. As the biomass contained in wild terrestrial animals has declined precipitously, the biomass contained in humans at ≈0.06 Gt C and domesticated animals at ≈0.1 Gt C has increased exponentially, now far exceeding that of all wild terrestrial mammals combined. This is also true for wild and domesticated birds, the biomass of domesticated poultry (mostly chickens) at ≈0.005 Gt C, is approximately two and a half times the biomass of all wild birds combined at ≈0.002 Gt C. The same goes for the biomass of marine mammals which has declined from ≈0.02 Gt C down to ≈0.004 Gt C, an 80% decline. Since humans started domesticating animals, the total biomass of marine and terrestrial wild mammals has decreased by approximately six times while the total biomass of land mammals has increased by approximately four times, entirely due to the vast increase of biomass contained in humans and our domesticated cattle, pigs and sheep. Human activity has also impacted global fish biomass with a decrease from ≈0.2 Gt C down to approximately ≈0.1 Gt C, a 50% decline. This decline in total fish biomass is directly linked to the gain in total terrestrial mammalian biomass as fish meal is a major source of feed protein for the livestock industry.

Footnote 17 in the report references a study entitled, *"Unexpectedly large impact of forest management and grazing on global vegetation biomass."* This study details how grazing and growing vast monocultures of maize and soybeans for animal feed have reduced the Earth's total plant biomass by more than half:

> *"Here we show, using state-of-the-art datasets, that vegetation currently stores around 450 petagrams of carbon. In the hypothetical absence of land use, potential vegetation would store around 916 petagrams of carbon, under current climate conditions. This difference highlights the massive effect of land use on biomass stocks. Deforestation and other land-cover changes are responsible for 53–58% of the difference between current and potential biomass stocks. Land management effects (the biomass stock changes induced by land use within the same land cover) contribute 42–47%, but have been underestimated in the literature. Therefore, avoiding deforestation is necessary but not sufficient for mitigation of climate change. Our results imply that trade-offs exist between conserving carbon stocks on managed land and raising the contribution of biomass to raw material and energy supply for the mitigation of climate change. Efforts to raise biomass stocks are currently verifiable only in temperate forests, where their potential is limited. By contrast, large uncertainties hinder verification in the tropical forest, where the largest potential is located, pointing to challenges for the upcoming stocktaking exercises under the Paris agreement."* ("Unexpectedly large impact of forest management and grazing on global vegetation biomass", Erb K H, et al., Nature 553 73–76 (Jan 2018)

In other words, the destruction of tropical forests around the world, particularly in the global south, to graze animals and grow their feed, has released enormous volumes of carbon into the Earth's atmosphere making animal agriculture a major source of the greenhouse gas emissions that are driving global warming. Preserving and restoring tropical forests shows the most promise for sequestering carbon to mitigate climate change.

Perhaps more than any other, the report, *"The biomass distribution on Earth,"* gives a broad overview of the impacts our animal-based diets have had on the Earth's biomass distribution. The conclusions to be drawn could not be starker: in the time since humans turned from a natural herbivore into an apex predator, there has been a nearly complete exchange of global biomass from a bewildering array of wild animals, to being dominated by five species – humans, cattle, pigs, sheep and chickens. As an unanticipated consequence of the global animal industrial complex, we humans and our associated livestock have largely replaced wild animals on this planet.

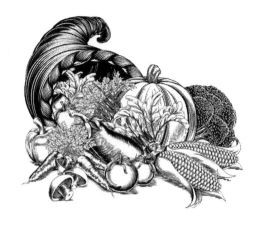

PART V

MAN EATING ANIMALS:

HOW ANIMAL-BASED DIETS ARE

DESTROYING OUR PLANET

• • •

"The truth is seldom welcome, especially at dinner."

– Margaret Atwood, novelist, (born in 1935)

20
GLOBAL ENVIRONMENTAL IMPACTS OF LIVESTOCK PRODUCTION

In the first two decades of the 21st century, while the corporate and alternative media largely ignored the devastation caused by animal agriculture, and governments were often complicit in it, independent scientists and non-governmental organizations (NGOs) began to issue science based reports that exposed the true environmental impacts of animal agriculture on the Earth's biosphere upon which all life depends. Below, I review in chronological order six of the most prominent of these reports:

"Livestock's Long Shadow – environmental issues and options" (2006)

In light of the rising demand for animal foods and the increasing pressure animal agriculture was exerting on natural resources, the *Food and Agriculture Organization (FAO) of the United Nations* formed the *Animal Production and Health Division* in 2005 to assess the environmental impacts of livestock production and to propose mitigations. This new division was to follow-up on the previous work of the FAO's multi-stakeholder *Livestock, Environment and Development (LEAD) Initiative.* In 2006, the FAO published the *Animal Production and Health Division's* comprehensive 390 page report on the environmental impacts of livestock production entitled, *"Livestock's Long Shadow – environmental issues and options,"* which included six chapters and dozens of maps, tables and citations. (FAO, Rome 2006).

Previous assessments of livestock/environment interactions by LEAD had focused exclusively on the livestock sector's effects on the natural resources used in animal food production. This new assessment, however, broadened its perspective to include the environmental impacts of animal agriculture on land use, climate change, soil and water pollution, and biodiversity loss. This broadened perspective on the environmental impacts of animal food production represented a major departure from the FAO's animal centric perspective of the past, and their findings were a wake-up call to the world of the shocking environmental impacts of animal agriculture. Segments gleaned from the *Executive Summary* of the report sum-up the enormous cumulative impacts of animal agriculture on land use, climate change, soil and water pollution, and biodiversity loss:

> *"Land degradation*
> *"The livestock sector is by far the single largest anthropogenic user of land. The total area occupied by grazing is equivalent to 26 percent of the ice-free terrestrial surface of the planet. In addition, the total area dedicated to feedcrop production amounts to 33 percent of total*

arable land. In all, livestock production accounts for 70 percent of agricultural land and 30 percent of the land surface of the planet.

Expansion of livestock production is a key in deforestation, especially in Latin America where the greatest amount of deforestation is occurring – 70 percent of previously forested land in the Amazon is occupied by pastures and feedcrops cover a large part of the remainder. About 20 percent of the world's pastures and rangelands, with 73 percent of rangelands in dry areas, have been degraded to some extent, mostly through overgrazing, compaction and erosion created by livestock action. The dry lands in particular are effected by these trends, as livestock are the only source of livelihoods for the people living in these areas."

"Atmosphere and climates

"With rising temperatures, rising sea levels, melting icecaps and glaciers, shifting ocean currents and weather patterns, climate change is the most serious challenge facing the human race.

The livestock sector is a major player, responsible for 18 percent of greenhouse gas emissions measured in CO2 equivalent. This is a higher share than transport.

The livestock sector accounts for 9 percent of anthropogenic CO2 emissions. The largest share of this derives from land-use changes – especially deforestation – caused by expansion of pastures and arable land for feedcrops. Livestock are responsible for much larger shares of some gases with far higher potential to warm the atmosphere. The sector emits 37 percent of anthropogenic methane (with 23 times the global warming potential (GWP) of CO2) most of that from enteric fermentation by ruminants. It emits 65 percent of anthropogenic nitrous oxide (with 296 times the GWP of CO2), the great majority from manure. Livestock are also responsible for almost two-thirds (64 percent) of anthropogenic ammonia emissions, which contribute significantly to acid rain and acidification of ecosystems."

"Water

"The world is moving towards increasing problems of fresh water shortage, scarcity and depletion, with 64 percent of the world's population expected to live in water stressed basins by 2025.

The livestock sector is a key player in increasing water use, mostly for the irrigation of feedcrops. It is probably the largest sectoral source of water pollution, contributing to eutrophication, "dead" zones in coastal areas, degradation of coral reefs, human health problems, emergence of antibiotic resistance and many others. The major sources of pollution are animal waste, antibiotics and hormones, chemicals from tanneries, fertilizers and pesticides used for feedcrops, and sediments from eroded pasture. Global figures are not available, but in the United States, with the world's forth largest land area, livestock are responsible for an estimated

55 percent of erosion and sediment, 37 percent of pesticide use, 50 percent of antibiotic use, and a third of the loads of nitrogen and phosphorus into fresh water sources.

Livestock also affect the replenishment of freshwater by compacting soil, reducing infiltration, degrading the banks of watercourses, drying up floodplains and lowering water tables. Livestock's contribution to deforestation also contributes to runoff and reduces dry season flows."

"Biodiversity

"We are in an era of unprecedented threats to biodiversity. The loss of species is estimated to be running 50 to 500 times background rates found in the fossil record. Fifteen out of 24 important ecosystem services are assessed to be in decline.

Livestock now account for about 20 percent of the total terrestrial animal biomass, and the 30 percent of the earth's land surface that they now pre-empt was once habitat for wildlife. Indeed, the livestock sector may well be the leading player in the reduction of biodiversity, since it is the major driver of deforestation, as well as one of the leading drivers of land degradation, pollution, climate change, overfishing, sedimentation of coastal areas and facilitation of invasions by alien species. In addition, resource conflicts with pastoralists threaten species of wild predators and also protected areas close to pastures. Meanwhile in developed regions, especially Europe, pastures had become a location of diverse long-established types of ecosystem, many of which are now threatened by pasture abandonment.

Some 306 of the 825 terrestrial ecoregions identified by the Worldwide Fund for Nature (WWF) – ranged across all biomes and all biogeographical realms, reported livestock as one of the current threats. Conservation International has identified 35 global hotspots for biodiversity, characterized by exceptional levels of plant endemism and serious levels of habitat loss. Of these, 23 are reported to be affected by livestock production. An analysis of the authoritative World Conservation Union (IUCN) Red List of Threatened Species shows that most of the world's threatened species are suffering habitat loss where livestock are a factor."

Before publication of *"Livestock's Long Shadow,"* who knew that livestock production accounted for 70% of agricultural land and 30% of the land surface of the planet, or that the livestock sector was responsible for 18% of greenhouse gas emissions measured in CO2 equivalents (CO2e), or that in the U.S. animal agriculture was responsible for an estimated 55% of erosion and sediment, 37% of pesticide use, 50% of antibiotic use, and 33% of eutrophication of fresh water sources, or that 23 of 35 global hotspots for biodiversity were being degraded by livestock production? The startling findings of this report shocked the world.

While the authors' of *"Livestock's Long Shadow,"* broke new ground in quantifying the staggering global environmental impacts of animal agriculture, when it came to exploring options to mitigate these impacts, they chose to stick with traditional mitigation measures that would make animal "husbandry" more efficient. The thought of reducing impacts by reducing demand for animal products was never seriously considered by the authors even as they acknowledge the health consequences of an animal-based diet:

> *"**While not being addressed by this assessment**, it may well be argued that environmental damage by livestock may be significantly reduced by lowering excessive consumption of livestock products among wealthy people. International and national public institutions (e.g. WHO and Tufts University, 1998) have consistently recommended lower intakes of animal fat and red meat in most developed countries."* (**Bold emphasis mine.**)

In fact, the entire report was geared around meeting the anticipated growth in demand for animal products into the foreseeable future. This expansionist approach stems from the authors' misconception that *"... proteins contained in animal products have higher nutritive values than those in the feed provided to animals."* Based on this misconception, the authors, all of whom had direct ties to the livestock industry, actually promoted an increase in consumption of animal products in underdeveloped countries:

> *"Because developing countries still have low intakes of animal foods the share of livestock products in the "global average diet" is expected to continue to rise to reach the OECD [Organization for Economic Co-operation and Development] country averages of about 30 percent of dietary energy and 50 percent of protein intake. **In terms of health and nutrition, therefore, livestock products are a welcome addition to the diets of many poor and under or malnourished people who frequently suffer from protein and vitamin deficiencies, as well as lack of important trace minerals.**"* (**Bold emphasis mine.**)

As we shall see in later reports reviewed below, this approach of expanding animal agriculture to mitigate the environmental impacts of animal agriculture is completely contrary to the authors stated goal that, *"The livestock sector... make a very significant contribution to reducing and reversing environmental damage."* It is impossible to mitigate the environmental impacts of animal agriculture through efficiencies while continuing to increase production; the only plausible mitigation that could actually contribute to reducing and reversing the environmental impacts of animal agriculture (i.e., reducing demand through dietary change) was deliberately excluded from this study.

"Livestock and Climate Change" (2009)

In the paper, *"Livestock and Climate Change,"* published in November 2009 by the U.S. think tank, *Worldwatch Institute*, environmental advisers at the *World Bank* disputed the FAO claim in *"Livestock's Long Shadow (2006)"* that 18% of global greenhouse gas emissions came from animal agriculture. The authors argue that the true figure was more like 51% and the FAO scientists had made several methodological errors that resulted in their gross underestimate, such as:

1) The FAO significantly underestimated emissions of methane expelled by livestock and they incorrectly extrapolated methane's impact over 100 years rather than the 20 years it actually stays in the atmosphere, diminishing the gases true impact. Correcting for this error added another 5 billion tons of CO_2e to livestock emissions.

2) The FAO failed to include CO_2 emitted by breathing animals. Correcting for this error added another 8.7 billion tons of CO_2 to livestock emissions.

3) On land use, the FAO did not consider returning the land currently used for livestock back to natural vegetation. This error discounted the 2.6 billion tons of CO_2e that could be removed from the atmosphere by regrowth of forests.

4) The FAO report failed to include the additional refrigeration required for processing and storage of animal products. This error led them to underestimate the additional energy and associated greenhouse gases emitted to get meat, dairy and eggs from farm to table.

5) The FAO grossly undercounted the global livestock herd, estimating it at 21.7 billion animals instead of the 50 billion estimated by *Worldwatch*. This error led them to underestimate all of the other environmental impacts related to livestock.

As mitigation against climate change, the World Banker advisors recommended investors steer away from livestock projects and toward more lucrative meat and dairy analog projects:

"Investors can be shown that it is in their self-interest to avoid new investments in the production of meat and dairy products and to seek investments in analogs instead. Compared with power and transportation projects, analog projects can be implemented quickly, with relatively low levels of incremental investment, larger amounts of GHGs mitigated for the same amount of investment, and faster returns on investment."

The all business *World Bank* even provided investors with a marketing plan for the meat and dairy analog industry:

"To achieve the growth discussed above will require a significant investment in marketing, especially since meat and dairy analogs will be new to many consumers. A successful campaign would avoid negative themes and stress positive ones. For instance, recommending that meat not be eaten one day per week suggests deprivation. Instead, the campaign should pitch the theme of eating all week long a line of food products that is tasty, easy to prepare, and includes a "superfood," such as soy, that will enrich their lives. When people hear appealing messages about food, they are listening particularly for words that evoke comfort, familiarity, happiness, ease, speed, low price, and popularity."

According to the *World Bank*, investing in meat and dairy analog projects would offer several other environmental impact mitigations:

"Meat and dairy analog projects will not only slow climate change but also help ease the global food crisis, as it takes a much smaller quantity of crops to produce any given number

of calories in the form of an analog than a livestock product. Analogs would also alleviate the global water crisis, as the huge amounts of water necessary for livestock production would be freed up. Health and nutritional outcomes among consumers would be better than from livestock products. Analog projects would be more labor intensive than livestock projects, so would create both more jobs and more skilled jobs. They would also avert the harmful labor practices found in the livestock sector (but not in analog production), including slave labor in some areas such as the Amazon forest region. Workers producing livestock products can easily be retrained to produce analogs."

While assessing the climate impacts of animal agriculture is a complex problem and far from an exact science, at the very least, *Worldwatch's* report *"Livestock and Climate Change"* did expose some of the weaknesses in the *"Livestock's Long Shadow"* by the FAO, and raised even further questions about the true size of those impacts. And at the very most, this report squarely focused on dietary change as our most effective mitigation measure against anthropogenic climate change.

"Tackling climate change through livestock –
A global assessment of emissions and mitigation opportunities"(2013)

In 2013, the FAO *Animal Production and Health Division* produced a second report that focused exclusively on the impacts of animal agriculture on climate change, entitled *"Tackling climate change through livestock – A global assessment of emissions and mitigation opportunities,"* (FAO, Rome, 2013). This report was written by coauthors of the 2006 FAO report, *"Livestock's Long Shadow,"* as well as other FAO staffers with direct ties to the livestock industry, and it suffers from the same industry bias.

In the *"Introduction"* to the report, the authors base their entire plan to mitigate the climate impacts of animal agriculture on the assumption that global demand for animal products *"will"* continue to grow through the year 2050:

*"World population will grow from 7.2 billion today to 9.6 billion in 2050. Population growth, growing incomes and urbanization combine to pose unprecedented challenges to food and agriculture systems, while the natural resources necessary to support global food and non-food production and provision of services from agriculture will not grow. Driven by strong demand from an emerging global middle class, diets **will** become richer and increasingly diversified, and growth in animal-source foods **will** be particularly strong; the demand for meat and milk in 2050 is projected to grow by 73 and 58 percent, respectively, from their levels in 2010 (FAO, 2011c)."* **(bold emphasis mine)**

Later in the *"Introduction,"* the authors explicitly ruled-out any effort to mitigate the climate impacts of animal agriculture through a reduction in demand for animal products:

"This report provides a snapshot of the current state of FAO's assessment work on livestock's contribution to climate change. It draws on three technical reports addressing emissions from dairy cattle (FAO, 2010a), ruminants (FAO, 2013a) and monogastrics (FAO, 2013b). It provides an overview of results and explores main mitigation potential and options on the production side. **It does not discuss possible mitigation options on the consumption side.***"* **(bold emphasis mine)**

By completely dismissing demand side mitigations, the authors have rejected up front the single most effective measure that could be taken to reduce climate impacts caused by animal agriculture. In their rejection of demand side mitigations, the authors have exposed their bias towards an animal-based diet and in so doing have seriously compromised the integrity of their report.

Most of this report is devoted to detailed analyses of animal "husbandry" techniques designed to make more efficient use of natural resources. But in their final analysis, the authors admit that even if all of their suggested mitigations were adopted globally, it would only result in a 30% reduction in greenhouse gas (GHG) emissions from animal agriculture:

"Technologies and practices that help reduce emissions exist but are not widely used. Their adoption and use by the bulk of the world's producers can result in significant reductions in emissions."

"A 30 percent reduction of GHG emissions would be possible, for example, if producers in a given system, region and climate adopted the technologies and practice currently used by the 10 percent of producers with the lowest emission intensity."

It is unclear whether the authors' projected 30% reduction in GHG emissions through more efficient animal "husbandry" techniques would be enough to offset the increase in GHG emissions from their projected 73% rise in global demand for meat and 53% rise for milk by the year 2050. Whether their proposed mitigations would actually result in a reduction in global GHG emissions from animal agriculture is a dubious proposition.

By summarily dismissing the benefits of a plant-based diet to mitigate the GHG emissions from animal agriculture, the report *"Tackling climate change through livestock – A global assessment of emissions and mitigation opportunities,"* completely missed tackling the only mitigation opportunity that could actually stave off the worst effects of climate change – that is, reducing consumer demand for animal products.

"Losses, inefficiencies and waste in the global food system"(2017)

Many studies have been conducted to assess how much of the world's food production gets lost or wasted in the global food system. But until the 2017 study, *"Losses, inefficiencies and waste in the global food system" (Agricultural Systems, May 2017)*, the sources and distribution of global food lost and wasted were ill defined. By making greater use of available empirical data than previous studies, the authors of this study were able to quantify food losses in terms of wet and dry biomass, protein and energy. Notably, this study was the first to distinguish between animal and plant food losses, and also the first to count overconsumption of calories as food system loss.

The authors' found that food system losses in terms of wet and dry mass, protein and energy, were surprisingly high:

> *"The absolute overall system losses are dominated by agricultural residues and other losses prior to harvest (both of cropland and grassland), with losses of 66–79% that account for around 80% of all losses (*Table 1*).* **However, the highest loss rate for the stages considered occurs for livestock production, with losses of 81–94% (*Table 1*)."**

> **"Livestock production therefore represents a major source of losses often not included in studies of losses and waste in the food system (*Gustavsson et al., 2011*, *Kummu et al., 2012*), and this difference in method contributes to the higher overall loss rates found here."** (**bold emphasis mine***)

In this study, food consumed in excess of nutritional needs was also considered wasted food production. By multiplying the average calorie and protein requirements for the average person by the 7.01 billion people alive in 2011, the authors calculated the food energy requirement for the world's population as 25.1 Exajoules (EJs)/year and the world's protein requirement as 133 metric tonnes/year. World food energy and protein production in excess of these requirements was considered wasted food production. By this method, the authors found:

> *"The results here suggest that system losses from over-consumption of food are at least as substantial as the losses from food discarded by consumers (Fig. 4), and therefore have comparable food security and sustainability implications…* **Changes to influence consumer behaviour, e.g. eating less animal products, reducing food waste, and lowering per capita consumption to be closer to nutrient requirements will all help to provide the rising global population with food security in a sustainable manner."** (**bold emphasis mine**)

This study shows that animal foods are lost at higher rates than plant foods on both the supply and demand sides of our global food system.

In their final analysis, the authors concluded:

> *"Both consumer behaviour and production practices play crucial roles in the efficiency of the food system. This study considers the interconnectedness of the food system and the losses occurring, using primarily empirical data.* **The results emphasise the substantial losses occurring during livestock production, and reveals the magnitude of losses from consumption of food in excess of human nutritional requirements. The greatest rates of loss were associated with livestock production, and consequently changes in the levels of meat, dairy and egg consumption can substantially affect the overall efficiency of the food**

system, and associated environmental impacts (e.g. greenhouse gas emissions) (Lamb et al., 2016). It is therefore regrettable from environmental and food security perspectives that rates of meat and dairy consumption are expected to continue to increase as average incomes rise (Kearney, 2010, Keyzer et al., 2005, McMichael et al., 2007), potentially lowering efficiency of the overall food system, as well as increasing associated negative health implications (e.g. diabetes and heart disease) (Hu, 2011, Tilman and Clark, 2014).*" (bold emphasis mine)

"Losses, inefficiencies and waste in the global food system," is the first study I have reviewed that actually laments the expected increase in meat and dairy consumption as average global incomes are expected to rise. The authors call for *"... eating less animal products... and lowering per capita consumption to be closer to nutrient requirements..."* was the first clear call for dietary change as a mitigation for food insecurity and climate change. This groundbreaking study would soon be followed by more studies detailing the human health and environmental impacts of animal based diets.

"The opportunity cost of animal based diets exceeds all food losses" (2018)

"Conventional food loss" refers to available food that is lost before consumption due to such factors as spoilage and inefficient supply chains. Reducing such losses is generally recognized as a vital strategy for combating hunger in food insecure regions of the world. But there is another source of food loss that these conventional sources do not take into account: when agricultural resources are used to produce resource intensive animal foods instead of resource conserving plant foods, those additional resources used to produce animal foods could have been used to produce more plant foods for human consumption. This loss of food production capacity is referred to as "opportunity food loss." It is the opportunity food loss of the U.S. animal based diet that the study *"The opportunity cost of animal based diets exceeds all food losses,"* (*Proceedings of the National Academy of Sciences* in April, 2018), was designed to assess.

Here, the authors explain how the opportunity food loss of an animal based diet impacts on food security and the environment:

*"Although the postproduction loss across the supply chain is similar for plant- and animal-based items, the production of **a gram protein (or calorie) from animal sources requires about an order of magnitude more resources and emissions than producing a gram of protein from plant sources** (1⇓–3, 18, 22, 23). Consequently, **shifting to plant-based diets confers substantial environmental savings, comparable to or even surpassing projected improvements in agricultural productivity** (1, 2, 24, 25). In other words, due to the disparate resource requirements of plant- and animal-based food items, **replacing animal-based items with more resource-efficient plant alternatives will increase food availability by permitting reallocation of production resources from feed to human food***

(8, 14⇊–17, 22, 26, 27). Favoring resource-intensive food items like beef and pork over plant alternatives thus carries a substantial opportunity cost." **(bold emphasis mine)**

To explain how they calculated a food's opportunity food loss, the authors worked through the example of cattle meat:

"To clarify the values presented in Fig. 3, *consider the example of beef. Its consumer level opportunity loss of 96% means that the land area that would deliver 100 g (after all processing and delivery losses) of human-edible protein when used for the production of the plant replacement diet can produce only 4 g of edible beef, resulting in an opportunity food loss of 96 g protein."*

Using this formula, the authors calculated the opportunity food loss percentage for other meats, dairy and eggs:

"We find that the opportunity food losses at the consumer level range from 40% for eggs to 96% for beef (the most and least efficient animal food categories). Put differently, nutritionally comparable plant-based diets optimized to nutritionally replace eggs and beef produce twofold and 20-fold more protein per acre than the eggs and beef they replace. Although eggs and beef bracket this range, poultry and eggs are comparable to each other, as are pork and beef, and dairy is between those extremes."

Here, the authors show that the nutritionally comparable plant-based diet they designed to replace eggs and beef easily provides adequate protein to meet our daily requirements:

"Melina et al. (32) argue that protein from a variety of plant sources successfully meets essential amino acid requirements when caloric requirements are met and that legumes and soy are reliable protein sources that also provide other essential nutrients. Our plant-based replacement diets include various sources of plants, and all include soy, which has a complete protein. Consequently, the plant replacements in this paper generally match or exceed the protein quantity and quality of the replaced items."

The nutritionally comparable plant-based diet designed by the authors to replace eggs and beef also took into account nutrients other than protein:

*"In our model (*Fig. 2*), plant-based replacement diets usually deliver 2–10, 3–10, and 1–2 times as much iron, calcium, and zinc as the animal items they replace, respectively (with the exception of zinc for beef and calcium for milk). These overwhelming additions offset any putative bioavailability differences. Moreover, traditional food preparation practices (e.g., fermentation and soaking) tend to increase bioavailability of some nutrients (*38, 40, 41*). In our calculations, we use nutritional values of raw vegetable items, but these might increase through cooking. In western diets with abundant supplies of micronutrients it is not clear if reduced bioavailability has any bearing on health. For example, despite lower iron stores, vegetarians do not appear to have greater incidence of iron deficiency anemia (*33*). Because*

excess iron is also a risk factor for such noncommunicable diseases as type 2 diabetes ([42](#)) or metabolic syndrome ([43](#)), lower iron ingestion among vegetarians may in fact prove protective ([44](#))."

The argument often made by animal food advocates that a plant-based diet is nutrient deficient is utter hogwash.

The authors found that the opportunity food loss of the U.S. meat-based diet is greater than all U.S. conventional food losses:

"[R]eplacing all animal-based products in the mean American diet using all feed croplands with nutritionally comparable or superior plant alternatives (Eq. 6) can sustain ≈350 million additional people or ≈120% of the US population for years 2000–2010. In comparison, production-to-consumer conventional food loss is ≈30–40% of total production (19⇓–21), and thus, the effect of recovering the opportunity food loss collectively is larger than completely eliminating all conventional food losses in the United States."

Effectively, what this means is that the opportunity food loss of the current U.S. animal-based diet is three to four times conventional food losses from spoilage and food chain inefficiencies.

The authors also noted that a change to a plant-based diet in the U.S. would free up land for wildlife habitat:

"Although our analysis concentrated on opportunity costs in terms of food gains or losses, the ramifications of consuming animals vs. plants include other considerations worth noting. For example, replacing milk and beef in the United States with plant-based alternatives liberates almost 700 million pastureland acres for wilderness preservation and reverses overgrazing induced ecosystem degradation (3, 23)."

In the study, *"The opportunity cost of animal based diets exceeds all food losses,"* the authors were careful to point out that in countries with less animal food consumption than in the U.S., the opportunity food loss resulting from animal agriculture is necessarily less than in the U.S. Nonetheless, this analysis represents a valuable contribution to the scholarship on how moving toward a plant-based diet could dramatically improve worldwide food security and mitigate environmental impacts over the coming decades.

"The carbon opportunity cost of animal-sourced food production on land" (2020)

The online-only monthly journal, *Nature Sustainability,* was launched in January 2018, to publish the best research about sustainability from the natural and social sciences, as well as from the fields of engineering and policy. In September, 2020, they published the report, *"The carbon opportunity cost of animal-sourced food production on land."* This report focuses exclusively on dietary change as a means to mitigate the climate impacts of animal agriculture.

The authors of this report modeled different dietary scenarios moving forward from the year 2015 to the year 2050. They calculated the net CO_2 balance for three different dietary scenarios: 1) a business-as-usual (BAU) diet; 2) the EAT-Lancet Commission (ELC) diet containing approximately 70% less meat than the BAU diet; 3) a vegan (VGN) diet containing no animal-sourced foods

Here the authors define each of these diet scenarios:

"In the 2050 BAU scenario in the main text, we used cropland expansion within each continent directly from Alexandratos and Bruinsma11. We assumed a global pasture expansion of 6% by 2050 25, consistent with a literature estimate that assumes optimistic grazing improvements. Pasture expansion was distributed proportionally over the same distribution potential vegetation biomes as the present day, a conservative assumption because expansion is presently occurring disproportionately in carbon-rich tropical areas 26.

"ELC requirements were derived from recent guidelines11. We calculated fractions of feed cropland and pastureland necessary for each animal-sourced food category in ELC relative to BAU diets, using crop11 and forage and pasture27 allocation parameters from the literature."

"In the VGN scenario, all permanent pastureland was taken out of production, as well as feed croplands minus land necessary to provide macronutrients of removed animal-sourced foods (with approximately 25% excess8 after wastes and losses; Supplementary Table 1)".

The authors then used the data generated from these three dietary scenarios, to calculate the potential for reducing anthropogenic GHG emissions by reducing or eliminating animal agriculture:

"The BAU diet results in land clearing, with land-use-change emissions of 86 (68–105) GtCO2 (Fig. 3) because optimistic future improvements in yields are insufficient to meet expected animal feed demands11.

"The ELC and VGN diets result in 332 (210 to 459) and 547 (358 to 743) total GtCO2 removal, respectively, approximately equal to the past 9 and 16 years of fossil fuel emissions. Ecosystem soil and litter could remove an additional 135 and 225 GtCO2 for ELC and VGN, respectively (Supplementary Table 6), but this estimate is highly uncertain.

"Ceasing fossil fuel use is necessary to limit global warming, but CO2 removal following plant-rich dietary shifts could substantially contribute to international greenhouse gas reduction targets... By contrast, most future scenarios of 1.5 °C warming rely on nascent bioenergy carbon capture and storage technology to remove 151 to 1,191 GtCO2 from the atmosphere13—an amount of CO2 comparable to plant-rich diets."

Most notable here is the authors' finding that a vegan diet could remove enough carbon from the atmosphere to keep global warming under the 1.5 °C called for in the international Paris Climate Accords of 2015. But rather than promote dietary change as a low tech mitigation for climate change that could be implemented immediately, world governments would rather rely on pie-in-the-sky "carbon capture" technologies that have yet to be invented.

Here, the authors quantify the *"carbon opportunity cost"* of producing animal-based foods relative to producing plant-based foods:

> *"Pastures for ruminant meat and dairy production represent the majority of the total carbon opportunity cost—72%—compared with animal feed croplands, which suppress the remaining 28% of native vegetation carbon (Supplementary Table 3)."*

> *"The cumulative potential of CO_2 removal on land currently occupied by animal agriculture is comparable in order of magnitude to the past decade of global fossil fuel emissions. The largest potential for negative emissions—74GtC or 48% of the global total—lies in upper-middle-income countries (Fig. 2), which will further increase as meat and dairy production expand. This is approximately equal to the past 19 years of fossil fuel emissions in these countries. In high-income countries, in which animal-sourced food demand is high but plateauing8, the total carbon opportunity cost of animal-sourced food production is 32GtC, approximately equal to the past 9 years of their domestic fossil fuel emissions.*

> *"Present-day pasturelands exist in areas of both native forests and grasslands within all continents (Supplementary Table 3). Pastures in native forest areas displace 72GtC—accounting for 68% of pastures' carbon opportunity cost but only 22% of total pasture area (Supplementary Table 3 and Supplementary Fig. 2). In native grasslands, vegetation may be partially restored by improved grazing management9, rather than removing animals altogether, although trade-offs remain with respect to non-CO_2 ruminant emissions. In addition, optimal grazing does not always promote restoration because ruminants selectively browse native species10 and translocate nutrients11."*

By quantifying native revegetation of former pasturelands in terms of years worth of carbonsequestration, the authors developed an innovative way to visualize the enormous carbon opportunity costs of an animal based diet.

The authors concluded:

> *"This analysis uses the most up-to-date and high-resolution data to map ecosystem carbon trade-offs associated with animal-sourced food production. Our results demonstrate substantial carbon opportunity costs incurred by resource-intensive diets, comparable to the remaining carbon budget to 1.5 °C. Animal agriculture across all continents and income categories represents a profound trade-off when compared with potential GHG mitigation. If future dietary shifts do not occur, carbon trade-offs are expected to grow, even with large improvements in yields and optimized cropland distribution. Our carbon accounting approach illuminates areas where policies could prioritize ecosystem restoration and CO_2 removal, including but not limited to tropical Latin American forests outside of the Amazon basin and temperate forests in Western Europe and East Asia, where carbon trade-offs are largest."*

"*Restoration of native ecosystems, including forests, is a land-based option for atmospheric carbon dioxide (CO2) removal1. Ecosystem restoration is constrained largely by land requirements of food production, the largest human use of land globally2. Food production therefore incurs a 'carbon opportunity cost', that is, the potential for natural CO2 removal via ecosystem restoration on land3,4. This cost can vary greatly depending on the 'potential' or 'native' vegetation of a given region and types of food produced. Animal-sourced foods such as meat and dairy have large land footprints because animals typically consume more food macronutrients than they produce5. Quantifying the spatial distribution of agriculture's cumulative carbon opportunity cost within this century can inform efforts to limit global warming to 1.5 °C.*"

In essence, what the authors are saying is that if we humans continue to dine at the top of the food chain, then we will miss our only opportunity to turn back the clock on global warming.

The clear message from the six reports and studies by independent scientists reviewed above is that the global animal industrial complex built to satisfy the insatiable desires of people to eat meat, dairy and eggs, is the primary driver of ecological collapse around the world today.

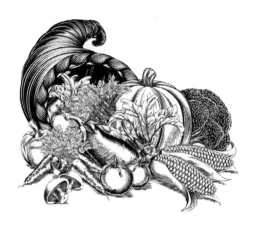

PART VI

MAN EATING PLANTS:

HOW A VEGAN DIET CAN SAVE THE

WORLD

• • •

"The greatest service which can be rendered any country is to add a useful
plant to its culture.
–The Fruit Hunters"

– Thomas Jefferson, statesman, third U.S. president (1743 – 1826)

21

NUTRITIONAL ADEQUACY AND ENVIRONMENTAL SUSTAINABILITY OF A PLANT-BASED DIET

As several of the reports cited in Part V made abundantly clear: if we humans do not reform our diets to conform to our natural place on the food chain as a plant-eating species, then any attempts we make to mitigate cataclysmic climate change are guaranteed to fail. Even the reports *"Livestock's Long Shadow (2006)"* and *"Tackling climate change through livestock (2013)"* authored by the FAO's own livestock industry specialists have acknowledged the extreme environmental impacts of animal agriculture. Yet, the FAO still insists that animal foods are a necessary part of the world food production system to provide food security for an ever growing human population. This assertion is demonstrably false. Let's now review six of the most prominent studies published between 2003 and 2021 that quantify the nutritional adequacy and environmental sustainability of a plant-based diet.

"Sustainability of meat-based and plant-based diets and the environment" (2003)

Dr. David Pimentel (1925 – 2019), PhD, was a Professor of Insect Ecology & Agricultural Sciences at Cornell University, Ithaca, New York, U.S.A. In his academic career, he published over 700 scientific papers including 37 books. He also served on many national and government committees including the *National Academy of Sciences*, the *President's Science Advisory Council*, the *Office of Technology Assessment* of the U.S. Congress, the U.S. State Department, the Departments of Agriculture, Energy, and Health, Education and Welfare and the Secretary's *Commission On Pesticides And Their Relationship To Environmental Health*. Dr. Pimentel was best known for his work in quantifying the effects of natural and human variables on crop yields and production. He wrote landmark papers on the energy intensiveness of modern agriculture, on losses due to soil erosion and invasive species, and on the net energy loss of making ethanol from maize. In September, 2003, *The American Journal of Clinical Nutrition*, published Dr. Pimentel's groundbreaking paper, *"Sustainability of meat-based and plant-based diets and the environment."* In this paper, he turns his expertise to quantifying the environmental sustainability of producing food for animal and plant-based diets in the United States.

To make this comparison between the environmental sustainability of these different diets, Dr. Pimentel analyzed the cost/calorie to produce the current U.S. animal-based diet and estimated the cost/calorie to produce the same number of calories in a theoretical no-meat diet.

It should be noted here that the no-meat, *"lactoovovegetarian,"* diet Dr. Pimentel chose to represent a "plant-based" diet includes dairy products and eggs which are animal foods, so the comparison does not fully account for the cost/calorie difference between producing animal and plant foods.

Here, Dr. Pimentel contrasts the current U.S. meat based diet with his theoretical lactoovovegetarian diet:

*"The meat-based diet differs from the vegetarian diet in that 124 kg of meat and 20.3 kg of fish are consumed per year (*Table 1*). Note that the number of calories is the same for both diets because the vegetarian foods consumed were proportionately increased to make sure that both diets contained the same number of calories. The total calories in the meat and fish consumed per day was 480 kcal. The foods in the meat-based diet providing the most calories were food grains and sugar and sweeteners—similar to the lactoovovegetarian diet."*

"In the lactoovovegetarian diet, the meat and fish calories were replaced by proportionately increasing most other foods consumed in Table 1 *in the vegetarian diet except sugar and sweeteners, fats, and vegetable oils. The total weight of food consumed was slightly higher (1002 kg per year) in the lactoovovegetarian diet than in the meat-based diet (995 kg per year). The most food calories consumed in both diets were associated with food grains, and the second largest amount of calories consumed was from sugar and sweeteners."*

It is interesting to note here that the second most calories in both diets came from sugar and sweeteners. This is reflective of the processed food diet of most Americans and does not truly represent the whole-food, plant-based diet that I advocate for in this book.

Here, Dr. Pimentel quantifies the production side of the current U.S. meat-based diet:

"The US food production system uses about 50% of the total US land area, approximately 80% of the fresh water, and 17% of the fossil energy used in the country (3)..."

*"In the United States, more than 9 billion livestock are maintained to supply the animal protein consumed each year (*11*). This livestock population on average outweighs the US human population by about 5 times. Some livestock, such as poultry and hogs, consume only grains, whereas dairy cattle, beef cattle, and lambs consume both grains and forage. At present, the US livestock population consumes more than 7 times as much grain as is consumed directly by the entire American population (*11*). The amount of grains fed to US livestock is sufficient to feed about 840 million people who follow a plant-based diet (*7*). From the US livestock population, a total of about 8 million tons (metric) of animal protein is produced annually. With an average distribution assumed, this protein is sufficient to supply about 77 g of animal protein daily per American. With the addition of about 35 g of available plant protein consumed per person, a total of 112 g of protein is available per capita in the United States per day (*11*). Note that the recommended daily allowance (RDA) for adults per day is 56 g of protein from a mixed diet. Therefore, based on these data, each American consumes about twice the RDA for protein. Americans on average are eating too much and are consuming about 1000 kcal in excess per day per capita (*12, 13*). The protein consumed per day on the lactoovovegetarian diet is 89 g*

per day. This is significantly lower than the 112 g for the meat-based diet but still much higher than the RDA of 56 g per day.

"About 124 kg of meat is eaten per American per year (6). Of the meat eaten, beef amounts to 44 kg, pork 31 kg, poultry 48 kg, and other meats 1 kg. Additional animal protein is obtained from the consumption of milk, eggs, and fish. For every 1 kg of high-quality animal protein produced, livestock are fed about 6 kg of plant protein. In the conversion of plant protein to animal protein, there are 2 principal inputs or costs: 1) the direct costs of production of the harvest animal, including its feed; and 2) the indirect costs for maintaining the breeding herds.

*"Fossil energy is expended in livestock production systems (**Table 2**). For example, broiler chicken production is the most efficient, with an input of 4 kcal of fossil energy for each 1 kcal of broiler protein produced. The broiler system is primarily dependent on grain. Turkey, also a grain-fed system, is next in efficiency, with a ratio of 10:1. Milk production, based on a mixture of two-thirds grain and one-third forage, is relatively efficient, with a ratio of 14:1. Both pork and egg production also depend on grain. Pork production has a ratio of 14:1, whereas egg production has a 39:1 ratio.*

*"The 2 livestock systems depending most heavily on forage but also using significant amounts of grain are the beef and lamb production systems (**Table 3**). The beef system has a ratio of 40:1, while the lamb has the highest, with a ratio of 57:1 (Table 2). If these animals were fed on only good-quality pasture, the energy inputs could be reduced by about half.*

*"The average fossil energy input for all the animal protein production systems studied is 25 kcal fossil energy input per 1 kcal of protein produced (Table 2). This energy input is more than 11 times greater than that for grain protein production, which is about 2.2 kcal of fossil energy input per 1 kcal of plant protein produced (**Table 4**). This is for corn and assumes 9% protein in the corn. Animal protein is a complete protein based on its amino acid profile and has about 1.4 times the biological value of grain protein (8). [Note: as we shall see in Part VII: A Diet for the 21ˢᵗ Century, Dr. Pimentel is mistaken about animal proteins being superior to plant proteins which also contain all 9 essential amino acids.]*

What stands out here is that the U.S. livestock population consumes more than 7 times as much grain as is consumed directly by the entire U.S. population and the amount of grains fed to U.S. livestock is sufficient to feed about 840 million people who follow the theoretical lactoovovegetarian diet. Since the 89 grams of protein/day consumed on the lactoovovegetarian diet is well above the U.S. RDA of 56 grams of protein/day, this means that a food production system that includes no meat products could easily provide enough protein to meet the nutritional needs of the U.S. population many times over. Another important fact cited above is that the fossil fuel energy expended to produce 1 kcal of animal protein is on average 11 times greater than that expended to produce 1 kcal of grain protein. This is one reason why animal-based diets emit so much more greenhouse gas than plant-based diets.

Here, Dr. Pimentel quantifies the production side of the dairy, egg and plant components of his theoretical **lactoovovegetarian diet:**

> *"The amount of feed grains used to produce the animal products (milk and eggs) consumed in the lactoovovegetarian diet was about half (450 kg) the amount of feed grains fed to the livestock (816 kg) to produce the animal products consumed in the meat-based diet (*Table 1*). This is expected because of the relatively large amount of animal products consumed in the meat-based diet (*7*). Less than 0.4 ha of cropland was used to produce the food for the vegetarian-based diet, whereas about 0.5 ha of cropland was used in the meat-based diet (*8*). This reflects the larger amount of land needed to produce the meat-based diet (*Table 1*).*

> ***"The major fossil energy inputs for grain, vegetable, and forage production include fertilizers, agricultural machinery, fuel, irrigation, and pesticides (8,9). The energy inputs vary according to the crops being grown (10). When these inputs are balanced against their energy and protein content, grains and some legumes, such as soybeans, are produced more efficiently in terms of energy inputs than vegetables, fruits, and animal products (8). In the United States, the average protein yield from a grain crop such as corn is 720 kg/ha (10). To produce 1 kcal of plant protein requires an input of about 2.2 kcal of fossil energy (10)."***

Of note in this analysis is that the feed grains grown for milk and egg production account for a substantial amount of the cropland used in the theoretical lactoovovegetarian diet; what this means is that a vegan diet would utilize significantly less land than the lactoovovegetarian diet. Also of note is that to produce 1 kcal of plant protein requires an input of about 2.2 kcal of fossil energy; as Dr. Pimentel pointed out in the "Introduction" to his report, *"The heavy dependence on fossil energy suggests that the US food system, whether meat-based or plant-based, is not sustainable."*

Here, Dr. Pimentel compares the environmental costs of producing the U.S. animal-based diet to the costs of producing the theoretical lactoovovegetarian diet:

> *"Each year about 90% of US cropland loses soil at a rate 13 times above the sustainable rate of 1 ton/ha/y (*28*). Also, US pastures and rangelands are losing soil at an average of 6 tons/ha/y. About 60% of United States pastureland is being overgrazed and is subject to accelerated erosion.*

> *"The concern about high rates of soil erosion in the United States and the world is evident when it is understood that it takes approximately 500 y to replace 25 mm (1 in) of lost soil (*28*). Clearly, a farmer cannot wait for the replacement of 25 mm of soil. Commercial fertilizers can replace some nutrient loss resulting from soil erosion, but this requires large inputs of fossil energy."*

"Agricultural production, including livestock production, consumes more fresh water than any other activity in the United States. Western agricultural irrigation accounts for 85% of the fresh water consumed (29). The water required to produce various foods and forage crops ranges from 500 to 2000 L of water per kilogram of crop produced. For instance, a hectare of US corn transpires more than 5 million L of water during the 3-mo growing season. If irrigation is required, more than 10 million L of water must be applied. Even with 800–1000 mm of annual rainfall in the US Corn Belt, corn usually suffers from lack of water in late July, when the corn is growing the most.

"Producing 1 kg of animal protein requires about 100 times more water than producing 1 kg of grain protein (8). Livestock directly uses only 1.3% of the total water used in agriculture. However, when the water required for forage and grain production is included, the water requirements for livestock production dramatically increase. For example, producing 1 kg of fresh beef may require about 13 kg of grain and 30 kg of hay (17). This much forage and grain requires about 100 000 L of water to produce the 100 kg of hay, and 5400 L for the 4 kg of grain. On rangeland for forage production, more than 200 000 L of water are needed to produce 1 kg of beef (30). Animals vary in the amounts of water required for their production. In contrast to beef, 1 kg of broiler can be produced with about 2.3 kg of grain requiring approximately 3500 L of water."

There are several facts that stand out here. First, about 60% of pastureland in the U.S. is being overgrazed and is subject to accelerated erosion. This indicates that grazing cattle is a major source of soil erosion and nutrient loss on U.S. rangelands. Second, commercial fertilizers that replace some of the nutrient loss resulting from soil erosion require large inputs of fossil energy. What this means is that industrialized agriculture using massive chemical fertilizer inputs is unsustainable, and to become sustainable U.S. farmers must adopt organic self-sustaining farming practices (more on this coming up in *Chapter 24: Growing Our Food, Healing Our Planet*). Third, agricultural production including livestock, consumes more fresh water than any other activity in the U.S., and western states irrigation of animal feed crops accounts for 85% of the fresh water consumed. What this means is that growing feed crops is a major cause of water depletion in the U.S. Fourth, producing 1 kg of animal protein requires about 100 times more water than producing 1 kg of grain protein. What this means is that feeding grains and beans directly to people instead of livestock would reduce water consumption for food production in the U.S. by trillions of liters/year (1 liter = 0.264 gallons).

Dr. Pimentel concludes with these remarks:

"Both the meat-based average American diet and the lactoovovegetarian diet require significant quantities of nonrenewable fossil energy to produce. Thus, both food systems are not sustainable in the long term based on heavy fossil energy requirements. However, the meat-based diet requires more energy, land, and water resources than the lactoovovegetarian

diet. In this limited sense, the lactoovovegetarian diet is more sustainable than the average American meat-based diet."

Dr. Pimentel's report, *"Sustainability of meat-based and plant-based diets and the environment,"* was published three years before the FAO report, *"Livestock's Long Shadow,"* and its focus on diet as an important factor in agricultural policy was revolutionary; following in the giant footsteps of groundbreaking diet researcher, Francis Moore Lappé, author of the 1971 bestselling book, *"Diet for a Small Planet,"* in which she first exposed the enormous environmental impacts of a meat-based diet. While Dr. Pimentel applied academic rigor to the quantification of the environmental impacts of animal and plant based diets in the U.S., his work is based on the same misconception as Lappé's was in the early 1970s: that animal proteins are "complete" and plant proteins are "incomplete." (Lappé would later recant her position in subsequent editions of *"Diet for a Small Planet."*) Based on this misconception, they both made the same mistake of including dairy and eggs in their "plant-based" diet, which effectively shortchanged the actual environmental advantages of a truly healthy and nutritious plant-based diet.

"Climate benefits of changing diet" (2009)

In March 1977, the science journal *Climatic Change* began to publish interdisciplinary research papers devoted to the description, causes and implications of climatic change. Unlike the FAO's *Animal Production and Health Division* that is run by representatives of the animal products industries, *Climatic Change* publishes the research of independent scientists who are dedicated to exposing the truth rather than punching their meal tickets. In February, 2009, *Climatic Change* published the groundbreaking report, *"Climate benefits of changing diet,"* that was the first major study to investigate the effects of different diets on climate change. As the authors of this report note, "…the effects of dietary changes in the context of mitigation scenarios and associated costs have yet to be studied quantitatively." The authors published their report to shine a light on this critical, yet unexplored aspect of our human response to anthropogenic climate change.

The authors explain their methodology:

"Here, we analyze how changes in the human diet may impact the technical and economic feasibility of ambitious climate stabilization targets. Using the integrated assessment model IMAGE 2.4 (MNP 2006), we compare four alternative dietary variants in terms of their greenhouse gas emissions and the corresponding costs for achieving stabilization of greenhouse gas concentrations at 450 ppm CO2-eq. to a reference and mitigation scenario without these dietary changes (Section 2, Methods)."

Here, the authors define the *"four alternative dietary variants"*:

"In order to explore the impact of dietary transitions, four variants of the reference scenario [i.e. current dietary patterns] were developed with partial or complete substitution of meat

by plant proteins. These four variants are (a) complete substitution of meat from ruminants (NoRM), (b) complete substitution of all meat (NoM), (c) complete substitution of all animal products (meat, dairy products and eggs) (NoAP) and finally (d) partial substitution of meat based on a healthy diet variant (HealthyDiet, HDiet). The stylized variants of complete substitutions should be regarded as analytical constructs allowing for a detailed assessment of the effects of specific food products on land use, carbon cycle, greenhouse gas emissions, and mitigation options."

To reiterate, the authors devised four dietary variants distinct from our current dietary patterns reference scenario: 1) no ruminant meats (NoRM), 2) no meat (NoM), 3) no animal products (NoAP), and 4) HealthyDiet (Hdiet). By including a no animal products (NoAP) diet as one of the options in their comparison, this report is a significant improvement over Dr. Pimentel's report, *"Sustainability of meat-based and plant-based diets and the environment."*

Here, the authors project the GHG emissions under the no dietary change *"reference scenario,"* for the years 2000 to 2050:

"Under the reference scenario, global population increases from 6 to 9 billion people between 2000 and 2050, and global average GDP per capita almost triples from 5.5 to 16 thousand US$ (Table 1)."

"In the same period, livestock production doubles (Fig. 1), mainly driven by population growth and increasing per capita meat consumption."

"[T]otal global methane emissions from enteric fermentation and animal waste increase steadily throughout the scenario period from about 100 Tg CH4 per year in 2000 to close to 170 Tg per year in 2050. It should also be noted that increasing (industrial) monogastric production will not only cause additional greenhouse gas emissions from manure, but also induces an increasing demand for feed crops, resulting in considerable greenhouse gas emissions associated with their production and fertilizer input."

Most notably, under the no dietary change *"reference scenario,"* methane emissions from animal agriculture would increase by 70% from 2000 to 2050!

Here, the authors quantify the GHG emissions of the four dietary variants from 2010 to 2050:

"In total, the global greenhouse gas emissions (CO2 and non-CO2) from agricultural production systems, calculated for the three stylized variants, show considerable reductions in relation to the reference scenario (Table 5). For the most extreme variant (NoAP), the cumulative emission reduction in the 2010–2050 period amounts to 17% for CO2 [carbon dioxide], 24% for CH4 [methane] and 21% for N2O [nitrous oxide] (Fig. 1). The largest reduction of greenhouse gas emissions by product category is caused by the substitution of ruminant meat (Fig. 2a), with a large terrestrial net CO2 sink of about 30 GtC over the whole period compared to a net source of 34 GtC in the reference case (Fig. 2b)." "Methane emission due to enteric

fermentation and from animal waste as well as the N2O emissions associated with animal waste are reduced significantly (in NoRM and NoM), or even dropping to zero (in NoAP). The contribution of the additional carbon sink and avoided deforestation contributes 65–75% to the total cumulative emission reduction." "The stylized dietary variants show a reduction of greenhouse gas concentrations of 57 to 76 ppm CO2-eq... compared to the reference scenario in 2050 (Fig. 1d)."

Relative to the reference scenario of a 70% increase in GHG emissions by 2050, the no animal products (NoAP) diet would actually decrease carbon dioxide (CO2) emissions from agriculture by 17%, methane (CH4) emissions by 24%, and nitrous oxide (N2O) emissions by 21%. Methane emission due to enteric fermentation from animal waste as well as the N2O emissions associated with animal waste would be reduced to zero under the no animal products diet.

Here, the authors come to some unheard-of, but inescapable conclusions:

"Our model experiment shows that changes in dietary patterns can be an effective means to decrease greenhouse gas emissions, in addition to more conventional strategies such as changes in the energy system, reforestation and the reduction of nonCO2 gases by add-on abatement technology."

"In addition to reductions in CH4 and N2O, the shift to low-meat diets induces a reduction in agricultural area, and subsequently leads to land availability for other purposes such as energy crops or nature reserves. The regrowth of vegetation on these abandoned areas leads to a substantial, though transient, uptake of CO2."

The publication of, *"Climate benefits of changing diet"* in 2009 was a watershed event in the study of the environmental impacts of the human diet. The authors' finding that between the years 2000 and 2050, a change from our prevailing dietary patterns of animal food consumption to a diet free of animal foods could reduce anthropogenic GHG emissions from a 70% increase to around a 20% decrease, is nothing short of a revelation. After publication of this landmark report, to be considered meaningful, all future studies on climate change mitigations required a serious reevaluation of the human place at the dining table of the Earth's ecosystems.

"Redefining agricultural yields: from tonnes to people nourished per hectare" (2013)

In August 2013, the study, *"Redefining agricultural yields: from tonnes to people nourished per hectare,"* was published in the *Environmental Research Letters* of the online science journal *IOPscience*. This study focused on the nutritional value of the food produced rather than simply its weight.

Here, the authors explain how redefining crop yields in terms of nutritional value helps identify opportunities to reduce the environmental impacts of agriculture while providing a healthy diet for the world's growing population:

"In this study, we consider how different systems of crop production and crop use are interwoven to actually feed people around the world. Specifically, we map global patterns of crop production as well as crop allocation (for human consumed food, animal feed, biofuels, and other non-food products) to determine the amount of human-consumable calories produced across the world. By comparing crop production (in terms of tonnes of crop per hectare) to actual food delivery (in terms of calories of human-consumable product per hectare), we illustrate where tremendous inefficiencies in the global food system exist today— and where opportunities to enhance food security exist by changing dietary preferences and biofuel policies."

In order to properly allocate global food calories/hectare produced for human consumption, the authors found four areas of calorie leakage in the global food production system that had to be accounted for:

- Calories lost in the conversion of animal feed to edible calories of meat, dairy and eggs for human consumption.
- Calories produced from crops that are processed for both human and livestock consumption.
- Crop calories lost to biofuels.
- Crop calories produced within a given nation that were not consumed domestically.

By correcting for these calorie leaks in the global food production system, the authors were able to develop a more accurate picture of global caloric production and consumption patterns.

Here, the authors summarize their findings on the crop calories produce around the world relative to the crop calories actually consumed by people:

*"From the 41 crops analyzed in this study, 9.46×10^{15} calories available in plant form are produced by crops globally, of which 55% directly feed humans. However, 36% of these produced calories go to animal feed, of which 89% is lost, **such that only 4% of crop-produced calories are available to humans in the form of animal products.** Another 9% of crop-produced calories are used for industrial uses and biofuels and so completely lost from the food system. Including both human-edible crop calories and feed-produced animal calories, only 5.57×10^{15} (59% of the total produced) calories are delivered to the world's food system (figure 1). Therefore, 41% of the calories available from global crop production are lost to the food system."* **(bold emphasis mine)**

In other words, the biggest leak in calories delivered from farm to table comes from the conversion of feed crops into animal products.

Here, the authors put these findings into perspective by calculating how many additional people could be fed with a shift of crop calories used for feed and other uses to direct human consumption:

"Put another way, shifting the crops used for feed and other uses towards direct human food consumption could increase calories in the food system by 3.89×10^{15} calories, from 5.57×10^{15} to 9.46×10^{15} calories, or a ~70% increase... Therefore, shifting the crop calories used for feed and other uses to direct human consumption could potentially feed an additional 4 billion people."

Put in yet another way, if everyone around the world today ate a plant-based diet, we could produce more than enough food calories to feed every human being on Earth using less than half the land now under cultivation. This analysis puts to rest the FAO's unsupported claim that animal foods are an essential source of calories to feed an ever growing human population.

The crop yields and consumption patterns cited above are worldwide averages, but actual yields and consumption patterns vary widely in different regions of the world. Here, the authors review the yields and consumption patterns of four of the world's major crop producing countries – India, China, Brazil and the U.S.:

"Because India dedicates land to mostly food crops and 89% of crop calories are used for direct human consumption, the calories produced on croplands and the calories delivered are similar: 90% of the calories produced in India are delivered to the food system. The number of people fed per cropland hectare on calories delivered on Indian croplands averages 5.9 people ha^{-1}, a result of a 90% rate of calorie delivery to the food system. If all produced calories were delivered as food, this figure would rise slightly to 6.5 people ha^{-1}. On delivered calories India is able to feed 5.9 people ha^{-1}, which is about the global average of 6 people fed ha^{-1}. This is a result of a high delivery fraction yet a low number of calories produced per hectare in India as compared to the global average.

"China produces one fifth of the world's meat, egg and dairy calories, and almost half of the world's pig meat. China uses 58% of its crop calorie production for food and 33% for feed. Of the total calories produced in China, 62% are delivered to the food system. China feeds more people than India per cropland hectare with 8.4 people fed with delivered calories, albeit with a lower calorie delivery fraction of 62%. If all produced calories were food, that number would rise substantially to 13.5 people ha^{-1}.

"Brazil directs 46% of calorie production to human food and 41% to animal feed. Of the calories produced in Brazil, 50% are delivered to the food system. Therefore, Brazil could feed twice as many people per hectare. Croplands in Brazil could feed 10.6 people ha^{-1}, but only feed 5.2 people. A high proportion of Brazil's calorie production goes to animal feed. Soybean production in Brazil accounted for 28% all calories produced, and over one-third of soybean

production was exported to other nations. Calorie delivery reflects the number of calories delivered to the global food system per calorie produced on croplands, regardless of where they are consumed. In the case of soybeans produced in Brazil, if they are exported to another country and used as feed, those calorie losses are reflected on Brazilian croplands, not in the importing nations that use them.

"The US uses 67% of total calorie production for animal feed. Because so much of the United States calorie production goes to animal feed, only 34% of the calories produced in the US are delivered to the food system. The US is the world's top producer of beef cattle, producing 22% of global beef supply. The number of domestically produced calories allocated to feed in the United States is 1.8 times the number allocated to feed in China. Yet when we look at the total of all meat, egg, and dairy calories produced, China produces 44% more than the United States [27]. However, because these numbers reflect allocation of only domestically produced feed crops, we are not fully capturing grain-fed livestock production in China. China's livestock production is more import dependent than the United States. This is especially the case for soybeans imported to China from Brazil [28]. For example, in 2000 45% of soybean supply in China was imported, and that proportion has increased over time to roughly 70% in 2009 [21].

The United States could feed almost three times as many people per cropland hectare on calories produced from major crops. US croplands feed 5.4 people ha^{-1} but could feed 16.1 people ha^{-1} if the current 34% efficiency rose to 100%. The US agricultural system alone could feed 1 billion additional people by shifting crop calories to direct human consumption."

The chart below summarizes the additional people who could be fed per hectare if the populations of these four major crop producing nations ate a 100% plant-based diet instead of their prevailing diet as of the year 2000:

	People fed/ha current diet (2000)	People fed/ha 100% plant-based diet	Additional People Fed/ha
India	5.9	6.5	0.6
China	8.4	13.5	5.1
Brazil	5.2	10.6	5.4
U.S.	5.4	16.1	10.7

The average diet in India was already the closest to plant-based, which means a switch to a 100% plant-based diet would have the least effect on people fed/ha. China, which has a fast growing animal agriculture sector, could increase people fed/ha by over 60% switching to a vegan diet. Brazil, which grows enormous quantities of corn, soy and sugarcane for livestock feed and biofuels, could more than double the people fed/hectare by feeding crops directly to people, and the U.S. which has the highest animal food consumption of any major crop producing nation and is a major biofuel producer, could nearly triple the people fed/hectare by feeding crops directly to people. These findings are illustrative of the *"... tremendous inefficiencies in the global food system [that] exist today—and where opportunities to enhance food security exist by changing dietary preferences and biofuel policies."*

The authors conclude with these prophetic remarks:

"While many efforts to address food security have focused primarily on improving crop yields [29, 30], it is also possible to dramatically increase the availability of food in the world by shifting the allocation of our crops from animal feed and biofuels towards more direct means of feeding the human population.

"In this study, we demonstrate that global calorie availability could be increased by as much as 70% (or 3.88×10^{15} calories) by shifting crops away from animal feed and biofuels to human consumption."

Several studies have modeled the effects of different human diets on the environmental impacts of agriculture, but the study, *"Redefining agricultural yields: from tonnes to people nourished per hectare,"* comes closest to quantifying how the actual caloric needs of the human population can most efficiently be met through a sustainable plant-based diet.

The fact that it takes many times more natural resources to raise animals than to grow plants has been known to humans since ancient times, and many wars have been fought over access to pasture land. The reason people have been so willing to lavish resources and resort to violence to secure animal foods is that these foods have been elevated to a superior status in most cultures around the world, and thus considered highly desirable. While these cultural belief systems persist to this day, we now know that not only are animal foods unhealthy for us to eat, but the Earth's ecosystems can no longer sustain themselves under the environmental burden imposed by animal agriculture.

This study brings the conflict between human caloric needs and the environmental impacts of animal agriculture into sharp focus. There can be no doubt: a plant-based diet that both meets our caloric needs and protects our environment is the only sustainable path forward for our out-of-control species.

"Cropland/pastureland dynamics and the slowdown of deforestation in Latin America" (2015)

As noted in some of the reports cited above: of all regions in the world, deforestation due to livestock production has been most pronounced in Latin America (i.e. Central America, South America and the Caribbean Islands). Since the introduction of synthetic fertilizers and pesticides with the "Green Revolution" of the 1960s, Latin American farmers have expanded agriculture faster than anywhere else on Earth. Agricultural production did stagnate in the 1990s, but the 2000s saw the greatest agricultural expansion in Latin American history. Deforestation resulted as farmers razed tropical forests to create pastureland for cattle and cropland for maize and soybeans used mostly to feed livestock.

Contemporary studies of this deforestation phenomenon in the early 21st century had analyzed changes in land cover as agriculture moved into forested areas, but they did not make the distinction between pastureland and cropland. In 2015, a group of international researchers sought to rectify this key omission with their report, *"Cropland/pastureland dynamics and the slowdown of deforestation in Latin America" (Environmental Research Letters, March, 2015).*

The authors used thirteen years (2001 – 2013) of the most advanced satellite imagery of the time to characterize cropland and pastureland expansion at multiple scales across Latin America. Here, the authors explain why the distinction between cropland and pastureland is important:

> *"Distinguishing between cropland and pastureland LUCC [land use/cover change] is important because the two systems vary in land use intensity and efficiency, particularly of food production. The manner in which the two agricultural systems produce food has important implications for food security and conservation.* **Cropland is typically a more efficient way to produce food than pastureland [57]. Pastures are often extensive systems whereas cropland is a more intensive land use; therefore, cropland produces more calories and protein per hectare.** *In contrast, pastureland expansion in Latin America has largely been for beef production, the most inefficient way to produce meat [58]. Moreover, during the twenty-first century pastureland expanded in frontier areas, often into intact forests, whereas cropland expanded into previously cleared pastureland. Given these modes of expansion, cropland expansion is relatively more favorable to forest conservation, as it requires less land to meet food demand. Thus, pastureland to cropland conversion intensifies production."* **(bold emphasis mine)**

In this study, the authors made no dietary recommendations for mitigating deforestation in Latin America, but by recognizing that cropland is a more efficient way to produce food than pastureland, they made the perfect argument for switching from a meat to a plant-based diet. In a practical sense, if people just ate the maize, soybeans and other fruit and vegetable crops instead of eating meat, billions of hectares of the most species diverse tropical forests on the planet could be spared from destruction.

"Reducing food's environmental impacts through producers and consumers" (2018)

In the study, *"Reducing food's environmental impacts through producers and consumers" (Science,* May, 2018), the authors explore the economics of food production and consumption. This ambitious study represented the most comprehensive metaanalysis of relevant studies to date attempting to quantify the environmental impacts of food producers and consumers.

The report goes on to quantify the various environmental impacts and possible mitigations of producers, but in their final analysis, the authors acknowledge that the most effective mitigations come from the consumer side of the food equation; that is, people moving away from an animal-based towards a plant-based diet:

"Producer mitigation limits and the role of consumers

"Though producers are a vital part of the solution, their ability to reduce environmental impacts is limited. These limits can mean that a product has higher impacts than another nutritionally equivalent product, however it is produced.

"In particular, the impacts of animal products can markedly exceed those of vegetable substitutes (Fig. 1), to such a degree that meat, aquaculture, eggs, and dairy use ~83% of the world's farmland and contribute 56 to 58% of food's different emissions, despite providing only 37% of our protein and 18% of our calories. Can animal products be produced with sufficiently low impacts to redress this vast imbalance? Or will reducing animal product consumption deliver greater environmental benefits?

"We find that the impacts of the lowest-impact animal products exceed average impacts of substitute vegetable proteins across GHG emissions, eutrophication, acidification (excluding nuts), and frequently land use (Fig. 1 and data S2). These stark differences are not apparent in any product groups except protein-rich products and milk."

"Although aquaculture can have low land requirements, in part by converting by-products into edible protein, the lowest-impact aquaculture systems still exceed emissions of vegetable proteins. This challenges recommendations to expand aquaculture (1) without major innovation in production practices first. Further, though ruminants convert ~2.7 billion metric tons of grass dry matter, of which 65% grows on land unsuitable for crops (34), into human-edible protein each year, the environmental impacts of this conversion are immense under any production method practiced today.

"Using GHG emissions (Fig. 3), we identified five primarily biophysical reasons for these results. These reasons suggest that the differences between animal and vegetable proteins will hold into the future unless major technological changes disproportionately target animal products. First, emissions from feed production typically exceed emissions of vegetable protein farming. This is because feed– to–edible protein conversion ratios are greater than 2 for most animals (13, 34); because high usage of low-impact by-products is typically offset by low digestibility and growth; and because additional transport is required to take feed to livestock. Second, we find that deforestation for agriculture is dominated (67%) by feed, particularly soy, maize, and pasture, resulting in losses of above- and belowground carbon.

Improved pasture management can temporarily sequester carbon (25), but it reduces life-cycle ruminant emissions by a maximum of 22%, with greater sequestration requiring more land. Third, animals create additional emissions from enteric fermentation, manure, and aquaculture ponds. For these emissions alone, 10th-percentile values are 0.4 to 15 kg of CO2eq per 100 g of protein. Fourth, emissions from processing, particularly emissions from slaughterhouse effluent, add a further 0.3 to 1.1 kg of CO2eq, which is greater than processing emissions for most other products. Last, wastage is high for fresh animal products, which are prone to spoilage."

The statistics that pop out from this part of the study are that meat, aquaculture, eggs, and dairy use ~83% of the world's farmland but provide only 37% of our protein and 18% of our calories. This disparity between high inputs and low outputs for animal foods is largely due to the high percentage of arable land devoted to feed crops and the low conversion rate of feed crops into edible animal foods. Feed crops were also found to be responsible for 67% of global deforestation. This study further confirms earlier studies that found animal agriculture and processing emit many times more GHGs than equivalent calorie and protein plant substitutes.

Here, the authors quantify how consumers adopting a plant-based diet could mitigate the environmental impacts of animal agriculture:

"Mitigation through consumers

"Today, and probably into the future, dietary change can deliver environmental benefits on a scale not achievable by producers. Moving from current diets to a diet that excludes animal products (table S13) (35) has transformative potential, reducing food's land use by 3.1 (2.8 to 3.3) billion ha (a 76% reduction), including a 19% reduction in arable land; food's GHG emissions by 6.6 (5.5 to 7.4) billion metric tons of CO2eq (a 49% reduction); acidification by 50% (45 to 54%); eutrophication by 49% (37 to 56%); and scarcity-weighted freshwater withdrawals by 19% (−5 to 32%) for a 2010 reference year. The ranges are based on producing new vegetable proteins with impacts between the 10th and 90th-percentile impacts of existing production. In addition to the reduction in food's annual GHG emissions, the land no longer required for food production could remove ~8.1 billion metric tons of CO2 from the atmosphere each year over 100 years as natural vegetation reestablishes and soil carbon re-accumulates, based on simulations conducted in the IMAGE integrated assessment model (17). For the United States, where per capita meat consumption is three times the global average, dietary change has the potential for a far greater effect on food's different emissions, reducing them by 61 to 73% [see supplementary text (17) for diet compositions and sensitivity analyses and fig. S14 for alternative scenarios]."

The statistics that pop out from this part of the study are that moving from current diets to a diet that excludes animal products has the potential to reduce food's land use by 76%, reduce food's GHG emissions by 49%, reduce ocean acidification by 50%, reduce fresh water eutrophication by 49%, and reduce scarcity-weighted freshwater withdrawals by 19%, relative to 2010 levels. These glaring statistics highlight the tremendous potential switching to a plant-based diet holds to mitigate the environmental impacts of animal agriculture.

"Reducing food's environmental impacts through producers and consumers," largely succeeded in its objective of consolidating huge data sets covering GHG emissions, agricultural production, and product life cycle assessments (LCAs), into a globally harmonized database on the variations of food's multiple environmental impacts. I do, however, have one major criticism of this report: it excludes any mention of the impacts on human health of an animal-based diet and the environmental impacts of treating those diseases. The damage to our environment of this pharmaceutically driven medical system is wreaking havoc on the endocrine systems of scores of animal species, especially aquatic animals.

"Food system impacts on biodiversity loss
Three levers for food system transformation in support of nature"(2021)

In February, 2021, the UK policy think tank, *Chatham House*, published the research paper, *"Food system impacts on biodiversity loss: Three levers for food system transformation in support of nature,"* that focused on the role of animal agriculture as the principal anthropogenic driver of mass species extinction.

The authors begin by identifying what they call the *"cheap food paradigm,"* as the main culprit in species extinction and biodiversity loss. Producing food cheaply is the primary objective of modern industrial agricultural by maximizing food production at the expense of natural habitat and ecosystems. As we have seen from studies cited above, industrial agriculture increases crop yields per acre by growing vast acreages of monocultures using enormous quantities of synthetic fertilizers and pesticides much of it to grow animal feed. This type of intensive industrial agriculture has fragmented ecosystems and resulted in accelerated biodiversity loss around the world.

To protect biodiversity from agricultural encroachment, the authors turn their attention to what they call *"Key levers for food system redesign,"* to make our food production and consumption systems more eco-friendly so humans and nature can coexist in harmony on this planet. Here the authors identify three key levers:

> *"The successful redesign of the food system in support of biodiversity and improved public health will depend on three key 'levers': **changing our diets; setting aside land for biodiversity; and adapting how we farm."* (**bold emphasis mine**)

As we shall see, setting land aside for biodiversity and adapting how we farm are both dependent on changing our diets.

The first key lever – changing our diets – identifies animal-based diets as driving land use patterns that *accelerate biodiversity loss:*

"... *the environmental footprint of food – its associated land use, GHG emissions, water use and biodiversity impact – varies significantly from one product to the next.* **In general, the largest differences occur between animal-sourced and plant-sourced foods, with the latter having smaller footprints; in some cases, substantially smaller (see Figure 7).**66 **[D]emand for the most environmentally damaging foods is both high and rising, a trend partly associated with nutrition transitions that are increasing demand for animal products.**67*"* (bold emphasis mine)

The second key lever – setting aside land for biodiversity – is inextricably tied to people moving towards a plant-based diet:

"*[A]ccording to a growing body of academic literature, setting aside land for biodiversity to the exclusion of other uses, including farming, and either protecting or restoring natural habitat would offer the most benefit to biodiversity across a given landscape.*74

"*The value of preserving undisturbed habitats and ecosystems – both for the sake of biodiversity and to support natural carbon sequestration and storage – has underpinned many of the global efforts to preserve primary forest cover, particularly in the tropics.*"

"*The greatest gains for biodiversity will occur when we preserve or restore whole ecosystems. With some exceptions, this will typically require significant areas of land to be left or managed for nature, primarily because the extinction risk for any species grows as its population size shrinks, and because many large animals require a large area of habitat to sustain an adequate population.* **Human dietary shifts are thus essential in order to preserve existing native ecosystems and restore those that have been removed or degraded.**" (bold emphasis mine)

The third lever – adapting the way we farm the land – is also inextricably tied to moving towards a plant-based diet:

"*There are many specific ways in which agriculture can become more nature-friendly and support biodiversity (including through agro-ecological farming and regenerative farming,*79 *of which organic farming is an example)... While some approaches may increase agricultural productivity,*81 *in general nature-friendly farming is less productive than conventional methods. For example, on a like-for-like comparison, organic farms typically yield 34 per cent less than intensively managed farms.*82

Even if farm-level incomes can be maintained via appealing to premium [organic] markets, **dietary change is still a necessary global enabler to allow widespread adoption of nature-friendly farming without increasing the pressure to convert natural land.**83 *(*bold emphasis mine*)*

There can be no mistaking the authors' message here: animal agriculture is the leading cause of biodiversity loss around the world, and the only practical way to mitigate these losses is the widespread adoption of a plant-based diet.

The authors end with a *"Technical annex"* that goes into great detail on specific biodiversity issues related to animal agriculture, such as:

"Loss of large herbivores through grazing of farmed animals

"Incentives to increase agricultural productivity and farm incomes in preference to preserving wildlife habitats are not limited to highly intensive agricultural systems. **Land degradation caused by overgrazing from extensively farmed herbivores is particularly acute in some countries, as illustrated in the example in Box 6 on pastoralist/grazer/wildlife conflict in Botswana."** (**bold emphasis mine***)*

"Box 6. *Pastoralist/grazer/wildlife conflict in Botswana*

*Conservation of African wildlife is often dependent on the interaction between conservation areas and adjacent pastoral areas. With human population densities, the size and number of settlements, and grazing pressure of farmed animals in communally managed pastoral areas all increasing, there is the potential for grazing land to become degraded, putting pressure on conservation areas. A study in the Kalahari Desert in 2019 looked at the interactions between farmed animals and wildlife.*140 **The study showed that while pastoral activities were largely confined to communally** *managed grazing areas within about 15 km of the main settlements, the free-ranging farmed animals reduced forage quality and quantity in wet and dry seasons. Large wild herbivores and carnivores avoided the communally managed grazing areas. Medium-sized wild herbivores and carnivores avoided areas of high grazing intensity, but used moderately grazed areas outside the conservation areas. Small wild herbivores, except springbok, foraged across the communally managed grazing areas. These results suggest that, even though pastoral lands near conservation areas are important as seasonal dispersal and breeding grounds for wildlife, intensified pastoral activities (such as increased intensity of farmed animal grazing) and pastoralist-induced risk are restricting the seasonal movements of medium-sized to large wildlife between the conservation areas and the adjacent communal grazing areas."*

It is always important to keep in mind that grazing livestock compete with native wildlife for food. Here, the authors quantify the land use savings of a plant-based diet in the U.S.:

*"Changing diets and reducing waste have greater potential to reduce environmental footprints and pressure on land than do supply-side interventions.*209 *For example, substituting beans for beef in the US diet could free up an area of 692,918 km2 – equivalent to 42 per cent of US cropland – which could then potentially be used for ecological purposes.*210 *Furthermore, one aspect of demand-side change likely to be helpful to biodiversity would be to shift towards*

healthier diets, rich in fruit and vegetables, and away from ultra-processed diets dependent on calorie-dense crops and animal products. A greater range of crops, coupled with reduced demand for animal products, would potentially allow for more diverse and regenerative farming landscapes to be maintained. Such landscapes would not only reduce nutrient leakage but would also, owing to greater spatial heterogeneity, support greater biodiversity." [211]

One relevant aspect of animal agriculture that received not a single mention in the *Chatham House* report was the immense suffering of the billions of sentient animals raised for food as well as the suffering of the wild animals they displace. Instead, the authors chose to stick strictly to quantifiable facts reported by the world's leading biological scientists. By checking their emotions at the door and only presenting objective evidence, the authors of this paper have demonstrated their commitment to objectivity that lends credence to their report.

The research paper, *"Food system impacts on biodiversity loss: Three levers for food system transformation in support of nature,"* is the most comprehensive study to date on the impacts of the human diet on the biodiversity loss that is leading to the sixth great mass extinction event in the 3.7 billion years since life began on Earth. Just as with mitigating climate change, the most effective mitigation for biodiversity loss is the worldwide adoption of a plant-based diet.

Each of the above six studies and reports received some mainstream media coverage upon publication, but as of the publication of *"Food system impacts on biodiversity loss"* in 2021, the world's major media outlets, national governments, and international health agencies have made little effort to encourage people to adopt a healthy and environmentally sustainable plant-based diet. If anything, these three influential social institutions have propped-up the myth that animal foods are part of a "healthy" diet, while governments have subsidized the production of animal products and socialized the environmental costs of production. As noted in the reports above, the consequence of this willful neglect and overt complicity has been that demand for animal foods is on the rise in many less developed countries around the world. Meanwhile, the clock keeps ticking with less than 30 years till 2050, when these modeled dietary scenarios play out.

The message from the six reports and studies by independent scientists reviewed above could not be clearer: to stave off extreme climate change and the sixth great mass extinction on Earth, we humans must return to our natural herbivorous roots.

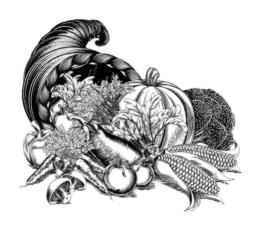

PART VII

A DIET FOR THE 21ST CENTURY

• • •

"Teaching kids how to feed themselves and how to live in a community
responsibly is the center of an education."

– Alice Waters, chef, restaurateur (born 1944)

22
THE OPTIMAL HUMAN DIET

Lions, wolves and zebras all still eat the same basic diets today they evolved to eat in the wild over millions of years, so it is easy to determine the optimal diet for these species. But because the modern human diet bears no resemblance to the natural herbivorous diet we evolved to eat, the optimal human diet is not so easy to discern. The human diet began to change around two million years ago when our earliest fruit eating ancestors came down out of tropical forests and began to cook and eat tubers that they dug-up on the open savanna. From around 60,000 years ago to around 10,000 years ago, as small bands of hunter/gatherers migrated into colder northern climates, meat became a more significant food source in the human diet. With the invention of agriculture in just the past 10,000 years, cultivated grains and tubers became staple foods which caused an explosion in the global human population. And in just the last 100 years, with the rise of the global animal industrial complex, the diet of billions of people now includes meat, dairy or eggs with virtually every meal.

With the possible exception of promotional flacks for the global food corporations, I know of no serious person who would argue that the modern Western diet of animal and processed foods is the optimal human diet. But this only begs the question: what is the optimal human diet? I am aware of no person better qualified to answer this questions than Dr. Michael Greger, MD. Dr. Greger is a physician who specializes in clinical nutrition, food safety, and public health issues, is a founding member and Fellow of the *American College of Lifestyle Medicine,* is founder of the website, *NutritionFacts.org,* which carefully reviews and places into scientific context the thousands of nutritional studies published in professional medical journals each year, and is author of the most authoritative book on the human diet written to date, titled *"How Not To Die."*

In *"How not to die,"* Dr. Greger explains the dietary causes of the top 15 causes of death in the U.S., the world's top animal and processed food consuming country. They are in order:

1. Coronary artery disease
2. Lung diseases (lung cancer, COPD, and asthma)
3. Iatrogenic causes (diseases induced inadvertently by a physician or surgeon or by medical treatment or diagnostic procedures
4. Brain diseases (stroke an Alzheimers)
5. Digestive cancers (colorectal, pancreatic, and esophagael)
6. Infections (respiratory and blood)
7. Diabetes
8. High blood pressure
9. Liver disease (cirrhosis and cancer)

10. Blood cancers (leukemia, lymphoma, and myeloma)

11. Kidney diseases

12. Breast cancer

13. Suicide

14. Prostate cancer

15. Parkinson's disease

In this passage, Dr. Greger explains the efficacy of a whole-food, plant-based diet to prevent and treat these diseases:

"Certainly there are prescription medications that can help with some of these conditions. For example, you can take statin drugs for your cholesterol to lower you risk of heart attack, pop different pills and inject insulin for diabetes, and take a slew of diuretics and other blood pressure medications for hypertension. But there is only one unifying diet that may help prevent, arrest, or even reverse each of these killers. Unlike with medications, there isn't one kind of diet for optimal liver function and a different diet to improve our kidneys. A heart-healthy diet is a brain-healthy diet is a lung-healthy diet. The same diet that helps prevent cancer just so happens to be the same diet that may help prevent type 2 diabetes and every other cause of death on the top-fifteen list. Unlike drugs – which only target specific functions, can have dangerous side effects, and may only treat the symptoms of disease – a healthy diet can benefit all organ systems at once, has good side effects, and may treat the underlying causes of illness.

"The one unifying diet found to best prevent and treat many of these chronic diseases is a whole-food, plant-based diet, defined as an eating pattern that encourages the consumption of unrefined plant foods and discourages meats, dairy products, eggs and processed foods. In this book, I don't advocate for a vegetarian diet or a vegan diet. I advocate for an evidence-based diet, and the best available balance of science suggests that the more whole plant foods we eat, the better – both to reap the nutritional benefits and to displace less healthful options." ("How Not To Die," pgs 9 - 10)

So what does a whole-food, plant-based diet look like? With Dr. Greger's encyclopedic knowledge of nutritional science, he created what he calls the *"Daily Dozen,"* that is, the eleven foods plus exercise that people should try to include in their regimen every day. Here, Dr. Greger explains the genesis of the *Daily Dozen*:

"The more I've researched over the years, the more I've come to realize that healthy foods are not necessarily interchangeable. Some foods and food groups have special nutrients not found in abundance elsewhere. For example, sulforaphane, the amazing liver-enzyme detox-boosting compound I profiled in chapters 9 and 11, is derived nearly exclusively from cruciferous vegetables. You could eat tons of other kinds of greens and vegetables on a given day and get

no appreciable sulforaphane if you don't eat something cruciferous. It's the same with flaxseeds and the anticancer lignan compounds. As I mentioned in chapters 11 and 13, flax may average one hundred times more lignans than other foods. And mushrooms aren't even plants at all; they may belong to an entirely different biological classification and may contain nutrients (like ergothioneine) not made anywhere in the plant kingdom. (So technically, maybe I should be referring to a whole-food, plant – and fungus-based diet, but that just sounds kind of gross.)

"It seems like every time I come home from the medical library buzzing with some exciting new data, my family rolls their eyes, sighs, and asks, 'What can't we eat now?' Or they'll say, 'Wait a second. Why does everything seem to have parsley in it all of a sudden?' My poor family. They've been very tolerant.

"As the list of foods I tried to fit into my daily diet grew, I made a checklist and had it on a dry-erase board on the fridge. We would make a game of ticking off the boxes. This evolved into the Daily Dozen (see figure 6).

"Daily Dozen

No. of servings	
XXX	Beans
X	Berries
XXX	Other Fruits
X	Cruciferous Vegetables
XX	Greens
XX	Other Vegetables
X	Flaxseed
X	Nuts
X	Spices
XXX	Whole Grains
XXXXX	Beverages
X	Exercise

Figure 6"

In the passages below that I gleaned from Dr. Greger's website, *NutritionFacts.org*, he explains how each whole plant food component of the *Daily Dozen* is an integral part of the optimal human diet:

Beans

"The most comprehensive analysis of diet and cancer ever performed was published by the American Institute for Cancer Research. Sifting through some half a million studies, nine independent research teams from around the globe created a landmark scientific consensus report reviewed by 21 of the top cancer researchers in the world. One of their summary cancer-prevention recommendations is to eat whole grains and/or <u>legumes</u> (beans, split peas, chickpeas, or lentils) with every meal. Not every week or every day. Every meal.

"The [U.S.] federal government's MyPlate campaign was developed to prompt Americans to think about building healthy meals. Most of your plate should be covered with <u>vegetables</u> and <u>grains</u>, preferably whole grains, with the rest of the plate split between <u>fruits</u> and the protein group. Legumes were given special treatment, straddling both the protein and the vegetable groups. They're loaded with protein, iron, and zinc, as you might expect from other protein sources like meat, but legumes also contain nutrients that are concentrated in the vegetable kingdom, including <u>fiber</u>, <u>folate</u>, and <u>potassium</u>. You get the best of both worlds with beans, all the while enjoying foods that are naturally low in saturated fat and sodium and free of <u>cholesterol</u>.

"Legumes comprise all the different kinds of beans, including soybeans, split peas, chickpeas, and lentils. While eating a bowl of pea soup or dipping carrots into hummus may not seem like eating beans, it is. We should all try to get three servings a day. A serving is defined as a quarter cup of hummus or bean dip; a half cup of cooked beans, split peas, lentils, tofu, or tempeh; or a full cup of fresh peas or sprouted lentils.

"Legume consumption is associated with a slimmer waist and lower blood pressure, and randomized trials have shown it may match or beat out calorie cutting for slimming tummy fat as well as improving the regulation of blood sugar, insulin levels, and cholesterol. Beans are packed with fiber, folate, and phytates, which may help reduce the risk of <u>stroke</u>, <u>depression</u>, and <u>colon cancer</u>. The phytoestrogens in <u>soy</u> in particular appear to both help prevent <u>breast cancer</u> and improve breast cancer survival. No wonder the cancer guidelines suggest you should try to fit beans into your meals—and it's so easy! They can be added to nearly any meal, easily incorporated into snack times, or served as the star attraction. The possibilities are endless." (https://nutritionfacts.org/topics/beans/)

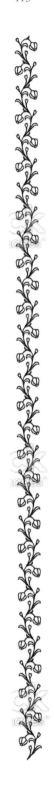

Berries

"I recommend one daily serving of berries (half cup fresh or frozen, or a quarter cup dried) and three daily servings of other fruit (a medium-sized fruit, a cup cut-up fruit, or a quarter cup dried). Why do I single out berries?

"Berries are the healthiest <u>fruits</u>—*due in part to their plant pigments. They evolved to have bright, contrasting colors to attract fruit-eating critters to help disperse their seeds, and the same molecular characteristics that give berries such vibrant colors may account for some of their* <u>antioxidant</u> *abilities. Berries are second only to herbs and spices as the most antioxidant-packed food category. As a group, they average nearly 10 times more antioxidants than other fruits and vegetables, and exceed 50 times more than* <u>animal-based foods</u>.

"Berries offer potential protection against <u>cancer</u>, *a boost to the immune system, and a guard for the liver and brain. An American Cancer Society study of nearly 100,000 men and women found that those who ate the most appeared significantly less likely to die of* <u>cardiovascular disease</u>. *Indeed, for disease prevention, berries of all colors have "emerged as champions," according to the head of the Bioactive Botanical Research Laboratory. The purported anticancer properties of berry compounds have been attributed to their apparent ability to counteract, reduce, and repair damage resulting from oxidative stress and inflammation. They may also boost our levels of natural killer cells, a type of white blood cell that's a vital member of the immune system's rapid-response team against virus-infected and cancerous cells.*

"Special antioxidant pigments in berries and <u>dark-green leafies</u> *may make them the brain foods of the fruit and vegetable kingdom. Harvard University researchers, using data from the Nurses' Health Study, which followed the diets and health of 16,000 women, found that women who consumed at least one serving of* <u>blueberries</u> *and two servings of* <u>strawberries</u> *each week had slower rates of cognitive decline by as much as two and a half years compared with those who didn't eat any. These results suggest that simply eating a handful of berries every day may slow our brain's aging by more than two years." (https://nutritionfacts.org/topics/berries/)*

Other Fruits

"It took years for nearly 500 researchers from more than 300 institutions in 50 countries to develop the 2010 Global Burden of Disease Study, the largest analysis of risk factors for death and disease in history. In the United States, the massive study determined that the leading cause of both death and disability was the American diet, followed by smoking. What did they find to be the worst aspect about our diet? Not eating enough fruit." (https://nutritionfacts.org/topics/fruit/)

Cruciferous Vegetables

"*The more commonly known cruciferous vegetables include broccoli, cauliflower, and kale, but there are many others in this family, such as collard greens, watercress, bok choy, kohlrabi, rutabaga, turnips, arugula, radishes (including horseradish), wasabi, and all types of cabbage.*

"*Cruciferous vegetables can potentially prevent <u>DNA damage</u> and metastatic cancer spread, activate defenses against pathogens and pollutants, help to prevent lymphoma, boost your liver detox enzymes, target breast cancer stem cells, and reduce the risk of prostate cancer progression. The component responsible for these benefits is thought to be sulforaphane, which is formed almost exclusively in cruciferous vegetables.*

"*Beyond being a promising anticancer agent, <u>sulforaphane</u> may also help protect your brain and your eyesight, reduce nasal allergy inflammation, manage type 2 diabetes, and was recently found to successfully help treat autism. A placebo-controlled, double-blind, randomized trial of boys with autism found that about two to three cruciferous vegetable servings' worth of sulforaphane a day improves social interaction, abnormal behavior, and verbal communication within a matter of weeks. The researchers, primarily from Harvard University and Johns Hopkins University, suggest that the effect might be due to sulforaphane's role as a "detoxicant."*

"*For all these reasons, cruciferous vegetables get their own spot on my <u>Daily Dozen</u>, which recommends at least one serving of cruciferous vegetables and at least two additional servings of other vegetables a day, cruciferous or otherwise.*

"*Indeed, if you were to add only one thing to your diet, consider cruciferous vegetables. Less than a single serving a day of broccoli, brussels sprouts, cabbage, cauliflower, or kale may cut the risk of cancer progression by more than half.*" (<u>https://nutritionfacts.org/topics/cruciferous-vegetables/</u>)

Greens

"*People may have <u>gained health benefits from wild greens</u> as long as <u>200,000 years ago</u>. Today, greens are considered one of the <u>healthiest vegetables</u>, and they're <u>inexpensive</u>. <u>Organic greens may be healthier</u> than non-organic greens due to their <u>defensive response to getting bitten by bugs</u>.*

"*The <u>calcium</u> in dark green leafy vegetables is <u>more effectively absorbed by the body</u> than that found in cow's <u>milk</u>. <u>Potassium</u> from greens may be <u>anti-inflammatory</u> and may <u>prevent strokes and heart disease</u>. Greens can also provide <u>iron and zinc</u>, <u>antioxidants</u>, and <u>magnesium</u>, a nutrient that may <u>lower the risk of a range of health concerns</u> including* *diabetes,* heart disease, *and* sudden cardiac death. *Green leafy vegetables are the* best source of plant-based nitrates. *Nitrates from a* plant-based *diet are* not considered harmful. *In fact, nitric oxide formed from plant-based nitrate may* play a role in the prevention of heart disease and high blood pressure. *Eating* whole plant foods *is likely better for your health than taking* supplements. *For example,* folate, which can reduce the risk of depression, *in greens appears* preferable to folic acid supplements. *Many nutrients found in greens are* fat *soluble, which means including some healthy whole food fats like* nuts *or* seeds, *in a meal can help you better* absorb the phytonutrients. Plant-based diets, *including greens, tend to be* alkaline-forming, *which may help protect muscle mass and reduce the risk of* gout *and* kidney stones. *High consumption in particular of* green leafy and cruciferous vegetables *may be linked to* lower rates of cognitive decline. *Greens can be an important part of a plant-based diet that could reduce risk for* cardiac disease *and* heart attack. *Some nutrients are destroyed by* cooking, *but some nutrients become more absorbable. So, a mix of* cooked and raw *vegetables, including greens, may be best.* Smoothies *may also be a* great source to get all of the nutrients *greens have to offer. Although make sure to* drink whole food smoothies *(not made from juice), and it may be better to use a straw to prevent enamel erosion.*

"Consuming at least one serving a month of greens appears to reduce the risk of glaucoma by 69%. *Lutein and* zeaxanthin, *nutrients found greens, also* appear to be protective against cataracts and macular degeneration. *Greens consumption is also associated with increased* physical attractiveness, reduced facial wrinkling, *improved* dental health, *better* immune system, *and may reduce* free radical DNA damage.

"Two or more daily servings of greens may help clear the human papilloma virus, *which can cause* cancer. Eating green leafy vegetables *may also reduce risk for* breast cancer, kidney cancer, *and* lymphoma, *and* overall cancer risk. *Adding mustard powder o cooked greens can boost* sulforaphane levels to help protect against cancer." *(https://nutritionfacts.org/topics/greens/)*

Other Vegetables

"The mammoth Global Burden of Disease Study identified the typical American diet as the primary cause of Americans' death and disability, and inadequate intake of vegetables as our fifth-leading dietary risk factor, nearly as bad as our consumption of processed meat.

"Indeed, a more plant-based diet *may help prevent, treat, or reverse some of our leading causes of death, including heart disease, type 2 diabetes, and high blood pressure, and may improve not only body weight, blood sugar levels, and ability to control cholesterol, but also*

our emotional states, including depression, anxiety, fatigue, sense of well-being, and daily functioning." (https://nutritionfacts.org/topics/vegetables/)

Flaxseed

"Flax seeds, known as one of the richest sources of essential <u>omega-3 fatty acids</u> *and having around one hundred times more cancer-fighting lignans than other foods, have also been demonstrated to prove helpful against* <u>breast</u> *and* <u>prostate cancers</u>*; controlling* <u>cholesterol</u>*, triglyceride, and blood sugar levels; reducing* <u>inflammation</u>*; and successfully treating constipation.*

"You can imagine how my skeptic red flag was raised by a review published in a medical journal titled 'Flaxseed: A Miraculous Defense Against Some Critical Maladies.' 'Miraculous'? Really? Well, a remarkable intervention trial published in the journal Hypertension suggests that, in this case, the term 'miraculous' may not be too far off.

"Researchers designed a prospective, double-blind, placebo-controlled, randomized trial so they could randomize subjects into two groups and secretly introduce tablespoons of ground flax seeds every day into the diets of half the participants to see if it made any difference. After six months, those who ate the placebo foods started out hypertensive and stayed hypertensive, despite the fact that many of them were on a variety of <u>blood pressure</u> *pills. What about the hypertensives who were unknowingly eating flax seeds every day? Their blood pressure dropped from 158/82 down to 143/75. A seven-point drop in diastolic blood pressure may not sound like a lot, but that would be expected to result in 46 percent fewer* <u>strokes</u> *and 29 percent less* <u>heart disease</u> *over time.*

"How does that result compare with taking drugs? The flax seeds managed to drop subjects' systolic and diastolic blood pressure by up to fifteen and seven points, respectively. Compare that result to the effect of powerful antihypertensive drugs, such as calcium-channel blockers (for example, Norvasc, Cardizem, Procardia), which have been found to reduce blood pressure by only eight and three points, respectively, or to ACE inhibitors (such as Vasotec, Lotensin, Zestril, Altace), which drop patients' blood pressure by only five and two points, respectively. Ground flaxseed may work two to three times better than these medicines, and they have only good side effects.

"'Miraculous'? Well, certainly super healthy, which is why a tablespoon of ground flaxseed every day gets its own spot on the Daily Dozen checklist I created to help inspire you to incorporate some of the healthiest foods into your daily routine." (https://nutritionfacts.org/topics/flax-seeds/)

Nuts

"The Global Burden of Disease Study, the most comprehensive and systematic analysis of the causes of death ever undertaken, involved nearly 500 researchers from more than 300 institutions in 50 countries and examined nearly 100,000 data sources. The study noted which foods, if added to the diet, might save lives. Eating more <u>vegetables</u> *could potentially save 1.8 million lives. How about more nuts and* <u>seeds</u>*? 2.5 million lives. The study calculated that not eating enough nuts and seeds was the third-leading dietary risk factor for death and disability in the world, killing more people than processed meat consumption, and potentially leading to the deaths of 15 times more people than all those who die from overdoses of heroin, crack cocaine, and all other illicit drugs combined.*

"<u>PREDIMED</u>*, one of the largest interventional dietary trials, randomized more than 7,000 men and women at high cardiovascular risk into different diet groups and followed them for years. One group received a free half-pound of nuts every week—the equivalent of eating about an extra half-ounce of nuts daily compared to what they had been consuming before the study even started. Without making major shifts in their diet, just the minor tweak of adding nuts appeared to cut stroke risk in half. Additionally, regardless of which group subjects had been assigned, those eating more nuts each day had a significantly lower risk of dying prematurely overall.*

Which nut is healthiest? Normally, my answer is whichever you'll eat regularly, but <u>walnuts</u> *really do seem to take the lead. They have among the highest* <u>antioxidant</u> *and* <u>omega-3</u> *levels, and beat out other nuts in vitro in terms of suppressing cancer cell growth.*

"One study found that a single serving of <u>Brazil nuts</u> *has been shown to lower your* <u>cholesterol</u> *levels faster than statin drugs and keep them down even a month after that single meal, and by eating three to four handfuls of pistachios a day for three weeks, men in one study reported significant improvement in blood flow through the penis, accompanied by significantly firmer erections.*

"Nuts are high in calories, but they can be a lifeline without expanding your waistline, as nut consumption has not been found to lead to the expected weight gain. They may also extend your lifeline: Your life span may be increased by two years by eating nuts regularly—one handful (or about a quarter of a cup) five or more days a week. Just that one simple and delicious act alone may extend your life." (<u>https://nutritionfacts.org/topics/nuts/</u>)

Spices

"Spices have been used in <u>medicine</u> *for thousands of years. Spices may provide multiple benefits to improve chronic health issues such as* <u>cancer</u>, <u>arthritis</u>, <u>Alzheimer's disease</u> *and even* <u>improve your overall mood</u>. *Today, researchers are discovering the ability of phytonutrients in spices such as* <u>ginger</u>, <u>rosemary</u>, <u>cilantro</u> *and* <u>turmeric</u> *to act as* <u>dietary restriction mimetics</u>, <u>multi-purpose drugs</u>, <u>chemopreventive agents</u> *and* <u>angiogenesis inhibitors</u>, *all which may help in the prevention and development of cancer. Saffron has been found to be just as effective in the treatment of Alzheimer's as the leading drug Aricept (see* <u>here</u>, <u>here</u>*).* <u>Black pepper</u> *has been found to be potentially protective against cancer and inflammation. Combining black pepper with turmeric boosts the bioavailability; this illustrates why* <u>diversity</u> *in the diet is very important.*

"Drinking <u>green tea</u> *every day may increase our lifespan. And* <u>chai tea</u> *has all the benefits of tea but also incorporates cloves and cinnamon, which makes it one of the healthiest beverages. The most antioxidant-packed food by weight is* <u>cloves</u> *(see also* <u>here</u>*).* <u>Cinnamon</u>, <u>oregano,</u> <u>lemonbalm, and majoram</u> *are also excellent sources of antioxidants (see also* <u>here</u>, <u>here</u>, <u>here</u>, <u>here</u>*). A yummy* <u>pumpkin pie</u> *is an excellent way to incorporate cloves and cinnamon into your diet. Cayenne pepper could help with* <u>Irritable Bowel Syndrome and Chronic Indigestion</u> *and may also help* <u>boost the fat burning properties</u> *of brown adipose tissue. Ginger* <u>may even help cure migraines</u>. *Spices may also replace common household supplements to aid in* <u>insomnia</u>, *improve* <u>muscle strength</u> *and even remove plaque better than typical* <u>mouthwash</u>.

"<u>Curcumin</u>, *the yellow pigment found in turmeric, has the greatest potential for acting as a* <u>multipurpose drug</u> *in* <u>treating</u> *and* <u>preventing</u> *Alzheimer's Disease, a* <u>variety of cancers</u> *such as* <u>skin cancer</u>, <u>pancreatic</u> *and* <u>colon cancer</u>, <u>osteoarthritis</u>, <u>MGUS and multiple myeloma</u>, *and for* <u>improving artery function</u> *(see also* <u>here</u>*).*

"However there is still a risk of toxicity and <u>side effects</u> *from over consuming spices such as* <u>turmeric</u>, <u>nutmeg</u> *and* <u>tarragon</u>.*" (*<u>https://nutritionfacts.org/topics/spices/</u>)

Whole Grains

"Consistent with recommendations from leading <u>cancer</u> *and* <u>heart disease</u> *authorities, my recommended* <u>Daily Dozen</u> *includes at least three servings of whole grains a day. Harvard University's preeminent twin nutrition studies—the Nurses' Health Study and the Health Professionals Follow-Up Study—have so far accumulated nearly three million person-years of data. A 2015 analysis found that people who eat more whole grains tend to live significantly longer lives independent of other measured dietary and lifestyle factors.*

"A diet rich in whole grains, for example, may yield the same benefits as taking <u>high blood pressure</u> *medications without the adverse side effects commonly associated with antihypertensive drugs, such as electrolyte disturbances in those taking diuretics; increased* <u>breast cancer</u> *risk for those taking calcium-channel blockers; lethargy and impotence for those on beta blockers; sudden, potentially life-threatening swelling for those taking ACE inhibitors; and an increased risk of serious fall injuries for apparently any class of these blood pressure drugs.*

"Indeed, eating whole grains appears to reduce the risk of heart disease, <u>type 2 diabetes</u>, <u>obesity</u>, *and* <u>stroke</u>. *Eating more whole grains could potentially save the lives of more than a million people around the world every year. Take note of the whole, however. While whole grains, such as oats, whole wheat, and brown rice, have been shown to reduce our risk of developing chronic disease, refined grains may actually increase risk.*

"People who ate the most whole grains had significantly slower narrowing of two of the most important arteries in our body: the coronary arteries that feed the heart and the carotid arteries that feed our brain. Since atherosclerotic plaque in the arteries is our leading killer, we should not just slow down the process but actually stop or even reverse it altogether, and eating more whole grains, whole vegetables, whole fruits, whole beans, and other whole plant foods can help with that." (<u>https://nutritionfacts.org/topics/grains/</u>)

Beverages

"The new <u>dietary guidelines</u> *and other studies on* <u>healthy beverages</u> *show that beverages can be a rich source of nutrients in the diet. In Asia, for example,* <u>green tea</u> *consumption may help explain comparatively low* <u>lung cancer</u> *and* <u>heart disease</u> *rates given the level of* <u>smoking</u>. *Green tea may also aid in* <u>stopping the malignant transformation of cultured breast cells</u> *and may even* <u>help prevent cavities</u>. *But, drinking too much green tea may pose the* <u>potential risk of dental fluorosis in children</u>. *Tea is a great* <u>low calorie source of nutrients</u> *that may also help* <u>modulate brain activity</u>. *Healthy herbal teas include* <u>tulsi</u>, <u>osmanthus</u>, <u>dandelion</u>, *and* <u>hibiscus</u>, *which may* <u>elevate antioxidant levels</u> *in the bloodstream within an hour, but some liquid supplements containing tropical fruit juices such as noni and mangosteen may be* <u>toxic to the liver</u>.

"<u>Cold water steeping</u> *of tea may lead to higher nutrient concentrations.* <u>Matcha tea</u> *(made from powdered tea leaves) is an excellent option. Avoid adding* <u>milk</u> *to tea to maximize nutrient absorption.* <u>10 cups</u> *of tea a day is probably the safe upper limit. Here are some other interesting comparisons:* <u>earl gray vs. black tea</u>, <u>green vs. white tea</u>, <u>coffee vs. tea</u>, *and* <u>bottled vs. tap water</u>.

"*Even light* <u>alcohol</u> *intake (up to a drink a day) is suspected to* <u>promote breast cancer</u>.

"*We may not be drinking enough fluids, evidenced by the fact that drinking* <u>water</u> *was found to* <u>boost children's' cognitive performance</u>. <u>Women should drink four to seven cups of water a day and men should drink six to eleven.</u>

"<u>Coffee</u> *has also been shown to be relatively* <u>health promoting</u>, *though there are* <u>concerns</u> *about its effect on coronary artery function, although it may help* <u>prevent liver cancer</u>. <u>Beet juice</u> *has been found to significantly* <u>Beet juice</u> *has been found to significantly* <u>improve athletic performance</u>. *Soymilk positively influences* <u>timing of puberty</u> *in girls and appears equal to cow's* <u>milk</u> *in terms of* <u>calcium absorption</u> *(as long as you shake it). Drinks to minimize include* <u>kombucha tea</u>, <u>yerba</u> <u>mate</u>, <u>noni juice</u>, <u>dairy</u>, *commercial* <u>carrot juice</u>, <u>artificially sweetened beverages</u>, *and* <u>soda</u>, *which may contain* <u>sodium benzoate</u> *and caramel coloring which* <u>may contribute to cancer</u> *risk. The media often bombards us with messages about what we should or shouldn't eat or drink so awareness of the* <u>source of funding</u> *and how it impacts the results of scientific findings is important.*

"*Smoothies may* <u>maximize nutrient absorption</u> *without risking* <u>overly rapid sugar absorption</u>. *As long as we drink them slowly, we* <u>don't risk weight gain</u>." *(*<u>https://nutritionfacts.org/topics/beverages/</u>*)*

Exercise

"*In addition to helping us enjoy a healthier body weight, exercise may also boost our* <u>immune system</u>. *Studies have found that if we let kids run around for just six minutes, the levels of immune cells circulating in their blood may increase by nearly 50 percent. At the other end of the life cycle, regular exercise may also help prevent age-related immune decline. One study found that while elderly, sedentary women have a 50 percent chance of getting an upper-respiratory illness during the fall season, those randomized to begin a half-hour-a-day walking program dropped their risk down to 20 percent.*

"*Physical activity is also considered a promising preventive measure against* <u>breast cancer</u>— *not only because it helps with weight control but because exercise tends to lower circulating estrogen levels. Five hours a week of vigorous aerobic exercise may lower estrogen and progesterone exposure by about 20 percent, and moderately intense activity may offer as much benefit as vigorous exercise; walking an hour a day or more appears to be associated with significantly lower breast cancer risk.*

"*Can exercise halt* <u>cognitive decline</u>? *Researchers took a group of people with mild cognitive impairment (for example, those starting to forget things or regularly repeating themselves) and had them engage in aerobic exercise for 45 to 60 minutes a day, 4 days a week, for 6 months.*

The control group simply stretched for the same time periods. Researchers found that in the control group, cognitive function appeared to continue to decline. But the exercising group not only didn't get worse, they seemed to get better, answering more test questions correctly after six months, indicating their memory *had improved. Indeed, aerobic exercise may actually reverse age-related shrinkage in the memory centers of the brain and help improve cerebral blood flow, improve memory performance, and help preserve brain tissue.*

"Exercise may also help prevent and treat high blood pressure, *and improve our* mood *and quality of* sleep. *If the U.S. population collectively exercised enough to shave just 1 percent off the national body mass index (BMI), 2 million cases of* diabetes, *1.5 million cases of* heart disease, *and up to 127,000 cases of* cancer *may be prevented.*

"I recommend 90 minutes of moderate-intensity activity, such as brisk (four miles per hour) walking or 40 minutes of vigorous activity (such as jogging or active sports) each day." (https:// nutritionfacts.org/topics/exercise/)

As Dr. Greger mentioned above, "the more whole plant foods we eat, the better – both to reap the nutritional benefits and to displace less healthful options." What this means is that it's not just what we eat that counts, it's also what we don't eat. There is a tendency for people to rationalize their meat and junk food habits by thinking that if they just eat some fruit and veggies, that will counteract the disease causing effects of the cholesterol, saturated fat and animal protein in animal foods. The reality is that the only way to truly immunize yourself against the chronic degenerative diseases of western culture is to kick the habit and to follow an optimal, high-fiber, whole-food, plant based diet.

The diet our herbivorous ancestors evolved to eat consisted entirely of wild plant species that had very different nutritional profiles than today's cultivated plants that Dr. Greger recommends in his Daily Dozen. But wild and cultivated plants are much more similar to each other than either is to meat, dairy or eggs. Most notably, wild and cultivated plants both contain health promoting complex carbohydrates, fiber, vitamin C, unsaturated fats and plant proteins, which are all virtually absent from animal foods. And disease causing cholesterol, saturated fats and animal proteins that are all virtually absent from plant foods are concentrated in animal foods. Cultivated plants still contain all the same phytochemical compounds as their wild plant derivatives; the same phytochemical compounds Dr. Greger identifies for their health promoting effects. The main difference between wild and cultivated plant foods is that wild plants tend to contain more fiber and less sugar than cultivated plants. But these differences do not mean that cultivated plants are less healthy than wild plants. It simply means that we modern humans do not have to spend all day eating in order to obtain enough food energy for our survival.

So, the answer to the question, "what is the optimal human diet?" is clear: a high-fiber, whole-food, plant-based diet. It is no coincidence this same diet that is optimal for human health is also optimal for restoring the health of our planet. If we humans were to assume our natural place in the trophic structure of the Earth's ecosystems, healthy people and a healthy planet is the predictable outcome.

Fiber and the Human Gut Microbiome

There are trillions of bacterial cells living within the human gut (small intestine and colon). In fact, there are many times more bacterial cells in our gut than there are human cells in our entire body. Only about 10% of the DNA in our body is actually human, most of the rest is in this community of bacteria in our gut called the "microbiome." How we digest our food is significantly influenced by the variety of bacteria that live in our gut microbiome as they metabolize, detoxify, and activate the nutrients in our diet.

There are around 1,000 different bacterial species that populate the human gut microbiome with an estimated 150 to 400 species residing in the gut of the average person, and each individual has their own unique bacterial assemblage. Until the second decade of the 21st century, however, the importance of the gut microbiome in regulating human health and disease was largely overlooked due to the inaccessibility of the intestinal habitat, the complexity of the microbiome itself and the fact that many of the bacterial species resist cultivation in a lab and were also new to science. This limited view of the gut microbiome began to rapidly change in the late 2000s with the introduction of rDNA genetic sequencing and high resolution imaging technologies for examining bacteria live in their natural habitat without the need to culture in a laboratory.

In 2011 and 2012 this new more advanced research lead to the publication of a series of studies in the journals *Science* and *Nature*, in which rDNA sequencing of bacteria taken from fecal samples of people living on different continents was compared to their individual food diaries (*"Linking Long-Term Dietary Patterns with Gut Microbial Enterotypes," Science*, Oct 2011) (*"Enterotypes of the human gut microbiome," Nature*, May 2011) (*"Human gut microbiome viewed across age and geography," Nature*, May 2012). The people surveyed included males and females of all ages and from rural and urban environments. Remarkably, these studies discovered that despite the uniqueness of each individual's gut microbiome, everyone they tested fit into one of two basic "enterotypes" (categories of microbiomes): those predominant in the "Bacteroides" species of bacteria, or those predominant in the "Prevotella" species of bacteria. The determining factor as to which enterotype people fit into was not their gender, age, race, body type or place of residence, it was their diet. Researchers looked at over 100 different food components and a pattern began to emerge: diets rich in animal protein and fat had a predominance of Bacteroides bacterial species with few Prevotella species, and diets rich in plant carbohydrates had a predominance of Prevotella bacterial species with few Bacteroides species.

The reason one or the other of these bacterial species predominates in our gut microbiome is because the food we eat is also the food they eat. What this means is that the bacteria that digest animal protein and fat proliferate in the gut of people who eat a largely animal-based diet, and the bacteria that digest carbohydrates proliferate in the gut of people who eat a largely plant-based diet. Since these two distinct enterotypes were first identified, the study of their long term health effects has been the focus of this rapidly advancing research on the human gut microbiome.

In the study, *"Diet, microbiota, and microbial metabolites in colon cancer risk in rural Africans and African Americans"* (*American Journal of Clinical Nutrition*, July, 2013), researchers measured differences in colonic bacteria and their metabolites between African Americans who have a high risk of colon cancer and rural native Africans who have a low risk. They found that rural Africans on a largely plant-based diet had a preponderance of Prevotella bacteria that metabolized plant fiber into the "short-chain fatty acid" called "butyrate," which is known to suppress and prevent colon cancer. Alternately, the African Americans consuming a largely animal-based diet had a preponderance of Bacteriodes bacteria that metabolized animal protein and fat into "secondary bile acids" which are a known carcinogen. The researchers concluded:

> *"Microbial composition was fundamentally different, with a predominance of Prevotella in native Africans (enterotype 2) and of Bacteroides in African Americans (enterotype 1). Total bacteria and major butyrate-producing groups were significantly more abundant in fecal samples from native Africans. Microbial genes encoding for secondary bile acid production were more abundant in African Americans, whereas those encoding for methanogenesis and hydrogen sulfide production were higher in native Africans. Fecal secondary bile acid concentrations were higher in African Americans, whereas short-chain fatty acids were higher in native Africans. Conclusion: Our results support the hypothesis that colon cancer risk is influenced by the balance between microbial production of health-promoting metabolites such as butyrate and potentially carcinogenic metabolites such as secondary bile acids."*

In the paper, *"Microbiota and diabetes: an evolving relationship"* (*Gut*, September, 2014), the authors reviewed studies on the association between gut bacteria and Type 2 diabetes. As with colon cancer, the studies reviewed found a connection between a deficiency in butyrate-producing bacteria and the incidence of Type 2 diabetes (T2D):

> *"First human metagenome-wide association studies demonstrated highly significant correlations of specific intestinal bacteria, certain bacterial genes and respective metabolic pathways with T2D. Importantly, especially butyrate-producing bacteria such as Roseburia intestinalis and Faecalibacterium prausnitzii concentrations were lower in T2D subjects. This supports the increasing evidence, that butyrate and other short-chain fatty acids are able to exert profound immunometabolic effects. Endotoxaemia, most likely gut-derived has also been observed in patients with metabolic syndrome and T2D and might play a key role in metabolic inflammation."*

In the study, *"Food, immunity, and the microbiome"* (*Gastroenterology*, May 2015), researchers found that the "short-chain fatty acids" metabolized from the abundant fiber in whole plant foods play an important role in our immune response:

> *"The microbiota and its metabolic machinery produce a myriad of metabolites that serve as important messengers between the diet, microbiota, and host. Short-chain fatty acids affect*

immune responses and epithelial integrity via G-protein-coupled receptors and epigenetic mechanisms. By increasing our understanding of interactions between diet, immunity, and the microbiota, we might develop food-based approaches to prevent or treat many diseases."

In the paper, *"The contributory role of gut microbiota in cardiovascular disease"* (*Journal of Clinical Investigation*, October 2014), the authors reviewed studies showing that the gut bacteria of people on an animal-based diet metabolized the nutrients "choline" and "L-carnitine" concentrated in meat and eggs into the chemical compound, "trimethylamine-N-oxide" (TMAO), which is a known risk factor for cardiovascular disease (CVD):

> *"Our group recently discovered that certain dietary nutrients possessing a trimethylamine (TMA) moiety, namely choline/phosphatidylcholine and L-carnitine, participate in the development of atherosclerotic heart disease. A meta-organismal pathway was elucidated involving gut microbiota-dependent formation of TMA and host hepatic flavin monooxygenase 3-dependent (FMO3-dependent) formation of TMA-N-oxide (TMAO), a metabolite shown to be both mechanistically linked to atherosclerosis and whose levels are strongly linked to cardiovascular disease (CVD) risks."*

In the paper, *"'The way to a man's heart is through his gut microbiota'--dietary pro- and prebiotics for the management of cardiovascular risk"* (*Proceedings of the Nutritional Society*, May 2014), the authors summarize studies showing that natural "probiotics" and "prebiotics" found in high fiber, whole-food, plant-based diets breed a gut microbiome that helps mitigate against the risk factors for cardiovascular disease (CVD):

> *"Diet, especially high intake of fermentable fibres and plant polyphenols, appears to regulate microbial activities within the gut, supporting regulatory guidelines encouraging increased consumption of whole-plant foods (fruit, vegetables and whole-grain cereals), and providing the scientific rationale for the design of efficacious prebiotics... Taken together such observations raise the intriguing possibility that gut microbiome modulation by whole-plant foods, probiotics and prebiotics may be at the base of healthy eating pyramids advised by regulatory agencies across the globe. In conclusion, dietary strategies which modulate the gut microbiota or their metabolic activities are emerging as efficacious tools for reducing CVD risk and indicate that indeed, the way to a healthy heart may be through a healthy gut microbiota."*

In the study, *"Strict vegetarian diet improves the risk factors associated with metabolic diseases by modulating gut microbiota and reducing intestinal inflammation"* (*Environmental Microbiology Reports*, October 2013), for one month researchers monitored the effects of a "strict vegetarian [vegan] diet" (SVD) on the microbiome of six obese subjects with Type 2 diabetes and/or hypertension, using blood biomarkers of glucose and lipid metabolisms and gene sequencing of faecal microbiota. They found that the vegan diet rapidly altered the ratio of bad bacteria (Bacteroides) to good bacteria (Prevotella) and improved all of their biomarkers for chronic diseases:

"This study underscores the benefits of dietary fibre for improving the risk factors of metabolic diseases and shows that increased fibre intake reduces gut inflammation by changing the gut microbiota."

Given what we already know about the health promoting properties of a whole-food, plant-based diet, the emerging picture of a healthy gut microbiome nourished on plant fiber is not the least bit surprising. Contrary to the popular belief that our Stone Age hunter-gatherer ancestors thrived by eating large quantities of meat, as modern promoters of the fad "paleo diet" would have you believe, for most of human existence, the staple food in their diet was highly fibrous wild plants. In the article, *"The "Paleo" Phenomena: Facing Facts"* (*Plant Based Health and Nutrition,* July 2015), by registered dietitian, award-winning and best-selling author, and former chair of the *Vegetarian Nutrition Dietetic Practice Group of the American Dietetic Association,* Brenda Davis, lays out the facts about the true Paleolithic diet:

*"Nutritional anthropologists have been estimating the nutrient intakes of cavemen for several decades. **As it turns out, vegan diets may actually come closer to matching the macro- and micronutrient intakes of Paleolithic diets than new paleo diets.***

"Table 1 (below) summarizes the results of a comparison among recommended paleo menus, recommended vegan menus, and a true Paleolithic diet eaten by early humans.

"The data compares three days of recommended paleo menus from a popular paleo website, three days of recommended vegan menus from Becoming Vegan: Comprehensive Edition, and the estimated average daily intakes of Paleolithic people. Table 1 also provides dietary reference intakes (DRIs) for adult males (M) and adult females (F) who aren't pregnant or lactating.

"The comparison shows that this recommended new paleo menu supplies protein, vitamin A, and zinc in amounts closer to a true Paleolithic diet than do the vegan menus. However, its fat and saturated fat levels are about double, cholesterol almost triple, and sodium five times as much as that of true Paleolithic diets. In addition, the new paleo menu contains about a third of the carbohydrates, and half the vitamin C, calcium, and fiber of true Paleolithic diets.

"Even the 100 percent plant-based vegan menus deliver fiber in amounts at the lowest end of the estimated Paleolithic intake range. Clearly, our preagricultural ancestors ate plenty of plants (the only source of fiber).

"The vegan menus do provide intakes of carbohydrate, fat, saturated fat, fiber, riboflavin, thiamin, vitamin C, vitamin E, iron, calcium, sodium, and potassium that are closer to the levels supplied by a true Paleolithic diet than do the new paleo menus." (**Bold emphasis mine.**)

Humans are one of the few mammals that must obtain vitamin C through our diet. This fact suggests that our evolutionary ancestors evolved to metabolize large quantities of plant fiber. Dr. Greger of NutritionFacts.org, explains how this unusual evolutionary adaptation probably occurred:

"[F]ruits and vegetables are not only just so good for us, but vital to our survival. We're actually one of the few species so adapted to a plant-based diet, that we could actually die from

not eating fruits and vegetables—from the vitamin C-deficiency disease, scurvy. Most other animals just make their own vitamin C. But why would our body waste all that effort when we evolved hanging out in the trees, just eating fruits and veggies all day long?

"It's presumably not a coincidence that the few other mammals unable to synthesize their own vitamin C (like guinea pigs, some bunny rabbits, and fruit bats) are all, like us great apes, strongly herbivorous. Even during the Stone Age, we may have been getting up to ten times more vitamin C than we get today. And ten times more dietary fiber, based on essentially rehydrated human fossilized feces."

All of the studies and papers cited above are but a small sample from the rapidly advancing field of nutritional research into fiber and the human gut microbiome; yet, in the 2020s, research on treating chronic degenerative diseases by changing our gut bacteria through a high fiber, whole-food, plant-based diet, has just barely begun.

Humans evolved from great apes, and more recently Paleolithic hunter-gatherers, who ate huge quantities of plant fiber, so it only stands to reason that our gut microbiome is well adapted to digest a high fiber, whole-food, plant-based diet.

Carbohydrates

Carbohydrates are biomolecules consisting of carbon, hydrogen and oxygen atoms that are primarily found in plant foods (although breast milk contains the simple carbohydrate, lactose). Carbohydrates come in different forms that include cellulose, starch and sugars.

Cellulose is the tough fibrous material found in the cell walls of all plants that allows them to hold erect their energy collecting solar arrays. The cellulose in plant foods is not digestible by humans, but this insoluble dietary fiber serves an important function in the digestive system by facilitating the slow and smooth transit of food through the intestines for maximum absorption of nutrients.

Starch consists of numerous glucose molecules bonded together and is the plants' primary source of stored energy. Starch is contained in large amounts in staple foods such as wheat, maize, potatoes and cassava; globally, it is the source of most of the food energy in the human diet.

Sugars are found in the tissues of most plants, but are particularly abundant in fruits, grains, sugar cane and sugar beets. Most of the sugar in the human diet is extracted from these plants and used in its refined form to sweeten processed foods. Refined sugars have no place in a healthy human diet.

As evidence mounted over recent decades that meat, dairy and eggs are the primary cause of the chronic degenerative diseases that plague Western cultures, an army of denialists was enlisted to defend these sacrosanct foods and to shift the blame for these diseases to anything else. From 1977 to 2010, added sugars consumed by American adults increased by more than 30% (from 228 calories/ day to 300 calories/ day) and added sugars consumed by children increased by approximately 20% (277 to 329 calories/ day), so sugar became the go to bogeyman for all our ills and sugar free diet books proliferated in the popular culture.

While it is certainly true that processed foods containing refined sugars are not healthy to eat, a blanket restriction of all sugars from the diet is not supported by nutritional science. When the sugar in fruit, fructose, is consumed in its whole food form, it not only does no harm, it actually has health benefits, as discussed here by Dr.Greger:

> *"There are a few popular diets out there that urge people to stop eating fruits because these natural sugars (fructose) are thought to contribute to weight gain. The truth is, only fructose from added sugars appears to be associated with declining liver function,9 high blood pressure, and weight gain.10 How could the fructose in sugar be bad but the same fructose in fruit be harmless? Think about the difference between a sugar cube and a sugar beet. (Beets are the primary source of sugar in the United States.11) In nature, fructose comes prepackaged with fiber, antioxidants, and phytonutrients that appear to nullify adverse fructose effects."*

> *"Consuming sugar in fruit form is not only harmless but actually helpful. Eating berries can blunt the insulin spike from high-glycemic foods like white bread, for example.15 This may be because the fiber in fruit has a gelling effect in your stomach and small intestine that slows the release of sugars16 or because of certain phytonutrients in fruit that appear to block the absorption of sugar through the gut wall and into your bloodstream.17 So eating fructose the way nature intended carries benefits rather than risks.*

> *"Low-dose fructose may actually benefit blood sugar control. Eating a piece of fruit with each meal could be expected to lower, rather than raise, the blood sugar response.18 What about people with type 2 diabetes? Diabetics randomized in a group restricted to no more than two daily pieces of fruit had no better blood sugar control than those randomized into a group told to eat a minimum of two pieces of fruit per day. The researchers concluded that 'the intake of fruit should not be restricted in patients with type 2 diabetes.'"19* (*How Not To Die*, pgs 290-291)

The demonization of sugar led others to conclude that all carbohydrates are bad and should be restricted in the diet while animal-based foods should be emphasized; this anti-carbohydrate bias spawned an entire industry of "low-carb" diet books. Of course, these low-carb dietary recommendations run completely contrary to the findings of nutritional science. Dr. T. Colin Campbell, Professor Emeritus of Nutritional Biochemistry at Cornell University, has been at the forefront of nutritional science for over 40 years and is one of the world's foremost authorities on human nutrition. In this passage from his groundbreaking book, *The China Study* (2006), Dr. Campbell clears up all this manufactured confusion about carbohydrates:

> *"An unfortunate outcome of the recent popularity of [low-carb] diet books is that people are more confused than ever about the health value of carbohydrates. As you will see in this book,*

there is a mountain of scientific evidence to show that the healthiest diet you can possibly consume is a high-carbohydrate diet. It has been shown to reverse heart disease, reverse diabetes, prevent a plethora of chronic diseases, and yes, it has been shown many times to cause significant weight loss. But it's not quite as simple as that.

At least 99% of the carbohydrates that we consume are derived from fruits, vegetables and grains. When these foods are consumed in the unprocessed, unrefined and natural state, a large proportion of the carbohydrates are in the so called 'complex' form. This means that they are broken down in a controlled, regulated manner during digestion. This category of carbohydrates includes the many forms of dietary fiber, almost all of which remain undigested – but still provide substantial health benefits. In addition, these complex carbohydrates from whole foods are packaged with generous amounts of vitamins, minerals and accessible energy. Fruits, vegetables and whole grains are the healthiest foods you can consume, and they are primarily made of carbohydrates.

On the opposite side of the spectrum, there are highly processed, highly refined carbohydrates that have been stripped of their fiber, vitamins and minerals. Typical simple carbohydrates are found in foods like white bread, processed snack items including crackers and chips made with white flour, sweets including pastries and candy bars and sugar-laden soft drinks. These highly refined carbohydrates originate from grains or sugar plants, like sugar cane or sugar beet. They are readily broken down during digestion to the simplest form of the carbohydrates, which are absorbed into the body to give blood sugar, or glucose.

Unfortunately, most Americans consume voluminous amounts of simple carbohydrates and paltry amounts of complex carbohydrates. For example, in 1996, 42% of Americans ate cakes, cookies, pastries or pies on any given day, while only 10% ate any dark green vegetables.46 In another ominous sign, only three vegetables accounted for half of the total vegetable servings in 1996,46: potatoes, which were mostly consumed as fries and chips; head lettuce, one of the least nutrient-dense vegetables, and canned tomatoes, which is probably only a reflection of pizza and pasta consumption. Add to that the fact that the average American consumed thirty-two teaspoons of added sugar per day in 1996,46 and it's clear that Americans are gorging almost exclusively on refined, simple carbohydrates, at the exclusion of healthful complex carbohydrates.

This is bad news, and this, in large measure, is why carbohydrates as a whole have gotten such a bad rap; the vast majority of carbohydrates consumed in America are found in junk food or grains so refined that they have to be supplemented with vitamins and minerals. On this point, the popular diet authors and I agree. For example, you could eat a low-fat, high-carbohydrate diet by exclusively eating the following foods: pasta made from refined flour, baked potato chips, soda, sugary cereals and low-fat candy bars. Eating this way is a bad idea. You will not derive the health benefits of a plant-based diet eating these foods, In experimental research, the health benefits of a high-carbohydrate diet come from eating the complex carbohydrates found in whole grains, fruits and vegetables. Eat an apple, a zucchini or a plate of brown rice topped with beans and other vegetables." (*The China Study*, Pgs 97-99)

Dr. Greger and Dr. Campbell are two of the most eminent nutritional scientists in the world today and their recommendations for a high-complex carbohydrate, whole-food, plant-based diet are based on the most advanced research on human nutrition to date. Take it from them, low-carb diets are health problems waiting to happen.

Fats

Fats are biomolecules consisting of carbon, hydrogen and oxygen atoms that come in different forms including "monounsaturated," "polyunsaturated," "saturated" and "trans fats." Fats are similar to carbohydrates in that they are both comprised of carbon, hydrogen and oxygen atoms, but fat molecules have a more compact structure and higher density than carbohydrates which translates into each fat molecule carrying more than twice the energy of a carbohydrate molecule as measured in calories (fat contains 9 calories/gram, carbohydrates contain 4 calories/gram).

Monounsaturated fats, found primarily in nuts, olives and avocados, and polyunsaturated fats found primarily in plant foods, serve many biological functions in our body including as a component of cell membranes, in the formation of hormones, for energy storage, in the absorption of fat-soluble vitamins A, D, E, and K, and to mediate our inflammatory response.

Saturated fat found primarily in animal foods (meat dairy and eggs), and trans fats found primarily in meat and partially hydrogenated vegetable oils, are not only unnecessary for healthy biological function, they are actually toxic to the human body.

Let's now take a closer look at these healthy and unhealthy fats.

Unsaturated Fats

Most naturally occurring unsaturated fats consist of carbon chains from 4 to 28 atoms long. These include:

- Short-chain fatty acids (SCFA) of five or fewer carbons
- Medium-chain fatty acids (MCFA) of 6 to 12 carbons
- Long-chain fatty acids (LCFA) of 13 to 21 carbons
- Very long-chain fatty acids (VLCFA) of 22 to 28 carbons

All of these fatty acids are necessary for healthy biological function, but only two of them that must be obtained through diet are considered essential, our liver can synthesize all the other fatty acids from other substances in sufficient quantities to maintain good health. The two essential fatty acids (EFAs) are linoleic acid (LA) and alpha-linolenic acid (ALA).

The chemical nomenclature for LA is 18:2ω6 meaning it has an 18 atom carbon chain with 2 double bonds and the first double bond is located between the sixth and seventh carbon atoms counting from the terminal end of the molecule, as denoted by ω (omega) which is the last letter in the Greek alphabet. LA is known as an ω6 fatty acid since its first double bonded carbon atoms appears between the sixth and seventh carbon atoms in the chain counting from the terminal end. LA, and its derivative arachidonic acid (AA), have pro-inflammatory properties.

The chemical nomenclature for ALA is 18:3ω3 meaning it has an 18 atom carbon chain with 3 double bonds and the first double bond is located between the third and fourth carbon atoms counting from the terminal end. ALA is known as an ω3 fatty acid since its first double bonded carbon atoms appear between the third and fourth carbon atoms in the chain counting from the terminal end. ALA and its ω3 derivatives, *e*icosapentaenoic acid (EPA) and *d*ocosahexaenoic acid (DHA*), have anti-inflammatory properties.*

LA and ALA mediate our body's inflammatory response to injury or infection. Our inflammatory response can result in varied outcomes including: resolution of the problem, or progression to chronic inflammation, scarring, and eventual loss of tissue function. When there is not enough of the anti-inflammatory ω3 fats in our cell membranes, a chronic state of inflammation can result that can lead to a range of chronic degenerative diseases including atherosclerosis, diabetes, cancers, brain wasting and autoimmune diseases.

Since the 1990s, essential fatty acids (EFAs) have been a hot topic in the field of nutritional research. Much of the study has focused on what is the best ratio of ω6 to ω3 fatty acids in the diet to achieve optimal health outcomes? Dr. Artemis Simopoulos, M.D., founder and President of the Center for Genetics, Nutrition and Health, evaluated the diets of our paleolithic ancestors for clues as to the natural ω6/ω3 ratio that humans evolved to eat. In his paper, "Evolutionary aspects of omega-3 fatty acids in the food supply," he expounded on his findings :

> *"Information from archaeological findings and studies from modern day hunter-gatherers suggest that the Paleolithic diet is the diet we evolved on and for which our genetic profile was programmed. The Paleolithic diet is characterized by lower fat and lower saturated fat intake than Western diets; a balanced intake of omega-6 and omega-3 essential fatty acids; small amounts of trans fatty acids [found in meat], contributing less than 2% of dietary energy; more green leafy vegetables and fruits providing higher levels of vitamin E and vitamin C and other antioxidants than today's diet and higher amounts of calcium and potassium but lower sodium intake. Studies on the traditional Greek diet (diet of Crete) indicate an omega-6/omega-3 ratio of about 1/1."* (Prostaglandins, Leukotrienes & Essential Fatty Acids, May-Jun 1999)

In his follow-up paper, *"The importance of the ratio of omega-6/omega-3 essential fatty acids"* (*Biomedicine & Pharmacotherapy*, October 2002), Dr. Simopoulos compares the natural ω6/ω3 ratio we humans evolved to eat with the ratio of the modern day Western diet:

> *"Several sources of information suggest that human beings evolved on a diet with a ratio of omega-6 to omega-3 essential fatty acids (EFA) of approximately 1 [1/1] whereas in Western diets the ratio is 15/1-16.7/1. Western diets are deficient in omega-3 fatty acids, and have excessive amounts of omega-6 fatty acids compared with the diet on which human beings evolved and their genetic patterns were established. Excessive amounts of omega-6 polyunsaturated fatty acids (PUFA) and a very high omega-6/omega-3 ratio, as is found in today's Western diets, promote the pathogenesis of many diseases, including cardiovascular disease, cancer, and inflammatory and autoimmune diseases, whereas increased levels of omega-3 PUFA (a low omega-6/omega-3 ratio) exert suppressive effects. In the secondary prevention of cardiovascular disease, a ratio of 4/1 was associated with a 70% decrease in total mortality. A ratio of 2.5/1 reduced rectal cell proliferation in patients with colorectal cancer, whereas a ratio of 4/1 with the same amount of omega-3 PUFA had no effect. The lower omega-6/omega-3 ratio in women with breast cancer was associated with decreased risk. A ratio of 2-3/1 suppressed inflammation in patients with rheumatoid arthritis, and a ratio of 5/1 had a beneficial effect on patients with asthma, whereas a ratio of 10/1 had adverse consequences. These studies indicate that the optimal ratio may vary with the disease under consideration. This is consistent with the fact that chronic diseases are multigenic and multifactorial. Therefore, it is quite possible that the therapeutic dose of omega-3 fatty acids will depend on the degree of severity of disease resulting from the genetic predisposition. A lower ratio of omega-6/omega-3 fatty acids is more desirable in reducing the risk of many of the chronic diseases of high prevalence in Western societies, as well as in the developing countries, that are being exported to the rest of the world."* (*Prostaglandins, Leukotrienes & Essential Fatty Acids*, May-Jun 1999)

As Dr. Simopoulos notes above, current study indicates that high ω6/ω3 ratios found in today's Western diets promote the pathogenesis of many diseases including cardiovascular disease, cancer, and inflammatory and autoimmune diseases, whereas low ω6/ω3 ratios exert suppressive effects on these degenerative diseases.

The modern Western food production system that concentrates on animal products and processed convenience foods is loaded with *ω6 and deficient in ω3 fatty acids. In this food culture, it is* hard to maintain a healthy ω6/ω3 ratio closer to 1/1. Terrestrial plants contain the ω3 fatty acid ALA which our liver converts into the ω3 fatty acid derivatives EPA and DHA that serve many important metabolic functions. But junk food vegans and vegetarians on a diet of processed convenience foods don't get enough ALA to synthesis into EPA and DHA, resulting in ω6/ω3 ratios around 20/1 rather than the 1/1 ratio of a whole-foods, plant-based vegan. Mortality studies have consistently shown that such junk food vegans receive none of the protective benefits against cancers and cardiovascular, inflammatory and autoimmune diseases that a whole-foods, plant-based vegan diet conveys.

People who eat fish regularly tend to have lower ω6/ω3 ratios than non-fish eaters since fish contain EPA and DHA they get from the algae which is at the bottom of the marine food chain. Junk food vegans and vegetarians and non-fisheating omnivores generally suffer from an ω3 deficiency and therefore should take an ω3 supplement containing preformed EPA and DHA. Adding EPA and DHA supplements to the diet has shown to be effective at improving the ω6/ω3 ratio and helping to relieve the symptoms of chronic inflammation. EPA and DHA supplements derived from fish oil are contaminated with the toxic chemicals from the polluted waters they live in, so to avoid exposure to these toxins it is recommended that EPA and DHA supplements derived directly from algae grown in pollution free tanks be taken instead, as noted here by the editors of *Nutritionfacts.org*:

> *"Thankfully, you can get the benefits without the risks by getting long-chain omega-3s from algae instead, which is where the fish primarily get it from to begin with. By getting EPA and DHA directly from the source at the bottom of the food chain, you don't have to worry about pollutant contamination. In fact, the algae used for supplements are just grown in tanks and never even come in contact with the ocean.*

People who eat a whole-food, plant-based vegan diet that includes ground flaxseed which is very high in the ω3 fat ALA, and who do not eat processed vegan junk foods, have an average ω6/ω3 ratio of around 1/1 which is the same ratio our Paleolithic ancestors had on a diet of wild plants, and for which we are genetically programmed. With an ω6/ω3 ratio of 1/1, our liver metabolizes plenty enough EPA and DHA from ALA to prevent chronic inflammation and to reduce our risk for chronic degenerative diseases. What this means is that whole-food, plant-based vegans who include daily ground flaxseed in their diet can probably get away without supplementation.

Over half the dry weight of the human brain is fat, and the ω3 derivatives EPA and DHA are particularly concentrated in the brain. Between the ages of 16 and 80, our brain loses about 1% of its volume every two to three years, such that by the time we are in our 70s, it has lost 26% of its size, and is smaller than when we were three years old. Also as we age, our ability to synthesize EPA and DHA from the ALA found in plant foods, declines.

In the epidemiological study, *"Red blood cell ω-3 fatty acid levels and markers of accelerated brain aging"* (*Neurology*, February 2012), researchers compared DHA blood levels to brain volumes in thousands of subjects and they found that lower DHA blood levels were associated with smaller brain volumes.

In the observational study, *"Higher RBC EPA + DHA corresponds with larger total brain and hippocampal volumes: WHIMS-MRI study"* (*Neurology*, February 2014), researchers found that over an eight year period, higher EPA and DHA levels correlated with larger brain volumes in the brains of 1,111 postmenopausal women.

Can supplementation with EPA and DHA slow down brain aging? The study, *"Long-chain omega-3 fatty acids improve brain function and structure in older adults"* (*Cerebral Cortex*, November, 2014), suggests yes. Researchers tested 65 healthy subjects 50-75 years old (35 males, 30 females) in an interventional study design to see whether higher levels of supplementary EPA and DHA would improve cognition. They concluded:

> *"This double-blind randomized interventional study provides first-time evidence that LC-n3-FA [long chain ω3 fatty acids EPA and DHA] exert positive effects on brain functions in healthy older adults, and elucidates underlying mechanisms. Our findings suggest novel strategies to maintain cognitive functions into old age."*

While the study of EPA and DHA on brain function is still in its infancy, there is already strong evidence that these ω3 derivatives are essential for the preservation of brain structure and function into old age.

Saturated Fat

Because Type 2 diabetes is a disease affecting sugar metabolism, it has long been assumed by the medical establishment and the lay public that the way to treat diabetes is to carefully regulate the ingestion of carbohydrates. But interventional dietary trials going back nearly 100 years have shown conclusively that Type 2 diabetes is actually a disease of fat metabolism.

In normal sugar metabolism, the pancreas produces the hormone "insulin" which ferries glucose from the bloodstream into our muscle cells to power our movement. In Type 2 diabetes, however, fat in the diet interferes with the insulin's ability to remove glucose from the bloodstream. This condition, known as "insulin resistance," can cause blood sugar levels to rise above 180 to 200 mg/dL which can lead to heart, nerve, kidney, and vision dysfunction, and over time, to coma and death. In 2020, the U.S. Center for Disease Control (CDC) estimated that **37.3 million** Americans suffered from Type 2 diabetes representing 11.3% of the U.S. population.

But not all dietary fats cause insulin resistance, as explained here by Dr. Greger:

> *"Not all fats affect our muscles in the same way. For example, palmitate, the kind of saturated fat found mostly in meat, dairy and eggs causes insulin resistance. On the other hand, oleate, the monounsaturated fat found mostly in nuts, olives and avocados, may actually protect against the detrimental effects of the saturated fat.38 Saturated fats can wreak all sorts of havoc in muscle cells and may result in the accumulation of more toxic breakdown products (such as ceramide and diacylglycerol)39 and free radicals and can cause inflammation and even mitochondrial dysfunction – that is, interference with the little power plants (mitochondria) within our cells.40 This phenomenon is known as lipotoxicity (lipo meaning fat, as in liposuction).41 If we take muscle biopsies from people, saturated fat buildup in the membranes of their muscle cells correlates with insulin*

resistance.47 Monounsaturated fats, however, are more likely to be detoxified by the body or safely stored away.43"

"… Those eating plant-based diets have been found to have better insulin sensitivity, better blood sugar levels, better insulin levels,45 and even significantly improved function of their beta cells – the cells in the pancreas that produce insulin in the first place.46

In other words, people eating plant-based diets appear to be better at both producing and using insulin." (*How Not To Die*, pgs 107-108)

That Type 2 diabetes is a disease of saturated fat intake associated with animal-based diets is no longer a matter of conjecture in nutritional science, yet you wouldn't know this fact by consulting the *American Diabetes Association* (ADA) website. According to the ADA, intake of carbohydrates (carbs) is what determines blood sugar levels:

"The main purpose of carbs in the diet is to provide energy as your body's main fuel source. The carbs plus the amount of insulin you have in your body determine your blood sugar levels and have a big impact on how you feel. Whether you're trying to lose weight or simply balance your blood sugar, carbs play a big role." https://www.diabetes.org/healthy-living/recipes-nutrition/meal-planning (4/8/2021)

The ADA advises Type 2 diabetics to follow their *"Diabetes Plate Method"* which recommends: *"To start out, you need a plate that is not too big. The size of our plate usually determines the size of our portions, so you want to start with a reasonably sized plate—we recommend about 9 inches across." "Fill half your plate with nonstarchy vegetables." "Fill one quarter of your plate with… [w]hole grains… [s]tarchy vegetables… [b]eans and legumes… [f]ruits and dried fruit… [and] [d]airy products…" "Fill one quarter of your plate with lean protein foods… foods high in protein such as fish, chicken, lean beef, soy products, and cheese…"* https://www.diabetesfoodhub.org/articles/what-is-the-diabetes-plate-method.html#:~:text=The%20Diabetes%20Plate%20Method%20is,you%20need%20is%20a%20plate*!*

Since this diet loaded with saturated animal fat does a poor job of controlling blood sugar levels in diabetes patients, much of the rest of the ADA website is devoted to treating the symptoms of diabetes with medications, insulin injections, and most importantly, by staying connected with the ADA for your diabetes management program.

Dr. Neal Barnard, MD, founder and president of the *Physicians' Committee for Responsible Medicine* (PCRM) and author of *"Dr. Neal Barnard's Program for Reversing Diabetes,"* takes a decidedly different approach to treating Type 2 diabetes with a high-carb plant-based diet:

"In our clinical research studies here at the Physicians Committee for Responsible Medicine, we've put a plant-based diet to the test with thousands of patients who have type 2 diabetes.

"In a 2003 study funded by the NIH, we determined that a plant-based diet controlled blood sugar three times more effectively than a traditional diabetes diet that limited calories and carbohydrates. Within weeks on a plant-based diet, participants saw dramatic health improvements. They lost weight, insulin sensitivity improved, and HbA1c levels dropped. In some cases, you would never know they'd had the disease to begin with." https://www.pcrm. org/health-topics/diabetes

In his study, *"A low-fat vegan diet elicits greater macronutrient changes, but is comparable in adherence and acceptability, compared with a more conventional diabetes diet among individuals with type 2 diabetes"* (*Journal of the American Dietetic Association*, February 2009), Dr. Barnard compared the adherence and acceptability of the *American Diabetes Association* diet versus a vegan diet among 99 Type 2 diabetes patients. He conducted a controlled trial between 2004 and 2006 with 50 participants randomly assigned to a diet following the 2003 *American Diabetes Association* guidelines, and 49 participants assigned to follow a low-fat, vegan diet for 74 weeks. At weeks 22 and 74 assessments were made of participants' attrition from the program, adherence to the diets, dietary behavior, diet acceptability, and cravings. The results were as follows:

"All participants completed the initial 22 weeks; 90% (45/50) of American Diabetes Association guidelines diet group and 86% (42/49) of the vegan diet group participants completed 74 weeks. Fat and cholesterol intake fell more and carbohydrate and fiber intake increased more in the vegan group. At 22 weeks, group-specific diet adherence criteria were met by 44% (22/50) of members of the American Diabetes Association diet group and 67% (33/49) of vegan-group participants (P=0.019); the American Diabetes Association guidelines diet group reported a greater increase in dietary restraint; this difference was not significant at 74 weeks. Both groups reported reduced hunger and reduced disinhibition. Questionnaire responses rated both diets as satisfactory, with no significant differences between groups, except for ease of preparation, for which the 22-week ratings marginally favored the American Diabetes Association guideline group. Cravings for fatty foods diminished more in the vegan group at 22 weeks, with no significant difference at 74 weeks.

"Conclusions: Despite its greater influence on macronutrient intake, a low-fat, vegan diet has an acceptability similar to that of a more conventional diabetes diet. Acceptability appears to be no barrier to its use in medical nutrition therapy."

The main reason the *American Diabetes Association* gives for including meat and dairy in their diet is their baseless assertion that Type 2 diabetes patients simply won't adhere to or accept a vegan diet. This study by Dr. Barnard clearly demonstrated that this need not be the case, finding little difference in adherence and acceptability between the omnivorous and low-fat vegan diets.

Saturated fat from an animal-based diet is also the leading cause of "nonalcoholic fatty liver disease" (NAFLD), as explained here by Dr, Greger:

"Some critics wrote off the film [Supersize Me by Morgan Spurlock] as overly sensational, but researchers in Sweden took it seriously enough to formally replicate Spurlock's one-man experiment. In their study, a group of men and women agreed to eat two fast food meals a day. At the start, their liver enzyme levels were normal, but after just one week of this diet, more than 75 percent of the volunteers' liver function test results became pathological.21 If an unhealthy diet can cause liver damage within just seven days, it should be no surprise that NAFLD [nonalcoholic fatty liver disease] has quietly become the most common cause of chronic liver disease in the United States, afflicting an estimated seventy million people.22 That's about one in three adults. Nearly 100 percent of those with severe obesity may be affected.23

Like alcoholic fatty liver, NAFLD starts with a buildup of fat deposits in the liver that cause no symptoms. In rare cases, this can progress to inflammation and, over years, end up scarring the liver into a state of cirrhosis, resulting in liver cancer, liver failure, and even death – as I saw in that endoscopy suite.24

Fast food is so effective at instigating the disease because NAFLD is associated with the intake of soft drinks and meat. Drinking just one can of soda a day appears to raise the odds of getting fatty liver disease by 45 percent.25 Meanwhile, those who eat the meat equivalent of fourteen chicken nuggets or more daily have nearly triple the rate of fatty liver disease compared to people who eat seven nuggets or less.26

NAFLD has been characterized as a "tale of fat and sugar,"27 but not all fat affects the liver similarly. People suffering from fatty liver inflammation were found to be consuming more animal fat (and cholesterol) but less plant fat (and fiber and antioxidants).28 This may explain why adherence to a Mediterranean style diet with plenty of fruits, vegetables, whole grains, and beans has been associated with less severe fatty liver disease even though it is not typically a low fat diet.29" (How Not To Die, pg 145)

In the study, *"Lipotoxicity: effects of dietary saturated and transfatty acids"* (*Mediators of Inflammation*, Epub, Jan 2013), researchers identified the role saturated fats and trans fats play in causing the chronic inflammation that is associated with insulin resistance and many other chronic degenerative diseases:

"The saturated and transfatty acids favor a proinflammatory state leading to insulin resistance. These fatty acids can be involved in several inflammatory pathways, contributing to disease progression in chronic inflammation, autoimmunity, allergy, cancer, atherosclerosis, hypertension, and heart hypertrophy as well as other metabolic and degenerative diseases. As a consequence, lipotoxicity may occur in several target organs by direct effects, represented by inflammation pathways, and through indirect effects, including an important alteration in the gut microbiota associated with endotoxemia. Interactions between these pathways may perpetuate a feedback process that exacerbates an inflammatory state. The importance of

lifestyle modification, including an improved diet, is recommended as a strategy for treatment of these diseases." ("*Lipotoxicity: effects of dietary saturated and transfatty acids*", *D Estadella, et al., Mediators Inflamm,* Jan 2013)

It is worth repeating here that in this study, researchers tied inflammation mediated by saturated fats and transfats to not just insulin resistance, but also to virtually every other chronic degenerative disease that plagues Western cultures. Their recommendation to stem this epidemic of chronic degenerative diseases is not to prescribe more drugs and surgeries, but rather to make dietary modifications.

Trans Fats

In 1897, French chemist, Paul Sabatier PhD, discovered how to turn unsaturated plant fats into something that resembled saturated animal fats, for which he won the Nobel Prize for Chemistry in 1912. Dr. Sabatier bubbled hydrogen gas through vegetable oil and introduced a trace amount of nickel as a catalyst which facilitated the addition of hydrogen atoms to the unsaturated plant fat molecules. This industrial process, now known as "hydrogenation," replaces all the double bonds between carbon atoms in unsaturated plant fat molecules with hydrogen atoms, turning them into "fully hydrogenated" saturated fat molecules similar to animal fat.

In unsaturated fat molecules, the double bonds cause a kink in the molecular structure giving it a curved shape that prevents unsaturated fat molecules from neatly lining up with each other. This structural instability causes unsaturated fats to remain liquid at room temperature. But when the unsaturated fat molecule becomes fully hydrogenated after hydrogenation, the kinks are all ironed out and the fat molecule becomes straight like a saturated fat molecule. This straight shape of hydrogenated fat molecules allows them to remain solid at room temperature like milk fat (butter), pig fat (lard) and cow fat (tallow).

In 1901, the German chemist, Wilhelm Normann PhD, while experimenting with the hydrogenation process, discovered the process of "partial hydrogenation." By stopping the catalyzing process midway through the chemical reaction, Dr. Normann found that some of the double bonds between carbon atoms remained intact, but because the hydrogen atoms that were added during the partial hydrogenation process bonded in to the carbon atoms in the so called "trans" position, the kinks normally caused by the remaining double bonds were flattened out to make these new "trans fat" molecules have a straight shape similar to fully hydrogenated fat molecules. Due to this stable molecular structure, trans fats, like hydrogenated fats, remain solid at room temperature.

With the invention of artificial trans fats, the food industry had a cheaper solid fat to make pie crusts and to fry potatoes. Soon, trans fats began to appear on grocery shelves in products such as Crisco, which arrived on the market in 1911. As doctors began to worry about the effects of saturated animal fat on heart health, Crisco, which was made from cottonseed oil, was marketed as a better alternative to lard. It was assumed that since trans fats were neither a saturated nor an animal fat, that it must be healthy.

Stable trans fats could sit on store shelves for months without going rancid, which made it very appealing to grocers.

In the 1980s, with the medical establishment's renewed concern about the health risks of saturated animal fats, the processed food industry in the U.S. voluntarily replaced the butter, lard and tallow in their products with cheaper trans fats which resulted in a tremendous increase in trans fats in the average American diet. By 1996, a national dietary survey indicated that people in the U.S were eating almost 0.2 ounces (6 grams) of trans fat per day, or nearly 10% of their recommended total daily fat limit.

In 1980, Dr. Walter Willett MD, of the famous *Nurses' Health Study*, and his colleagues set out to examine the relationship between trans fats intake and the risk of coronary heart disease (CHD). They included trans fats in a comprehensive assessment of diet in the *Nurses' Health Study* cohort of over 100,000 women and developed a regularly updated database of the trans fats content of foods. After eight years of follow-up, and after accounting for known risk factors for heart disease, they found that women with the highest intake of trans fats had a 50% greater risk of hospitalization or death due to CHD. Margarine, the primary source of trans fats in 1980, was directly implicated as a health risk. In a 2013 article in the journal *Scientific American* (*"The Scientific Case for Banning Trans Fats, The FDA's new policy on these deadly artificial fatty acids is long overdue"*, December 13, 2013), Dr. Willett wrote:

> *"I was particularly concerned about the process of partial hydrogenation itself: the vegetable oils being processed are primarily composed of linoleic acid and alpha-linolenic acid, precursors of molecules with many critical biological functions in the human body. But the process of partial hydrogenation changes the shape of those molecules, which almost certainly alters their function in unpredictable ways."*

Also in the 1980s, the Dutch researcher Martijn Katan and colleagues investigated the metabolic effects of trans fats on healthy volunteers, conducting carefully controlled feeding studies lasting several weeks. They found that trans fats and saturated fat increased LDL cholesterol (the so called "bad" cholesterol) to a similar degree, but unlike any other type of fat, trans fats also reduced HDL cholesterol (the so called "good" cholesterol).

By 2003, the U.S. Food and Drug Administration (FDA) found evidence of health risks from trans fats consumption compelling enough to require that trans fats be included on food labels. Soon thereafter New York City banned the use of trans fats in restaurants, and other cities nationwide followed suit. Many processed food manufacturers responded by eliminating trans fats from their product lines and by 2012, approximately 75% of the trans fats had been removed from the U.S. food supply.

In 2009, at the age of 94, Dr. Fred Kummerow, professor emeritus at the University of Illinois at Urbana-Champaign Department of Food Science and Human Nutrition, filed a petition with the FDA for a federal ban on artificial trans fats. Dr. Kummerow 's petition stated explicitly, *"Artificial trans fat is a poisonous and deleterious substance, and the FDA has acknowledged the danger."* The FDA did not act on his petition for four years, so in March 2013, Dr. Kummerow filed a lawsuit against the FDA seeking to compel them to respond to his petition. Three months later, the FDA issued its ruling that trans fats were not *"generally recognized as safe"* (GRAS) and *"could no longer be added to food after June 18, 2018, unless a manufacturer could present convincing scientific evidence that a particular use was safe."* After over 40 years of advocacy to ban trans fats, Dr. Kummerow cheered the FDA's decision saying, *"Science won out."*

Cholesterol

Cholesterol is a waxy, fat-like substance naturally synthesized by our liver out of dietary fat that is circulated through our blood to every cell in our body. We need cholesterol to build cell structure and to make hormones, vitamin D, and digestive substances. Our liver produces all the cholesterol we need for optimal metabolic function, but people who eat animal foods get an additional load of cholesterol in their diet as all animal foods (meat, dairy and eggs) contain residual cholesterol made by the animal. Plant foods contain no cholesterol.

Over the course of the 1950s, in the now famous *Framingham Heart Study,* researchers found that high blood cholesterol, high blood pressure, obesity and cigarette smoking were highly correlated with elevated risk of coronary artery disease (CAD), the single largest cause of death in the U.S. Based on these findings, in 1961 the *American Heart Association* (AHA) established elevated blood cholesterol as the gold standard for diagnosing patients at high risk for CAD. Further observational study would later contradict this AHA determination, however, finding that more than half of heart attacks occurred in patients with normal cholesterol levels in their blood. This disparity between the AHA guidelines for cholesterol and the actual data on CAD patients had been observed since the 1980s, and by the 1990s research teams from around the world began to take a closer look at the biomarkers used to predict heart disease.

What they found was that cholesterol is carried through the blood by molecules called "lipoproteins" that are made out of fat (lipid) and protein. There are two types of lipoproteins: low-density lipoprotein (LDL), and high-density lipoprotein (HDL). LDL molecules are the main carriers of cholesterol in the bloodstream, and HDL carries the LDL back to the liver where it is broken down and excreted from the body. In 2001 a series of studies began to hone in on elevated levels of LDL, particularly LDL that had been "oxidized," as an accurate biomarker for diagnosing patients at high risk for CAD.

In the study, *"Circulating oxidized LDL is a useful marker for identifying patients with coronary artery disease"* (*Arteriosclerosis Thrombosis Vascular Biology,* May 2001), a research team headed by Dr. Paul Holvoet, PhD, Department of Cardiovascular Sciences, Experimental Cardiology, KU Leuven University, Leuven, Belgium, found that high levels of oxidized LDL in the blood had a strong correlation with CAD patients:

> *"Thus, circulating oxidized LDL is a sensitive marker of CAD. Addition of oxidized LDL to the established risk factors may improve cardiovascular risk prediction."*

In another study, "*Elevated levels of oxidized low density lipoprotein [cholesterol] show a positive relationship with the severity of acute coronary syndromes*" (*Circulation*, April 2001), a team of researchers headed by Dr. Shoichi Ehara, MD and PhD, Osaka City University Department of Cardiovascular Medicine, Osaka, Japan, also found that high levels of oxidized LDL in the blood had a strong correlation with CAD patients:

> "*This study demonstrates that ox-LDL levels show a significant positive correlation with the severity of acute coronary syndromes and that the more severe lesions also contain a significantly higher percentage of ox-LDL-positive macrophages. These observations suggest that increased levels of ox-LDL relate to plaque instability in human coronary atherosclerotic lesions.*"

The two studies cited above clearly identify oxidized LDL as a sensitive biomarker for risk of CAD, but neither explains how oxidized LDL causes heart disease. A third team of researchers headed by Dr. Fred Kummerow, PhD biochemist and professor of comparative biosciences at the University of Illinois at Urbana-Champaign, Illinois, USA, attempted to bridge this gap in their study, "*Changes in the phospholipid composition of the arterial cell can result in severe atherosclerotic lesions*" (*Nutritional Biochemistry*, October, 2001).

Dr. Kummerow teamed up with surgeons at the University of Illinois Hospital to retrieve and examine tissues from the arteries of heart bypass patients. He and his colleagues first reported that the arteries of people who had undergone bypass operations contained elevated levels of "sphingomyelin," which is one of several fats that make up the membranes of cell walls. They also found that a high influx of calcium was noted in the cells of bypass patients, but not in the control patients without heart disease. Calcium is often a constituent of the arterial plaques that clog the arteries of heart disease patients. From these experiments, Dr. Kummerow's team hypothesized the pathology of coronary artery disease:

> "*The higher level of oxysterol [oxidized LDL] in the plasma of patients suffering from severe atherosclerosis could increase the concentration of sphingomyelin in the arterial cell membrane and thereby increase calcium influx required for producing the calcific type VII lesions in the coronary arteries.*"

In 2013, at the age of 94, Dr. Kummerow wrote a review published in the *American Journal of Cardiovascular Disease* entitled, "*Interaction between sphingomyelin and oxysterols contributes to atherosclerosis and sudden death*," in which he expounded on his theory of heart disease:

> "*Oxidized cholesterol (oxysterols) enhances the production of sphingomyelin, a phospholipid found in the cellular membranes of the coronary artery. This increases the sphingomyelin content in the cell membrane, which in turn enhances the interaction between the membrane and ionic calcium ($Ca2+$), thereby increasing the risk of arterial calcification.*"

> *"Oxidized low-density lipoprotein (OxLDL) further contributes to heart disease by increasing the synthesis of thromboxane in platelets, which increases blood clotting."*
>
> *"Levels of oxysterols and OxLDL increase primarily as a result of three diet or lifestyle factors: the consumption of oxysterols from commercially fried foods such as fried chicken, fish, and french fries; oxidation of cholesterol in vivo [in the living body] driven by consumption of excess polyunsaturated fatty acids [trans fat] from [hydrogenated] vegetable oils; and cigarette smoking."*

While Dr. Kummerow had positively identified oxidized LDL as a plausible culprit in the pathology of heart disease, he firmly believed that cholesterol and saturated fat found in animal foods were healthy nutrients for humans to include in their diet, and he continued to eat animal products throughout his long life. But when he died in 2017 at the ripe old age of 102, he was found to have atherosclerotic plaques in his arteries. What Dr. Kummerow overlooked was that it's not just fried chicken or fish that contain oxidized LDL; the process of cooking meat, dairy and eggs oxidizes the cholesterol found in these foods making cooked animal foods the primary source of oxidized LDL in the bloodstream. In this post from NutritionFacts.org, Dr. Michael Greger MD explains:

> *"[I]f you take a step back, only foods that start out with cholesterol can end up with oxidized cholesterol. So, the primary method, in terms of reducing cholesterol oxidation in foods, may be to 'reduce the total cholesterol content of the food'—not just by avoiding adding extra with butter, but instead, centering one's diet around whole plant foods, which don't have any cholesterol to get oxidized in the first place."*

Proteins

Proteins are large biochemical molecules comprised of varying assemblages of 21 different amino acids which are chemical compounds made of hydrogen, oxygen, carbon and nitrogen atoms. The cellular structure of all living organisms is constructed out of proteins. Through digestion, our body breaks down the proteins in our food into its component amino acids and circulates them through the bloodstream to be used by our body to construct new cells or repair damaged cells.

There is a common misconception among the general public that proteins from animal foods are superior in quality to proteins from plant foods since the amino acid profile of animal proteins more closely resembles that of our own bodies. This misconception dates all the way back to 1914 when Yale biochemists Lafayette Mendel and longtime collaborator Thomas Osborne first demonstrated that rats grew better on animal protein sources than on plant protein sources. From these experiments they surmised that plant foods are deficient in some of the amino acids essential for normal cellular growth in rats. Due to this and other similar animal experiments, protein from meat, dairy and eggs were classified as superior, or "Class A" protein sources, and proteins from plant sources were deemed inferior, or "Class B" proteins.

But the protein requirements for rats are considerably different than those of humans, mainly due to the fact that rats grow to adult size much faster than people. Since all mammals grow fastest during infancy suckling breast milk, this difference in protein requirements is most obvious when comparing the protein content of rat breast milk to human breast milk. Rat breast milk has a 10 times more protein content than human breast milk. This is because infant rats double in size in 4.5 days while it takes human infants 6 months. Rats mature to adult size in 6 months while it takes humans 17 years. That rats grow so much faster than humans necessarily requires more protein in their diet than humans.

At the turn of the 20th century the most esteemed nutritional scientists of the day, including German biochemists Carl Voit and Max Rubner, and American chemist Wilbur Atwater, recommended a protein intake of up to 127 grams/day for adults, and as high as 165 grams/day for soldiers doing hard physical labor. To achieve these recommended daily protein intakes required people to eat lots of Class A animal proteins.

But even as these rather arbitrary protein recommendations were accepted without serious question among most biochemists of the day, Dr. Russell Chittenden, Professor of Physiological Chemistry at Yale University, came to a radically different conclusion. In 1905 he published his scientific findings on human protein needs in his classic book, *Physiological Economy in Nutrition.* Dr. Chittenden's data included his own personal daily dietary and urine history for nine months to determine nitrogen excretion as a measure of protein utilization. He also recorded his body weight. His daily protein intake was one third of what Voit recommended to maintain nitrogen equilibrium and although he lost weight, his health remained excellent without compromising physical vigor or muscular tone. Thereafter, Dr. Chittenden conducted a year-long study on athletic men in excellent health on a low protein diet of less than 1 gram/kilogram of body weight/day. These subjects also experienced no deterioration of health or ability to perform physical tasks. Dr. Chittenden had proven that even without a large protein intake, individuals could maintain their health and fitness, but his findings were largely ignored by the nutritional science community.

In subsequent studies on rats using purified diets, Dr. William Rose, Professor of Physical Chemistry at the University of Illinois, and his colleagues were able to identify ten amino acids that were essential for the rats' survival. Considering the differences between rat and human metabolic function, Dr. Rose realized that his rat experiments were not satisfactory to determine human amino acid requirements, so he and his team set out in 1942 to determine which amino acids were essential in the human diet to maintain good health. By making note of symptoms of nervousness, exhaustion, and dizziness when subjects were deprived of a particular amino acid, Dr. Rose was able to distinguish the amino acids that are absolutely essential for survival from those that are necessary only for optimal growth. An unexpected finding of Rose's experiments was that the active young men remained in good health at surprisingly low levels of amino acid intake, equivalent to only 24 grams (0.85 ounces) of crude protein/day. In 1949, Dr. Rose published the book, *"Amino Acid Requirements of Man,"* where he announced that the list of eight essential amino acids required by human adults was now complete, since in the absence of even one, good health could not be obtained at any level of intake. Through his experiments, Dr. Rose also determined a minimum level of intake for each of the eight essential amino acids. He found that there were small amounts of unexplained variation in individual needs among his test subjects, so he included a large margin of safety in his final minimum requirement for each amino acid. His formula for establishing a minimum "recommended requirement" for each amino acid was to take the highest recorded level of need in any subject and double it.

An amino acid is considered essential if it cannot be synthesized by the body at a rate commensurate with its demand, so must be supplied by diet. There are 21 amino acids that are common to all life forms, eight of which are essential to humans: isoleucine, leucine, lysine, methionine, phenylalanine, threonine, trytophan and valine. A ninth amino acid, histidine, is considered essential for infants. Six other amino acids are considered conditionally essential in the human diet, meaning their synthesis can be limited under certain conditions, such as prematurity in an infant or individuals in severe catabolic distress. These six are: arginine, cysteine, glycine, glutamine, proline and tyrosine. The remaining six amino acids are non-essential in humans meaning they can be synthesized in sufficient quantities by the body. These six are: alanine, aspartic acid, asparagine, glutamic acid, serine and selenocysteine.

It is important to note here that Dr. Rose's requirements for all eight essential amino acids are easily met by a plant-based diet. In Dr. Rose's classic series on protein requirements published in *The Journal of Biological Chemistry* in 1955, he presented a chart comparing the human requirement for each of the eight essential amino acids to the amino acid profile of a number of plants: maize, brown rice, oatmeal flakes, wheat flour, white beans, potatoes, sweet potatoes, taro, asparagus, broccoli, tomatoes and pumpkin. The amino acid profile of every plant exceeded the human requirement for all eight essential amino acids. What this means is that as long as caloric needs are met, all of a person's essential amino acid requirement can be met by eating a single starchy vegetable. While such a limited diet is not recommended, it would not cause a protein deficiency.

Animal Proteins and Cancer

Nutritional biochemist, Dr. T. Colin Campbell, wrote his Ph.D. dissertation at Cornell University (1958 – 1961) on finding ways to make cattle and sheep grow faster to supply more of what he firmly believed at the time to be high quality animal protein for people to eat. Early in his career, while working in the Philippines to improve nutrition by increasing intake of protein, especially animal protein, Dr. Campbell made a startling discovery; in his own words:

> "Children who ate the highest-protein diets were the ones most likely to get liver cancer! They were the children of the wealthiest families." "(The China Study, by T. Colin Campbell and Thomas M. Campbell II, pg 5, 2006)

At that same time, Dr. Campbell came across a study conducted in India in which researchers fed rats varying amounts of protein in their diet. Astonishingly, 100% of the rats fed a diet containing 20% protein showed evidence of liver cancer while 0% of the rats fed a diet containing 5% protein showed any evidence of liver cancer. Both groups also received equivalent doses of the powerful carcinogen, aflatoxin, so this experiment showed definitively that protein intake trumped chemical carcinogens in controlling cancer in rats. Again, in Dr. Campbell's own words:

> *"This information countered everything I had been taught. It was heretical to say that protein wasn't healthy, let alone say it promoted cancer. It was a defining moment in my career. Investigating such a provocative question so early in my career was not a very wise choice. Questioning protein and animal based foods in general ran the risk of my being labeled a heretic, even if it passed the test of 'good science.'"(The China Study, by T. Colin Campbell and Thomas M. Campbell II, pgs 5–6, 2006)*

So it was at this point that Dr. Campbell decided to conduct in-depth animal feeding experiments in his lab at Cornell University, in Ithica, New York, to investigate the role of protein in the development of cancer. In order to get funding for this project from the *National Institute of Health (NIH)*, the *American Cancer Society* and the *American Institute for Cancer Research*, Dr. Campbell and his colleagues were careful to focus their research at a very basic level, studying the biochemical details of cancer formation, since any hint that they were studying the link between protein and cancer would have doomed funding for the project. All of the results of Dr. Campbell's lab experiments were subsequently published in top peer reviewed scientific journals. Dr. Campbell was astounded by their results:

> *"What we found was shocking. Low-protein diets inhibited the initiation of cancer by aflatoxin, regardless of how much of this carcinogen was administered to these animals. After cancer initiation was completed, low-protein diets also dramatically blocked subsequent cancer growth. In other words, the cancer producing effects of this highly carcinogenic chemical were rendered insignificant by a low-protein diet. In fact, dietary protein proved to be so powerful in its effects that we could turn-on and turn-off cancer growth simply by changing the level consumed.*

> *"Furthermore, the amounts of protein being fed were those that we humans routinely consume. We didn't use extraordinary levels, as is so often the case in carcinogen studies.*

> *"But that's not all. We found that not all proteins had this effect. What protein consistently and strongly promoted cancer? Casein, which makes up 87% of cow's milk protein, promoted all stages of the cancer process. What type of protein did not promote cancer, even at high levels of intake? The safe proteins were from plants, including wheat and soy. As this picture came into view, it began to challenge and then to shatter some of my most cherished assumptions."* (The China Study, T. Colin Campbell and Thomas M. Campbell II, pg 6, 2006)

In the early 1980s, to study the nutritional effects of dietary protein on humans, Dr. Campbell conducted the now famous "China Study" which is still the largest observational nutritional study of its kind. The country of China offered a unique opportunity for Dr. Campbell since at that time the population was ethnically homogeneous (87% Han) and up to 94% of the people lived in the same geographic area all their lives and consumed the same diets unique to their region. Also, while the great majority of rural Chinese people consumed a low-protein, low-fat, high-fiber plant-based diet, there did exist significant variations in diet between different geographical areas within China. As Dr. Campbell noted:

> *"Crucial to the importance of the China Study was the nature of the diet consumed in rural China. It was a rare opportunity to study health related effects of a mostly plant-based diet."*
> (*The China Study,* T. Colin Campbell and Thomas M. Campbell II, pg 73, 2006)

Dr. Campbell teamed up with Dr. Junshi Chen, the deputy director of China's premier health research laboratory, Dr. Junyao Li, who was one of the authors of China's massive *Cancer Atlas Survey* and a key scientist in China's *Academy of Medical Sciences,* and Dr. Richard Peto of Oxford University, U.K., considered one of the premier epidemiologists in the world. This all-star team of scientists constructed the *China Study* to take snapshots in time of the dietary and environmental conditions in rural China including what they ate, how they lived, what was in their blood and urine, and how they died. They decided to make the study as comprehensive as possible covering over four dozen different kinds of diseases including individual cancers, vascular diseases and infectious diseases. Upon detailed analysis of the reams of data collected in the *China Study*, Dr. Campbell's team found over 8,000 statistically significant correlations between diet and disease.

The correlations between animal-protein intake and breast and prostate cancer were particularly striking. Though the Chinese consumed much less animal protein than Americans, even small differences in intake between different geographical regions of China resulted in significant differences in cancer incidence, as explained here by Dr. Campbell:

> *"Diet and disease factors such as animal protein consumption or breast cancer incidence lead to changes in the concentrations of certain chemicals in our blood. These chemicals are called biomarkers... We measured six blood biomarkers that are associated with animal protein intake. Do they confirm the finding that animal protein intake is associated with cancer in families? Absolutely. Every single animal protein-related blood biomarker is significantly associated with the amount of cancer in a family.*
>
> *"In this case, multiple observations, tightly networked into a web, show that animal-based foods are strongly linked to breast cancer. What makes this conclusion especially compelling are two kinds of evidence. First the individual parts of this web were consistently correlated and, in most cases, were statistically significant. Second, this effect occurred at unusually low intakes of animal-based foods.* (*The China Study,* T. Colin Campbell and Thomas M. Campbell II, pgs 88–89, 2006)

Subsequent to the China Study, researchers identified one of the fundamental biochemical pathways by which animal proteins cause prostate cancer, as explained here by Dr. Campbell:

> *"In effect, there are many reactions acting in a coordinated and mutually consistent way to cause disease when a diet high in animal protein is consumed. When blood levels of 1,25 D [vitamin D] are depressed, IGF-1 [the growth hormone 'Insulin-like Growth Factor 1'] simultaneously becomes more active. Together, these factors increase the birth of new cells while simultaneously inhibiting the removal of old cells, both favoring the development of cancer (seven studies cited by 28). For example, people with higher-than-normal blood levels of IGF-1 have been shown to have 5.1 times the risk of advanced-stage prostate cancer. 28 If combined with low blood levels of a protein that inactivates IGF-1 (i.e. more IGF-1 activity), there is 9.5 times the risk of advanced-stage prostate cancer.28 This level of disease risk is alarming. Fundamental to it all is the fact that animal-based foods like meat and dairy 30-32 lead to more IGF-1 and less 1,25 D, both of which increase cancer risk."* (*The China Study,* by T. Colin Campbell and Thomas M. Campbell II, pgs 367–368, 2006)

As it turns out, the common misconception among the general public that proteins from animal foods are superior in quality to proteins from plant foods could not be more wrong. Plant proteins contain all of the essential amino our body needs to build a healthy cell structure, while animal proteins promote biochemical conditions favorable to the growth of cancer cells.

Vitamin B_{12}

Vitamin B_{12} is an essential nutrient meaning that if we don't obtain it from our diet, we will die. Vitamin B_{12} is not synthesized by plants or animals, but rather by bacteria that are ubiquitous in the soil and in fresh water rivers, streams and springs. Our evolutionary ancestors got all the vitamin B_{12} they needed by drinking water from these natural sources, but in the modern era of chlorinate water supplies which kills water borne bacteria, drinking water is no longer a reliable source of vitamin B_{12}.

While animals don't make vitamin B_{12} themselves, there is a residual amount of B_{12} in the organ and muscle tissue of terrestrial, aquatic and avian animals and to a lesser extent in the milk of mammals, but there is no residual vitamin B_{12} in plants. In the modern world of purified drinking water, people who consume animal products with residual vitamin B_{12} still get all they need through diet, but people on a vegan diet are at significant risk of developing a vitamin B_{12} deficiency, and lacto-ovo vegetarians are also at some increased risk. Indeed, multiple observational studies of people from around the world have shown that about a quarter of the vegetarians and nearly three-quarters of the vegans tested were vitamin B_{12} deficient or depleted.

Vitamin B_{12} plays an essential role in red blood cell formation, cell metabolism, nerve function and the production of DNA, and a vitamin B_{12} deficiency is a risk factor for many of the chronic degenerative diseases that plague Western cultures including cardiovascular diseases.

When researchers measured the amount of atherosclerotic plaques in the carotid arteries (the main arteries supplying blood to the brain) of omnivores, vegetarians and vegans, they found no significant difference between them despite the vegetarians and vegans having lower cardiovascular disease risk factors such as lower blood pressure and cholesterol. This is the opposite of what would be expected: lower blood pressure and cholesterol should predispose vegans and vegetarians to have less atherosclerosis than omnivores. Researchers then turned their attention to the vitamin B_{12} deficiency of vegans and vegetarians as the likely explanation for this apparent contradiction.

Multiple studies have identified a build-up of the amino acid, "homocysteine," in the bloodstream, called "hyperhomocysteinemia," as a biomarker for vitamin B_{12} deficiency. In a normal metabolism, vitamin B_{12} is integral to the metabolic process of breaking down homocysteine into other substances our body needs, but a vitamin B_{12} deficiency prevents this break down process from occurring which causes homocysteine to build-up in the bloodstream. High levels of homocysteine in the blood makes the epithelial cells lining the artery walls more prone to injury which leads to inflammation in the blood vessels which leads to atherosclerosis which leads to heart attacks and strokes.

In the paper, *"Is vitamin B12 deficiency a risk factor for cardiovascular disease in vegetarians?"* (*American Journal of Preventive Medicine*, June 2015), author Dr. Roman Pawlak, PhD., Associate Professor, Department of Nutrition Science, East Carolina University, Greenville, North Carolina, reviewed studies connecting the vitamin B_{12} deficiency of vegetarians to their increased risk of cardiovascular disease:

> *"The goal of this paper is to describe the role of vitamin B12 deficiency in cardiovascular disease development among vegetarians. Vegetarians have a high prevalence of vitamin B12 deficiency. Deficiency of this vitamin is associated with a variety of atherogenic processes that are mainly, but not exclusively, due to vitamin B12 deficiency-induced hyperhomocysteinemia... Compared with non-vegetarians, vegetarians have an improved profile of the traditional cardiovascular disease risk factors, including serum lipids, blood pressure, serum glucose concentration, and weight status. However, not all studies that assessed cardiovascular disease incidence among vegetarians reported a protective effect. Among studies that did show a lower prevalence of circulatory health problems, the effect was not as pronounced as expected, which may be a result of poor vitamin B12 status due to a vegetarian diet. Vitamin B12 deficiency may negate the cardiovascular disease prevention benefits of vegetarian diets. In order to further reduce the risk of cardiovascular disease, vegetarians should be advised to use vitamin B12 supplements."*

In the interventional study, *"Vitamin B-12 supplementation improves arterial function in vegetarians with subnormal vitamin B-12 status"* (*The Journal of Nutritional Health & Aging*, March 2012), researchers investigated the efficacy of vitamin B_{12} supplementation using vitamin B_{12} supplements derived directly from bacteria, to improve the arterial function of vitamin B_{12} deficient vegetarians. The results were that vitamin B_{12} supplementation significantly increased blood vitamin B_{12} levels and lowered homocysteine levels. Vitamin B_{12} supplementation also significantly improved blood flow in the brachial artery and reduced thickness in layers of the carotid artery. The researchers concluded that:

> *"Vitamin B-12 supplementation improved arterial function in vegetarians with subnormal vitamin B-12 levels, proposing a novel strategy for atherosclerosis prevention."*

The last refuge of omnivores to defend their dietary practice of meat eating is that the only reliable dietary source of the essential nutrient, vitamin B_{12}, is meat. But as the study above makes clear, supplementation with bacteria derived vitamin B_{12} supplements is a highly efficacious therapy for vegetarians and vegans to reduce their risk of cardiovascular disease without taking on the additional risk factors associated with meat consumption.

Vitamin D

Vitamin D is not really a vitamin at all, true vitamins must be obtained from food, whereas vitamin D is synthesized by our own body. Vitamin D was misnamed because it was first discovered as a nutrient in cod liver oil that prevented the bone deforming disease rickets in children, a few years before it was discovered that vitamin D is synthesized by our own bodies when our skin is exposed to UV light from the sun, but the substance was never reclassified as the hormone that it truly is.

When our skin is directly exposed to UV light rays, cholesterol in our skin is changed into a form of vitamin D called "cholecalciferol," which is also known as vitamin D_3. Cholecalciferol is transported in our blood to our liver where it is metabolized into a storage form of vitamin D called "calcifediol." Calcifediol is stored in our liver until it is released to our kidneys where kidney enzymes metabolize it into another form of vitamin D called "calcitriol." Calcitriol, also known as 1,25-dihydroxycholecalciferol or simply as 1,25 D, is 1,000 times more biologically active than its precursors.

Vitamin D in its most biologically active form, calcitriol, is a hormone that circulates in our blood and binds to receptors in the nucleus of every cell in our body which increases the expression of many genes. Calcitriol only survives for six to eight hours after it is made, so our stores of vitamin D must constantly be replenished through exposure to sunlight (or through oral supplementation).

The mineral calcium is essential in our body for nerve, muscle and bone function, and our blood level of circulating calcium must be tightly regulated within a narrow range for healthy cellular metabolism. Calcitriol (the activated form of vitamin D) works in conjunction with another hormone secreted into our blood by the parathyroid gland in our neck, called parathyroid hormone or PTH, to keep our calcium levels balanced within this narrow range. In the paper, *"PTH and Vitamin D,"* published in the journal, *Comprehensive Physiology,* (March 15, 2016), researchers were finally able to piece together how this extremely complex balancing act works:

> *"PTH and Vitamin D are two major regulators of mineral metabolism. They play critical roles in the maintenance of calcium and phosphate homeostasis as well as the development and maintenance of bone health. PTH and Vitamin D form a tightly controlled feedback cycle, PTH being a major stimulator of vitamin D synthesis in the kidney while vitamin D exerts negative feedback on PTH secretion. The major function of PTH and major physiologic regulator is circulating ionized calcium. The effects of PTH on gut, kidney, and bone serve to maintain serum calcium within a tight range. PTH has a reciprocal effect on phosphate metabolism. In contrast, vitamin D has a stimulatory effect on both calcium and phosphate homeostasis, playing a key role in providing adequate mineral for normal bone formation. Both hormones act in concert with the more recently discovered FGF23 and klotho, hormones involved predominantly in phosphate metabolism, which also participate in this closely knit feedback circuit. Of great interest are recent studies demonstrating effects of both PTH and vitamin D on the cardiovascular system. Hyperparathyroidism and vitamin D deficiency have been implicated in a variety of cardiovascular disorders including hypertension, atherosclerosis, vascular calcification, and kidney failure. Both hormones have direct effects on the endothelium, heart, and other vascular structures. How these effects of PTH and vitamin D interface with the regulation of bone formation are the subject of intense investigation."*

If our bare skin is exposed to UV rays from direct sunlight for enough time each day, it produces all the vitamin D we need to maintain a healthy calcium and phosphorus balance. But, if for any reason our skin does not get sufficient solar exposure, this can lead to a vitamin D deficiency which can completely throw off our calcium balance. Every cell in our body uses calcium to send messages and communicate with the different parts of the cell. Our nerve cells use calcium to send signals throughout our nervous system to our muscles and organs, that is why a calcium imbalance can cause so many neurological symptoms, including tiredness, anxiety, depression, poor sleep and poor concentration. Our muscles cells use calcium to flex, that is why a calcium imbalance can cause our muscles to either cramp or get weak. Our bones act as a storage area for calcium, they are constantly absorbing, remodeling, and giving away calcium when the rest of the body needs it, that is why a calcium imbalance can cause bone deformations like rickets. Ultimately, if left untreated, a long term calcium imbalance can become a contributing co-factor in the pathology of cardiovascular diseases, cancers, autoimmune diseases, kidney diseases, and bone diseases.

Living conditions in modern times preclude many people in the world today from receiving adequate skin exposure to direct sunlight, and as a result billions live in a chronic state of vitamin D deficiency. There are many contributing factors as to why people don't get enough sunlight exposure. Most notably, the farther from the Earth's equator one lives, the less sunlight there is during the winter months, and also the sun's rays are coming in at such a severe angle as to not effectively stimulate vitamin D production. Everyone living north or south of 20 degrees latitude is at risk for vitamin D deficiency during the winter months. Dark pigmented skin is also less efficient at metabolizing vitamin D than white skin, so people of color are at additional risk. As we age our skin becomes less efficient at metabolizing vitamin D, so seniors are also at additional risk. Clothing, sunscreen and indoor living further reduce people's direct exposure to sunlight putting them at increased risk for a vitamin D deficiency.

What is the optimal blood level of vitamin D to maintain healthy cellular function throughout our body? Should people who get inadequate solar exposure take vitamin D supplements and if so, how much? These questions have been the subject of great debate within the medical establishment since the discovery of vitamin D in the early 20th century, and the prevailing view in the early 21st century is much the same as it was back then: that the optimal level of vitamin D in the blood should be pegged at the amount required to prevent rickets, and since most people in the world attain this level through solar exposure, they don't need to take vitamin D supplements. But the study of bone biology and calcium and vitamin D physiology has come a long way since the rickets model for deficiency was developed, and this recommendation is completely outdated and no longer supported by the evidence.

Dr. Robert Heaney, MD, is a Professor of Clinical Endocrinology specializing in nutrition at Creighton University, Omaha, Nebraska. For over 50 years he has been one of the world's leading researchers in the field of bone biology and calcium and vitamin D physiology. In his paper, "*Lessons for nutritional science from vitamin D*" (*The American Journal of Clinical Nutrition*, May 1999), Dr. Heaney gave his take on the appropriate blood levels of Vitamin D and the need for supplementation:

> "*The compound we call vitamin D can no longer properly be considered a vitamin, and for most mammals, it is not in any sense even a nutrient. Nevertheless, vitamin D resembles true vitamins inasmuch as humans—who are cut off from the critical solar ultraviolet wavelengths by reason of latitude, clothing, or shelter—depend on an exogenous source of the substance just as they do for the true essential nutrients. In any event, vitamin D is inextricably imbedded in nutritional science and the matter of discerning how much we need for health offers instructive general lessons for the setting of nutrient requirements.*
>
> "*Rickets and osteomalacia were recognized as being caused by vitamin D deficiency ≈75 y ago; their prevention and cure with fish liver oil constituted one of the early triumphs of nutritional science. The requirement for vitamin D has been pegged to these disorders ever since. Despite the explosion in understanding how vitamin D operates, vitamin D sufficiency continues, implicitly at least, to be equated with the absence of rickets or osteomalacia. Many developments have made it clear that that is no longer a tenable position. The shift away from this approach is reflected, for example, in the tripling of the vitamin D recommendation for the elderly in the most recent dietary reference intakes from the Food and Nutrition*

Board of the Institute of Medicine (1), arguably the largest increase in the history of dietary recommendations.

"There is now a consensus that serum 25-hydroxyvitamin D [25(OH)D] concentration is the correct functional indicator. What is less certain is what the optimal concentration of 25(OH) D should be and how much we must produce or ingest to achieve it. In this issue of the Journal, Vieth (2) marshalls an impressive array of evidence relating to both questions. Vieth stresses that early humans would have produced far more vitamin D daily than the amount needed simply to prevent rickets or osteomalacia—production on the order of several thousands of IUs per day. And although this abundance has reassuring implications for safety, it also raises questions about the functional significance of this seeming surplus."

"As Vieth notes, total daily intake, production, or both, amounting to 2.5–5 µg (100–200 IU) and serum 25(OH)D concentrations >20–25 nmol/L, suffice to prevent HVOiii [rickets]. But the mere absence of clinical rickets can hardly be considered an adequate definition either of health or of vitamin D sufficiency. This is particularly important in view of the worldwide epidemic of osteoporosis which, although a multifactorial disorder like hypertension and coronary artery disease, can nevertheless also be produced by milder degrees of vitamin D insufficiency (ie, HVOi and HVOii).

"The key questions then are as follows: What serum 25(OH)D concentration is needed to prevent HVOi [osteoporosis]? How much vitamin D must we make (or ingest) each day to reach that concentration? Clearly, the laboratory reference ranges are of no help here. Vitamin D insufficiency is prevalent in higher latitudes (4); hence, population distributions, although undoubtedly typical, cannot be considered normative. Published lower reference values are in the range of 40–45 nmol/L, but Vieth argues for a lower limit of 100 nmol/L and there is a well-established body of evidence extending back over 20 y that has pointed to a value ≥80 nmol/L (5). Moreover, Dawson-Hughes et al (6) and Kinyamu et al (7) reported recently that the evidence of HVOi persists with serum 25(OH)D concentrations as high as 100–120 nmol/L. Not all studies support values that high and the reasons for discrepancies between them are not always clear [although analytic differences in measurement of serum 25(OH)D have been a factor]. Thus, careful studies are still needed to define the optimal 25(OH)D concentration. Nevertheless, it will almost certainly be higher than was previously thought. Vieth makes a point that should help us with the needed mental adjustment: individuals exposed to the sun for much of the year in lower latitudes always have blood 25(OH)D concentrations values >100 nmol/L. So, if the true lower limit of the acceptable normal range is, in fact, ≈100 nmol/L, it could hardly be considered 'high.'

"The issue of how much vitamin D must be ingested to reach 100 or even 80 nmol/L will require even greater conceptual readjustment as well as careful studies specifically designed *to answer the question. Part of the difficulty here lies in the fact that the response to orally administered vitamin D is nonlinear (8); the achieved increment in serum 25(OH)D per unit dose varies as some inverse function of the baseline 25(OH)D concentration. Vieth's estimate of the daily requirement from all sources is 100 µg (4000 IU), an order of magnitude higher than the current dietary reference intakes. Whatever the value turns out to be, it seems inescapable that it will be substantially higher than the current values and possibly higher than nutritional policymakers may be prepared to accept. Nevertheless, the adequacy of even the newly elevated dietary reference intakes, still released only in draft form, has already been questioned (9).*

The experience with vitamin D may offer several lessons for nutrition generally. Significant dysfunction occurs at exposures far short of those needed to evoke the index disease. It would be surprising if something similar were not to occur with other nutrients.

"Far from being a "chronic condition" that may be helped by intake of a nutrient above the requirement, osteoporosis occurring as HVOi and HVOii is as truly a deficiency disease as is scurvy or beriberi. The fact that it takes 30 or more years to manifest itself makes it no less a deficiency condition than a disorder that develops in 30 d. It is easy to understand how long-period deficiency diseases could never have been recognized in the early days of nutritional science, but with modern methods and a better grasp of the relevant physiology, failing to recognize a slowly developing condition as a true deficiency state can no longer be justified.

"Finally, better understanding of the prevailing availability of various nutrients during hominid evolution challenges the privileged position accorded to contemporary exposures. Primitive environmental availability of a nutrient does not ipso facto establish the requirement, but primitive exposures would have influenced the evolution of the relevant physiology and such concentrations should at least be considered presumptively acceptable. Rather than have all the burden fall on establishing their efficacy, one would think that the burden would be on establishing the safety and adequacy of the often much lower contemporary exposures."

To summarize, Dr. Heaney is saying that while most people receive enough vitamin D through solar exposure to prevent rickets, they do not receive enough to prevent osteoporosis or many of the other chronic degenerative diseases that are epidemic in Western cultures, so most people in the world today should do some amount of supplementation. Though the current recommendation for minimum vitamin D blood level is 40 – 45 nmol/L, there is convincing evidence that for maximum health benefits, the minimum level of vitamin D in the blood should be closer to 100 nmol/L. The amount of supplementation needed to achieve this blood level of vitamin D is highly variable depending on each person's individual circumstance.

While vegans are somewhat more at risk of vitamin D deficiency than lacto ovo vegetarians or meat eaters since there is some residual vitamin D in meat, milk and eggs, vitamin D deficiency is also prevalent among people who eat animal foods. Remember, we evolved getting our vitamin D through solar exposure, not depending on dietary sources, so supplementation with food is no more natural than taking an oral supplement. Vitamin D_3 oral supplements are widely sold over-the-counter without prescription. Vitamin D_3 supplements are mostly derived from two sources: isolated from "lanolin," a fatty byproduct of the wool industry, or from "lichen" (which is neither plant nor animal) exposed to UV light rays. As for determining your own personal optimal dose to achieve and maintain your blood level of vitamin D at around 100 nmol/L, that requires experimentation with dosing and having regular vitamin D blood tests to adjust your dose accordingly.

The World's Healthiest People

Beginning in 1999, journalist and explorer Dan Buettner led a series of expeditions with *National Geographic* and a team of anthropologists, demographers, and scientists to discover the world's longest-living populations and to see if there were commonalities between these diverse cultures. In 2008, *National Geographic* published Buettner's book based on this research entitled, *"The Blue Zones: Lessons for Living Longer From the People Who've Lived the Longest."* By way of these expeditions, the researchers identified five regions of the world with the largest percentage of individuals 100 years of age or older. Buettner called these regions *"Blue Zones"* because when he and his colleagues located one of these areas, they drew a blue circle around it on a map. Residents of these zones also suffered a fraction of the chronic diseases that commonly afflict people in the developed world. The five regions identified by Buettner's team were: Loma Linda, California, U.S.; Nicoya Peninsula, Costa Rica; Sardinia, Italy; Ikaria, Greece; Okinawa, Japan.

The researchers also found that residents of all five Blue Zones engaged in similar lifestyle habits, what Buettner referred to as the "Power Nine." Three of the Power Nine related to diet: moderate caloric intake, moderate alcohol intake (especially of red wine), and a plant-based diet. People living in the Blue Zones primarily ate a 95% plant-based diet though few were strictly vegan. Diets in the Blue Zone were typically rich in legumes, fruits, vegetables, whole grains and nuts, with meat consumed only around once a week. This shared dietary pattern between people living in these Blue Zones is pretty close to the whole-food, plant-based – optimal human diet – prescribed above by Dr. Michael Greger.

Along with a long lifespan and freedom from chronic disease, physical fitness is a third metric often used to access a person's degree of health. As research in the 1980s began to elucidate the health advantages of a plant-based diet, some world class athletes who were looking for a competitive edge in their sport were some of its earliest adopters.

Track and field star Carl Lewis was one such athlete. Lewis's long career spanned from 1979 to 1996, over which time he dominated the world's number one rankings in the individual 100 and 200 meter sprint events and the long jump. In his career he won nine Olympic gold medals, winning gold medals in the same individual event in four consecutive Olympic Games. He also won eight gold medals at the World

Track and Field Championships. His athletic accomplishments led to numerous accolades, including being voted "World Athlete of the Century" by the *International Association of Athletics Federations*, "Sportsman of the Century" by the *International Olympic Committee*, "Olympian of the Century" by *Sports Illustrated* magazine, and three times "Athlete of the Year" by *Track & Field News*. In the introduction to the book "Very Vegetarian" (2001) by vegan chef Jannequin Bennett, Lewis wrote, *"I've found that a person does not need protein from meat to be a successful athlete."*

Professional basketball is one of the most physically demanding of all professional sports and *National Basketball Association* (NBA) players are some of the most well conditioned athletes in the world. Another early adopting vegan athlete was Hall of Fame NBA superstar Bill Walton. Walton won NBA championships in 1977 and 1986 and the NBA Finals Most Valuable Player (MVP) award. A Walton contemporary, Hall of Fame NBA superstar Robert Parish, was also an early vegan adopter who won four NBA championships and played 21 seasons in a still standing record of 1,611 regular season games. Both Walton and Parish were centers, with Walton measuring in at 6 feet 11 inches tall and 210 pounds (211 centimeters, 95 kilograms), and Parish at 7 feet 1 inch and 230 pounds (216 centimeters, 104 kilograms). Since the 2000s there have been a number of vegan NBA players including superstars Kyrie Irving and Chris Paul.

Another one of the most physically demanding of all professional sports is football (called soccer in America). Vegan football player Lionel Messi is widely regarded as one of the greatest players of all time. Messi has won a record 6 *Ballon d'Or* awards regarded as the most prestigious individual award for football players. He also won a record 6 *European Golden Shoes* awards presented each season to the leading goalscorer in league matches. Messi holds numerous goal scoring records and in 2020 was named to the *Ballon d'Or Dream Team*. Another vegan superstar football player is Alex Morgan. Morgan played on the USA women's team that won the gold medal at the 2012 Olympic Games in London. That year she became the youngest woman to score 20 goals in a season. She played on the U.S. women's teams that won *Fédération Internationale de Football Association (FIFA)* world cup titles in 2015 and 2019. She was named to the *Dream Team* for both tournaments, and took home the *Silver Boot Award* for second most goals scored in 2019.

Tennis superstar Venus Williams credits her vegan diet with extending her career as a competitive player. Williams has won 7 Grand Slam singles titles including 5 Wimbledon championships. She has also won 14 Grand Slam Women's doubles titles, all with her sister Serena, and two Mixed Doubles Grand Slam titles. Her combined total of 23 Grand Slam titles across all disciplines has her tied for fourth-most by a woman player in the Open Era (since 1968). Williams also has won 4 Olympic gold medals and been ranked No. 1 in the world by the *Women's Tennis Association* for a total of 19 weeks. Tennis superstar Novak Djokovic follows a vegan diet. To date, Djokovic has been ranked No. 1 by the *Association of Tennis Professionals* (ATP) for a record 328 weeks, he has won 19 Grand Slam men's singles titles including a record nine Australian Opens, and 84 ATP singles titles overall. He is also the only player in the Open

Era to complete two Grand Slams, that is win all four Major tournaments in a row – the Australian Open, French Open, Wimbledon and the U.S. Open.

Even in that bastion of male virility, American pro football, players have turned to a plant-based diet for a competitive edge. National Football League (NFL) superstar Tom Brady is the most celebrated quarterback in NFL history. To date, Brady has played in the NFL for 21 years and led his teams to a record 10 Super Bowl title game appearances and 7 NFL championships. In 2017 at age 40, he was the oldest player to win the NFL's Most Valuable Player (MVP) award and in 2020 at age 43, he was the oldest player to win a Super Bowl as starting quarterback and to be named Super Bowl MVP. Brady holds virtually every career record for NFL quarterbacks including total passing yards, pass completions, touchdown passes, games started, regular-season wins and playoff wins. In 2017 Brady went public with his diet regimen in his book, *"The TB12 Method: How to Achieve a Lifetime of Sustained Peak Performance."* While not strictly vegan, Brady's *TB12 Diet* centers around whole fruits and vegetables, whole grains, beans, protein powders and bars, and so called lean proteins (mostly fish). Brady's TB12 diet, like the Blue Zone diet, is strikingly similar to Dr. Greger's whole-food, plant-based optimal human diet described above. NFL running back Theo Riddick went vegan in 2017. That year he told *The Detroit News, "I turned vegan over the summer. I've noticed a difference just with my energy level."* In 2018 Riddick told *Mlive, "I just think my recovery level was just phenomenal. I think when I was younger, to be honest I wouldn't really feel better until probably Friday. And then you go back out there and play on Sunday. I can say last year I was feeling good by Tuesday. And to have that recovery level on my side and working with me, instead of against me, has given me the chance to play all 16 games."* Other vegan NFL stars include 6 foot 1 inch, 301 pound defensive lineman Jurrell Casey, and 6 foot 4 inch, 320 pound defensive lineman DaQuan Jones.

Vegan ultramarathon runner Scott Jurek is considered one of the best endurance athletes of all time. To date, Jurek has won many of the sport's most prestigious races multiple times including the 153-mile Spartathlon in Greece, the 135 mile Badwater Ultramarathon (considered the world's toughest foot race), and the Western States 100-Mile Endurance Run seven times in a row. In 2015 he ran the entire 2,200 mile (3,500 kilometer) length of the Appalachian Trail in 46 days, eight hours, and seven minutes, breaking the speed record by over three hours.

There are now world class vegan athletes performing in virtually every competitive sport from surfing to body building to martial arts who were attracted to a plant-based diet by its performance enhancing qualities.

That people can compete as athletes at the highest level and can live into old age in good health on a diet of plant foods does not in itself prove that a plant-based diet is the optimal human diet, after all, there are plenty of people who eat animal foods who are also champion athletes and who live into old age. What it does prove, however, is that not only is it possible to live a healthy active life on a plant-based diet, it is highly probable.

(Note to readers: living as I do in early 21ˢᵗ century USA, in a culture where animal food consumption has been tightly woven into the social fabric for generations, I am acutely aware of the false narratives upon which this self destructive behavior is based. One of the most pernicious of these false narratives goes something like this: to be strong and healthy, animal foods are a necessary component of the human diet, therefor we must produce meat, dairy and eggs to feed the human population. If anything, nutritional science has proven beyond doubt that animal foods are the primary cause of chronic degenerative diseases, and that whole plant foods provide all the nutrients we need to live long, active, healthy lives. These facts alone totally refute the most compelling argument the animal products industries have to justify their very existence.)

23

GROWING OUR FOOD, HEALING OUR PLANET

"Eating is an agricultural act."
– Wendell Berry, philosopher farmer

In Chapter 20, we reviewed six 21ˢᵗ century studies that quantified the enormous global environmental impacts of animal agriculture. In Chapter 21, we reviewed six 21ˢᵗ century studies that quantified the sustainability of a plant-based diet. In Chapter 22, we explored the efficacy of a whole-food, plant-based diet to prevent disease and promote vigorous health. Here in Chapter 23, we will now take a closer look at the sustainable farms of the future: who should grow our food and how our food should be grown to renew the Earth's soil fertility?

Smallholders

In 2018, the most comprehensive study to date on farm size, *"How much of the world's food do smallholders produce?" (Global Food Security, June 2018), was published. The authors* compiled the first open source dataset to estimate crop production by farm size derived from actual farmer surveys of crop production cross-referenced with farm size classes from 1 to over 1,000 hectares (2.5 to 2,500 acres). Their dataset included 154 crop types from 55 countries, which represented 51.1% of global agricultural area. Using this data the authors estimated total global food production by crop type within each farm size class. This study was also the first to evaluate how the crop macro-nutrient (carbohydrates, proteins and fats) conrents varied by farm size.

From their exhaustive research, the authors found that crop yields were the highest on the smallest class of farms:

"The smallest two farm size classes (0–1 ha and 1–2 ha) are the greatest contributors to global food production compared to all other classes. Farms less than 2 ha produce 28–31% of total crop production and 30–34% of the global food supply (by calories; Fig. 2A-H) as extrapolated from the 55 countries in our dataset. Their contribution is slightly higher than their areal coverage of 24% of gross harvested area, suggesting small farmers have greater cropping intensity or higher yields than larger farms. We found smallholders (farms < 2 ha) also allocate the largest percentage (55–59%) of their crop production to food compared to all other farm size classes (Fig. 2G). Generally, larger farms devote more of their production towards feed and processing. Farms between 200 and 500 ha have the largest allocation of their production to feed (16–29%) compared to farms < 2 ha who allocate 12–16% to feed. Farms >1000 ha allocated 12–32% of their production to processing."

What these findings tell us is that smallholder farms < 2 hectares (under 5 acres) produce one third of the world's food supply on less than one quarter of the world's agricultural lands. This means that not only do smallholder farmers already produce a significant portion of the world's food supply, they are also much more efficient at coaxing food from the ground than larger farms. Theoretically, these findings suggest that if all farms over 1,000 hectares were converted to farms under 2 hectares, smallholder farmers could easily feed the world's entire human population.

The authors also found that species diversity declined as farms got bigger:

"We found that species richness declined with increasing farm size (Fig. 3A). Diversity also scaled differently with area within different farm size classes, with greater turnover in unique species in small farms than in land allocated to larger farms (Fig. 3B) Between farm size dissimilarity in species shows that larger farms, while harboring less diversity, and lower turnover in crop diversity across space, show greater specialization in certain crop groups than other farm sizes... The crop portfolio of each farm size class shows that smaller farms (< 2 ha) produce a greater share of the world's fruits, pulses, and roots and tubers, while medium sized farms produce more vegetables and nuts, and large farms produce more oil crops and 'other' (Fig. 5). While all farm sizes contribute a large proportion to cereals, smaller farms devote a greater percentage of their overall production to cereals compared to other farm size classes."

What these findings tell us about the diversity of crops by farm size is that farms < 100 ha (under 250 acres) produce a greater share of the world's fruits, nuts, vegetables, pulses, roots and tubers, and farms > 100 ha (over 250 acres) produce a greater share of the world's oil, feed and biofuel crops. This means that the healthiest foods for people to eat (whole plant foods) are mostly produced on small and medium sized farms, and the unhealthiest foods for people to eat (animal products and processed foods) are mostly produced on large farms > 100 ha (over 250 acres).

All of the calories in our diet come from the macro-nutrients – carbohydrates, proteins and fats. This study found that there were *"no significant differences in the percentage of macro-nutrients produced within each farm size class.*" This tells us that if all the world's arable land was divided into farms < 100 ha (under 250 acres), they could easily supply all the calories necessary to provide food security for the world's entire human population.

Veganic Farming

Animal agriculture is so pervasive in the world today that its byproducts, mainly manure, blood meal and bone meal, are commonly used as soil amendments on fruit and vegetable crops. If, as I advocate in this book, the human population was to transition back to our natural plant-based diet, animal agriculture would cease to exist and these animal-based soil amendments would no longer be available. The elimination of animal agriculture would necessitate growing fruits and vegetables without these animal-based soil amendments which begs the question: can fruits and vegetables be grown in the abundance necessary to feed the world without these animal-based inputs?

Tolhurst Organic Farm

In the 1970s, to test out the feasibility of animal free agriculture, a group of vegans in England who wanted their food grown without animal byproducts, formed the *Vegan Organic Network* (VON), and together with local farmer Iain Tolhurst developed the world's first set of "*veganic standards,*" which they initially called "*stockfree standards.*" In the over 40 years since, certified veganic farms in England following these standards have proven to be both highly productive and eco-friendly.

Veganic standards as defined by VON are basically the same as "organic standards" with the added standard that no animals are raised for food and no animal byproducts are used to grow produce, as denoted in this VON statement of Veganic Standards (*Veganic-Standards-September-2018.pdf*):

"*Produce attaining the Veganic Symbol utilises organic production techniques. The term "organic" refers to a method of producing food by promoting soil fertility and soil life through the addition of biological (non-synthetic) substances to the soil to replenish any organic matter lost through cropping. Veganic growers minimise their reliance on imported inputs and utilise all the resources on the registered holding.*

"*No inputs, as the sole source of fertility, are allowed into an organic system that may adversely affect the soil ecosystem. Soluble fertilisers are not permitted, as they by-pass the soil and feed the crops directly. Synthetic fertilisers, synthetic pesticides and weedkillers are not permitted in an organic agricultural or horticultural system. The registered grower is not permitted to use genetically modified organisms (GMOs) or any products derived from such GMOS.*

"*The organic production system makes a positive ecological impact on the registered holding by conserving wildlife habitats as well as attempting to prevent harmful impacts on the wider environment. Reliance on non-renewable resources like fossil fuels is discouraged.*

"Produce attaining the Veganic symbol is additionally certified free from deliberate animal inputs. The term "veganic" refers to a method of producing plant-based foods. Growers must not keep animals for food production or commercial gain on the registered holding and must not use animal manures or slaughterhouse by-products of animal or fish origin."

It is important to emphasize here that veganic farming is not just about growing crops without animal inputs, but equally about integrating farms into the natural environment so as to preserve habitat for native wild flora and fauna.

The VON Veganic Standards identify17 different aspects of farming and goes into considerable detail about what is allowed and what is forbidden for each. The 17 farming practices addressed are:

1. Keeping of animals on the registered holding

2. Protecting soil life and soil structure

3. Primary sources of soil fertility

4. Composting procedures

5. Supplementary nutrients

6. Propagation

7. Crop rotations

8. Environmental Pollution

9. Practices promoting environmental conservation

10. Weed control

11. Disease, mollusc and insect pest control

12. Competing birds and mammals

13. Harvesting and storage

14. Packaging materials

15. Labelling for box schemes / packers selling to third parties using multi-sourced produce

16. Transportation of Veganic produce

17. Record keeping

While the veganic standards are very specific and exacting from seed to sales, the basic concept of veganic farming is relatively simple: to maintain the nutrient cycle of the soil by regularly replenishing the organic matter in the soil with annual crops of nitrogen fixing "green manures" (i.e. clovers and legumes), and by applying compost made from organic plant material that is gathered on site. By minimizing inputs from outside sources, veganic farming is resource conserving and sustainable.

The first farm to be certified veganic in 1976 was the *Tolhurst Organic* farm located in south Oxfordshire, England, near the banks of the Thames River. At 7.7 hectares (19 acres) of land under cultivation, *Tolhurst Organic* is classified as a small farm. *Tolhurst Organic* markets its produce directly to consumers by way of a "box scheme" where customers place orders with local reps in a delivery area and pick up orders at local collection points in their delivery area.

The *Tolhurst Organic* website (*What is Stockfree Organic? - Tolhurst Organic*) gives an overview of the farm's operation and energy savings:

"*Our aim is not to supply every family in the south but to farm with an emphasis on education and conservation. Our farming system not only helps to minimise harmful effects on the environment but feeds you and your family as well.*"

"*We started to look at our carbon footprint several years ago, before it became fashionable. We had always felt that we were reasonably energy efficient, so we worked out how much energy the business produced over a year and then calculated the carbon footprint that this gave.*"

"*We have a very low carbon footprint. Compared with supermarket conventional produce, we are 90% more efficient.* Our whole farm produces the same amount of carbon as the average household and supplies 400 families, so we are probably one of the greenest box schemes available. *As verified by Prof. Tim Jackson, BBC Climate Change special programme March 2007.*"

"*Our total energy usage for the year is mostly in the form of fuel for tractors, delivery vehicles and other machinery. This comes to 2,030 litres, around 5 litres per family that we supply for the whole year. Electricity is used to light buildings, provide some facilities for plant raising and other odd jobs. We use 6,400 units per year, about the same as the average household.*"

"*The total carbon footprint for our business comes to around 8 tonnes, which is the same as an average house in the UK.*"

Here, the *Tolhurst Organic* website reports on their annual production:

"*We produce and distribute around 120 tonnes of vegetables every year direct from the farm. Our system of production utilising* stockfree methods, *growing all of our own plants (over 140,000 per annum) ensures that we are operating as near as possible to a closed system. This means that we do not have to import fertility and plants produced on other farms. This reduces energy inputs quite considerably.*"

"*We grow a high percentage of our own vegetables, whereas many large box schemes buy from other producers, often from overseas. Wherever possible we only use local UK produce when we do have to buy in during the "hungry gap".*

Here, the *Tolhurst Organic* website describes how they integrate the farm into the natural environment:

"*Our farm is situated in a very beautiful part of the country, right on the edge of the Chiltern Hills with the river Thames passing close to our land. We are surrounded by a diverse range of habitats – river meadow, chalk downland, arable fields, pastoral fields with beech and oak woodland.*"

"*It is classed as an area of outstanding natural beauty AONB. We aim to preserve this unique habitat with our farming methods. We have planted the only new farm hedges in our parish for over 100 years, in two sections totalling almost 500 m. These are planted with mixed indigenous species of trees and shrubs. Some of the trees will eventually grow on to produce timber in future generations, and many of them are producing fruits and nuts for wildlife now. Within our 17 acres of field vegetables we now have over 1800 m of hedgerow, which have completely changed the way that our crops interact with their local environment."*

"The hedges are just a part of our bio-diversity and habitat management. There are many other features that we have implemented on our fields to improve the chances for wildlife. We have had to give up small areas of land to do this, but it has enabled us to reduce the problems of pest attacks on our vegetables. The creation of a diverse and dynamic habitat within the fields is all part of our 'systems approach' to managing potential pest problems. Increased bio-diversity has ensured that we have a healthy balance of predators feeding on pests and maintaining nature's equilibrium. Working with Nature has proved to be easier that battling against it. We have not sprayed any crops at all even with organic sprays, so successful has our predator management become."

"We have had several surveys done to asses our bio-diversity and it has been most encouraging to see the way that the number of species has grown over the past 20 years."

The farmers at *Tolhurst Organic* are optimistic about the future of veganic farming:

"We see a big future in stockfree organic systems as they use considerably less land than livestock dependent systems, have a much lower carbon footprint and lower energy requirements."

The 40+ year experiment in veganic farming at *Tolhurst Organic* has been an unqualified success at providing organic fruits and vegetables to the local market at a fraction of GHG emissions of commercial produce while also preserving local habitat for native wild flora and fauna.

What lessons for small farms around the world does the *Tolhurst Organic* farm experience hold? Clearly, farms in sub-Saharan Africa or Southeast Asia have very different environmental conditions than a farm in Northern Europe, but the basic concepts of veganic farming to maintain the nutrient cycle of the soil by regularly replenishing the organic matter with annual nitrogen fixing crops and by applying compost made from organic plant material gathered on site, can be applied anywhere in the world. Yields will vary depending on the climate, water and soil resources available in a given area, but whatever the resources available, veganic farming will yield the most fruits and vegetables possible while causing the least amount of environmental harm.

Common Ground Mini-Farm

In the coastal mountains of Northern California not 25 miles from my home, is another small experimental stockfree fruit and vegetable farm called the Common Ground Mini-Farm, in Willits, California, USA, which has gained worldwide recognition for its GROW BIOINTENSIVE® Sustainable Mini-Farming method of growing more food with less resources. The mini-farm was the brainchild of

John Jeavons, Executive Director of the globally active non-profit Ecology Action, and a leader in the field of biointensive agriculture since the early1970s. Jeavons comes with an impressive resume:

> *"He developed the small-scale, high-yielding, resource-conserving GROW BIOINTENSIVE® Sustainable Mini-Farming method—an approach that allows small farmers to increase yields, build fertile soil up to 60x faster than nature, and use 66% less water per pound of food, compared with conventional practices. This comprehensive cropping system enables people everywhere to grow a complete, balanced diet, significant income, and sustainable soil fertility using very little land. As a result of Ecology Action's demonstration, teaching and research activities in biologically intensive farming over the last 43 years, John's methods are now being used in 143 countries in virtually all climates and soils where food is grown."*

> *"He is the author of the best-selling sustainable farming handbook How to Grow More Vegetables and Fruits, Nuts, Berries, Grains, and Other Crops Than You Ever Thought Possible With Less Water On Less Land Than You Can Imagine, now in its 9th edition in eight languages, plus Braille, with over 600,000 copies in print worldwide. He has authored, co-authored or edited over 40 publications on Biointensive agriculture, including a five-part, peer-reviewed article that appeared in The Journal of Sustainable Agriculture.[1]"*

> *"He has given numerous presentations and workshops in the U.S., and has taught in Kenya, Mexico, South Africa and Canada. This year [2014] he will teach at the 1st World Meeting on "Family Organic Agriculture with the Biointensive Method" in the Dominican Republic, with representatives from 50 countries present; in 2015 he will present a 5-day Biointensive workshop at the "Feeding the Planet, Energy for Life", Expo in Milan, Italy with 20 million visitors from 144 countries expected; and a 3-day workshop for a farmer's cooperative in southern France." (https://johnjeavons.org)*

In December 2011, Jeavons was interviewed by *ACRES U.S.A*, North America's oldest publisher on production-scale organic and sustainable farming. In this extended interview, Jeavons makes such an eloquent case for his beautiful vision of sustainable mini-farming that I will leave it to him to tell his own story. We pick up the narrative with Jeavons explaining the primary technique of biointensive agriculture – "double digging":

> ***ACRES U.S.A.*** *What did you do to make the work more manageable?*
>
> ***JEAVONS.*** *In terms of easier, we use a process called double digging, where manually we prepare the soil 24 inches deep. This is really important, because if you have good soil structure down 24 inches deep you've got nutrient cycling 24 inches deep. In farming, whether it's organic or chemical, currently the soil is only prepared about 6 inches deep, and unless you have a really good soil already you only have ease of nutrient cycling one quarter as deep. When you make it deeper, then you*

can put all the plants closer together so there's about four times the plants per unit of area per unit of time, and the nutrient cycling in the soil to support that. Using the double digging technique in 1972 certainly was strenuous. Over time I've found ways to make it easier, so now we have a Grow Biointensive DVD that shows how to dig with almost no effort. I once taught one of the best market gardeners in California how to double dig, and she learned how to do it without any effort. She came back to me two minutes later and said, "John, I just realized something. I really like to work." John Dromgoole was the Southwest region representative for Rodale when I taught in Austin, Texas. After seeing the way we double dig, he said, "John, I now realize nobody's ever really taught us how to dig. You don't really need to use much effort. You can just use your body weight; you shift your body weight and you let gravity and the tool do the rest." If you're digging, you're not digging right. If you're letting the process do it for you, you're digging right.

ACRES U.S.A. *It's tempting to wonder how many other techniques were developed and forgotten and are ripe for revival.*

JEAVONS. The French gardeners, who developed over a 300-year period peaking in the early 1900s, broke into guilds. These were like extended families, and they had a cradle-to-grave social system because their farming was so effective and made a good income. But they had different ways of growing crops that enabled them to bring cantaloupe, for example, to market four to six weeks earlier than anybody else. That's where they made most of their net income. They used all sorts of special tricks and pieces of knowledge. What Ecology Action has been doing is relearning how people 5,000 years ago in Ethiopia, 4,000 years ago in China, 2,000 years ago in Greece, and 1,000 years ago in the Mayan culture structured their biologically intensive forms of raising food. Along the way we've found tricks and little processes that make a big difference. For instance, if you transplant your carrots you can get double the yield that you get if you directly sow them. We've replicated this more than once.

ACRES U.S.A. *Why is that?*

JEAVONS. I don't know all the reasons why, but I think it's because the soil is looser at the point where you transplant the seedling. When you put a seed in, it doesn't germinate for about two to three weeks, and the soil is more compacted by then. Some of the nutrients are less available. And it takes you a fair amount of time to thin a carrot bed that's been broadcast, but it doesn't take much longer to transplant than it does to thin. For many people around the world who want to eat, a little bit of extra time isn't an issue while a lot more food is wonderful. What we found out is that there are lots of economies of small scale. One of them is that we use three to eight times less water per pound of food produced with this biologically intensive system. We use 50 to 100 percent less purchased nutrient in organic fertilizer form. We use 94 to 99 percent less energy in all forms in producing food."

"**ACRES U.S.A.** How long did it take to develop the fundamentals of biointensive growing?

JEAVONS. *We spent the first seven years breaking the code of economic mini-farming. We worked on everything — economics, diet, and sustainable soil fertility — but we focused particularly on income mini-farming. During the second seven years we worked on complete diet mini-farming, and I'll come back to that. Then for the last 26 years we've worked on sustainable soil fertility, which has been the most challenging code to break. Organic farming is not fully sustainable because it imports 50 to 84 percent of its inputs — composts, manures and organic fertilizers — from other soils. Even though we're building up our soils with organic farming, we're depleting other soils. Worldwide there are as few as 34 to 49 years of farmable soil left.*

ACRES U.S.A. *Not to mention challenges like the droughts hitting many parts of the world currently, including part of the U.S.?*

JEAVONS. *It's more than challenging. Biointensive has the potential of using as little as 88 percent less water per pound of vegetable produced, and it has the potential of using as little as 67 percent less water per pound of grain produced. We've found that by growing seedlings in flats and transplanting them, the amount of water you save if you choose the right crops is enough to feed half a person to a whole person for an entire year compared with direct sowing.*

"ACRES U.S.A. Can you cite some extended benefits of those savings?

JEAVONS. *There's a human side to all this that's just terrific and I'll mention one of those sides. In India there are millions of children who have eyesight problems and brain development issues because they don't get enough vitamin A and iron during the first six years of their life. You can grow the missing vitamin A and iron in just a few square feet with dark green vegetables such as collards or parsley. It's so simple that once the children are older, like 4, 5 and 6, they can actually grow their own food."*

"ACRES U.S.A. Let's return to the diet component you mentioned.

JEAVONS. *You asked about how my systems analysis experience helps in farming area and food raising. One of the things we discovered is that special root crops, and there are seven of them, produce a tremendous amount of calories per day per unit of area compared with grains and compared with soybeans. These special root crops can produce as much as five times the calories and more compared with soybeans per unit of area, per unit of time. Here's another way of looking at it. If you have just 100 square feet of wheat and Grow Biointensive intermediate yields, you produce about 15,000 calories. But if you have potatoes, you're going to be producing something like about 70,000 calories. That seems fantastic, and it is. But the wheat takes eight months to grow and the 65-day maturing potato takes only two months to grow, so when you figure out the effectiveness on a per-month basis the potato is incredible! Now, we're not trying to encourage another Irish potato famine because you should have more crops than just potatoes, and we do. Potatoes or sweet potatoes, leeks, garlic, salsify, Jerusalem artichoke, and a few others — if they're part of your diet, they're going to greatly reduce the amount of area it takes to grow your food. Growing the food for the average U.S. diet takes* *an average of about ¾ of an acre, about 30,000 square feet. With a different diet and with biological intensity, we're able to grow all of the nutrients you need for one person for all year in 4,000 square feet. That is seven-and-a-half times the area efficiency. It's not the same diet. It's got a lot of root crops in it. It has some grain crops in it, but in an increasingly desertified world with less farmable land it's the type of diet design that is healthy. And people just may have enough land to grow it.*

ACRES U.S.A. *What are your thoughts about the heavy reliance on soybean and grains in this country?*

JEAVONS. *I think I have one way that will make the challenge clear for people. Certainly it did for me. If you grow soybeans at the kind of yield that they normally produce, which is not a high yield, it takes about 12,000 square feet to grow all of your calories. But if you grow using a cropping plan like we do, then 60 percent of the area is in what we call compost and calorie crops. That's your grain and seed crops such as wheat, corn, and amaranth. They grow a significant amount of calories and a very large amount of compost material. Then in 30 percent of our area the goal is to grow the special root crops that produce so many calories per unit of area per unit of time. In 10 percent of our area we grow vegetable crops for any vitamins or minerals that are not in the other two kinds of crops, and also for income. With this particular kind of combination you can grow all your calories for one person for all year in about six beds — 600 square feet not 12,000 square feet. If you grow a mixed diet plan with 40 beds, then that would be 4,000 square feet rather than 12,000 square feet. Many of the people in the world, especially low income people, are only going to have about 4,500 square feet of farmable land.*

ACRES U.S.A. *Have these ideas been implemented in India, for example?*

JEAVONS. *There are currently people in 142 countries using Grow Biointensive sustainable mini-farming practices. These aren't giant projects, though sometimes large numbers of people are affected. It's reported that there's as many as 2.5 million farmers in Kenya using biointensive practices, and over 2 million people in Mexico have been taught biointensive. In India we had a wonderful experience. In 1976 we got a list of alternative technology agriculture locations around the world. We sent out a letter saying we're doing this ages old but new-to us biologically intensive practice of food raising. It produces higher yields and uses less water, and if you're interested we'll send you a free manual showing how to do it. Only one person in the whole world answered, and that was Dr. Seshadri in Madras, India. We sent him a book, and they ran the test with 22 low-income families who had never farmed before. They had sandy soil, and the only fertilizer they had was fresh manure. By the end of their third season these farmers were getting 75 percent to 100 percent of the yields of the good farmers in India. Now good farmers there average about double the regular average. These formerly* *inexperienced people were in the upper 15th percentile of yields in India. I don't attribute it just to biointensive. I attribute it to the great teaching of the late Dr. Seshadri and his wife Chitra."*

"ACRES U.S.A. *Nature takes many, many years to create rich topsoil. How do you address this reality?*

JEAVONS. *The thing that excites me tremendously is the result of a master's thesis at the University of California at Berkeley in the Soil Science department.*

We discovered that Grow Biointensive has the capacity to build the soil up to 60 times faster than happens in nature, and in fact for every pound of food eaten it can produce up to 20 pounds of farmable soil. This is in contrast to conventional practices in the United States, which result in six pounds of farmable soil getting lost. In developing countries on average 12 pounds of farmable soil are lost.

In China 18 pounds of farmable soil are lost. We're talking about just the reverse being possible, potentially, with biointensive practices. At a time of increasing desertification, at a time in which there is less and less farmable soil left per capita in the world, this is exciting. When I teach workshops, one of the things that I say is, "Here's the most important thing I want everyone here to do for a better world and a better future and a better diet. I want everyone to stop growing crops and I want instead for everyone to grow soil."

ACRES U.S.A. *What do you say next?*

JEAVONS. *If you grow soil, you have to grow crops, so you didn't lose anything. The reason for growing crops isn't just to eat; it's to grow soil. If you grow soil, the soil will provide for you abundantly. This is something we all need to start focusing on — growing soil. To do that we use the recipe I mentioned earlier — 60 percent compost and calorie crops, 30 percent special root crops, and 10 percent vegetable and income crops. It is a goal. There are other percentages that can work. In the tropics it's 50 percent, 30 percent, 20 percent for a 12-month tropical growing season. The important thing is to realize that we've got to feed the soil. Too much of what we're doing now is like milking a cow every day and not feeding it. The cow here that's nurturing us is the soil and what a wonderful opportunity. I'm thinking of a quote from Voltaire in his book Candide. On the last page Candide says, "The whole earth is a garden, and what a wonderful place it would be if each one of us just took care of our part of the garden." I would say our mini-farm, because we need to realize our gardens are powerful farms. There are a lot of challenges happening in the world. There's peak water — it's incredible the degree to which people aren't having enough water, but you're experiencing that in Texas right now. And people are experiencing that in different locations globally. But Ecology Action has a theme, a philosophy, of changing scarcity into abundance. If normally it takes one unit of water to grow a certain amount of food, with Grow Biointensive — if it's practiced properly — you can grow the same amount of food with 1/3 to 1/8 a unit of water. You've just changed from a situation* *where you didn't have enough water to where you have more than enough water. Rain has to come down of course — some.*

ACRES U.S.A. *What happens if it's not practiced properly?*

JEAVONS. *If you don't use Grow Biointensive properly, because it's so productive — it has the capacity for higher yields — you can deplete the soil 2 to 6 times faster than other techniques."*

*"***ACRES U.S.A.** *Is there an upper limit to how far you can scale your techniques?*

JEAVONS. *In 1911 the Chinese were farming their whole country in biologically intensive agriculture. There's no upper-scale limit in that way — China's a big country. However, if we're talking about a single-family farm, is there an upper limit? I have a friend who farmed three acres biointensively in Pennsylvania with just four people, and it was a production farm. It uses more people if you begin to get into the acre range, but what I'd like to encourage people to do is think about income range. If you choose your crops right, you can have a good income on less than an acre. You can even have a good income on a quarter-acre or halfacre. Marketing is half of it. It isn't just growing it."*

John Jeavons' Common Ground Mini-Farm in the U.S. and Iain Tolhurst's Tolhurst Organic farm in the UK are both stockfree, but they differ in two significant respects: first, Jeavons' mini-farm is under 1 acre and Tolhurst's farm, while still small, is much bigger at 19 acres, and second, Jeavons' mini-farm is an experimental farm designed to research the smallest possible plot necessary to sustainably produce all the food one person needs for a healthy diet, whereas Tolhurst's farm is a market farm designed to sustainably produce food for a community of people. While Jeavons' approach is more oriented towards subsistence farming than market farming, it can also be scaled up to where a collective of people could make a good income from marketing their produce.

As a research farm, Jeavons meticulously recorded all the inputs and outputs from his mini-farm, and as he noted in the interview above, by using his biointensive farming techniques, one person can sustainably meet all their nutritional requirements on 4,000 square feet, which is less than one tenth of an acre. Of course, for these numbers to add up, the mini-farmer must eat a plant-based diet that contains a lot of root crops and some grain crops. Between anthropologist Richard Wrangham's cooked tuber diet of H. erectus and John Jeavons' root crop dependent mini-farm diet, we have come full circle in a return to the natural human diet we evolved to thrive on.

The secret to biointensive farming is deep cycling of soil nutrients by first double digging the garden beds to a 24 inch depth, and then by growing 50% to 60% "compost and calorie crops" like wheat, corn, and amaranth that grow a significant amount of calories and a very large amount of compost material. The compost made from crop residues is continuously folded back into the beds. This deep cycling of soil nutrients allows for very close spacing of plants and continuous harvesting and transplanting year-round. As Jeavons noted above, farming biointensively uses 94% to 99% less energy in all forms to produce food, and potentially uses 88% less water/pound of vegetables and 67% less water/pound of grain than traditional organic farming.

Perhaps the most exciting development in Jeavons' biointensive mini-farm experiment is that he has replicated his experimental results with farmers in 142 countries around the world, including as many as 2.5 million in Kenya and over 2 million in Mexico. In an increasingly food insecure world, Jeavons' remarks about a sustainable diet become ever more prescient, "*It's not the same diet. It's got a lot of root crops in it. It has some grain crops in it, but in an increasingly desertified world with less farmable land it's the type of diet design that is healthy. And people just may have enough land to grow it.*" Biointensive mini-farming will be key to food security for hundreds of millions of people over the coming decades of the 21st century.

Humanure

The Vegan Organic Network (VON) Veganic Standards reviewed above prohibit the use of "*Human faeces and urine*" as soil amendments. Considering that human excretions are animal byproducts the same as cattle or chicken excretions, there's a clear logic to their reasoning. But banning this valuable source of soil nutrients also runs afoul of the VON principle of operating a veganic farm as near as possible to a "*closed system*," since soil nutrients leaving the farm as produce must be replaced with soil nutrients taken from somewhere else.

In this instance where two principles of veganic farming come into direct conflict, I would argue that closing the soil nutrient cycle should take precedence over the ban on human feces and urine. In the wild, animal excreta are a natural part of the soil nutrient cycle; the veganic total ban on animal excreta is not due to its unsuitability as a soil amendment, rather it is because the manures available on the market are derived from factory farmed livestock operations that are environmental sacrifice zones. But if humans were to transition back to our natural plant-based diet and stop raising livestock, we would become the single most populous large domesticated animal on the planet, and recycling our manure would become the missing link in closing the soil nutrient cycle. With over 7.7 billion people and counting on Earth, humanure is a vast untapped resource that is literally being flushed away and polluting and depleting trillions of gallons of fresh water in the process. This unsustainable system of "waste disposal" is the height of human folly.

One of the least heralded but most consequential books of the early 21st century was self-published by Joseph Jenkins in 2005 entitled "*The Humanure Handbook.*" Now in its third addition, Jenkins began writing the book in the early 90s as a thesis for his Masters of Science in Sustainable Systems from Slippery Rock University, Slippery Rock, Pennsylvania, USA. Later he converted his thesis into a book format that has since been translated into a dozen languages, and sold thousands of copes worldwide. Jenkins cuts through all the squeamishness people have about their own crap (what he calls "*fecophobia*"), and presents the most comprehensive analysis ever written on recycling human manure (and urine) into a nutrient rich soil amendment.

Jenkins deals with all aspects of composting humanure starting with "*The Human Nutrient Cycle*":

"When crops are produced from soil, it is advisable that the organic residues resulting from those crops, including animal excrements, be returned to the soil where the crops originated. This recycling of organic residues for agricultural purposes is fundamental to sustainable agriculture. Yet, spokespersons for sustainable agriculture movements remain silent about using humanure for agricultural purposes. Why?

"Perhaps the silence is because there is currently a profound lack of knowledge and understanding about what is referred to as the "human nutrient cycle" and the need to keep the cycle intact. The human nutrient cycle goes like this: a) we grow food, b) we eat it, c) we collect and process the organic residues (feces, urine, food scraps and agricultural materials) and d) we then return the processed organic material back to the soil, thereby enriching the soil and enabling more food to be grown. This cycle can be repeated, endlessly. This is a process that mimics the cycles of nature and enhances our ability to survive on this planet. When our food refuse materials are instead discarded as waste, the natural human nutrient cycle is broken, creating problems such as pollution, loss of soil fertility and abuse of our water resources."

Jenkins devotes in depth chapters to how sewer water and sewage sludge contaminated with feces and urine are breeding grounds for antibiotic resistant disease causing bacteria, and how beneficial bacteria in humanure promote breaking down organic materials into nutrient rich, pathogen free *"humus"* that is safe to apply to food crops. He estimates that in the U.S. alone, around 1,000 pounds of humanure/person/year is wasted, which amounted to approximately 150 million tons/year in the late 1990s.

Jenkins goes on to discuss every manner of humanure collection device being used in different cultures around the world; he then describes the very simple, elegant and easy to use, self-built toilet that he and his family have used at home for years, which is far more practical to operate for the average backyard composter:

"How it works is a model of simplicity. One begins by depositing one's organic refuse (feces and urine) into a receptacle intended for that purpose, with about a five-gallon (20 liter) capacity. Food scraps should be kept in a separate receptacle, but can also be deposited into the toilet receptacle, if necessary. A five gallon capacity is recommended because a larger size would be too heavy to carry when full.

"The contents of the toilet are always kept covered with a clean, organic cover material such as rotted sawdust, peat moss, leaf mould, rice hulls or grass clippings, in order to prevent odors, absorb urine and eliminate any fly nuisance. Urine is deposited into the same receptacle, and as the liquid rises, more cover material is added so that a clean layer of organic material covers the toilet contents at all times.

"A lid is kept on the toilet receptacle when not in use. The lid need not be air tight; a standard, hinged toilet seat is quite suitable. The lid does not necessarily prevent odor from escaping, and it does not necessarily prevent flies from gaining access to the toilet contents. Instead, the cover

material does. The cover material acts as an organic lid or biofilter, the physical lid or toilet
seat is used primarily for convenience and aesthetics."

"Full receptacles are carried to the composting area and deposited on the pile (you'll know that
a receptacle is full enough to empty when you have to stand up to take a shit)."

"It is best to dig a slight depression in the top of the center of the compost pile in the outdoor
compost bin, then deposit the fresh toilet material there, in order to keep the incoming humanure
in the hotter center of the pile. This is easily achieved by raking aside the cover material on top
of the pile, depositing the toilet contents in the resulting depression, and then raking the cover
material back over the fresh deposit. The area is then immediately covered with additional
clean, bulky, organic material such as straw leaves or weeds, in order to eliminate odors and
to trap air as the pile is built."

(Personal note: I myself have been using this system to compost my own humanure for years
and I can personally attest to its safety, functionality, and beneficial effects in my garden. If readers
are interested in recycling their own humanure, I would strongly recommend getting your own copy
of *"The Humanure Handbook,"* **since there are very important sections about proper sanitation that**
you should study before trying this at home.)

The humanure recycling system Jenkins describes above is designed for single family use for people
living in rural or suburban areas where they have enough room for a garden and a compost pile. But
Jenkins has a much bigger vision for large centralized recycling systems to compost everyone's humanure
the world over. In a dialogue with himself, Jenkins lays out his vision for how to close the soil nutrient
cycle around the globe:

"MS [Myself]: I predict… that composting toilets and toilet systems will continue to be designed
and redesigned in our lifetimes. Eventually, entire housing developments or entire communities
will utilize composting toilet systems. Some municipalities will eventually install composting
toilets in all new homes.

"M [Me]: You think so? What would that be like?

"MS: Well, each home would have a removable container made of recycled plastic that would
act as both a toilet receptacle and a garbage disposal.

"M: How big a container?

"MS: You'd need about five gallons of capacity per person per week. A container the size of
a 50-gallon drum would be full in about two weeks for an average family. Every household
would deposit all of its organic material except graywater into this receptacle, including maybe
some grass clippings and yard leaves. The municipality could provide a cover material for
odor prevention, consisting of ground leaves, rotted sawdust, or ground newsprint, neatly
packaged for each household and possibly dispensed automatically into the toilet after each

use. This would eliminate the production of all organic garbage and all sewage, as it would all be collected without water and composted at a municipal compost yard.

"M: Who'd collect it?

"MS: Once every couple of weeks or so, your municipality or a business under contract with your municipality would take the compost receptacle from your house. A new compost receptacle would then replace the old. This is already being done in the entire province of Nova Scotia, Canada, and in areas of Europe where organic kitchen materials are collected and composted.

"When toilet material is added to the system, your manure, urine and [organic] garbage, mixed together with ground leaves and other organic refuse or crop residues, would then be collected regularly, just like your garbage is collected now. Except the destination would not be a landfill, it'd be the compost yard where the organic material would be converted, through thermophilic composting, into an agricultural resource and sold to farmers, gardeners, and landscapers who'd use it to grow things. The natural cycle would be complete, immense amounts of landfill space would be saved, a valuable resource would be recovered, pollution would be drastically reduced, if not prevented, and soil fertility would be enhanced. So would our long-term survival as human beings on this planet."

In China, Korea and Japan, where civilizations have thrived for millennia and human populations have grown immense, farmers managed to grow bountiful crops continuously on the same plots of land for thousands of years. In 1905, Dr. F. H. King, who had been Professor of Agricultural Physics at the University of Wisconsin, USA, and Chief of the Division of Soil Management of the U.S. Department of Agriculture, wanted to know how these Eastern farmers kept their soils fertile without all the inputs of Western agriculture, so he traveled to Asia to find out for himself. When he returned, he wrote a book about his experience entitled, "Farmers of Forty Centuries or Permanent Agriculture in China, Korea and Japan," which was published posthumously by his wife in 1911. In "The Humanure Handbook," Jenkins quotes this passage from Dr. Kings book:

"One of the most remarkable practices adopted by any civilized people is the centuries long and well nigh universal conservation and utilization of all [humanure] in China, Korea and Japan, turning it to marvelous account in the maintenance of soil fertility and in the production of food. To understand this evolution it must be recognized that mineral fertilizers so extensively employed in modern Western agriculture have been a physical impossibility to all people alike until very recent years. With this fact must be associated the very long unbroken life of these nations and the vast numbers their farmers have been compelled to feed.

When we reflect upon the depleted fertility of our own older farm lands, comparatively few of which have seen a century's service, and upon the enormous quantity of mineral fertilizers which are being applied annually to them in order to secure paying yields, it becomes evident that the time is here when profound consideration should be given to the practices the

Mongolian race has maintained through many centuries, which permit it to be said of China that one sixth of an acre of good land is ample for the maintenance of one person, and which are feeding an average of three people per acre of farm land in the three southern most islands of Japan.

[Western humanity] is the most extravagant accelerator of waste the world has ever endured. His withering blight has fallen upon every living thing within his reach, himself not excepted; and his besom of destruction in the uncontrolled hands of a generation has swept into the sea soil fertility which only centuries of life could accumulate, and yet this fertility is the substratum of all that is living."

As also noted by Dr. King, in these Asian countries, so called "night soil" was collected and sold back to farmers where it was applied raw to the fields. While this practice did complete the soil nutrient cycle and sustained soil fertility, it also provided a vector for disease organisms in the food supply; organisms that are destroyed when properly composted as prescribed by Jenkins in "The Humanure Handbook." Most revealing in Dr. King's book is that it was already known by the early 1900s that Western agricultural practices were depleting soil fertility in the U.S.

Modern industrialized agriculture in which soil nutrients that leave the farm in the form of food products are replaced with synthetic nitrogen fertilizers and mined mineral soil amendments, and in which human excreta is dumped into the ocean or landfills, is not a sustainable system of agriculture. If we continue down this path, it is not a question of if, but when this unsustainable system will collapse causing crop failures, famine and pestilence. In *"The Humanure Handbook,"* Joseph Jenkins offers a visionary, plausible, alternative for a sustainable system that closes the human nutrient cycle and ensures the perpetuation of food production indefinitely. The only remaining question is whether or not we humans can get over our collective case of fecophobia and return to our natural place in the soil nutrient cycle.

In 2019 the UN Population Division estimated that by 2050 the human population of the world will increase by two billion people bringing the total to 9.7 billion mouths to feed. Feeding this unprecedented number of people a healthy diet on less arable land with less predictable weather patterns over the coming decades is going to be the greatest challenge in the history of agriculture.

As we have seen, producing an animal-based diet is the most inefficient and environmentally destructive way to grow food that is unhealthy for people. The livestock sector of the agricultural economy is responsible for enormous GHG emissions, mass species extinctions and epidemics of chronic degenerative diseases.

The exact opposite is true of producing a plant-based diet: it is the most efficient and environmentally sustainable way to grow healthy food for people. If the vast tracks of agricultural land devoted to raising livestock were broken-up into small and medium sized farms (from 1 to 250 acres) growing fruits, vegetables, nuts, grains and tubers, overall farm efficiency and crop diversity would increase dramatically. If humanure were reintroduced back into the soil nutrient cycle, farmers could grow abundant healthy food for everyone in the world while stabilizing the environment and preserving soil fertility for generations to come. And if people were to adopt a plant-based diet, the scourge of chronic degenerative diseases could be banished forever.

24

FOOD SECURITY AND THE GLOBAL FOOD TRADE

Food Security

In 1996 the Food and Agriculture Organization (FAO) of the United Nations (UN) held a *"World Food Summit"* in Rome, Italy, attended by high level governmental delegations from 186 participating countries. In its final report the summit defined *"food security"* as *"when all people, at all times, have physical, social and economic access to sufficient, safe and nutritious food to meet their dietary needs and food preferences for an active and healthy life."* At a subsequent *"World Summit of Food Security"* held in 2009, the FAO added the *"four pillars of food security: availability, access, utilization, and stability,"* to its definition of food security. Food security has been a top priority of the FAO for decades and in 2015, in its ambitious *2030 Agenda for Sustainable Development*, the UN codified 17 *Sustainable Development Goals* including the goal of zero hunger by 2030.

The main measure of food security used by the FAO is the percentage of a given population that has a caloric intake sufficient to meet the minimum energy requirements defined as necessary for that population. By this measure, the FAO's world food security survey for 2017 found that 663 million people globally (8.8% of the world population) were undernourished. While this number was well down from the 883 million undernourished people (13.4%) in 2001, it began to trend up again after 2013 when it stood at 643 million people. Reducing food insecurity for over 200 million people in less than two decades is no small feat and lends credence to the effectiveness of many FAO programs that have relieved chronic undernourishment in some food insecure regions of the world. Yet, in 2017 there were still a staggering 663 million people going to bed hungry every night and that number is likely to increase as climate change, loss of arable land and fresh water depletion exact their toll on agricultural food production in the years to come.

In 2017, FAO data indicated that globally more than 50% of people suffering from severe food insecurity lived in Asia, nearly 40% lived in Africa, and the remaining 10% were divided among the Americas, Europe and Oceania. As a percentage of national population, food insecurity was highest in Sub-Saharan African countries where nearly one third of the people were defined as severely insecure. In these regions of the world where food insecurity is most pronounced, smallholder farms are the primary food producers, but while the average yield per hectare for smallholder farms worldwide is higher than that of medium and large sized farms, smallholder farms in food insecure regions have much lower yields per hectare, such that historically they have not met the caloric needs of their population.

There have been numerous studies conducted by the FAO, WHO, World Bank and other public and private institutions to investigate why food insecurity is so prevalent in these regions and to find solutions that improve people's access to sufficient quantities of healthy food. Many of these studies have focused on increased production and marketing of fruits and vegetables. The 2015 study, *"How does the Fruit and Vegetable Sector contribute to Food and Nutrition Security?"* (Wageningen University and Research Centre, Netherlands, Belgium, June 2015), summarized the findings to date of the best research on this tragic prevalence of systemic hunger.

To begin, the authors report on the growth in recent decades of the fruit and vegetable sector of the agricultural economy in these food insecure regions:

> *"Strong growth rates in fruit and vegetable cultivation have also been recorded in food-insecure and low-income regions such as Sub-Saharan Africa and Southern Asia. Especially countries like Kenya, Ethiopia, Ghana, Rwanda, Uganda, Indonesia and Viet Nam have expansion of fruit and vegetable production (Figure 3.2). In particular high-value crops, like fruit and vegetables, have been identified as one of the fastest growing agricultural sub sectors in Sub-Saharan Africa in the past two decades (Afari-Sefa, 2007)."*

These facts suggest that much of the reduced food insecurity in Africa and Asia between 2001 and 2017 was due to increased production from the fruit and vegetable sector.

The authors go on to discuss the contribution of the fruit and vegetable sector to the agricultural economy in food insecure countries:

> *"The fruit and vegetable sector compares favourably with cereals and other food crop sectors in terms of employment and income generation. The production of vegetables has a comparative advantage particularly under conditions where arable land is scarce and labour is abundant."*

> *"Fruit and vegetable crops generate more income for farmers compared to traditional staple crops. In addition they generate employment for the rural workers, and therefore improve access to food (Weinberger and Lumpkin, 2007). This positive correlation between vegetable commercialisation and household income is confirmed by various researchers. For example, Muriithi and Matz (2015) found a positive welfare effect for vegetable producers in Kenya. Afari-Sefa (2007) identified positive income effects for fruit producers in Ghana. Also English et al. (2004) indicate that vegetable production is more profitable for a smallholder than the traditional maize-bean intercropping system often found in Kenya."*

> *"The figures indicate that fruit and vegetable producers [in Kenya] are much better off than non-horticulture smallholders, with a mean income that is four times larger. Also workers on exporter-owned farms and independent commercial farms do better than non-horticulture*

smallholders. As a result poverty rates are much lower among workers employed in the fruit and vegetable sector. Most of these workers are paid a wage that is above the government-mandated minimum agricultural wage."

In other words, the fruit and vegetable sector of the agricultural economy employs more people, provides more income, is more profitable and lifts more people out of poverty than cereals and other food crop sectors.

The authors found that fruit and vegetable farmers were better integrated into the food economy:

"[V]egetable producers are better integrated into markets. For instance in Bangladesh, farmers on average sell 96% of their vegetable products but only 19% of their cereal output (Weinberger and Genova, 2005). The same pattern is reported for other countries in Southeast Asia and East Africa. A study from Tanzania that analysed the significance of traditional African vegetables in agricultural production showed that the degree of commercialisation is high for fruits as well as traditional African vegetables (i.e. amaranth and African eggplant) and exotic vegetables (i.e. tomato and cabbage). In this study, 100% of farmers who grew fruits, 98% of farmers who grew exotic vegetables, and 88% of farmers who grew traditional African vegetables marketed their output. In comparison, only 49% of farmers who grew cereals marketed their output (Weinberger and Msuya, 2004)."

"Minot (2002) found that both fruit and vegetable production in Viet Nam is highly commercialised, with about 70% of fruit and vegetable farmers selling their output. Minot compared the degree of commercialisation for wealthy and poor farmers. The market integration of the highest income quintile is higher at 75%, while in the poorest income quintile, 56% sell their output to the market."

In effect, this means that fruits and vegetables are much more marketable commodities than cereal grains in the food economy of food insecure countries.

The authors found that the fruit and vegetable sector made the largest contribution to the welfare of women and children:

"Women in particular have been able to capitalise on these new labour market opportunities. In Africa, Asia, and Latin America, high-value crop [fruits and vegetables] exports are female intensive industries, with women dominating most aspects of production and processing. Evidence suggests that women occupy at least 50% or more of the employment in these industries (Dolan and Sorby, 2003). Often these farm workers are landless women who have few other opportunities for earning an income (McCulloch and Ota, 2002)."

"In Ethiopia we found that a medium-scale farm of about 10 ha can employ 38–50 women a day to weed, pick, and grade. In addition about 17 men are employed to spray and irrigate the fields, transporting and loading. Many farm labourers typically own little or no land of their own and tend to be poorer than most smallholders, especially those engaged in fruit and

vegetable production. Consequently, their employment in the fruit and vegetable sector has a direct effect on poverty reduction."

"Women tend to invest in their families by providing more food, preventative health care and education for their children (Hoddinott and Haddad, 1995). As a result female-headed households appear to spend more on fruit and particularly vegetables than male-headed households (Ruel et al., 2005). They found that in Rwanda, female-headed households allocated a large share of their budget to fruit and vegetable consumption. Also in Kenya where more female-headed households were found in the highest fruit and vegetables expenditure quintile (Ayieko et al., 2005)."

These finding indicate that growing fruits and vegetables empowers women to earn a better living and to better care for their children.

The authors note that the fruit and vegetable sector contributes to the overall health of the population:

"It is widely accepted that fruit and vegetables are important component of a healthy diet and that the consumption can help prevent a wide range of diseases. The WHO/FAO recommends a minimum of 400g of fruit and vegetables per day (excluding potatoes and other starchy tubers) for the prevention of chronic diseases such as heart disease, cancer, diabetes and obesity, as well as for the prevention and alleviation of several micronutrient deficiencies, especially in less developed countries."

In essence, the fruit and vegetable sector of the agricultural economy provides the biggest nutritional bang for the buck of any other food crop sector.

In order for the fruit and vegetable sector in food insecure countries to thrive, the authors indicate certain macro and micro economic preconditions that are necessary:

"At the macro level, crucial factors of the FNS [Food and Nutrition Security] system include macro-economic stability, inclusive economic growth, public spending, and governance and quality of institutions. The state and related institutions play an important role in ensuring that public services are provided effectively and efficiently to citizens and that a good business climate attracts domestic and foreign private investments. Such investments, in addition to advances in productivity, are critical for accelerating economic growth and income generation. Whether economic growth improves FNS depends on a number of factors (Ecker and Breisinger, 2012). Research confirms that economic growth is good for improving food and nutrition security, especially at early stages of development. Economic growth and agricultural growth in particular are crucial for reducing undernourishment and thus for improving people's calorie sufficiency.

Here, the authors throw in the caveat that in order for smallholder fruit and vegetable farmers to have access to the marketplace there must be a responsive government, a peaceful business climate and a functional supply chain infrastructure.

The authors note that simply producing more fruits and vegetables is not enough to reduce food insecurity. Demand for fruits and vegetables must also be stimulated through nutritional education programs:

> *"Of at least equal importance are nutrition and awareness and education campaigns that educate the malnourished population about the importance of good nutritional habits. Lack of this understanding will severely limit the potential impact of growth and policies aimed at improving people's economic access to improved sources of nutrition (Ecker et al., 2011)."*

People living in food insecure regions, just like people living in food secure regions, need to be educated as to what constitutes a healthy diet. The authors of this study did not specify teaching the health advantages of a whole-food, plant-based diet, but as we have seen, that is clearly what is called for in food insecure and secure regions alike.

The authors of *"How does the Fruit and Vegetable Sector contribute to Food and Nutrition Security?"* concluded their report with these remarks:

> *"When comparing to other crop production sectors, the F&V [Fruit & Vegetable] sector is far more labour intensive. The traditional small-scale fruit and vegetable production and marketing sector is still the most important sector in terms of employment, income and scale of production. However, informal and inefficient supply chain arrangements provide low income and offer little incentives for growers and their families to improve their production and marketing activities. Smallholders could alter their market focus and target markets where more value is added and supply chain arrangements are more efficiently organised and implemented.*
>
> *"More opportunities are provided for F&V growers to link with upcoming small and medium-sized enterprises in the African agri-food sector that invests in logistics, wholesale, warehousing, cold storage, processing, local fast food and retail. Another important trend is the upcoming supermarket sector in Asia and Sub-Saharan Africa. Surveys in Kenya and Indonesia show that F&V growers who participate in these higher value supply chain arrangements for the domestic and regional markets (preferred suppliers) receive a higher income. Improving the level of organisation among F&V growers and creating economies of scale in the smallholder sector is a precondition for their inclusion in these emerging F&V supply chains."*

In their final analysis, the authors found that while the fruit and vegetable sector offers the best opportunity for smallholder farms in food insecure regions to integrate into the agricultural economy and to become food secure, there are institutional barriers that prevent them from fully realizing their potential. The authors call for smallholders to organize together to create economies of scale is basically a blueprint for a co-operative economic model of agriculture in which smallholders' join together to share production and marketing resources to create better working relations with large retailers. This study is a road map for how the fruit and vegetable sector of the agricultural economy can lead the way to food security in food insecure regions of the world.

The study did not compare the contribution to the agricultural economy of the fruit and vegetable sector to the animal products sector in these food insecure regions. But as we have seen throughout this book, animal agriculture does not compare favorably to growing fruits and vegetables in terms of yields per hectare, calories provided, micro nutrient content, or land use. Most livestock operators in food insecure regions of the world graze sheep or goats on marginal land and do not use imported feed to quickly bring animals to slaughter weight, so meat production is limited. Dairy and egg production are also inefficient relative to fruit and vegetable production, so expanding animal food production to reduce food insecurity in food insecure countries just doesn't add up.

The Global Food Trade

According to the *World Bank*, in 2016 food products accounted for 8.9% of the world's total exports of merchandise. According to the *World Atlas* website, worldatlas.com, in 2016 the U.S. was by far the world's largest food exporter at $72.7 billion. The top importers of U.S. food exports were Canada, Mexico, Japan and Germany, and the main foods exported from the U.S. were maize, soybeans, milk, wheat, sugar beet, sugar cane, potatoes, and chicken. Germany was the second largest food exporter at $34.6 billion. The top importers of German food exports were the U.S., France, the UK, and China, and the main exports from Germany were sugar beets, milk, wheat, and potatoes. The UK was the third largest food exporter at $29.5 billion. The top importers of UK food exports were the European Union, the U.S. and China, and the UK's main exports were milk, wheat, sugar beets, and barley. China was the fourth largest food exporter at $25.1 billion. The top importers of Chinese food exports were the U.S., Hong Kong, Japan, and South Korea, and China's main exports were maize, rice, fresh vegetables, and wheat. The next 5 through 10 top food exporters were France, Netherlands, Japan, Canada, Belgium and Italy. One observation is clear from this blur of economic data: most of the world food trade takes place between food secure countries, and most of the food traded is in staple foods.

In the report, "*Countries Most Dependent On Others For Food*" (*World Atlas*, December 5 2017), the authors explain why it is that the world's most food secure countries import the most food:

> "*Continued population and/or income increase have pushed the United States, China, Germany, Japan and the United Kingdom up the list of the Countries Who Import the Most Food.*"

> "*The United States, being one of the world's largest economies, imports a total of $133 billion USD worth of food and food products, followed by China at $105.26 billion USD, Germany at $98.90 billion USD, Japan at $68.86 billion USD, the United Kingdom at $66.54 billion USD,*"

the Netherlands at $64.38 billion USD, France *at $62.29 billion USD,* Italy *at $51.34 billion USD,* Belgium *at $40.87 billion USD, and the* Russian Federation *at $38.60 billion USD.*

"*However, importing a high amount of food does not necessarily mean that a country is food insecure. In fact, many of the world's largest food importing countries also happen to be among the world's wealthiest. It is important to note that majority of the countries importing the most food in the world have the potential to become completely food sufficient if they choose to do so. In these cases, where food insecurity is not of concern, food is imported to create more variety for the consumer, not to prevent starvation within the population. Importing a large amount of food does not mean that a country is food insecure.*"

What this means is that most of the world's food exports or imports are not to relieve hunger in food insecure countries, but rather to expand food choices in food secure countries.

In 2016, food exports from food secure countries to food insecure countries amounted to only a small fraction of the world food trade, but if the following prediction by the *World Atlas* comes true, this situation will change dramatically by the mid 21st century:

"*By year* 2050*, more than half of the world's population is expected to rely on food sourced from other countries. A comprehensive study conducted by Marianela Fader of Potsdam Institute for Climate Impact Research shows that population pressures will push many nations to make maximizing their domestic food production capacity a top priority. This conclusion was made after the research team computed the growing capability of each and every country to do so, and differentiated their respective production capacities with their current and future food requirements. The team's model made use of soil categories, climate information, and patterns of land utilization for each country, which were then translated into yields for numerous kinds of crops. By using the information on hand regarding the respective populations and water and food intakes of each nation, the team was able to closely evaluate what percentage of its food requirement each country could produce on their own in the future.*

"*Significant issues with food security will continue to trouble the world in coming years if the aforementioned study plays out to be an accurate projection. One way to combat such concern is for each country, rich or poor, to focus its resources on improving their agricultural productivity, which can play an important role in alleviating food shortages. Another possible solution is diet modifications geared towards the consumption of crops that are already produced locally, although further studies will have to be conducted to determine the viability of this option.*"

While it is notable that the authors of this *World Atlas* report made mention of "*diet modifications*" as one possible solution to world food insecurity, to hedge their bets on the "*viability*" of this option was unwarranted. As we have seen in many of the studies presented above, a plant-based diet containing no animal products would in fact go a long way to improving food security in food insecure countries while also improving overall nutrition and helping to mitigate the environmental impacts of animal agriculture.

The remark above by the *World Atlas* that the "*majority of the countries importing the most food in the world have the potential to become completely food sufficient if they choose to do so,*" indicates that most of the world's international food trade is completely unnecessary to relieve food insecurity in wealthy countries. And the *World Atlas*' recommendation for "*consumption of crops that are already produced locally*" as a possible solution to hunger in food insecure countries, suggests that food importation is not a long term solution to food insecurity in poor countries. While both of these statements are manifestly true, if these economic scenarios were to play out to their expected conclusions, there would be no need for any international food trade at all. But of course, eliminating the world food trade is neither a practical nor feasible approach to ending world food insecurity in a future where fully half the human population is expected to be reliant on food imports from other countries, (that is, if people don't shift towards a plant-based diet).

Local production and consumption of fruits, vegetables and staple crops is the single most effective strategy to relieving hunger in food insecure countries, but regional famines caused by hot and cold spells, long term droughts, more powerful storms and frequent floods, and incessant wars, are becoming more common with progression of climate change. Food imports under these adverse conditions will be essential to avoid mass starvation. Also, the export and import of specialty fruits, vegetables and spices native to specific geographic regions and climates can provide a valuable source of income to farmers and a valuable source of variety and nutrition to distant consumers. With widespread adoption of a plant-based diet, the mass export and import of maize and soybeans used for animal feed could be eliminated, and local farms could supply these staple crops for local human consumption.

Facilitation of the international food trade requires a vast network of transportation infrastructure to move the food from place to place, and to transport large quantities of food over long distances requires burning large amounts of greenhouse gas (GHG) emitting fossil fuels. Since transportation of food contributes to the GHG emissions of agriculture, the question must be asked: does the positive contribution to world food security of the international food trade outweigh its negative contribution to global warming? In the report, "*Environmental impacts of food production*" (*OurWorldInData.org.*, January 2020), the authors attempt to answer this question:

> "*You want to reduce the carbon footprint of your food? Focus on what you eat, not whether your food is local*"
>
> "*'Eating local' is a recommendation you hear often – even from prominent sources,* <u>including the United Nations</u>. *While it might make sense intuitively – after all, transport does lead to emissions – it is one of the most misguided pieces of advice.*
>
> "*Eating locally would only have a significant impact if transport was responsible for a large share of food's final carbon footprint. For most foods, this is not the case.*

"GHG emissions from transportation make up a very small amount of the emissions from food and what you eat is far more important than where your food traveled from."

Here the authors break down the sources of GHG emissions from agriculture:

"In this study, the authors looked at data across more than 38,000 commercial farms in 119 countries.[16]

"In this comparison we look at the total GHG emissions per kilogram of food product. CO2 is the most important GHG, but not the only one – agriculture is a large source of the greenhouse gases methane and nitrous oxide. To capture all GHG emissions from food production researchers therefore express them in kilograms of 'carbon dioxide equivalents'. This metric takes account not just CO2 but all greenhouse gases.[17]

"The most important insight from this study: there are massive differences in the GHG emissions of different foods: producing a kilogram of beef emits 60 kilograms of greenhouse gases (CO2-equivalents). While peas emits just 1 kilogram per kg.

"Overall, animal-based foods tend to have a higher footprint than plant-based. Lamb and cheese both emit more than 20 kilograms CO2-equivalents per kilogram. Poultry and pork have lower footprints but are still higher than most plant-based foods, at 6 and 7 kg CO2-equivalents, respectively."

As we have seen time and again, the production of animal foods emits many times more greenhouse gases than does the production of plant foods, so eating less animal foods, even if locally produced, cuts GHG emissions many times more than boycotting foreign grown fruits and vegetables.

Here the authors factor in the GHG emission from transportation into the overall GHG emission from agricultural production in the European Union (EU) and the U.S.:

"[H]ere we show the results of a study which looked at the footprint of diets across the EU. Food transport was responsible for only 6% of emissions, whilst dairy, meat and eggs accounted for 83%.[18]

"In a study published in Environmental Science & Technology, Christopher Weber and Scott Matthews (2008) investigated the relative climate impact of food miles and food choices in households in the US.[19]

"They estimated that if the average household substituted their calories from red meat and dairy to chicken, fish or eggs just one day per week they would save 0.3 tCO2eq. [But if] they replaced it with plant-based alternatives they would save 0.46 tCO2eq. In other words, going 'red meat and dairy-free' (not totally meat-free) one day per week would achieve the same as having a diet with zero food miles."

"There are also a number of cases where eating locally might in fact increase emissions. In most countries, many foods can only be grown and harvested at certain times of the year. But consumers want them year-round. This gives us three options: import goods from countries where they are in-season; use energy-intensive production methods (such as greenhouses) to

produce them year-round; or use refrigeration and other preservation methods to store them for several months. There are many examples of studies which show that importing often has a lower footprint. Hospido et al. (2009) estimate that importing Spanish lettuce to the UK during winter months results in three to eight times lower emissions than producing it locally.21 The same applies for other foods: tomatoes produced in greenhouses in Sweden used 10 times as much energy as importing tomatoes from Southern Europe where they were in-season.22"

Easily missed in this presentation is the calculation that if people in the U.S. were to adopt a plant-based alternative diet seven days per week, they would save over 26 times more GHG equivalents than by forgoing red meat and dairy just once per week. This amounts to 1.12 tons of CO_2 equivalents/household/week; with over 120 million households in the U.S. in 2021, the total savings would be well over 120 million tons of CO_2 equivalents/week in the U.S. alone.

Here the authors point out how air-freight is the exception to the rule when buying imported foods:

"Avoid the small share of foods that are air-freighted

"The impact of transport is small for most products, but there is one exception: those which travel by air.

"Many believe that air-freight is more common than it actually is. Very little food is air-freighted; it accounts for only 0.16% of food miles.23 But for the few products which are transported by air, the emissions can be very high: it emits 50 times more CO_2eq than boat per tonne kilometer.24

"Many of the foods people assume to come by air are actually transported by boat – avocados and almonds are prime examples. Shipping one kilogram of avocados from Mexico to the United Kingdom would generate 0.21kg CO_2eq in transport emissions.25 This is only around 8% of avocados' total footprint.26 Even when shipped at great distances, its emissions are much less than locally-produced animal products.

"Which foods are air-freighted? How do we know which products to avoid?

"They tend to be foods which are highly perishable. This means they need to be eaten soon after they've been harvested. In this case, transport by boat is too slow, leaving air travel as the only feasible option.

"Some fruit and vegetables tend to fall into this category. Asparagus, green beans and berries are common air-freighted goods.

To avoid air-freighted foods, people should stick to local fresh fruits and vegetables when they are in season locally, and switch to preserved fruits and vegetables in the off-season.

Here the authors show that no matter where or how animal foods are produced, they almost always give off more GHG emissions than plant foods:

"Many argue that this overlooks the large variation in the footprints of foods across the world. Using global averages might give us a misleading picture for some parts of the world or some

producers. If I source my beef or lamb from low-impact producers, could they have a lower footprint than plant-based alternatives?

"The evidence suggests, no: plant-based foods emit fewer greenhouse gases than meat and dairy, regardless of how they are produced.

"Let's take a look at the full range of footprints for protein-rich foods.

"Protein-rich foods account for the bulk of our dietary emissions. In European diets, meat, dairy and eggs account for 83%. That's why I focus on them here.

"The median footprint for beef is 25 kgCO2eq.30 But some producers have a much higher footprint: ten percent emit more than 105 kgCO2eq per 100 grams. At the other end, some are much lower. Ten percent emit less than 9 kgCO2eq. We see from the height of the curve that most beef production lies in the range between 17 to 27 kgCO2eq."

"How do the distributions between plant-based and meat-based sources compare?"

"Plant-based protein sources – tofu, beans, peas and nuts – have the lowest carbon footprint. This is certainly true when you compare average emissions. But it's still true when you compare the extremes: there's not much overlap in emissions between the worst producers of plant proteins, and the best producers of meat and dairy.

"Let's compare the highest-impact producers (the top ten percent) of plant-based proteins with the lowest-impact producers (the bottom ten percent) of meat and dairy.

"The pea producers with the highest footprint emit just 0.8 kgCO2eq per 100 grams of protein.31 For nuts it is 2.4 and for tofu, 3.5 kgCO2eq. All are several times less than the lowest impact lamb (12 kgCO2eq) and beef (9 kgCO2eq). Emissions are also lower than those from the best cheese and pork (4.5 kgCO2eq); and slightly lower or comparable to those from the lowest-footprint chicken (2.4 kgCO2eq).32

"If you want a lower-carbon diet, eating less meat is nearly always better than eating the most sustainable meat."

The more relevant message here is that eating a plant-based diet is always more sustainable than eating the most sustainably produced meat even if it was produced by your friendly local rancher.

The problem of feeding the world's human population over the next three decades between 2020 and 2050 faces two formidable challenges: 1) we are currently adding 82 million more mouths to feed every year, and 2) resources needed to grow food such as arable land and fresh water are diminishing. As we have seen in previous chapters, reverting back to our natural human diet of fruits, vegetables, tubers, nuts and seeds is the only realistic way to meet both of these challenges, and to also help mitigate against climate change and species extinction. But even if every country were to adopt plant-based dietary and agricultural practices that maximized its potential to feed itself, the international food trade will remain integral to mitigating food insecurity around the world over the coming decades.

25

Changing Back to a Plant-based Diet

Modern day humans evolved over millions of years from a long line of primates that specialized in eating the reproductive parts of plants which are high in nutritive value. As a result, our bodies are perfectly adapted to thrive on a whole-food, plant-based diet of fruits, vegetables, tubers, nuts and seeds. But in just over a few thousand years' time, meat, dairy and eggs have come to take an increasingly prominent place on the plates of billions of people, and the consequences to human and planetary health have been catastrophic. Diseases of excess are endemic in affluent countries while diseases of deficiency afflict the world's poor, and animal agriculture is leading the way to runaway climate change and the sixth great mass species extinction on Earth.

In the first quarter of the 21st century, as we close in on 8 billion mouths to feed, our life sustaining planet is rapidly losing its capacity to indulge our unnatural dietary habits. If our species does not kick this life threatening addiction to animal foods and revert back to our natural plant-based diet over the next two generations, we will end up eating ourselves into oblivion. The question is not should we change back to our natural plant-based diet, but how do we do it?

Setting Goals

Several of the studies I have reviewed above project the environmental impacts of different dietary scenarios forward to 2050 and 2100. While they all found animal-based diets to have substantially more environmental impacts than plant-based diets, the studies' authors all recommended a human diet of reduced animal food consumption rather than ending animal food consumption altogether. These researchers made this recommendation knowing full well that animal foods are unhealthy to eat, unnecessary to feed our growing population, and environmentally destructive. The reason they invariably gave for taking this halfway measure approach to dietary reform is that they considered the goal of ending animal food consumption as impractical, and in order for their studies to be taken seriously, they had to recommend a diet that included "moderate consumption" of animal foods.

I would argue that just the opposite is true: recommending a reduced animal foods diet only gives people an excuse to continue their consumption of unhealthy foods and practice unsustainable agriculture indefinitely into the future. I would also argue against the assumption that dietary recommendations should be based on practicality. The goal of changing back to a plant-based diet is aspirational; whether it is entirely achievable or not is beside the point. If we set goals for dietary change that are insufficient to change the course of our imperiled future, then surely we shall fail. It is only by setting our standards high enough to achieve our goals, that we have any realistic chance of actually achieving them.

False Promise of Improved Efficiency

All of the studies I have reviewed above that quantify the environmental impacts of animal agriculture, suggested mitigations that involved improved efficiency of animal "husbandry," so that meat, dairy and eggs could be produced using fewer natural resources. In this way, so they say, animal foods can be produced sustainably. This improved efficiency approach to natural resource conservation was shown to be counterproductive back in the mid-1800s when English economist William Jevons observed that technological improvements that increased the efficiency of coal extraction actually led to an increase in demand for coal.

Due to this so called "Jevons' Paradox," increased efficiency of animal foods production is more likely to lead to an increase in animal food consumption and the associated environmental impacts from animal agriculture. Indeed, despite decades of improvements that have increased the efficiency of animal foods production, global demand for animal foods has continued to rise, as has the global environmental impacts of animal agriculture.

The Jevons' Paradox is another reason why setting a dietary goal of no animal foods makes more sense as a practical strategy to mitigate the global environmental impacts of animal agriculture than does the counterproductive strategy of producing animal foods more efficiently.

Taxing Animal Foods

I did come across one interesting study that actually proposed a practical strategy for reducing the global consumption of animal foods through taxation, entitled, *"Mitigation potential and global health impacts from emissions pricing of food commodities"* (*Nature Climate Change,* November, 2016*).* This analysis modeled the effects on consumer demand for food of levying a tax on food commodities based on the greenhouse gasses (GHGs) emitted in its production cycle. Such a tax would make high GHG emitting animal foods much more expensive relative to low GHG emitting plant foods. By levying this tax on the consumption side rather than the production side, demand for expensive high GHG emitting animal foods would be expected to shift over to relatively less expensive low GHG emitting plant foods, thereby improving health outcomes in the bargain. The study's authors concluded:

> *"Our analysis suggests that levying GHG taxes on food commodities could, if appropriately designed, be a health-promoting climate change-mitigation policy in high-income, middle-income, and most low-income countries (except possibly for some very low income countries in Sub-Saharan Africa; Supplementary Table 23)."*

In other words, these researchers found that levying a tax on food commodities based on a food's production cycle GHG emissions is a viable approach to reducing global demand for animal foods and to improve human health. But the social impacts of rationing animal foods by making them more expensive might produce consequences unforeseen by the study's authors.

Expensive animal foods would become less affordable to the masses of middle and low income people, while a relative few corporate elites would continue to consume animal foods as desired. Since animal foods would retain their high status value, this disparity in distribution would likely inflame social tensions between economic classes that are already strained to a breaking point around the globe. I bring up this point not in criticism, but rather in support of a carbon tax on food; if managed skillfully, this animal food envy could result in extreme pressure on corporate elites to give up this most conspicuous symbol of their affluence.

One difficulty I foresee with this strategy of levying GHG taxes on food commodities is that under the world's prevailing economic system of corporate capitalism, any attempt by national governments to levy such taxes would be vetoed by the politically powerful global animal industrial complex.

A Moral Imperative

"It is easier to change a man's religion than to change his diet."
– Margaret Mead, anthropologist (1901 – 1978)

Over the past 10,000 years since the invention of agriculture led to the development of large human population centers, there has been a constant evolution of governmental and economic institutions to manage the affairs of these burgeoning civilizations. As we enter the 21st century, the most advanced stages of this social evolution that have come to dominate the globe are the governmental institutions of "liberal democracy," and the economic institutions of "corporate capitalism." Ostensibly, liberal democracy is supposed to represent the political will of the people, and corporate capitalism is supposed to be the most efficient means of utilizing natural resources to meet the material needs of the people. But as we have seen in countless examples throughout this book, the overwhelming power of corporate capital has so corrupted popularly elected national governments that the extreme inequality of wealth and the destruction of our natural environment have reached epic proportions.

One prime example of this sorry state of world affairs is the annual *Conference of Parties* (COP) international meeting held under the auspices of the *United Nations Framework Convention on Climate Change* (UNFCCC), to address the existential threat of global warming. The first COP, COP 1, was held in Berlin, Germany in March, 1995, and the most recent COP 26, attended by 197 countries, was held in Glasgow, Scotland, in November, 2021. At these COP meetings, the fossil fuel industries have had larger delegations than any of the participating countries, and the resulting agreements to reduce GHG emissions have been nonbinding and the national pledges for GHG reductions have fallen far short of what is necessary to mitigate climate change. The fossil fuel industries have promoted the policy of "net zero" emissions rather than setting a target of reducing GHG emissions to absolute zero. The idea behind net zero is that GHG emissions from industry be offset by sequestering carbon in forests and by developing technologies in the future that remove carbon from the atmosphere so that "net" emissions will total zero. In effect, net zero is a prescription designed to allow for the burning of fossil fuels indefinitely into the future. The real world effect of this net zero approach to climate change has been a steady increase in atmospheric carbon dioxide (CO2) levels from 350 parts per million (ppm) in 1995 to 412 ppm in 2020, and fast rising. The last time atmospheric CO2 levels were this high was more than 3 million years ago, during the Mid-Pliocene Warm Period, when global temperatures averaged 3.6° – 5.4°F (2° – 3°C) above the pre-industrial era (before 1750 AD), and the sea level was 50 – 80 feet (15 – 25 meters) higher than it is today (*"Climate Change: Atmospheric Carbon Dioxide,"* NOAA, Climate.gov, August, 2020). As for the unequaled contribution of animal agricultural to global GHG emissions, this matter has never even been raised at any of the 26 COP meetings.

What these facts indicate is that the social institutions of liberal democracy and corporate capitalism have utterly failed to meet the existential threat that climate change represents to life as we've known it since the first H. sapiens walked the Earth some 200,000 years ago. While the vast majority of climate scientists have been issuing increasingly dire warnings on the urgency of reducing GHG emissions, and mass popular movements around the world have pleaded with national governments to take action on climate change, these pleas have fallen on deaf ears and corporate capital has continued to plunder the planet apace as if there were no tomorrow. Since our prevailing political and economic institutions have shown themselves to be incapable of making the reforms necessary to meet this existential threat at this critical juncture in human history, it is now incumbent upon us to consider other social institutions to confront this unprecedented global challenge.

As secular institutions, governments and corporations are ill equipped to respond to a crisis that is felt most profoundly as a moral imperative: do we want to save this planet for future habitation by our progeny, or not? While identifying the causes and mitigations of climate change are scientific pursuits, the human response to climate change is deeply rooted in our moral capacity to take a stand against wantonly destructive behaviors. For better or for worse, religious institutions have assumed the mantle of moral arbiters in human affairs.

As we have seen, the change from our natural human diet of plant foods to our current diet laden with animal foods, is the single largest anthropogenic contributor to global climate change and species extinction. With history as our guide, let's take a look at some historical precedents where the moral authority of religion was wielded to influence diet during existential crises of the past.

Judaism

When the Israelites were wandering in the desert east of the Jordan River after leaving Egypt around 3,400 years ago (1400 BC), many restrictions were put on the eating of meat. In the Old Testament Book of Exodus, the eating of rams (adult male sheep) was restricted to priests (*Exodus* 29:29-34). In the Book of Leviticus, the eating of rabbit, pig, all water creatures that do not have fins and scales, all birds of prey, bats, weasels, rats, lizards and snakes was prohibited (*Leviticus* 11:1-47). *Leviticus* 17:1-6 required that all ox, lamb and goats must be slaughtered by priests in front of the holy tabernacle with transgressors punished by banishment from the tribe; *Leviticus* 7:19-20 prohibits eating meat that is "ceremonially unclean" or by persons who are "unclean" with transgressors also punished by banishment.

These restrictions undoubtedly had a depressing effect on the consumption of meat at a time of food insecurity. The Biblical proscriptions against eating pig meat and shellfish were codified in the "Kosher" food laws that are still practiced by devout Jews today.

Hinduism

On the Indian Subcontinent between 1500 BC and 500 BC, the Ganges River Valley was filling up with people and livestock. The earliest unequivocal reference to the idea of nonviolence to animals was written in the Hindu philosophical text, *Chandogya Upanishad*, dated to the 8th century BC, which bars violence against animals except in the case of ritual sacrifice. This same view was expressed later in the epic poem *Mahabharata* and the sacred text *Bhagavata Purana*. When the famous Chinese Buddhist monk, Faxian, visited the Magadha region of the Ganges Valley in the early 5th century AD, he observed that the people there abstained from taking life and they did not breed pigs or poultry or sell any animal foods. Cattle originally introduced to the Indian Subcontinent by Aryan herders in the first millennium BC, were turned to pulling plows and providing milk.

Fueled largely by a vegetarian diet, India was able to sustain a continuous growth rate for the past 2,000 years despite periodic wars, famines and disease epidemics. By the year 2000 AD its population had reached 1.06 billion people.

Buddhism

By the 1st century AD (2000 years ago) the human population of East Asia had reached 60 million and meat eating had become unsustainable. Over the next two hundred years the Buddhist religion in the Mahāyāna tradition began to spread in China, which discouraged the killing of sentient beings and encouraged a vegetarian diet. In the Mahāyāna sacred text, Aṅ gulimālīya Sūtra, there is a dialogue on meat eating between Gautama Buddha and Mañjuśrī, who was the oldest and most significant bodhisattva (enlightened being) in Mahāyāna literature:

> Mañjuśrī asked, *"Do Buddhas not eat meat because of the tathāgata-garbha [the Buddha Nature within all beings]?"*

Gautama Buddha replied, *"Mañjuśrī, that is so. There are no beings who have not been one's mother, who have not been one's sister through generations of wandering in beginningless and endless saṃsāra. Even one who is a dog has been one's father, for the world of living beings is like a dancer. Therefore, one's own flesh and the flesh of another are a single flesh, so Buddhas do not eat meat.*

"Moreover, Mañjuśrī, the dhātu [primitive matter] of all beings is the dharmadhātu, so Buddhas do not eat meat because they would be eating the flesh of one single dhātu."

In the Mahāyāna sacred text, *Mahaparinirvana Sutra*, which purports to be the final definitive Mahāyāna teachings of the Buddha before his death, the Buddha states, *"...the eating of meat extinguishes the seed of Great Kindness."*

Due to its largely plant-based diet, China was able to sustain the fastest growth rate of any country on Earth over the past 2,000 years, and despite periodic wars, famines and disease epidemics, its population had reached 1.3 billion people by the year 2000.

Christianity

In the Dark Ages of Europe from the 5th to the 10th century AD (1,500 to 1000 years ago), the Catholic Church realized that raising animals greatly limited the amount of food they could produce which in turn placed severe limits on population growth. As a way of reducing the amount of meat people ate, the Church proclaimed every Wednesday and Friday to be meat-fasting days and they also made meat-fasting a requirement for the 40 days of the holy period known as Lent. In effect, these proscriptions on meat eating for over one third of the days each year significantly reduced overall meat consumption.

In the 11th through the 13th centuries, a vegetarian Christian sect called Catharism flourished in France, Germany, Belgium and Italy. The Cathars refused to eat anything that was the result of "coition" which to their understanding eliminated meat, dairy and eggs. Believing that fish reproduced asexually, they were considered eatable.

In more recent times, the Seventh Day Adventist sect of Christianity established in 1860, advises a vegetarian diet. Many adherents settled in Loma Linda California where they have been the subject of many health studies due to their unusual longevity.

Islam

In the 7th century AD, eating pig meat was prohibited by the *Quran*, the central religious text of Islam (*Quran* 2:173). Ostensibly this prohibition was because pigs were considered unclean animals under Islamic dietary laws. But more likely, the reason for this prohibition was that pigs were not well adapted to living in the desert environment where Islam was founded, so in order to keep wealthy people from using scarce resources to raise pigs thus creating dissension among the people, they simply banned eating pig meat altogether.

Tikopia

While all of the major world religions above at one time or another have called on their adherents to restrain meat eating, one example of dietary restrictions on meat eating as a means of self preservation that has global implications today, took place on the tiny remote Pacific island of Tikopia with a total land area of 1.8 square miles (5 square kilometers), located in the Southwest Pacific Ocean. First inhabited by humans around 900 BC (2,900 years ago), the problem faced by the pioneers of Tikopia for the next three millennia was how to sustainably feed its population without importing food from outside the island? The Earth itself is like a tiny remote island hurtling through the vastness of space, and all of humanity now faces much the same problem as the Tikopians did: how do we sustainably feed our population without importing food from outside our planet? In a very real sense, the island of Tikopia was a natural lab experiment on how to create a long-term sustainable food supply with finite resources.

Dr. Jared Diamond, Professor of Geography at the University of California, Los Angeles, has estimated that from an initial group of perhaps 25 colonists, the population of Tikopia grew to around 1,200 people in under 300 years, which works out to a population density of 800 people/square mile (309 people/square kilometer), (*"Collapse, How Societies Choose To Fail Or Succeed," Viking*, 2005). For comparison, in 2021 the densely populated island of Japan had 864 people/square mile.

To sustain this initial population growth the Tikopians first drove the native wildlife to extinction, severely depleted native fish and shellfish populations, and resorted to slash-and-burn agriculture which severely depleted the native forest cover on the island. As food production on the tiny island could no longer sustain continued population growth, the Tikopians resorted to population control through abortion, infanticide, suicide and inter-clan warfare to stabilize the population at around 1,200 people.

Archaeological remains indicate that over the period from 100 BC to 900 AD, the Tikopians abandoned slash-and-burn agriculture in favor of maintaining orchards of native almond trees and micromanaging the island to utilize virtually every plant species for continuous sustainable food production. This included the introduced tree species of coconuts, breadfruit, and sago and betelnut palms. Under this tall fruit and nut tree canopy they grew yams, bananas and swamp taro. This form of multistory gardening that mimics the structure of a natural rainforest has been compared to the modern day practice of "permaculture." To protect diminishing populations of aquatic animals, permission to catch fish and shellfish was required from the four clan chiefs who held positions of moral authority. During this period, the Tikopians also imported and intensively raised pigs which came to account for around half of their protein consumption.

Around 1,200 AD, Polynesian settlers from Fiji, Samoa and Tonga arrived who introduced the technique of fermenting breadfruit in pits to preserve food for the annual dry season of May and June and for times when periodic cyclones would destroy their crops.

Oral tradition and archaeological remains indicate that around 1,600 AD, the Tikopians made the conscious decision to killed every pig on the island since the pigs required 10 pounds of edible plants to produce 1 pound of pig meat which had become a luxury food for the clan chiefs creating dissension among the population (*"We the Tikopia: A Sociological Study of Kinship in Primitive Polynesia,"* 1936) (*"Tikopia, the Prehistory and Ecology of a Polynesian Outlier,"* June 1984). This was the state of the Tikopian food economy when Europeans began to permanently settle on the island in the 1800s. This tale of survival of a people densely packed on a tiny remote island for nearly three millennia is truly remarkable.

In two significant ways, the Tikopian experience mimics that of the larger human experience on Earth. First, as humans spread around the globe, our first order of business to insure survival was to wipe out vulnerable native animal species for food, and second, after the native fauna was extirpated, non-native animal species were introduced to replace the animal component of the diet. But this is where the Tikopian experience and the larger human experience diverged. The Tikopians made the conscious decision to eliminate animal agriculture as a means of sustaining themselves on their tiny island, whereas in the world at large, even as it has become increasingly clear that animal agriculture is decimating our planet, we are mindlessly plowing ahead with increasing the animal component of the human diet around the globe.

In his book *"Collapse, How Societies Choose To Fail Or Succeed,"* Dr. Jared Diamond makes the case that the Tikopians were able to choose to succeed because their society was not highly stratified with clan chiefs working in the garden just like everyone else. Also, since the perimeter of the island could be walked in under 12 hours, every person was familiar with the entire island. Dr. Diamond may be right about this, but the only way we humans will be able to save ourselves from ultimate destruction is by coming together as one species to change our relationship with this tiny island planet of ours. To achieve this planetary unity of purpose, the world's major religious institutions must be fully engaged in what can only be described as a moral imperative.

Are the world's major religions up to this task? Probably not, but sometimes they can surprise you. Joseph Jenkins, author of *"The Humanure Handbook"* (3rd edition, 2005) tells a wonderful story of his personal experience with an order of Catholic nuns that gives a sign of hope. The story begins with a phone call he received from a convent soon after he self-published the first edition of his book:

> *"'Mr. Jenkins, we recently bought a copy of your book, Humanure, and we would like to have you speak at our convent.'*
>
> *'What do you want me to talk about?'*
>
> *'About the topic of your book.'*
>
> *'Composting?'*
>
> *'Yes, but specifically, humanure composting.' At this point I was at a loss for words. I couldn't understand exactly why a group of nuns would be interested in composting human crap. Somehow, I couldn't imagine standing in front of a group of nuns speaking about turds. But I kept the stammering to a minimum and accepted the invitation.*

It was Earth Day, 1995. The presentation went well. After I spoke, the group showed slides of their gardens and compost piles, then we toured their compost area and poked around in the worm boxes. A delightful lunch followed, during which I asked them why they were interested in humanure, of all things.

'We are the Sisters of Humility,' they responded. 'The words 'humble' and 'humus' come from the same semantic root, which means 'earth.' We also think these words are related to the word 'human.' Therefore, as part of our vow of humility, we work with the earth. We make compost, as you have seen. And now we want to learn how to make compost from our toilet material. We're thinking about buying a commercial composting toilet, but we want to learn more about the overall concepts first. That's why we asked you to come here.' This was deep shit. Profound.

A light bulb went off in my head. Of course, composting is an act of humility. The people who care enough about the earth to recycle their personal by-products do so as an exercise in humility, not because they're going to get rich and famous for it. That makes them better people. Some people go to church on Sunday, others make compost. Still others do both. Others go to church on Sunday, then throw all their garbage out into the environment. The exercising of the human spirit can take many forms, and the simple act of cleaning up after oneself is one of them. The careless dumping of waste out into the world is a self-centered act of arrogance – ignorance.

Humanure composters can stand under the stars at night gazing at the heavens, and know that when nature calls, their excretions will not foul the planet. Instead, those excretions are humbly collected, fed to microorganisms and returned to the Earth as healing medicine for the soil."

If an order of Catholic nuns can come to terms with their own excrement, then that gives me a glimmer of hope that anyone is capable of changing their dietary habits to conform to our natural place on the food chain.

The End Times?

Through the pages of this book, we have traveled together on a long journey from the origins of one precocious species of ape 2,000,000 years ago, to the invention of agriculture and civilization 10,000 years ago, to the ecological crises we are now experiencing in the 21st century. Along the way we have seen how this one species rather abruptly changed from its natural diet of fruits, vegetables, tubers, nuts and seeds to a diet containing large quantities of meat, dairy and eggs, and how this unnatural diet has harmed human health, induced climate chaos and decimated our fellow inhabitants with whom we share this precious life sustaining planet. We have seen the human population grow from a relative few vulnerable individuals scavenging for food on the savannas of Africa to a population of well over seven billion people plundering the entire planet to satisfy our insatiable desires for animal foods while driving the Earth's ecosystems to the brink of collapse. We have also seen how the world's dominant governmental and economic institutions have failed to control our most destructive impulses. But above all, we have seen how returning to our natural whole-food, plant-based, vegan diet, can be our saving grace.

Climate scientists tell us that our window of opportunity to stabilize our planet's climate within a temperature range suitable for human habitation is rapidly closing. Will it be possible for us to alter our unsustainable trajectory in time to stave-off our untimely demise? I submit that if we do not change back to the plant-based diet our species evolved to eat, then surely we shall perish from this Earth.

· · ·

"The world will not be inherited by the strongest, it will be inherited by those most able to change."
– Charles Darwin, naturalist (1809 – 1882)

Jonathan Spitz is an environmental and animal rights activist. In 1990, after reading *Diet for a New America* by John Robbins, he realized that humans lacked the anatomy or physiology of apex predators and our true role in a sustainable ecosystem is as a plant-eating species. With this new understanding of the human place on the food chain, at the age of thirty-seven he adopted a plant-based vegan diet and began defending the rights of all animals to live free from human exploitation.

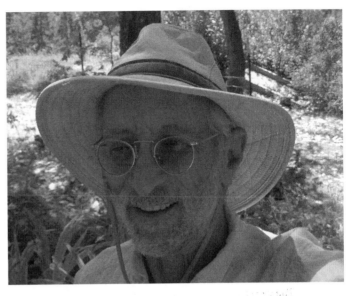

Through the 1990s, he served on the Board of Directors of the *Willits Environmental Center* to thwart the relentless destructive forces of local economic development. In the 2000s and 2010s, he authored an op/ed column, *Connecting the Dots*, that focused on environmental and animal rights issues for his hometown newspaper, *The Mendocino County Observer*.

For thirty years, Jonathan kept abreast of the most current studies on the complex relationship between the human food niche and the Earth's ecosystems. When he realized there were no books in the ecological canon telling the story of how humans evolved from an obscure herbivorous species to become the world's most populous carnivorous apex predator species, and how this change in human diet has led to epidemics of chronic degenerative disease, runaway climate change and mass species extinction, he decided to write it himself.

Jonathan has lived on California's North Coast since the 1980s.
He can be reached at: plantbased.js@gmail.com